MRI for Orthopaedic Surgeons

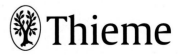

MRI for Orthopaedic Surgeons

Edited by

A. Jay Khanna, MD, MBA

Associate Professor
Departments of Orthopaedic Surgery and Biomedical Engineering
The Johns Hopkins University School of Medicine

Co-Director
Division of Spine Surgery
Johns Hopkins Orthopaedic Surgery at Good Samaritan Hospital
Baltimore, Maryland

Thieme
New York • Stuttgart

Thieme Publishers, Inc.
333 Seventh Ave.
New York, NY 10001

Editorial Director: Michael Wachinger
Executive Editor: Kay Conerly
Editorial Assistant: Dominik Pucek
International Production Director: Andreas Schabert
Production Editor: Print Matters, Inc.
Vice President, International Marketing and Sales: Cornelia Schulze
Chief Financial Officer: James W. Mitos
President: Brian D. Scanlan
Compositor: The Manila Typesetting Co.
Printer: Everbest Printing Co.

Library of Congress Cataloging-in-Publication Data

MRI for orthopaedic surgeons / [edited by] A. Jay Khanna.
    p. ; cm.
Includes bibliographical references and index.
ISBN 978-1-60406-022-5 (alk. paper)
1. Musculoskeletal system—Diseases. 2. Magnetic resonance imaging. I. Khanna, A. Jay.
[DNLM: 1. Musculoskeletal Diseases—diagnosis. 2. Magnetic Resonance Imaging—methods. WE 141 M9388 2009]
RC925.M75 2009
617.4'707548—dc22
                    2009016354

Important note: Medical knowledge is ever-changing. As new research and clinical experience broaden our knowledge, changes in treatment and drug therapy may be required. The authors and editors of the material herein have consulted sources believed to be reliable in their efforts to provide information that is complete and in accord with the standards accepted at the time of publication. However, in view of the possibility of human error by the authors, editors, or publisher of the work herein or changes in medical knowledge, neither the authors, editors, or publisher, nor any other party who has been involved in the preparation of this work, warrants that the information contained herein is in every respect accurate or complete, and they are not responsible for any errors or omissions or for the results obtained from use of such information. Readers are encouraged to confirm the information contained herein with other sources. For example, readers are advised to check the product information sheet included in the package of each drug they plan to administer to be certain that the information contained in this publication is accurate and that changes have not been made in the recommended dose or in the contraindications for administration. This recommendation is of particular importance in connection with new or infrequently used drugs.

Some of the product names, patents, and registered designs referred to in this book are in fact registered trademarks or proprietary names even though specific reference to this fact is not always made in the text. Therefore, the appearance of a name without designation as proprietary is not to be construed as a representation by the publisher that it is in the public domain.

Printed in China

5 4 3 2 1

ISBN 978-1-60406-022-5

*To my parents, Mona and Surinder, who have
always helped me achieve my dreams.*

To my wife, Roma, the woman of my dreams.

*To my children, Rajan and Priya, for whom
I have so many dreams.*

Contents

Foreword ix
Frank J. Frassica

Preface xi

Acknowledgments xiii

Contributors xv

Abbreviations xix

I Initial Concepts

1. **Essentials of MRI Physics and Pulse Sequences** 3
   Rick W. Obray, Douglas P. Beall, John D. Reeder, John A. Carrino, and Laura M. Fayad

2. **Normal MRI Anatomy of the Musculoskeletal System** 17
   J. Dana Dunleavy, A. Jay Khanna, and John A. Carrino

3. **A Systematic Approach to the Review of Musculoskeletal MRI Studies** 77
   A. Jay Khanna

II Upper Extremity

4. **The Shoulder** 97
   Adam J. Farber, A. Jay Khanna, Laura M. Fayad, Timothy S. Johnson, and Edward G. McFarland

5. **The Elbow** 118
   Lance M. Brunton, Mark W. Anderson, and A. Bobby Chhabra

6. **The Wrist and Hand** 129
   Lance M. Brunton, Mark W. Anderson, and A. Bobby Chhabra

III Lower Extremity

7. **The Hip** 147
   Michael K. Shindle, Bryan T. Kelly, Luis E. Moya, and Douglas N. Mintz

8. **The Knee** 164
   Brett M. Cascio, A. Jay Khanna, Sergio A. Glait, Andrew J. Cosgarea, Timothy S. Johnson, and John D. Reeder

9. **The Foot and Ankle** 202
   Daniel J. Durand, John A. Carrino, Meena W. Shatby, Ali Moshirfar, and John T. Campbell

IV Spine

10. The Cervical Spine 229
Lukas P. Zebala, Jacob M. Buchowski, Aditya R. Daftary, Joseph R. O'Brien, John A. Carrino, and A. Jay Khanna

11. The Lumbar and Thoracic Spine 269
Gbolahan O. Okubadejo, Aditya R. Daftary, Jacob M. Buchowski, John A. Carrino, and A. Jay Khanna

12. Tumors of the Spine 316
Daniel M. Sciubba, Bruce A. Wasserman, and Ziya L. Gokaslan

13. The Pediatric Spine 338
A. Jay Khanna, Bruce A. Wasserman, and Paul D. Sponseller

V Special Considerations

14. Articular Cartilage 353
Michael K. Shindle, Li Foong Foo, Bryan T. Kelly, and Hollis G. Potter

15. Soft-Tissue and Bone Tumors 370
Derek F. Papp, A. Jay Khanna, Edward F. McCarthy, Laura M. Fayad, Adam J. Farber, and Frank J. Frassica

16. Advanced Techniques in Musculoskeletal MRI 397
Douglas E. Ramsey, Rick W. Obray, Priya D. Prabhakar, and John A. Carrino

17. Correlation of MRI with Other Imaging Studies 414
Uma Srikumaran, Laura M. Fayad, and A. Jay Khanna

18. MRI Safety 425
Monica D. Watkins and Bruce A. Wasserman

Index 431

Foreword

The ability to accurately interpret an MRI study of a given anatomic region is essential to the practice of orthopaedic surgery. Until now, we have taught orthopaedic surgeons-in-training how to evaluate such studies in a rather informal manner: in the office, in conferences, and in the operating room. In most cases, the orthopaedic surgeon learns the skill of interpreting MRI studies through his or her own experience, through interaction with the radiologists who interpret the studies, and perhaps by attending a continuing medical education conference or reviewing a textbook on the topic. At our institution, the orthopaedic surgeons work closely with the Department of Radiology and, specifically, the Division of Musculoskeletal Imaging. For example, for a patient with a musculoskeletal tumor, I review all of the imaging studies with an experienced musculoskeletal radiologist and pathologist before proceeding with a treatment plan of observation, biopsy, or resection. This interaction occurs in our daily clinic sessions and during our weekly MRI conference, at which orthopaedic surgeons, musculoskeletal radiologists, pathologists, and other clinicians evaluate the studies and review the clinical history together. We make fewer mistakes when we work together.

MRI for Orthopaedic Surgeons is written by orthopaedic surgeons and radiologists for the purpose of providing a more formal process of teaching the technique and the fund of knowledge necessary to accurately interpret various MRI pulse sequences. This textbook is edited by Dr. Jay Khanna, who is a passionate educator and clinician with a background in radiology and orthopaedic surgery. His knowledge comes from seeing patients every day and teaching students and residents. Dr. Khanna has assembled an experienced team of orthopaedic surgeons and radiologists from within our institution and throughout the country who have the expertise and passion to make this book the standard for educating individuals interested in the musculoskeletal system.

The book is organized into five focused sections: initial concepts, upper extremity, lower extremity, spine, and special considerations. The region-specific chapters have a common format that very effectively teaches the reader how to evaluate imaging studies of that section of the musculoskeletal system. The many MR images are of superb quality, and the numerous line drawings illustrate key anatomy and pathology principles very clearly.

This text will not only benefit orthopaedic surgeons and radiologists but will also serve as an excellent resource for everyone who cares for the musculoskeletal system: primary care physicians, emergency department physicians, physiatrists, neurologists, physical therapists, and nurses. This wonderful textbook will be well worn with daily use.

Frank J. Frassica, MD
Chairman and Robert A. Robinson Professor
Department of Orthopaedic Surgery
The Johns Hopkins University
School of Medicine
Baltimore, Maryland

Preface

Although the ability to evaluate MRI studies is critical to the practice of orthopaedic surgery, most orthopaedic surgeons learn this skill in an informal fashion and with experience throughout their training and in clinical practice. As a result, we may not have a thorough understanding of the science and physics of MR imaging and the various pulse sequences that are available for obtaining the images. Many of us—those in general orthopaedic surgery practice as well as those in subspecialties such as sports medicine, spine surgery, hand and upper extremity surgery, foot and ankle surgery, and orthopaedic oncology—prefer to read our patients' MR imaging studies ourselves rather than rely solely on the "official" radiologist's report. We learn to make preoperative, intraoperative, and postoperative decisions based on those readings. However, unlike radiologists who are trained to evaluate MRI studies in a systematic fashion, we may be more likely to rely on our anatomic expertise and experience, which may not be the most effective method.

MRI for Orthopaedic Surgeons will help teach orthopaedic surgeons how to systematically evaluate and interpret MR imaging studies of the musculoskeletal system. Although there are many excellent books that focus on MR imaging of the musculoskeletal system, this one is unique in that it is written by orthopaedic surgeons and radiologists specifically for orthopaedic surgeons. As such, it is clinically oriented and presents the information from a perspective and at a level that an orthopaedic surgeon will appreciate. It is also an excellent reference for radiologists and others—such as physical medicine and rehabilitation clinicians, rheumatologists, and nonoperative musculoskeletal care specialists—who read musculoskeletal MR images and who would like to gain a better appreciation of the associated clinical aspects.

My desire to create this book stems from my interest and background in musculoskeletal imaging and from my recognition of the fact that the ability to accurately evaluate MR imaging studies is critical to the practice of orthopaedic surgery. Along these lines, my colleagues and I have developed instructional materials and lectures for the orthopaedic surgery residents at our institution to teach them how to systematically evaluate MR imaging studies of the musculoskeletal system. In doing so, we realized that many of the textbooks and other resources on the topic of musculoskeletal MRI are written by radiologists and directed toward radiologists and radiologists in training. This perceived void of imaging resources for orthopaedic surgeons led me to compile and edit this textbook.

MRI for Orthopaedic Surgeons is organized into five sections: 1) core concepts, 2) upper extremity, 3) lower extremity, 4) spine, and 5) special considerations. Each of these five sections, or each chapter, can be read independently, but the textbook is best read in sequential chapter order. In particular, before reading the chapters on individual anatomic areas, the clinician should review Chapter 2, Normal MRI Anatomy of the Musculoskeletal System. That chapter provides a moderately comprehensive evaluation of the key anatomic structures and concepts with which one should be familiar when reviewing an MR imaging study of a particular region; it also serves as a reference point when evaluating the pathology images in a region-specific chapter.

The book features two different types of chapters: region-specific and concept-specific. The region-specific chapters (for example, The Shoulder and The Cervical Spine) share a common organization, with sections on specialized pulse sequences and protocols, traumatic pathology, degenerative pathology, infectious conditions, and postoperative findings. The concept-specific chapters (for example, Advanced Techniques in Musculoskeletal MRI) are organized in a fashion that best suits the individual chapter's content and the goal of providing orthopaedic surgeons with the information they need to maximize their proficiency in evaluating and interpreting MR imaging studies.

MRI for Orthopaedic Surgeons contains more than 700 MR images and 130 artist's drawings that have been carefully selected and created to help illustrate and teach the essential anatomy and pathology that an orthopaedic surgeon, other clinician, or radiologist should be able to recognize and define when evaluating an MRI study of the musculoskeletal system. As such, much of the material can be learned effectively by reviewing the images and illustrations along with the associated figure legends.

Most of the chapters have been authored by both orthopaedic surgeons and radiologists. Some, such as the region-specific chapters, have orthopaedic surgeons as the primary authors, with radiologists as co-authors for accuracy and clarity from their standpoint. Others (for example, Essentials of MRI Physics and Pulse Sequences) have been written solely by radiologists, but the presentation of the material has been specifically designed with an orthopaedic surgeon audience in mind. The collaboration between orthopaedic surgeons and radiologists that we have used to produce this textbook emulates the optimal relationship between these two subspecialties in clinical practice.

This book was envisioned to be a practical aid to develop and/or refine the skills needed to effectively and systematically evaluate MR imaging studies of the musculoskeletal system. I hope that it accomplishes this goal for you.

A. Jay Khanna, MD, MBA

Acknowledgments

First and foremost, I would like to thank the many contributors to this text for their time, patience, and hard work. They have made this undertaking infinitely easier and allowed all of us to benefit from their years of experience.

Special thanks go to Kay Conerly, Dominik Pucek, and Torsten Scheihagen at Thieme for their expertise and outstanding efforts in bringing this book through the publishing process. Thanks also go to Tony Pazos, medical illustrator extraordinaire, for his skill, attention to detail, and willingness to work through many rounds of revisions.

Finally, I would like to express my greatest appreciation to Elaine Henze, Medical Editor for The Johns Hopkins University's Department of Orthopaedic Surgery. She, with the support of Sara Cleary, has spent countless hours at work and on her own time helping me edit the first and second (and fifth!) iterations of every chapter, table, image, and legend. Without her commitment to accuracy, focus on quality, and resolution in handling innumerable e-mails, telephone calls, and personal visits with me and the contributors, this book would never have been completed.

Contributors

EDITOR

A. Jay Khanna, MD, MBA
Associate Professor
Departments of Orthopaedic Surgery
  and Biomedical Engineering
The Johns Hopkins University School of Medicine
Baltimore, Maryland

Co-Director
Division of Spine Surgery
Johns Hopkins Orthopaedic Surgery at Good
  Samaritan Hospital
Baltimore, Maryland

CONTRIBUTORS

Mark W. Anderson, MD
Professor
Departments of Radiology and Orthopaedic Surgery
University of Virginia
Charlottesville, Virginia

Chief
Division of Musculoskeletal Radiology
University of Virginia
Charlottesville, Virginia

Douglas P. Beall, MD
Chief of Radiology Services
Clinical Radiology of Oklahoma
Oklahoma City, Oklahoma

Clinical Professor
Department of Orthopaedic Surgery and Rehabilitation
University of Oklahoma College of Medicine
Oklahoma City, Oklahoma

Lance M. Brunton, MD
Assistant Professor
Department of Orthopaedic Surgery
University of Pittsburgh School of Medicine
University of Pittsburgh Medical Center
Division of Hand, Upper Extremity, and Microsurgery
Pittsburgh, Pennsylvania

Jacob M. Buchowski, MD, MS
Assistant Professor of Orthopaedic and Neurological
  Surgery
Washington University in St. Louis
St. Louis, Missouri

Director
Center for Spinal Tumors
Washington University in St. Louis
St. Louis, Missouri

John T. Campbell, MD
Attending Orthopaedic Surgeon
Institute for Foot and Ankle Reconstruction
Mercy Medical Center
Baltimore, Maryland

John A. Carrino, MD, MPH
Associate Professor
Russell H. Morgan Department of Radiology
  and Radiological Science
Department of Orthopaedic Surgery
The Johns Hopkins University School of Medicine
Baltimore, Maryland

Section Chief
Musculoskeletal Radiology
Russell H. Morgan Department of Radiology
  and Radiological Science
The Johns Hopkins Hospital
Baltimore, Maryland

Brett M. Cascio, MD
Head Team Physician
McNeese State University
Lake Charles, Louisiana

Medical Director
Lake Charles Memorial Sports Medicine
Lake Charles, Louisiana

Gratis Faculty
Louisiana State University
Baton Rouge, Louisiana

Major
U.S. Army Reserve

A. Bobby Chhabra, MD
Associate Professor and Vice Chair
Department of Orthopaedic Surgery
University of Virginia Health System
Charlottesville, Virginia

Chief
Division of Hand and Upper Extremity Surgery
University of Virginia Health System
Charlottesville, Virginia

Andrew J. Cosgarea, MD
Professor
Department of Orthopaedic Surgery
The Johns Hopkins University School of Medicine
Baltimore, Maryland

Division Chief
Sports Medicine and Shoulder Surgery
The Johns Hopkins Hospital
Baltimore, Maryland

Aditya R. Daftary, MBBS
Consultant Radiologist
Innovision Imaging
Mumbai, India

J. Dana Dunleavy, MD
Resident
Russell H. Morgan Department of Radiology
  and Radiological Science
The Johns Hopkins University School of Medicine
The Johns Hopkins Hospital
Baltimore, Maryland

Daniel J. Durand, MD
Senior Resident
Russell H. Morgan Department of Radiology
  and Radiological Science
The Johns Hopkins University School of Medicine
Division of Musculoskeletal Radiology
The Johns Hopkins Hospital
Baltimore, Maryland

Adam J. Farber, MD
Orthopaedic Surgeon
Arizona Orthopedic Surgical Specialists
Chandler, Arizona

Laura M. Fayad, MD
Associate Professor
Russell H. Morgan Department of Radiology
  and Radiological Science
Department of Orthopaedic Surgery
The Johns Hopkins University School of Medicine
Baltimore, Maryland

Radiologist
The Johns Hopkins Hospital
Baltimore, Maryland

Li Foong Foo, MD
Assistant Professor
Radiology
Weill Medical College
Cornell University
New York, New York

Assistant Attending Radiologist
New York Presbyterian Hospital
New York, New York

Frank J. Frassica, MD
Chairman and Robert A. Robinson Professor
Department of Orthopaedic Surgery
The Johns Hopkins University School of Medicine
Baltimore, Maryland

Sergio A. Glait, MD
Resident
Department of Orthopaedic Surgery
New York University Hospital for Joint Diseases
New York, New York

Ziya L. Gokaslan, MD, FACS
Donlin M. Long Professor
Professor of Neurosurgery, Oncology, and Orthopaedic
  Surgery
Vice-Chair
Department of Neurosurgery

Director
Neurosurgical Spine Program
Department of Neurosurgery
The Johns Hopkins University School of Medicine
Baltimore, Maryland

Timothy S. Johnson, MD
Assistant Professor
Department of Orthopaedic Surgery
The Johns Hopkins University School of Medicine
Baltimore, Maryland

Orthopaedic Surgeon
National Sports Medicine Institute
Lansdowne, Virginia

Bryan T. Kelly, MD
Assistant Professor
Orthopaedic Surgery
Weill Medical College
Cornell University
New York, New York

Assistant Attending
Department of Orthopaedic Surgery
Hospital for Special Surgery
New York Presbyterian Hospital
New York, New York

Edward F. McCarthy, MD
Professor
Departments of Pathology and Orthopaedic Surgery
The Johns Hopkins University School of Medicine
Baltimore, Maryland

Attending Orthopaedic Surgeon and Pathologist
The Johns Hopkins Hospital
Baltimore, Maryland

Edward G. McFarland, MD
Wayne H. Lewis Professor of Orthopaedics
   and Shoulder Surgery
Vice-Chairman
Department of Orthopaedic Surgery
The Johns Hopkins University School of Medicine
Baltimore, Maryland

Douglas N. Mintz, MD
Associate Professor
Clinical Radiology
Weill Medical College
Cornell University
New York, New York

Attending Physician
Hospital for Special Surgery
New York Presbyterian Hospital
New York, New York

Ali Moshirfar, MD
Assistant Professor
Department of Orthopaedic Surgery
The Johns Hopkins University School of Medicine
Baltimore, Maryland

Director
Center for Advanced Orthopaedics and Pain Management
Ashburn, Virginia

Luis E. Moya, MD
Clinica Alemana de Santiago
Santiago, Chile

Rick W. Obray, MD
Fellow
Interventional Pain Medicine
Mayo Clinic
Rochester, Minnesota

Joseph R. O'Brien, MD, MPH
Assistant Professor
Departments of Orthopaedic Surgery and Neurosurgery
The George Washington University School of Medicine
Washington, District of Columbia

Associate Director of Orthopaedic Spine Surgery
The George Washington University Hospital
Washington, District of Columbia

Gbolahan O. Okubadejo, MD
Orthopaedic Spine Surgeon
Active Joints Orthopaedics
Englewood Hospital
Englewood, New Jersey

Orthopaedic Spine Surgeon
Holy Name Hospital
Teaneck, New Jersey

Orthopaedic Spine Surgeon
Meadowlands Hospital
Secaucaus, New Jersey

Derek F. Papp, MD
Chief Resident
Department of Orthopaedic Surgery
The Johns Hopkins University School of Medicine
The Johns Hopkins Hospital
Baltimore, Maryland

Hollis G. Potter, MD
Chief
MRI Division
Department of Radiology and Imaging
Hospital for Special Surgery
New York, New York

Professor
Radiology
Weill Medical College
Cornell University
New York, New York

Priya D. Prabhakar, MD, MPH
Clinical Assistant Professor
Department of Radiology
Jefferson Medical College
Thomas Jefferson University
Philadelphia, Pennsylvania

Staff Radiologist
Albert Einstein Medical Center
Philadelphia, Pennsylvania

Douglas E. Ramsey, MD
Instructor
Diagnostic Radiology
Russell H. Morgan Department of Radiology
    and Radiological Science
The Johns Hopkins University School of Medicine
Baltimore, Maryland

Fellow
Musculoskeletal Radiology
Russell H. Morgan Department of Radiology
    and Radiological Science
The Johns Hopkins Hospital
Baltimore, Maryland

John D. Reeder, MD, FACR
Director of Imaging
Proscan Imaging Columbia
Columbia, Maryland

Daniel M. Sciubba, MD
Assistant Professor
Department of Neurosurgery
The Johns Hopkins University School of Medicine
Baltimore, Maryland

Director
Minimally Invasive Spine Surgery
Department of Neurosurgery
The Johns Hopkins Hospital
Baltimore, Maryland

Director
Spine Research
Department of Neurosurgery
The Johns Hopkins Hospital
Baltimore, Maryland

Meena W. Shatby, MD
The Woodlands Sports Medicine
The Woodlands, Texas

Michael K. Shindle, MD
Orthopaedic Fellow
Hospital for Special Surgery
New York, New York

Paul D. Sponseller, MD, MBA
Professor and Executive Vice Chair
Pediatrics Division Chief
Department of Orthopaedic Surgery
The Johns Hopkins University School of Medicine
The Johns Hopkins Hospital
Baltimore, Maryland

Uma Srikumaran, MD
Chief Resident
Department of Orthopaedic Surgery
The Johns Hopkins University School of Medicine
The Johns Hopkins Hospital
Baltimore, Maryland

Bruce A. Wasserman, MD
Associate Professor
Russell H. Morgan Department of Radiology
    and Radiological Science
The Johns Hopkins University School of Medicine
Baltimore, Maryland

Director of Diagnostic Neurovascular Imaging
The Johns Hopkins Hospital
Baltimore, Maryland

Monica D. Watkins, MD
Fellow
Neuroradiology
The Johns Hopkins Hospital
Baltimore, Maryland

Radiologist
American Radiology
Baltimore, Maryland

Lukas P. Zebala, MD
Chief Resident
Department of Orthopaedic Surgery
Washington University in St. Louis School of Medicine
Barnes-Jewish Hospital at Washington University Medical
    Center
St. Louis, Missouri

Abbreviations

Abbreviation	Definition	Abbreviation	Definition
2D	two-dimensional	MCP	metacarpophalangeal
3D	three-dimensional	MFH	malignant fibrous histiocytoma
AC	acromioclavicular	MGHL	middle glenohumeral ligament
ACL	anterior cruciate ligament	MR	magnetic resonance
AIDS	acquired immune deficiency syndrome	MRI	magnetic resonance imaging
		MTP	metatarsophalangeal
AP	anteroposterior	OCD	osteochondritis dissecans
CSF	cerebrospinal fluid		OR osteochondral defect
CT	computed tomography	PCL	posterior cruciate ligament
CVJ	craniovertebral junction	PVNS	pigmented villonodular synovitis
ECU	extensor carpi ulnaris	RA	rheumatoid arthritis
FDA	Food and Drug Administration	RCL	radial collateral ligament
FHL	flexor hallucis longus	RF	radiofrequency
FSE	fast spin echo	SE	spin echo
HAGHL	humeral avulsion of the glenohumeral ligament	SLAP	superior labrum anterior and posterior (lesions)
HIV	human immunodeficiency virus	SPONK	spontaneous osteonecrosis of the knee
IGHL	inferior glenohumeral ligament		
IP	interphalangeal	STIR	short tau inversion recovery
ITB	iliotibial band	TE	echo time
LCL	lateral collateral ligament	TFCC	triangular fibrocartilage complex
LUCL	lateral ulnar collateral ligament	TR	repetition time
MCL	medial collateral ligament	UCL	ulnar collateral ligament

Initial Concepts

1 Essentials of MRI Physics and Pulse Sequences

Rick W. Obray, Douglas P. Beall, John D. Reeder, John A. Carrino, and Laura M. Fayad

MRI is an essential tool in the accurate diagnosis and treatment of musculoskeletal disease. The number of MRI applications has increased dramatically over the past two decades and will likely continue to increase. A detailed understanding of the fundamentals of MRI physics is not required to review images, although a basic working knowledge of certain key principles is important for the accurate utilization of the technology. This chapter provides the reader with a basic understanding of the physics behind MRI by addressing specific applications of MRI within musculoskeletal radiology and emphasizing how an MR image is generated and what basic sequences are important for optimally showing musculoskeletal anatomy. The intent is to provide the reader with a sufficient working knowledge of the technology to allow for the acquisition of high-quality images in a reasonable amount of time. This chapter is only a brief introduction to what most would consider a complex technology, and the reader is referred to additional sources for more detailed explanations.[1–6]

■ Fundamentals of MRI

Magnetization of Nuclei and Tissues and the Larmor Equation

Understanding how an MR image is generated requires some knowledge of the basic physical properties of the nucleus of an atom and its components, that is, neutrons and protons. All neutrons and protons within the nucleus spin about their axes and generate a magnetic field called a magnetic dipole (**Fig. 1.1**). The magnetic dipoles of protons and neutrons of even-numbered nuclei cancel each other out. However, odd-numbered nuclei generate a magnetic moment, which can be represented as a vector. When placed in a magnetic field, odd-numbered nuclei, because of their magnetic moments, align parallel to the external magnetic field in one of two orientations: spin-up or spin-down (**Fig. 1.2**). A small excess of nuclei align in a spin-up orientation (slightly greater stability) and generate an overall small net magnetization vector (**Fig. 1.3**). Conveniently, the human body is replete with hydrogen, a ubiquitous atom with odd-numbered nuclei (hydrogen has one proton and no neutrons) and, to a lesser extent, with fluorine. It is the manipulation within an exter-

nal magnetic field of this small number of excess spin-up, odd-numbered nuclei that is the basis for the signal that ultimately generates an MR image.[1,2]

When spinning nuclei are exposed to an external magnetic field, the magnetic fields of the spinning nuclei and the external magnetic field interact and cause the nuclei to precess, or "wobble" (**Fig. 1.4**). The frequency of precession can be described by the Larmor equation:

$$\omega_0 = B_0 \times \gamma$$

where ω_0 is the precessional frequency, B_0 is the external magnetic field strength measured in tesla (T) units, and γ is the gyromagnetic ratio measured in megahertz per tesla unit. Conveniently, the ω_0 is constant for every atom at a particular magnetic field strength, and it is key for the localization of the MRI signal within space (see details below).

When an RF pulse (at the Larmor frequency for hydrogen at a given field strength) is applied within an external magnetic field, the net magnetization vector flips from its

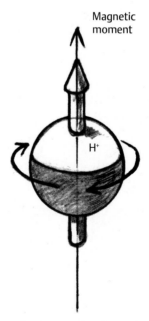

Fig. 1.1 Neutrons and protons within the nucleus spin about their axes and generate a directional magnetic field called a magnetic dipole. In this illustration, the dipole is pointing upward.

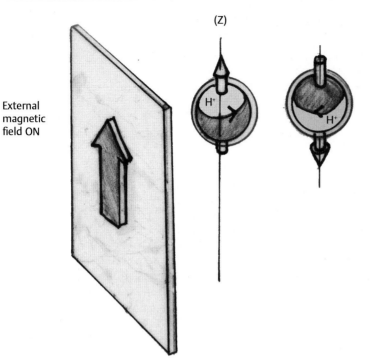

External magnetic field ON

(Z)

Fig. 1.2 Odd-numbered nuclei may exist in one of two energy states when placed in an external magnetic field: spin-up or spin-down orientation, that is, parallel to and aligned with the external magnetic field (*large arrow*) or parallel to and in an opposite direction to the external magnetic field. The spin-up orientation (*z*), is a slightly more stable energy state.

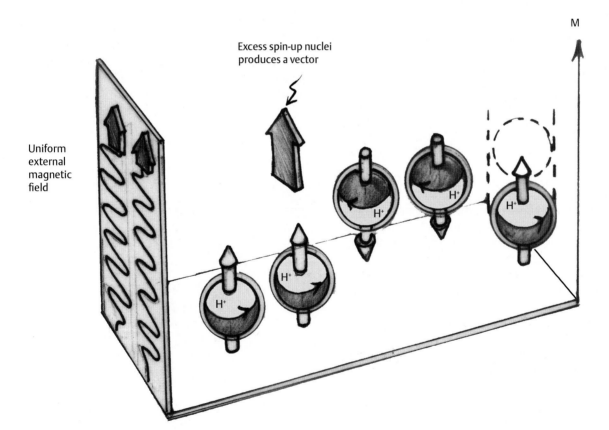

Uniform external magnetic field

Excess spin-up nuclei produces a vector

M

Fig. 1.3 The slight excess nuclei in the spin-up orientation is the result of the increased stability of the spin-up orientation relative to the spin-down orientation, and it produces a net magnetization vector (*large arrow*) that can be manipulated to create an RF signal, which in turn can be used to create an MR image. The two *smaller arrows* depict the direction of the external magnetic field (*M*).

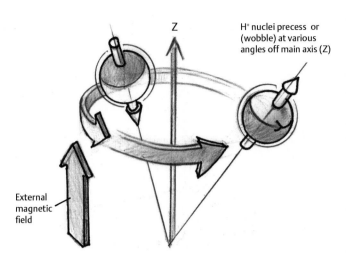

Fig. 1.4 All nuclei, including hydrogen nuclei, precess about their axes when placed in an external magnetic field, which is similar to a "spinning top." The frequency of precession is related to the strength of the external magnetic field as determined by the Larmor equation ($\omega_0 = B_0 \times \gamma$).

longitudinal direction by a certain angle (flip angle). This flipping process produces a transverse magnetization vector (perpendicular to the external magnetic field) and a longitudinal magnetization vector (parallel to the external magnetic field) (**Fig. 1.5**). The magnitude of the flip angle is determined by the strength and duration of the RF pulse applied. A 90-degree RF pulse, for instance, aligns the magnetization vector in a plane perpendicular to the external magnetic field, whereas a 180-degree RF pulse aligns the magnetization vector in a plane parallel to but in a direction opposite to that of the external magnetic field. After the RF pulse, the precessing nuclei initially are also "in phase" with one another; that is, they are precessing in synch with one another. This synchronized precession maximizes the transverse magnetization vector (additive effect). Once the RF pulse is turned off, the precessing nuclei relax, the longitudinal vector returns, and the transverse vector dissipates (**Fig. 1.6**). The transverse magnetization vector produces a signal as it precesses around a receiver coil; this signal can be optimized, recorded, and ultimately transformed into MRI images by Fourier analysis.[1]

In summary, by using an RF pulse to flip the excess spin-up hydrogen nuclei and ultimately transform the longitudinal magnetization vector within a sample or tissue into a transverse magnetization vector, an RF signal can be generated and subsequently used to create an image.

T1, T2, and T2*

The transverse and longitudinal magnetization vectors and the generation of the MRI signal should be addressed in terms of how they relate to T1, T2, and T2*. When an RF pulse that is interacting with nuclei in an external magnetic field is turned off, the precessing nuclei return to their original equilibrium state and realign with the external magnetic field. As one might expect, the longitudinal magnetization vector returns to equilibrium value before the RF pulse does. The return or recovery of the longitudinal magnetization is known as *T1 recovery,* with T1 being defined as the time constant representing 63% recovery of the equilibrium longitudinal magnetization vector.[2] Conversely, after the RF pulse is turned off, the transverse magnetization vector decays exponentially, with a decay rate constant, or T2. The T2 decay relates to spin dephasing secondary to the interaction of the local magnetic fields of the individual nuclei. The time necessary for T2 decay quantitatively represents the time in which the transverse magnetization vector has decayed by 63% of its maximum. The T1 relaxation time is also known as the longitudinal or spin-lattice relaxation, and T2 is also known as the transverse or spin-spin relaxation. The T2* relaxation time represents the loss of the transverse magnetization vector secondary to T2 effects and the spin dephasing secondary to local magnetic field inhomogeneities. Therefore, the T2* relaxation time is always shorter than T2. As would be expected, T1, T2, and T2* differ for individual tissues. Tissues with a long T1 include water and large protein molecules, and tissues with a short T1 include fats and intermediate-size molecules. Tissues with a long T2 include liquids, whereas large molecules and solids generally have short T2 times. The T2* relaxation time usually is short for fat and water.[2,3]

In summary, individual tissues, such as fat and water, have reasonably well-defined T1, T2, and T2* time constants related to the recovery of the longitudinal magnetization signal (T1) and the decay of the transverse magnetization signal (T2, T2*) after an RF pulse. These differences in T1, T2, and T2* directly impact the strength of the RF signal emitted from a particular type of tissue (e.g., fat or water) at a given time and ultimately can be converted to visual differences in tissue contrast on the final image.[2,3] It is MRI's ability to resolve subtle differences in the T1, T2, and T2* characteristics of various tissues and assign the differences to a discrete location (pixel/voxel, see below) within the patient that allows MRI to produce images of such high spatial resolution and to provide information about the anatomy and pathology within the musculoskeletal system.

Gradient Coils and Signal Localization

The transverse magnetization signal is localized within tissue via the use of gradient coils. Nuclei in an external magnetic field precess at a particular frequency when subjected to an RF pulse, as described by the Larmor equation. By altering the external magnetic field and creating gradients in the x, y, and z planes, it is possible to identify the location

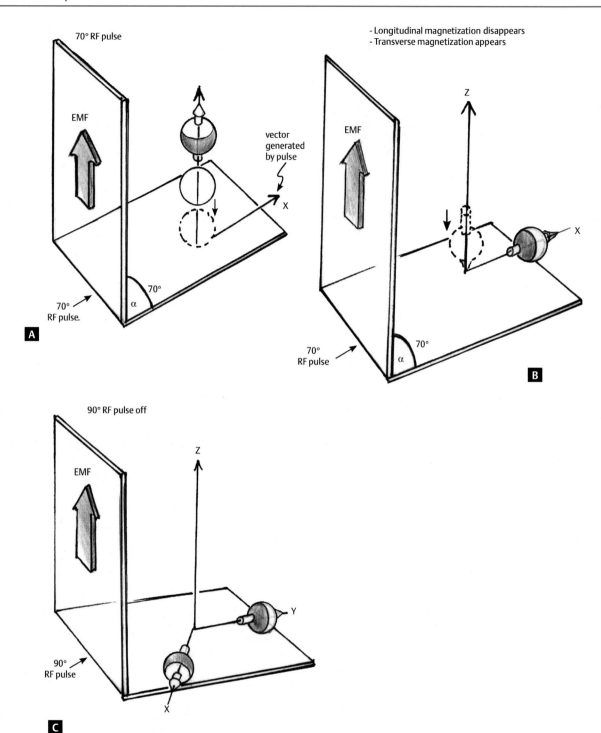

Fig. 1.5 Manipulation of the magnetization vector (*EMF*, external magnetic field). **(A)** An external RF pulse administered at the Larmor frequency can flip the direction of the magnetization vector from the longitudinal to the transverse direction. **(B)** The longitudinal component of the magnetization vector decreases and the transverse component of the magnetization vector increases, based on the strength and duration of the applied RF pulse. The angle the net magnetization vector makes with the longitudinal axis, that is, the external magnetic field, is called the flip angle. **(C)** A 90-degree RF pulse, for instance, will flip the direction of the net magnetization vector 90 degrees relative to the external magnetic field.

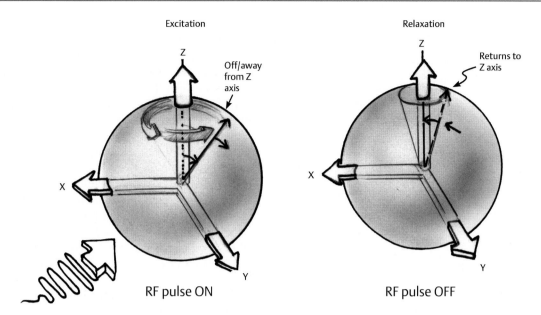

Fig. 1.6 After the discontinuation of an RF pulse, the net magnetization vector will relax, or return, to a more stable energy state, with recovery of the longitudinal component and loss of the transverse component of the magnetization vector. The strength of the transverse component of the magnetization vector is what is ultimately used to generate the MR image.

of signal within tissue based on its emitted RF and phase. Gradient coils superimpose small field gradients in the x, y, and z directions on the main magnetic field and include section-selection gradients, phase-encoding gradients, and frequency-encoding gradients.[1] Section-selective gradients select the section to be imaged.[1] The phase-encoding gradient causes a phase shift that allows for localization of the signal by its phase. A frequency-encoding gradient causes a frequency shift, allowing for localization by frequency.[1] The determination of which plane (i.e., x, y, z) each gradient is applied depends on the orientation of the image (i.e., axial, sagittal, coronal).[1,4] Data within the MR image are divided into pixels and voxels, which localize the signal in two or three dimensions, respectively. A pixel is a 2D unit in the x-y, x-z, or y-z planes, whereas a voxel is a 3D unit, representing a unit of volume within the data set/image.

MRI Pulse Sequence and TE, TR, and Inversion Time

An MRI pulse sequence is the sequence of RF pulses and magnetic field gradients used to generate an image, and several concepts in addition to those discussed above are important when interpreting an MRI pulse sequence: TE, TR, and inversion time.

In conventional SE and gradient-echo sequences, the TE is the time from the initial RF pulse (used to flip the longitudinal magnetization vector into the transverse plane/transverse magnetization vector) to the center of the echo signal (time when signal is at its maximum) (**Fig. 1.7**). In conventional

SE sequences, a phase-encoding gradient is applied at TE/2 to allow for spin rephasing at TE. This technique maximizes the recorded signal at readout (**Fig. 1.7**). In gradient-echo sequences, gradients are used to "recall the echo" at TE and use a negative gradient followed by a positive gradient (gradient

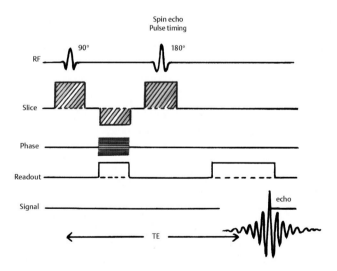

Fig. 1.7 In this example of a conventional SE pulse sequence, the top line shows an RF pulse sequence, a 90-degree pulse followed by a 180-degree refocusing pulse. Section-selection gradients, a phase-encoding gradient, and a readout or frequency-encoding gradients are also shown. The bottom line depicts the RF signal or "echo" recorded at TE. The 180-degree pulse is responsible for the echo at a specific time, that is, TE.

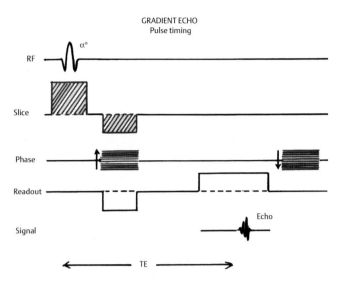

GRADIENT ECHO
Pulse timing

Fig. 1.8 In this example of a standard gradient-echo pulse sequence, the top line shows the RF pulse resulting in a predetermined flip angle. Section-selection gradients, a phase-encoding gradient, and readout or frequency-encoding gradients also are shown. A refocusing gradient (readout or frequency selection gradient sequence), which refocuses signal, produces an echo at TE, hence the name gradient echo.

echo) to refocus the signal at readout (**Fig. 1.8**). One might question why it is necessary to refocus at all. The transverse magnetization degrades secondary to dephasing effects, as described above, and is represented quantitatively by T2 and T2*. Dephasing weakens the transverse magnetization vector/signal, and rephasing (using a perfectly timed gradient echo) rephases, or resynchronizes, the precessing nuclei. When all the nuclei are in phase, or precessing in synch (i.e., vectors pointing in the same direction), the recorded signal is at a maximum. TE primarily affects T2 in conventional SE sequences and T2* in gradient-echo sequences.[1,2]

TR is the time interval between the initial RF pulse of the basic pulse sequence and the subsequent repetition of the initial RF pulse.[1] In conventional SE sequences, TR primarily affects T1 or the recovery of the longitudinal magnetization vector.

TE and TR can be manipulated to visualize the inherent differences in T1 and T2 among tissues on MRI sequences. For example, in conventional SE sequences, a short TE (<30 ms) and a relatively short TR (<1000 ms) result in T1-weighted images (T1 effects maximized and T2 effects minimized). A relatively long TE (>60 ms) and a relatively long TR (>2000 ms) result in T2-weighted images on the T2 SE sequences (i.e., T2 effects maximized and T1 effects minimized). An intermediate TR (>1000 ms but <2000 ms) and a short TE (<30 ms) minimize differences in T1 and T2 within tissues and result in an image based primarily on the density of the protons within that tissue on conventional SE sequences. This minimalization of the differences in T1 and T2 effects

within tissue when creating an MR image is known as proton-density weighting. In gradient-echo sequences, TR varies and is related to the flip angle and the TE. A larger flip angle (70 to 110 degrees) and a short TE favor T1 weighting, whereas a smaller flip angle (5 to 20 degrees) and a larger TE favor T2* weighting. A low flip angle and a short TE result in a proton-density-weighted image.[1-3]

Inversion time is the time to inversion used in inversion recovery MRI pulse sequences, such as STIR and fluid-attenuated inversion recovery. More specifically, it represents the time interval between the initial 180-degree pulse used to invert the longitudinal magnetization vector and the subsequent 90-degree pulse used to convert the longitudinal magnetization vector into the transverse plane. A second 180-degree pulse is used at TE/2 that generates an echo at TE, at which time the signal is recorded. Why use a 180-degree pulse followed by a 90-degree pulse? By applying a 90-degree pulse as the longitudinal vector of a certain tissue (e.g., water) crosses from a negative to a positive value (near zero), the transverse magnetization vector generated by the RF pulse from that type of tissue is very small or zero,[1,2,4] which essentially nulls the signal from that tissue. The most common tissue that is suppressed is fat, and STIR sequences are commonly used in musculoskeletal radiology for this purpose.[1-3]

In summary, it is important to note that occasionally there is confusion regarding the terms T1, T2, TR, and TE. T1 and T2 are characteristics of a given tissue and are intrinsic to that tissue. Conversely, TR and TE are parameters of the pulse sequence and, as such, are extrinsic to the tissue and may be modified by the radiologist. By altering the TE and TR in a pulse sequence, it is possible to manipulate the visually perceived differences within tissue and the MRI generated from that tissue. MR pulse sequences are, in fact, designed to take advantage of the intrinsic differences within tissue, that is, differences in T1, T2, and T2*, to create an image that allows these differences to be perceptible visually. The fact that disease processes often alter the intrinsic properties of the affected tissue and subsequently alter the T1, T2, and T2* effects is the reason that MRI is helpful in the detection of disease.

■ MRI Applications

Standard Sequences

Standard MRI pulse sequences used in musculoskeletal radiology include T1-weighted, T2-weighted, and proton-density-weighted SE (and FSE) sequences, STIR-weighted sequences, T2* gradient-echo sequences, 3D imaging techniques, and contrast-enhanced imaging techniques. For the purposes of this text, the authors have simplified the nomenclature as it relates to the "standard" pulse sequences used for most musculoskeletal MRI by using the following terms:

- T1-weighted image
- T2-weighted image
- Intermediate-weighted or proton-density–weighted image
- Fluid-sensitive sequence, such as STIR or fat-suppressed T2-weighted image
- Gradient-echo image
- Postgadolinium T1-weighted image

Various other proprietary terms and acronyms (e.g., FLASH, GRASS, FLAIR, etc.) commonly used primarily in the radiologic literature have been avoided.

Unlike imaging techniques based on electron absorption, such as conventional radiography and CT, the appearance of biologic tissue with MRI, that is, its relative brightness or darkness, is determined to a great extent by the operator-chosen parameters of the MR pulse sequence used to acquire the images. Thus, a joint effusion may appear bright, dark, or intermediate in signal intensity, depending on the MR pulse sequence and the selective parameters in that sequence. Each MR pulse sequence has its own specific strengths and weaknesses, and typically a combination of pulse sequences is used in a standard examination.

Conventional SE (and FSE) sequences make up the bulk of sequences in the MRI assessment of musculoskeletal anatomy. Proton-density-weighted sequences are useful because they produce images with the highest signal-to-noise ratio and, therefore, provide better resolution than do T2-weighted FSE images. T1-weighted images, which provide nearly as high a signal-to-noise ratio, are also useful in showing musculoskeletal anatomy. T2-weighted sequences tend to have the poorest signal-to-noise ratio, and therefore the poorest resolution, but they are used primarily for their fluid

sensitivity and their ability to detect pathology that has a high fluid content (e.g., tendon or ligament tears, tumors). T2 sequences can also give a rough depiction of anatomy, although it is inferior to that of proton-density-weighted and T1-weighted sequences.

Fluid-sensitive sequences include T2, fat-suppressed T2-weighted, and STIR sequences. Depending on the clinical situation, each specific MRI sequence has some optimal and some less than optimal characteristics (**Table 1.1**).

T1-Weighted SE

Standard T1-weighted SE sequences use a short TR (250 to 700 ms) and a short TE (10 to 25 ms) to maximize T1 differences of the tissues being imaged.[1] The ability to depict anatomic detail, bone marrow abnormalities (including marrow infiltrating processes and fractures), meniscal pathology, blood products, melanin, and enhancement after the administration of gadolinium are the strengths of T1-weighted SE sequences.[3] Proton-poor substances, such as air, and substances that do not have mobile protons, such as cortical bone or other calcified structures (e.g., calcific tendinitis), produce no detectable signal and produce a relative signal void. Fast-flowing blood may generate a flow void and appear dark on T1-weighted sequences, mostly because of a lack of refocusing of the blood, which is excited by the 90-degree pulse but not by the 180-degree pulse. Other tissues, such as fat, melanin, fatty bone marrow, and certain blood products (intracellular and extracellular methemoglobin), appear bright on T1-weighted images (**Fig. 1.9**). Collagenous tissue, such as ligaments, tendons, hyaline cartilage, and fluids (urine, simple cysts, edema), show low signal on standard T1-weighted sequences (**Fig. 1.10**). Tissue with mixed characteristics (with some fluid and some collagenous tissue), such as abscesses, synovium, and complex cysts, tend

Table 1.1   **Basic Pulse Sequences for MRI**

Image Type	TR	TE	Signal Intensity		Advantages	Disadvantages
			Fat	**Water**		
T1	Short	Short	Bright	Dark	Best anatomic detail; rapid acquisition	Poor visualization of pathology/edema
T2	Long	Long	Intermediate	Bright	Moderately sensitive for pathology/edema	Poor spatial resolution, time-consuming
Fat-suppressed T2	Long	Short	Very dark	Very bright	Most sensitive for pathology/edema	Susceptible to artifacts related to magnetic field inhomogeneity
Gradient echo	Short	Short	Intermediate	Intermediate/high	Excellent for evaluation of articular cartilage, PVNS, and blood	Very susceptible to metallic artifacts (prostheses)
Proton density	Long	Short	Intermediate/high	Intermediate	Excellent for evaluation of meniscal pathology	

Source: Adapted from Khanna AJ, Cosgarea AJ, Mont MA, Andres BM, Domb BG, Evans PJ, Bluemke DA, Frassica FJ. Magnetic resonance imaging of the knee: current techniques and spectrum of disease. J Bone Joint Surg Am 2001;83(suppl 2, part 2):128–141. Adapted by permission.

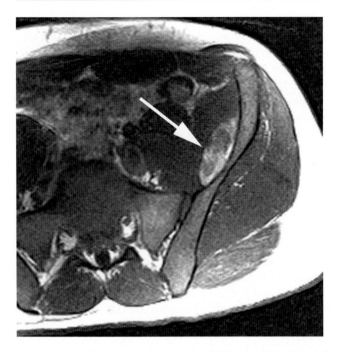

Fig. 1.9 An axial T1-weighted conventional SE image through the left pelvis shows a lesion in the iliac fossa with areas of increased signal *(arrow)*, which represent a hematoma in a patient with hemophilia. The differential diagnosis for T1 hyperintense material includes fat, hemorrhage in the form of methemoglobin, gadolinium-based contrast material, proteinaceous material, some forms of calcium (when in solution), and melanin (as may be seen in melanoma).

sions (**Fig. 1.12**). The T2-weighted SE and FSE sequences also are good for evaluating ligaments and tendons, cartilage, and fluid-filled structures such as cysts. As on T1-weighted SE sequences, air, cortical bone, calcified structures, and fast-flowing blood appear dark on T2-weighted sequences. Hyperacute blood (oxyhemoglobin) and subacute blood (extracellular methemoglobin) are bright on T2-weighted SE and FSE sequences. These sequences also have been shown to be useful for differentiating between fluid and tissue with a high fluid content, such as articular cartilage. The T2-weighted sequences (especially the FSE sequences) may be used in evaluating for articular cartilage defects.

One of the limitations of standard T2-weighted SE sequences is the relatively long image acquisition times. FSE imaging represents a technical innovation that permits much more rapid imaging with T2 contrast[7] with the use of multiple 180-degree RF pulses to create multiple echoes during a single TR period. The series of echoes is called the echo train, and the number of echoes produced in a single TR period is known as the echo train length. Because of their fast acquisition times, T2-weighted FSE sequences largely have replaced standard T2-weighted SE sequences.[1,8]

The major weakness of T2-weighted SE and T2-weighted FSE sequences is their inability to detect marrow pathology when not combined with fat-suppression techniques (**Fig. 1.13**). This limitation is secondary to the fact that both fat and water are bright on non–fat-suppressed T2-weighted FSE and SE sequences.[3]

to show intermediate signal intensity that is somewhere between that of collagenous tissue and fat. Usually, the higher the protein content of the fluid, the brighter the fluid appears on T1-weighted images. For the assessment of tumors or musculoskeletal infection, fat-suppressed T1-weighted imaging after gadolinium contrast administration represents the sequence of choice because the high signal from fat is suppressed, making enhancement of abnormal tissue more conspicuous (**Fig. 1.11**). Short scan times (because of the relatively short TRs) and excellent spatial resolution and depiction of anatomic detail are the major advantages of a T1-weighted pulse sequence. Its major weakness is the relative lower sensitivity for detecting soft-tissue edema compared with fluid-sensitive sequences such as fat-suppressed T2-weighted and STIR sequences.[3]

T2-weighted SE and T2-weighted FSE

T2-weighted SE and FSE sequences use a relatively long TE and long TR to maximize the T2 differences in the tissues. Both sequences, when combined with fat suppression, are excellent for detecting edema/fluid, which appears bright and is often associated with pathologic processes such as tumors, infection, fractures, tenosynovitis, and bone contu-

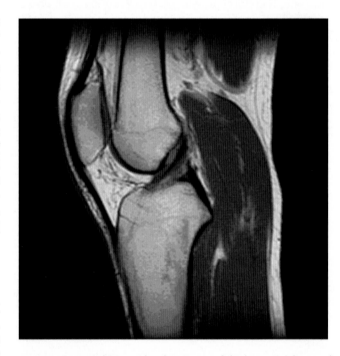

Fig. 1.10 A sagittal T1-weighted SE image of the knee. Tendons and ligaments appear dark, fat is predominantly bright, and muscle has an intermediate signal.

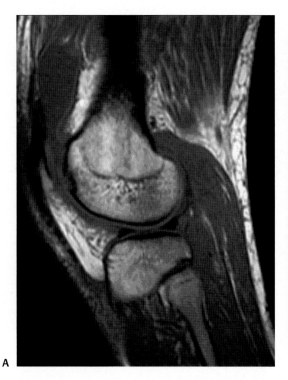

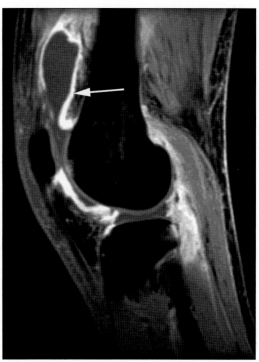

A

B

Fig. 1.11 Sagittal T1-weighted SE images after the intravenous administration of a gadolinium-based contrast material without **(A)** and with **(B)** fat suppression. The diffuse enhancement of the synovium (*arrow on* **B**) is much more apparent with fat suppression in this patient with septic arthritis. The improved conspicuity is a major benefit of using fat suppression.

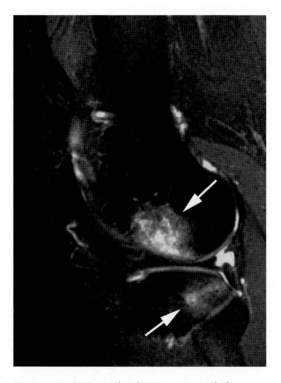

Fig. 1.12 A sagittal T2-weighted FSE image with fat suppression through the lateral compartment of the knee shows high signal within the distal femur and proximal tibia related to bone contusions (*arrows*).

Proton-Density SE and Proton-Density FSE

Proton-density SE sequences and proton-density FSE sequences are excellent for depicting anatomic detail[3] because of the high signal-to-noise ratio of proton-density–weighted images. Proton-density SE sequences also are used to evaluate regions obscured by high signal on T2-weighted images. Fat-suppressed proton-density imaging is often used for the MRI evaluation of meniscal and articular cartilage (**Fig. 1.14**).[9]

The major weakness of proton-density–weighted images is that tissue contrast is not as pronounced as with T1-weighted or T2-weighted images because proton-density–weighted images are a combination of T1 and T2 weighting.[3] Therefore, proton-density–weighted SE sequences are not as sensitive for the detection of fluid and marrow pathology.[3]

Fat Suppression with T1-Weighted, T2-Weighted, and Proton-Density SE and FSE

Fat suppression commonly is achieved by spectral fat suppression or a STIR technique.[10] Spectral fat-suppression imaging is restricted to MRI systems with midlevel and high magnetic field strength because of the necessity for identifying distinct fat and water resonance peaks and selectively suppressing the signal arising from adipose tissue, a process dependent on the presence of a relatively strong magnetic

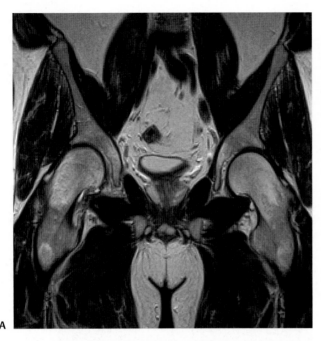
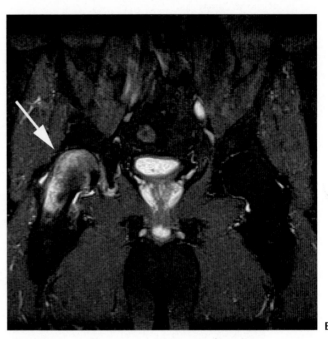

A

B

Fig. 1.13 Coronal T2-weighted FSE images of the pelvis and hips without **(A)** and with **(B)** fat suppression. Increased signal within the right proximal femur related to transient osteoporosis (transient bone marrow edema syndrome) is seen much more easily with fat suppression (*arrow on B*) and is inconspicuous on the FSE image that is not fat suppressed.

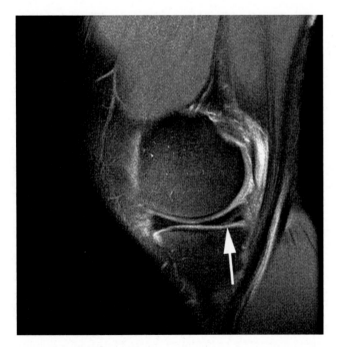

Fig. 1.14 A sagittal proton-density (intermediate)-weighted FSE image with fat suppression through the medial compartment of the knee, showing an arthroscopically proven meniscal tear. Linear signal is present in the posterior horn of the medial meniscus extending obliquely to the undersurface *(arrow)*. This type of sequence is very useful for evaluating the internal derangement of joints.

field. When combined with T2-weighted or proton-density-weighted imaging, this technique is particularly useful in detecting bone bruises and osseous stress injury; the hyperintense intraosseous fluid that accumulates secondary to osseous contusion and microtrabecular fractures appears particularly conspicuous in contrast to the adjacent suppressed normal marrow fat signal.[11]

On T1-weighted images, fat suppression can allow for the differentiation of fat-containing masses, for example, lipoma/liposarcoma, from other tissue that may contain elements of increased signal (e.g., hemorrhage within tissue). Additionally, it can be used to verify the presence of fat within a lesion and to increase the conspicuity of enhancing masses on contrast-enhanced T1-weighted images.

One of the disadvantages of T2, T1, and proton-density fat-suppression sequences is incomplete suppression of the signal from fat secondary to local magnetic field inhomogeneities and susceptibility effects (**Fig. 1.15**).[3] This effect is most prominent with images of curved surfaces, such as in the shoulder and ankle, or of any body part in the presence of metal or air. Additionally, as mentioned above, fat suppression requires higher strength magnets (>1 T) to ensure proper fat suppression than is generally required for non–fat-suppression MRI. STIR sequences often are used to overcome the effects of magnetic field inhomogeneities seen with fat-suppression techniques (see the section below).

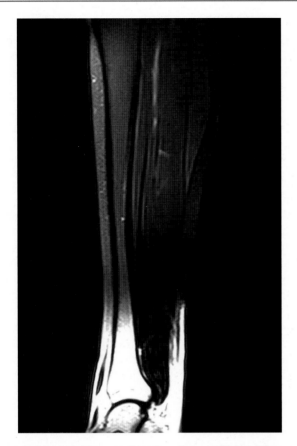

Fig. 1.15 A sagittal T1-weighted SE image of the leg shows suppression of the signal from fat; the distal leg shows bright signal in the marrow and subcutaneous regions. One of the weaknesses of chemically selective fat-suppression techniques is this incomplete fat suppression, which results from local field heterogeneity. This incomplete fat suppression may arise if the imaging is off isocenter (outside of the "sweet spot" of the magnet), such as in the wrist or elbow, when there are noncylindrical structures with materials of substantially different magnetic susceptibilities next to each other (soft tissue and air), such as the foot, or with large field of views.

STIR

STIR is another MRI pulse sequence commonly used in musculoskeletal imaging and, like T2-weighted sequences with fat suppression, is excellent for detecting fluid and edema when administered with a long TE. STIR can be used as an alternative to T2-weighted imaging. On fluid-sensitive-images such as STIR, fluid appears bright and makes the edema and fluid associated with certain types of pathology more conspicuous (**Fig. 1.16**) than they are on non–fluid-sensitive sequences. Such pathology includes osteomyelitis, fasciitis, abscesses, metastases, primary bone tumors, fractures, tenosynovitis, tendon tears, and bone contusions. Unlike T1-weighted and T2-weighted fat-suppression sequences, STIR uses a 180-degree RF inversion pulse, followed by a 90-degree

RF pulse after inversion time to nullify the signal from fat. Because of this phase-refocusing inversion pulse, STIR sequences are less susceptible to magnetic field inhomogeneities and subsequent susceptibility effects that often result in inhomogeneous fat suppression on SE and FSE sequences. One of the major weaknesses of the STIR sequence, however, is that it suppresses the signal from all tissue with T1 signal characteristics similar to those of fat. Therefore, STIR pulse sequences should not be used with gadolinium contrast because gadolinium has relaxation properties similar to those of fat tissue, and thus all tissue with the same inversion time as fat (e.g., certain types of hemorrhage, melanin, and proteinaceous fluid) also will have its signal suppressed.[3]

Gradient Echo, 3D Gradient Echo

As indicated above, gradient-echo MRI pulse sequences use gradients to recall the echo at TE. Specifically, a negative gradient is followed by a positive gradient to refocus the signal at readout. As described above, in gradient-echo sequences, the TR varies and is related to the flip angle and the TE. A large flip angle (70 to 110 degrees) and a short TE favor T1 weighting, whereas a small flip angle (5 to 20 degrees) and a large TE favor T2* weighting. A low flip angle and a short TE result in a proton-density–weighted image.

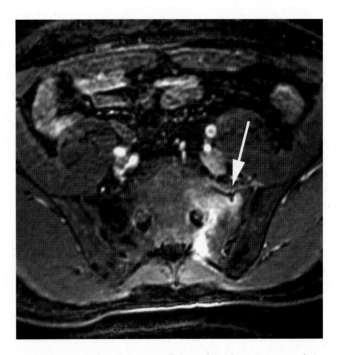

Fig. 1.16 An axial STIR image of the pelvis shows increased signal within the left side of the sacrum. A small incomplete fracture line is present within the anterior cortex *(arrow)*. These findings represent an insufficiency-type stress fracture. Note that the signal from fat is very uniformly suppressed with the use of this pulse sequence.

Gradient-echo sequences are more sensitive than SE sequences to local magnetic field inhomogeneities. These inhomogeneities can be created by blood, air, or calcium within tissue or can be intrinsic to the MRI unit itself. As a result, gradient-echo sequences are very sensitive for the detection of certain types of tissue, such as calcification, focal air collections, and blood products, that produce magnetic field inhomogeneity. Similarly, gradient-echo sequences of tissue that contains surgical instrumentation (metal) tend to produce substantial artifact secondary to the disturbance in the local magnetic field created by that instrumentation. Because of the susceptibility effects of the trabecular bone, gradient-echo images also tend to overestimate the size or prominence of osteophytes within the spine and marrow pathology when the trabecular bone is not destroyed.[3]

Susceptibility artifacts seen on gradient-echo sequences can be helpful in identifying diseases such as PVNS because the hemosiderin deposits that are characteristic of the disease produce local magnetic field inhomogeneities that result in focal susceptibility artifacts.

Gradient-echo sequences also can be used to detect abnormalities involving the glenoid labrum and menisci of the knee; however, the contrast between other soft tissues (such as muscle and fat) is relatively poor compared with that of other pulse sequences. Gradient-echo sequences may be T2* weighted, T1 weighted, or proton-density weighted, depending on what tissue is being evaluated.

In 3D gradient-echo sequences, signal from an entire volume of tissue (i.e., in the x, y, and z planes) is acquired at the same time. This volume of tissue then may be partitioned into sections in any plane. These sections obtained from the 3D volume data set may be isotropic, or nearly so, and can be oriented in any way that is helpful for interpreting the data set. In general, 3D sequences (also known as volume acquisitions) have a higher signal-to-noise ratio because an entire volume of tissue is sampled rather than a single thin section. This optimal signal-to-noise ratio makes the 3D acquisition pulse sequences especially useful at low field strengths.[4] Additionally, relatively high resolution and the high signal-to-noise ratio make the 3D gradient-echo sequences good for detecting abnormalities within small structures, such as the ligaments in the wrist[3] and the articular cartilage.[3,4,12] The major disadvantages of 3D gradient-echo pulse sequences are the relatively long acquisition times and the tendency toward susceptibility and motion artifacts.

Contrast-Enhanced Imaging

Gadolinium is commonly used as an intravenous and intraarticular contrast agent in musculoskeletal imaging. Its function in intravenous imaging is analogous to that of the iodinated contrast agent used in CT, and tissues that show increased vascularity generally show enhancement on postcontrast T1-weighted images. Fat-suppression techniques are commonly used with gadolinium because of their sensitivity to detecting gadolinium.[12] Areas in which there is breakdown of the blood–brain barrier also show enhancement. Specific uses for intravenous contrast include the evaluation of spinal lesions and differentiation of the following[3,12]:

- Solid from cystic lesions
- Soft-tissue phlegmon from inflammation from abscess
- Surgical scars from disc fragments

Intravenous administration also can be used in indirect MR arthrography.

MR arthrography and the intraarticular administration of gadolinium involve the direct injection of a gadolinium contrast solution into the joint. MR arthrography has the advantage of being able to provide joint distention and is especially helpful in delineating labral tears in the hip and shoulder, ligamentous injuries, and TFCC tears in the wrist (**Fig. 1.17**). In the knee, MR arthrography has also been proposed as a technique that may improve sensitivity and specificity in detecting articular cartilage pathology, loose bodies, and meniscal tears, particularly in the postoperative knee.[13,14] Disadvantages include the relatively invasive

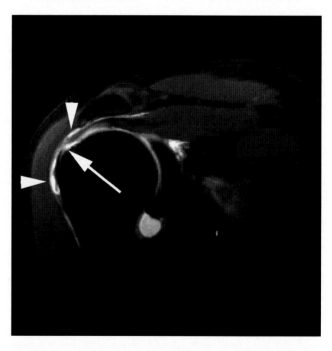

Fig. 1.17 This coronal T1-weighted SE image through the right shoulder with fat suppression after the intraarticular administration of a dilute gadolinium-based contrast material shows a full-thickness rotator cuff tear as a defect involving the supraspinatus tendon *(arrow)*. Note that the hyperintense contrast material extends from the full-thickness defect and is present within the subacromial/subdeltoid bursa *(arrowheads)*.

nature of the procedure, the potential for introducing air bubbles that could simulate loose bodies, and leakage of paramagnetic contrast material into the periarticular tissues that could obscure or mimic pathology.

Indirect arthrography involves the intravenous injection of gadolinium contrast material and imaging the joint approximately 5 to 10 minutes after injection, following movement of the joint through its range of motion. An alternative technique images the joint immediately after injection, focusing on the enhancement of abnormal periarticular tissue or hyperemia rather than using the arthrographic effect provided by direct and indirect MR arthrography. With this technique, contrast material rapidly diffuses into the synovial fluid, facilitated by joint movement, providing an arthrographic appearance without directly violating the joint.[15,16] In patients with inflammatory arthritis, this technique proves particularly useful in evaluating synovial thickening.

■ Artifacts

Common artifacts seen in MRI include motion artifacts, truncation artifacts, the *magic angle effect*, and susceptibility effects.

Motion artifacts in MRI are common and are directly related to patient motion within the scanner. Patient motion results in misregistration of the MR signal and subsequent blurring of the MR image. Motion from the pulsation of arteries results in a particular type of motion artifact or pulsation artifact. This type of artifact produces partial reproductions of the pulsating vessel in the phase-encoding direction.

Truncation artifacts occur in MRI and are related to the way the MR signal is processed during image creation and, in particular, to the Fourier transformation method used to process the MR signal data.[17] Truncation artifacts that can be seen include ring artifacts, artificial edge widening at parallel high-contrast interfaces, interface edge enhancement, and distortion of adjacent tissues at parallel high contrast interfaces.[17]

Susceptibility artifacts seen in MRI, briefly discussed above, are the result of local field inhomogeneities within the scan field, which create areas of focal signal loss. These magnetic field inhomogeneities can be related to the magnet or to metal, air, calcium, or blood products within the tissues being imaged.[3,4]

The magic angle effect is the result of the prolongation of T2 within tissues with highly ordered structures that are at a 55-degree angle relative to the main magnetic field.[12] This effect can simulate pathology by producing increased signal, such as that seen within a normal supraspinatus tendon. To avoid overtreating a normal patient or structure, care should be taken when evaluating highly structured tissues such as tendons and cartilage when they are oriented at or near 55 degrees to the main magnetic field.

■ Summary

A fundamental knowledge base of MRI physics is important for the optimal use of MRI technology. This imaging modality is well suited for evaluating musculoskeletal disease because it provides an accurate anatomic assessment, which is of paramount importance. RF pulses, appropriately applied within a graded magnetic field, can localize the tissue of interest, and the signal produced can be Fourier-transformed into an image. This image is defined not only by the T1, T2, and T2* relaxation time constants of the specific tissue, but also by the parameters that are used to assess the region of interest.

The primary pulse sequence parameters in MRI are TE, TR, and inversion time, and these values determine the weighting of the image (e.g., T1, T2, or proton-density), the strength of the signal, and whether a certain type of tissue (e.g., fat) is suppressed. Each of the standard pulse sequences used in musculoskeletal imaging (SE, FSE, STIR, and gradient echo) has its own strengths and weaknesses, and a combination of various sequences is typical for evaluation of the joints and spine. T1-weighted images are optimal for showing anatomic detail, bone/bone marrow abnormalities, and cartilage tears, and they are excellent, when combined with fat suppression, for showing abnormal contrast enhancement. Conversely, T1-weighted images are not optimal for showing soft-tissue edema. T2-weighted images are excellent for detecting edema/fluid and processes associated with an increased fluid content, such as trauma and tumors. They also may be useful for articular cartilage evaluation but are relatively insensitive to marrow fluid unless combined with a fat-suppression technique. Proton-density images provide the highest signal-to-noise ratio and are excellent for showing anatomic detail. The primary disadvantage of proton-density sequences is the lack of pure contrast compared with that of T1-weighted and T2-weighted images. Gradient-echo sequences are useful for detecting fibrocartilage tears and for identifying tissue such as blood or metal that causes magnetic inhomogeneity. 3D gradient-echo sequences can be obtained in one sequence and examined in any plane as a volume of tissue. The primary disadvantage of 3D gradient-echo imaging is the long acquisition time; the same susceptibility to magnetic field inhomogeneity that may be useful is also a disadvantage when it obscures the tissue of interest. Fat suppression may be accomplished by frequency-specific suppression or by inversion recovery techniques. Frequency-specific suppression is useful but may be affected by magnetic field heterogeneity. Inversion recovery fat suppression is homogeneous but also suppresses tissue with the same inversion time as fat. Gadolinium is used as a contrast agent, most often with frequency-specific fat suppression (because inversion recovery techniques may suppress the signal from the gadolinium). Intravenous injections also may be used for indirect arthrography, although direct injection of gadolinium often may be necessary to achieve optimal joint distention and visualization of the appropriate anatomy.

It is often said that MRI is a compromise and that no gain in image quality is obtained without sacrificing some other portion of the sequence or the examination. A clear understanding of the basic elements of MRI, along with how these elements interact, allows the imager to adjust the scanning techniques and image protocols to obtain the highest quality images possible. This optimization is important in all subspecialty imaging but is especially so in musculoskeletal imaging, where elucidating the anatomy is fundamental to analyzing the structure for the presence of pathology.

References

1. Bitar R, Leung G, Perng R, et al. MR pulse sequences: what every radiologist wants to know but is afraid to ask. Radiographics 2006;26:513–537

2. Huda W, Slone RM. Review of Radiologic Physics. 2nd ed. Philadelphia: Lippincott William & Wilkins; 2003

3. Kaplan PA, Helms CA, Dussault R, Anderson MW, Major NM. Basic principles of musculoskeletal MRI. In: Kaplan PA, et al., eds. Musculoskeletal MRI. Philadelphia: WB Saunders; 2001:1–21

4. Runge VM, Nitz WR, Schmeets SH, Faulkner WH Jr, Desai NK. The Physics of Clinical MR Taught Through Images. New York: Thieme; 2005

5. Lejay H, Holland BA. Technical advances in musculoskeletal imaging. In: Stoller DW, ed. Magnetic Resonance Imaging in Orthopaedics and Sports Medicine. 3rd ed. Baltimore: Lippincott Williams & Wilkins; 2007:1–28

6. Wehrli FW, Shaw D, Kneeland JB. Biomedical Magnetic Resonance Imaging: Principles, Methodology, and Applications. New York: VCH Publishers; 1988

7. Mirowitz SA. Fast scanning and fat-suppression MR imaging of musculoskeletal disorders. AJR Am J Roentgenol 1993;161:1147–1157

8. Escobedo EM, Hunter JC, Zink-Brody GC, Wilson AJ, Harrison SD, Fisher DJ. Usefulness of turbo spin-echo MR imaging in the evaluation of meniscal tears: comparison with a conventional spin-echo sequence. AJR Am J Roentgenol 1996;167:1223–1227

9. Potter HG, Linklater JM, Allen AA, Hannafin JA, Haas SB. Magnetic resonance imaging of articular cartilage in the knee. An evaluation with use of fast-spin-echo imaging. J Bone Joint Surg Am 1998;80:1276–1284

10. Delfaut EM, Beltran J, Johnson G, Rousseau J, Marchandise X, Cotten A. Fat suppression in MR imaging: techniques and pitfalls. Radiographics 1999;19:373–382

11. Kapelov SR, Teresi LM, Bradley WG, et al. Bone contusions of the knee: increased lesion detection with fast spin-echo MR imaging with spectroscopic fat saturation. Radiology 1993;189:901–904

12. Stoller DW. Magnetic Resonance Imaging in Orthopaedics and Sports Medicine. 3rd ed. Philadelphia: Lippincott Williams & Wilkins; 2007

13. Brossmann J, Preidler KW, Daenen B, et al. Imaging of osseous and cartilaginous intraarticular bodies in the knee: comparison of MR imaging and MR arthrography with CT and CT arthrography in cadavers. Radiology 1996;200:509–517

14. Magee T, Shapiro M, Rodriguez J, Williams D. MR arthrography of postoperative knee: for which patients is it useful? Radiology 2003;229:159–163

15. Drapé JL, Thelen P, Gay-Depassier P, Silbermann O, Benacerraf R. Intraarticular diffusion of Gd-DOTA after intravenous injection in the knee: MR imaging evaluation. Radiology 1993;188:227–234

16. Winalski CS, Aliabadi P, Wright RJ, Shortkroff S, Sledge CB, Weissman BN. Enhancement of joint fluid with intravenously administered gadopentetate dimeglumine: technique, rationale, and implications. Radiology 1993;187:179–185

17. Czervionke LF, Czervionke JM, Daniels DL, Haughton VM. Characteristic features of MR truncation artifacts. AJR Am J Roentgenol 1988;151:1219–1228

2 Normal MRI Anatomy of the Musculoskeletal System

J. Dana Dunleavy, A. Jay Khanna, and John A. Carrino

To evaluate effectively an MRI examination of a particular joint or region in the musculoskeletal system, it is essential to have at least a basic understanding of the normal MRI anatomy of that region. Many excellent texts and atlases have been written to serve this need for clinicians and radiologists.[1,2] This chapter provides a brief overview of the most clinically important anatomy for each major region of the musculoskeletal system. The figures and line drawings in this chapter serve to highlight the structures with which the musculoskeletal medicine provider should be familiar before interpreting an imaging examination of the region. Reviewing the normal anatomy images pertinent to a specific anatomic region before reading the corresponding region-specific chapter will enhance the clinician's understanding of the relevant pathologic conditions and facilitate recognition and differentiation of the subtle regional anatomic alternations that represent various pathologic conditions.

■ Shoulder

Axial Images

Axial images are obtained from the superior aspect of the AC joint through the inferior glenoid margin. Axial plane images are best used for evaluating the glenoid labrum (anterior and posterior portions) (**Fig. 2.1**) and capsular structures as well as the long head of the biceps tendon in the bicipital groove.[3] In addition, these images provide good visualization of the subscapularis muscle and tendon, the humeral head, and the glenoid (**Fig. 2.2**). On superior axial images, the normal oblique course of the supraspinatus muscle is displayed with intermediate signal intensity, and the supraspinatus tendon is low in signal intensity. In cross-section, the tendon of the long head of the biceps is seen as a low signal intensity structure within the bicipital groove. Glenoid articular cartilage follows the concave shape of the glenoid cavity and shows intermediate signal intensity on T1-weighted and T2-weighted images. Articular cartilage of the glenohumeral joint is best evaluated on gradient-echo or fat-suppressed T2-weighted sequences.[4–6] The glenohumeral ligaments, best visualized on axial images, have low signal intensity on all pulse sequences. The superior glenohumeral ligament is identified at the level of the coracoid and the biceps tendon. The MGHL is highly variable and may

be identified as a thin band or a cord between the anterior labrum and subscapularis or may not be visualized at all without capsular distention. The anterior band of the IGHL is visualized more inferiorly between the anterior inferior labrum and the subscapularis tendon.

Coronal Oblique Images

Coronal oblique images are obtained in a plane that is parallel to the course of the supraspinatus tendon; they tend to show shoulder anatomy and pathology in a plane that is familiar to most. The osseous structures of the shoulder are easily recognized (**Fig. 2.3A**) as they would be seen on an AP shoulder radiograph. Similarly, the sagittal oblique images show the osseous structures as they would be seen from a lateral view (**Fig. 2.3B**). The coronal oblique images should include the subscapularis muscle anteriorly and the infraspinatus and teres minor muscles posteriorly. Coronal oblique images are best used to evaluate the supraspinatus muscle and tendon (**Fig. 2.4**), the subacromial and subdeltoid bursa, and the AC joint. The long head of the biceps tendon and biceps attachment, the infraspinatus muscle and tendon, the glenoid labrum (superior and inferior portions), and the glenohumeral joint space can also be visualized in the coronal oblique plane. Each coronal oblique image should be evaluated systematically from anterior to posterior. On anterior coronal oblique images, the subscapularis muscle and tendon can be identified as the tendon courses from its origin in the subscapularis fossa to its insertion on the lesser tuberosity. However, the subscapularis muscle and tendon can be seen more clearly on axial images (**Fig. 2.2**). The long head of the biceps tendon is best seen in its intraarticular location on coronal oblique images. On anterior and midcoronal oblique images, the supraspinatus muscle and tendon are seen in continuity (**Fig. 2.5**). The supraspinatus originates in the supraspinatus fossa of the scapula and inserts on the superior facet of the greater tuberosity of the humerus. On coronal oblique images, the anatomy of the AC joint is best displayed at the level of the supraspinatus tendon. The AC joint should be evaluated for the shape of the acromion (**Fig. 2.4**) and the various ligaments around the shoulder (**Fig. 2.6**). The superior and inferior portions of the glenoid labrum, as well as the axillary pouch, are also clearly shown on coronal oblique

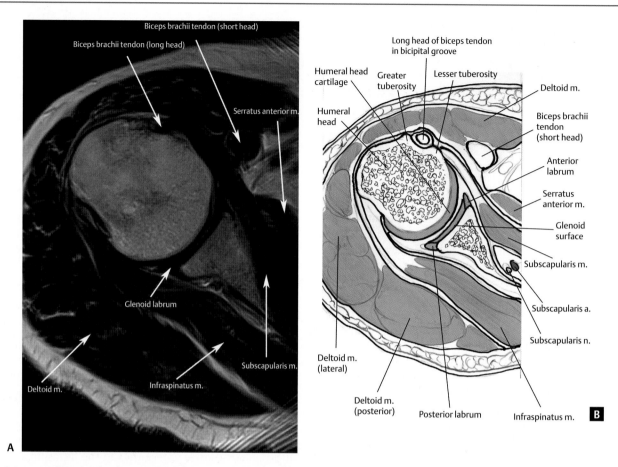

Fig. 2.1 An axial T2-weighted image **(A)** and artist's sketch **(B)** of the right shoulder at the level of the glenoid labrum showing the long head of the biceps tendon as it courses along the bicipital groove.

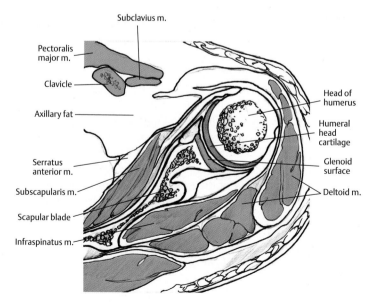

Fig. 2.2 An axial illustration of the left shoulder showing the anterior position of the subscapularis muscle and the articular cartilage of the glenoid and humeral head.

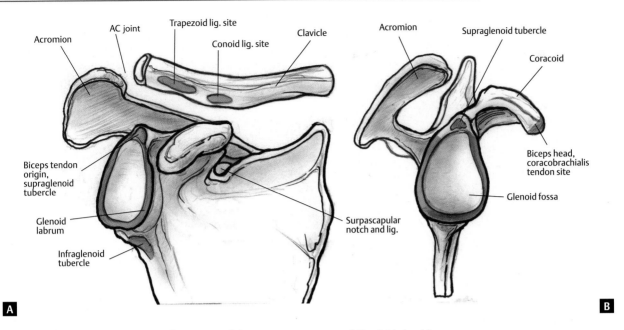

Fig. 2.3 Anterior **(A)** and lateral **(B)** 3D illustrations of the osseous structures of the right shoulder.

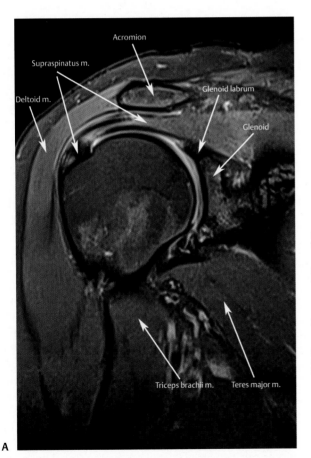

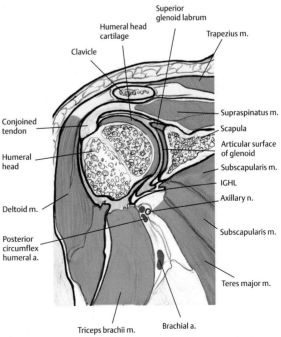

Fig. 2.4 A coronal proton-density fat-suppressed image **(A)** and artist's sketch **(B)** of the right shoulder at the level of the supraspinatus muscle and the insertion of the conjoined tendon, a site that is very prone to rotator cuff injury. The normal, flat acromion is also seen at this level, without evidence of supraspinatus impingement.

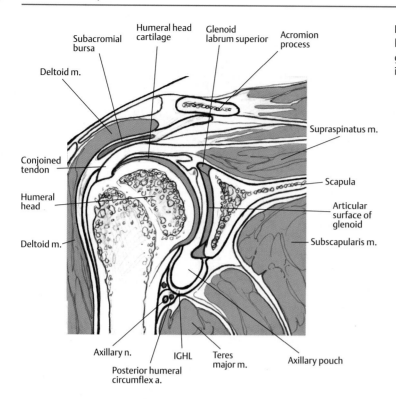

Deltoid m.

Subacromial bursa

Humeral head cartilage

Glenoid labrum superior

Acromion process

Supraspinatus m.

Conjoined tendon

Humeral head

Scapula

Articular surface of glenoid

Deltoid m.

Subscapularis m.

Axillary n.

IGHL

Teres major m.

Axillary pouch

Posterior humeral circumflex a.

Fig. 2.5 A coronal illustration of the right shoulder at the level of the supraspinatus muscle and tendon showing the glenoid and humeral head cartilage and the superior and inferior glenoid labrum.

images. The superior and inferior glenoid labrum are seen as low signal intensity structures, in contrast to high signal intensity fluid on T2-weighted images. The axillary pouch usually is collapsed or has a small amount of fluid in the recess (**Fig. 2.5**). Humeral head articular cartilage, intermediate in signal intensity on T1-weighted and T2-weighted images, is

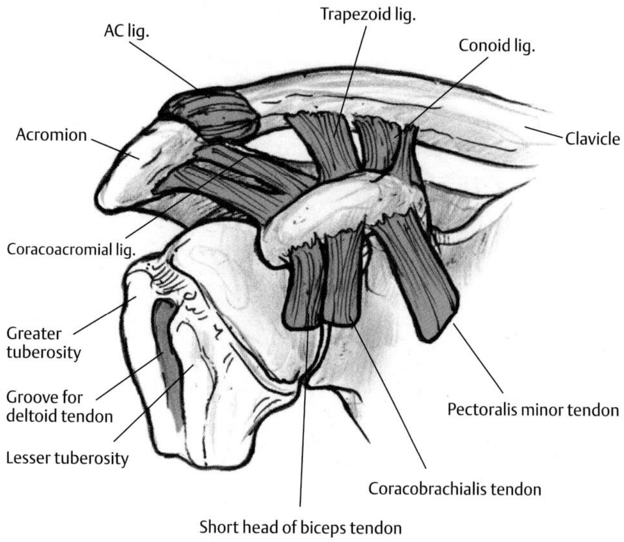

AC lig.

Trapezoid lig.

Conoid lig.

Acromion

Clavicle

Coracoacromial lig.

Greater tuberosity

Groove for deltoid tendon

Lesser tuberosity

Pectoralis minor tendon

Coracobrachialis tendon

Short head of biceps tendon

Fig. 2.6 A 3D coronal illustration of the right shoulder, identifying the insertion locations of the rotator cuff tendons at the greater and lesser tuberosities of the humerus. Also shown are the coracoclavicular and coracoacromial ligaments and other ligaments that stabilize the shoulder.

interposed between the low signal intensity supraspinatus tendon superiorly and the cortex inferiorly.

The subclavian artery courses laterally between the anterior scalene and middle scalene muscles. The axillary artery continues from the subclavian artery at the lateral border of the first rib. Branches of the axillary artery are the supreme thoracic artery, thoracoacromial artery, lateral thoracic artery, subscapular artery, and anterior and posterior humeral circumflex arteries. The brachial artery continues from the axillary artery at the lateral border of the teres major muscle (**Fig. 2.7**). The brachial artery passes posterior to the bicipital aponeurosis, and its branches provide arterial flow to the forearm and hand.

Sagittal Oblique Images

Sagittal oblique images, obtained in a plane that is perpendicular to the supraspinatus tendon, should extend from the most lateral aspect of the humeral head to the midscapula (to evaluate rotator cuff muscle atrophy). The osseous structures (**Fig. 2.3B**) can be used to orient oneself to the location of the rotator cuff muscles, tendons, and other nonosseous structures (**Fig. 2.8**). These oblique images are well suited for evaluating the rotator cuff muscles and tendons (**Fig. 2.9**), coracoacromial arch, rotator interval, and acromial morphology.[3] The glenoid labrum and the long head of the biceps can also be evaluated on the sagittal oblique images. However, both structures are better visualized on axial and coronal oblique images. Sagittal oblique images should be

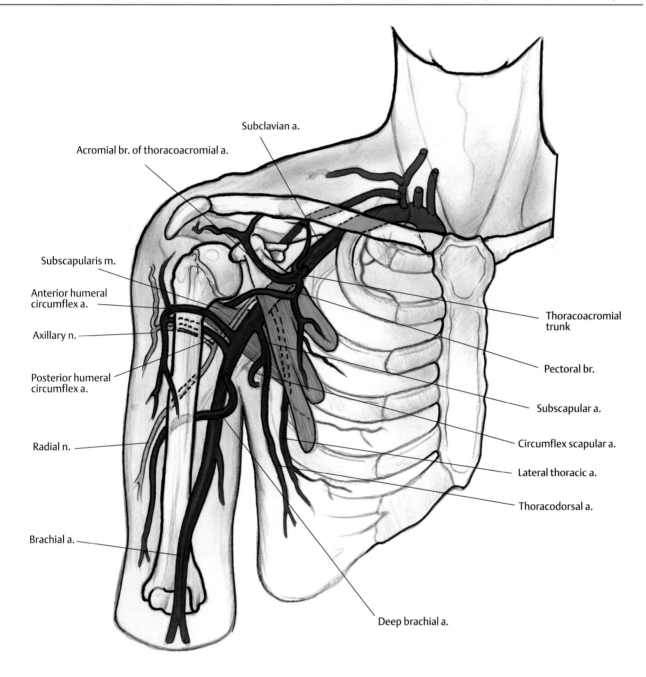

Subclavian a.

Acromial br. of thoracoacromial a.

Subscapularis m.

Anterior humeral circumflex a.

Axillary n.

Posterior humeral circumflex a.

Radial n.

Brachial a.

Thoracoacromial trunk

Pectoral br.

Subscapular a.

Circumflex scapular a.

Lateral thoracic a.

Thoracodorsal a.

Deep brachial a.

Fig. 2.7 A 3D coronal illustration of the neurovascular structures of the right shoulder and arm showing the subclavian, axillary, and brachial arteries, as well as smaller branch vessels such as the anterior humeral circumflex artery, a tributary of the axillary artery, which is seen coursing anterior to the surgical neck of the humerus.

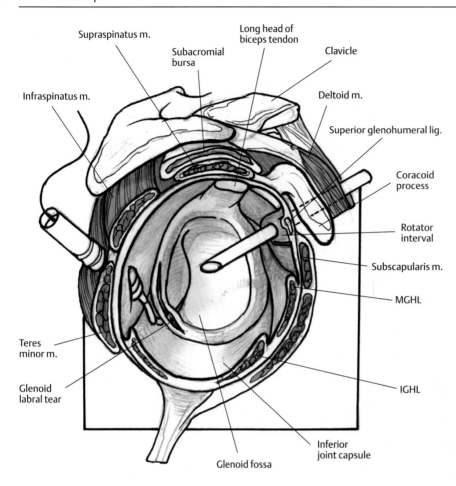

Supraspinatus m.

Long head of biceps tendon

Clavicle

Subacromial bursa

Infraspinatus m.

Deltoid m.

Superior glenohumeral lig.

Coracoid process

Rotator interval

Subscapularis m.

MGHL

Teres minor m.

Glenoid labral tear

IGHL

Inferior joint capsule

Glenoid fossa

Fig. 2.8 A 3D sagittal illustration of the right glenoid showing a labral tear.

reviewed systematically from medial to lateral. Medial sagittal sections display the clavicle and AC joint in profile. On midsagittal and lateral sagittal images, the supraspinatus, the infraspinatus, and the confluence of the cuff tendons are visualized between the acromion and the superior articular surface of the humeral head. The supraspinatus originates from the supraspinatus fossa of the scapula, and the infraspinatus originates from the infraspinatus fossa of the scapula. The teres minor originates from the posterolateral aspect of the scapula. All three of these rotator cuff structures (the supraspinatus, infraspinatus, and teres minor) insert at the greater tuberosity of the humerus: the supraspinatus, along the most superior aspect of the greater tuberosity; the infraspinatus, along the middle facet of the greater tuberosity; and the teres minor, along the inferior facet of the greater tuberosity. The subscapularis is the most anterior rotator cuff muscle, and it originates from the subscapularis fossa of the scapula. It is unique in that it is the only rotator cuff structure to insert along the lesser tuberosity of the humerus rather than the greater tuberosity (**Fig. 2.6**). The biceps tendon can be followed from medial to lateral as it courses from its in-

traarticular origin within the synovial sheath to its more lateral extracapsular location in the bicipital groove. The long head of the biceps originates from the supraglenoid tubercle, and the short head of the biceps originates from the coracoid (**Fig. 2.3**).

■ Elbow

Axial Images

Axial images of the elbow should extend from above the humeral epicondyles (**Fig. 2.10**) to a level distal to the radial tuberosity. The tendons related to the elbow are best evaluated in the axial plane. The major muscles in the anterior compartment of the arm are the biceps brachii and the brachialis; the major muscle in the posterior compartment is the triceps brachii. Ventrally, the biceps tendon is seen as a low signal intensity structure, which courses from its musculotendinous junction, beneath the lacertus fibrosis, to its insertion on the radial tuberosity (**Fig. 2.11**). Some fibers of

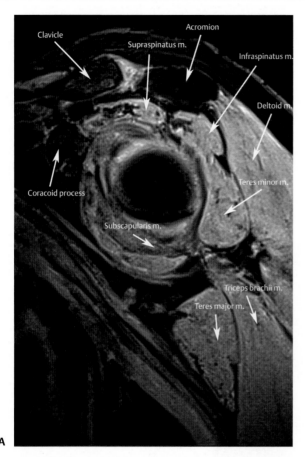

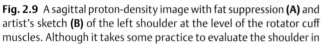

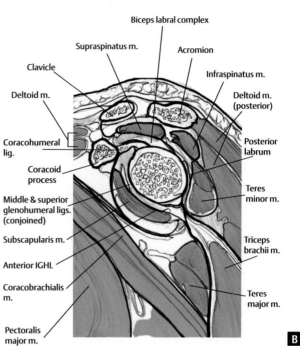

Fig. 2.9 A sagittal proton-density image with fat suppression **(A)** and artist's sketch **(B)** of the left shoulder at the level of the rotator cuff muscles. Although it takes some practice to evaluate the shoulder in the sagittal plane, the rotator cuff muscles are often best visualized on this view.

the distal biceps brachii also contribute to the bicipital aponeurosis. The aponeurosis extends from the myotendinous junction of the biceps to the fascia overlying the anteromedial muscles (flexors and pronators) and is identified as a thin, black, low signal intensity line on an axial image. The biceps brachii spans the shoulder and elbow joints and has a short and long head. The brachialis originates from the anterior aspect of the distal humerus, and its tendon courses immediately deep and slightly medial to the biceps and inserts on the ventral surface of the coronoid process of the ulna. The brachialis muscle is intermediate in signal intensity. Posteriorly, the triceps brachii has three heads with three separate origins; the distal triceps tendon attaches to the olecranon process of the ulna (**Figs. 2.12** and **2.13**).

Axial images also show the muscle architecture well. Because of the relative complexity of the forearm musculature compared with the arm musculature, forearm muscles are often grouped by location (superficial or deep) or by compartment (anterior, lateral, or posterior). Both classification

schemes are acceptable, although individual radiologists or clinicians may have a preference; it may be helpful to review both classification schemes.

Muscle Classification by Location

There are seven superficial muscles within the dorsal aspect of the proximal forearm:

- Extensor carpi radialis brevis
- Extensor carpi radialis longus
- Brachioradialis
- Extensor digitorum
- Extensor digiti minimi
- ECU
- Anconeus (not always present)

Five superficial muscles are found within the volar aspect of the proximal forearm:

- Pronator teres
- Flexor carpi radialis
- Flexor carpi ulnaris
- Flexor digitorum superficialis
- Palmaris longus (absent in approximately 15% of the population[7])

In the proximal forearm, there is only one superficial muscle within the dorsal aspect, the supinator, and one deep muscle within the volar aspect, the flexor digitorum profun-

dus (for the superficial and deep muscles within the distal forearm, see Wrist, below).

Muscle Classification by Compartment

The anterior compartment of the forearm contains the following five muscles:

- Pronator teres
- Flexor carpi radialis

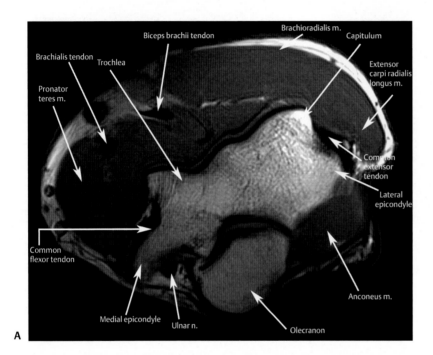

A

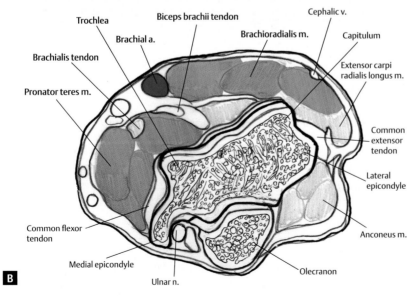

B

Fig. 2.10 An axial proton-density image **(A)** and artist's sketch **(B)** of the left elbow at the level of the humeral epicondyles illustrating the muscle architecture of the distal arm. The biceps brachii tendon, the common flexor tendon, and the common extensor tendon show normal thickness and low signal intensity.

- Flexor digitorum superficialis
- Flexor carpi ulnaris
- Flexor digitorum profundus

There are four muscles in the lateral compartment of the forearm:

- Brachioradialis
- Extensor carpi radialis longus

- Extensor carpi radialis brevis
- Extensor digitorum

Two muscles are found in the posterior compartment of the forearm:

- Anconeus
- ECU

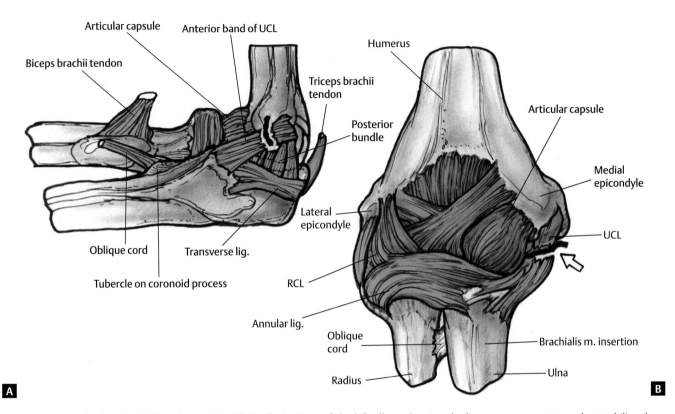

Fig. 2.11 Lateral (ulnar side) **(A)** and posterior **(B)** 3D illustrations of the left elbow showing the ligamentous structures that stabilize the elbow joint and a tear of the UCL (*arrow* on **B**).

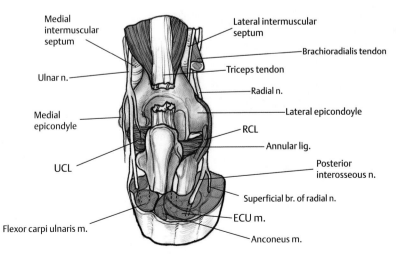

Fig. 2.12 A posterior 3D illustration of the right elbow showing the insertion of the triceps tendon (cut) onto the olecranon process of the ulna. Also seen are other neural and ligamentous structures.

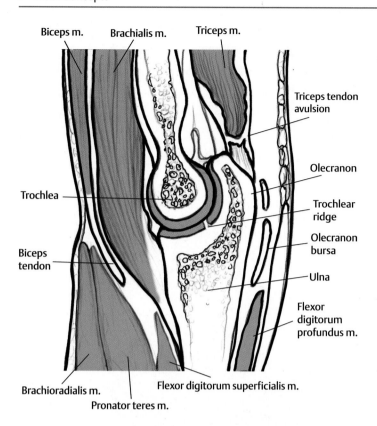

Biceps m. Brachialis m. Triceps m.

Triceps tendon avulsion

Olecranon

Trochlea

Trochlear ridge

Olecranon bursa

Biceps tendon

Ulna

Flexor digitorum profundus m.

Brachioradialis m. Flexor digitorum superficialis m.

Pronator teres m.

Fig. 2.13 A sagittal illustration of the elbow at the ulnotrochlear articulation showing an avulsion of the distal triceps tendon near its insertion.

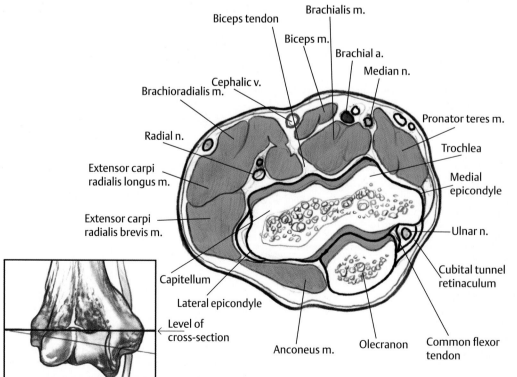

Brachialis m.

Biceps tendon

Biceps m.

Brachial a.

Median n.

Cephalic v.

Brachioradialis m.

Pronator teres m.

Radial n.

Trochlea

Extensor carpi radialis longus m.

Medial epicondyle

Extensor carpi radialis brevis m.

Ulnar n.

Capitellum

Cubital tunnel retinaculum

Lateral epicondyle

Level of cross-section

Anconeus m. Olecranon Common flexor tendon

Fig. 2.14 An axial illustration of the elbow at the level of the medial and lateral epicondyles (see inset) showing the radial and ulnar nerves and the common flexor and common extensor tendons.

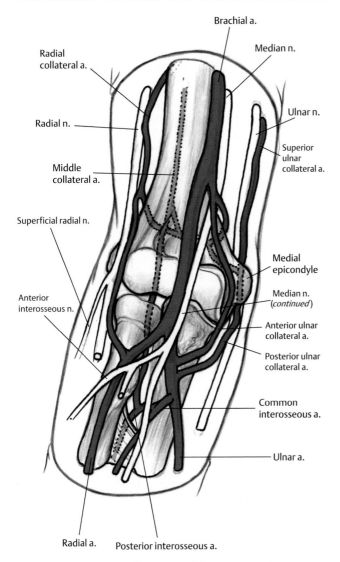

Radial collateral a.

Brachial a.

Median n.

Radial n.

Ulnar n.

Middle collateral a.

Superior ulnar collateral a.

Superficial radial n.

Medial epicondyle

Median n. (*continued*)

Anterior interosseous n.

Anterior ulnar collateral a.

Posterior ulnar collateral a.

Common interosseous a.

Ulnar a.

Radial a.

Posterior interosseous a.

Fig. 2.15 An anterior 3D illustration of the neurovascular structures about the right elbow.

Tendons, Ligaments, and Neurovascular Structures

It is helpful to identify the origin and insertion sites of forearm tendons that involve the elbow because these locations are often the sites of tears and avulsions. Medially, the common flexor tendon is seen on axial images in cross-section as an ovoid, low signal intensity structure originating from the medial epicondyle of the humerus (**Fig. 2.14**). It is shared by several superficial flexor muscles in the forearm:

- Pronator teres
- Flexor carpi radialis
- Palmaris longus
- Flexor digitorum superficialis
- Flexor carpi ulnaris

Not surprisingly, given their shared origin at the medial epicondyle via the common flexor tendon, the pronator teres and flexor carpi radialis are both involved in medial epicondylitis.

The medial epicondyle is not only the origin of the common flexor tendon, but also the origin of the MCL (or UCL). The common flexor tendon is superficial to the MCL, which also attaches to the sublime tubercle, the most proximal and medial portion of the ulna. The sublime tubercle is a helpful landmark, which can be used to easily identify the MCL, especially given that the common flexor tendon and the MCL are similarly low in signal intensity.

The LUCL and RCL are low signal intensity structures originating along the lateral epicondyle in the lateral compartment of the elbow (**Fig. 2.11**). The common extensor tendon is located more posteriorly but also attaches to the lateral epicondyle (**Fig. 2.14**). It is seen in cross-section on axial images and is low in signal intensity. The common extensor tendon is shared by several extensor muscles in the forearm, including the following:

- Extensor digitorum
- Extensor carpi radialis brevis
- ECU
- Extensor digiti minimi

The anconeus is fairly isolated from other musculature, located posterolateral to the elbow. Normal muscles are usually intermediate in signal intensity, so the isolation of the anconeus from other structures with similar signal intensity makes it more easily identifiable. The anconeus is a short muscle, spanning only the elbow joint, with its origin at the lateral epicondyle and its insertion along the proximal ulna. The anconeus is a weak extensor, but it also functions to tighten the joint capsule. The supinator is also seen in this general region, although it originates directly from the lateral epicondyle and the olecranon, rather than attaching to the lateral epicondyle via the common extensor tendon. The supinator runs along the radius laterally and inserts along the lateral aspect of the proximal radius.

The axial plane allows for evaluation of the neurovascular structures (**Fig. 2.15**). The median nerve, which lies in close association with the pronator teres and flexor carpi radialis, can often be identified as a thin, intermediate signal structure located between the ulnar and humeral heads of the pronator teres. The brachial artery, seen in close association with the origin of the pronator teres, lies lateral to the median nerve.

The ulnar nerve is well visualized posterior to the medial epicondyle within the cubital tunnel (**Fig. 2.14**), just deep to the cubital tunnel retinaculum, where it is surrounded by high-signal fat on non–fat-suppressed images. The ulnar nerve is normally intermediate in signal intensity. Although not present in most individuals, the anconeus epitrochlearis muscle is a normal variant structure that may overlie the cubital tunnel and ulnar nerve, extending from the posterior aspect of the medial epicondyle to the medial aspect of the ulna. Proximal to the elbow, the ulnar nerve is located along the medial border of the triceps muscle. Distal to the elbow, the ulnar nerve is seen between the two heads of the flexor carpi ulnaris muscle.

The radial nerve runs between the brachioradialis and brachialis muscles. At the level of the biceps myotendinous junction, the radial nerve can be seen dividing into its superficial and deep branches within the radial tunnel (**Fig. 2.12**). The posterior interosseous nerve (deep branch of the radial nerve) is located between the two origins of the supinator. The median nerve lies centrally but is difficult to distinguish from the adjacent brachial vessels.

Coronal Images

Coronal images of the elbow are obtained in a plane parallel to the interepicondylar line. Although the common flexor and common extensor tendons are seen on axial images,

these structures are also well visualized in the coronal plane. The collateral ligament complexes (**Fig. 2.16**) are best evaluated on coronal images. Starting with the medial aspect of the elbow, the common flexor tendon is seen as it arises from the medial epicondyle. Just deep to this tendon, the anterior band of the UCL courses from the distal margin of the medial epicondyle to its attachment on the sublime tubercle of the proximal ulna. The posterior and oblique bands of the UCL are generally not evaluated well on MRI examinations.

The ulnar nerve can be identified posterior to the medial epicondyle and is shown in long axis on the coronal images, allowing for large segments of the ulnar nerve to be visualized on a single image. When evaluating the lateral aspect of the elbow, the common extensor tendon can be identified arising from the lateral epicondyle of the humerus. The RCL lies deep to the common extensor tendon and extends from the anterior aspect of the lateral epicondyle to the radial head, where it inserts onto the annular ligament. The LUCL is also deep to the common flexor tendon but is more posteriorly located relative to the RCL; the LUCL extends from

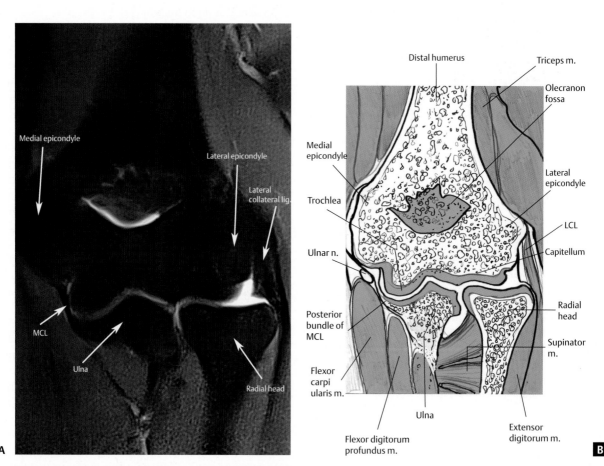

Fig. 2.16 A coronal proton-density fat-suppressed image **(A)** and artist's sketch **(B)** of the left elbow showing the MCL and LCL in the long axis at the level of the radiocapitellar and ulnotrochlear articulations.

the tubercle of the supinator crest of the ulna to the postero-lateral aspect of the radius. The LCL complex comprises the following:

- RCL
- LUCL
- Annular ligament

The articular cartilage of the radiocapitellar and ulnotrochlear joints is well visualized in the coronal plane, but a "pseudodefect" is often identified on the capitellum on more posterior coronal images. This appearance in the coronal plane relates to the fact that the surface of the posterior capitellum is not covered with articular cartilage, often resulting in the appearance of a dark, thin line at the junction of the distal humerus and the capitellum; fluid accumulation in this region may accentuate the appearance of a defect because of its high signal intensity. Awareness of the normal appearance of this pseudodefect is critical: the dark line at the junction of the distal humerus and capitellum could otherwise be misinterpreted as an impacted fracture,

and the accumulation of fluid in this region could be confused with an OCD. Another area that may mimic a cartilage defect is along the lateral aspect of the radial head, where the articular cartilage is generally thinner than the cartilage in other areas of the elbow.

Sagittal Images

The sagittal plane is useful for evaluating osseous architecture and relationships, especially the humerotrochlear and radiocapitellar articulations (**Fig. 2.17**). Intraarticular bodies are occasionally difficult to identify because they may have signal characteristics similar to those of joint fluid. The brachialis muscle can be followed to its insertion on the ulnar tuberosity and is seen just anterior to the joint capsule. The biceps muscle can be followed distally to its tendinous insertion on the radial tuberosity. The triceps is best seen on the midline image as it inserts onto the olecranon. Each of these structures can usually be visualized on several images in the sagittal plane. The lateral images show the components of the common

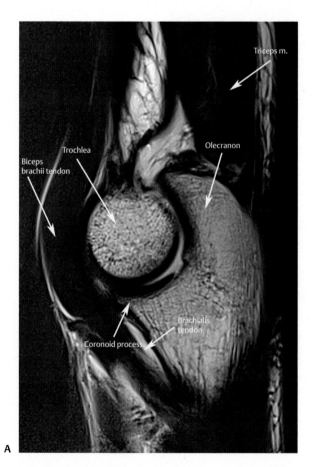

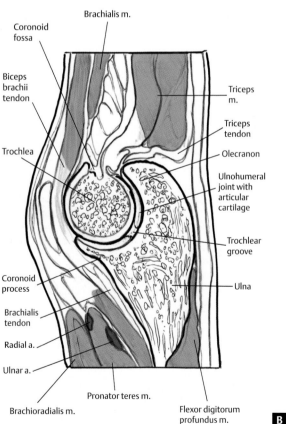

Fig. 2.17 A sagittal T2-weighted image **(A)** and artist's sketch **(B)** of the elbow showing the ulnotrochlear joint and articular cartilage, and the normal appearance of the biceps and triceps muscles in long axis. The normal appearance of the trochlear groove as shown should not be misinterpreted as a cartilaginous defect.

extensor tendon originating from the lateral epicondyle, and the medial images show the components of the common flexor tendon originating from the medial epicondyle. In the sagittal plane, the ulnar nerve is often well visualized running posterior to the medial epicondyle. The common flexor tendon lies in close association with the ulnar nerve, and both structures can often be visualized on the same sagittal image.

■ Wrist/Hand

Axial Images

The best use of axial images is for evaluating the median and ulnar nerves (**Fig. 2.18**) and the contents of the carpal tunnel and Guyon canal. Additionally, the flexor and extensor tendons crossing the wrist joint are best visualized in this plane (**Fig. 2.19**). Many of the muscles in the forearm exert

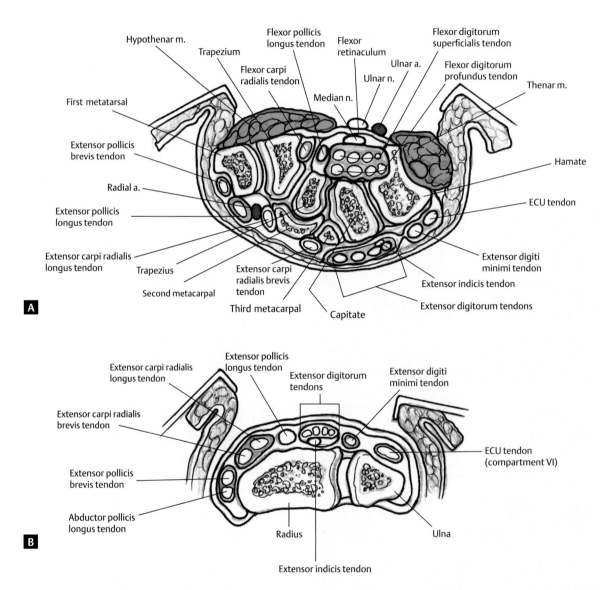

Fig. 2.18 Axial illustrations of the musculotendinous units and neurovascular structures of the wrist with retraction of the skin and subcutaneous tissues along the volar **(A)** and dorsal **(B)** aspect of the wrist.

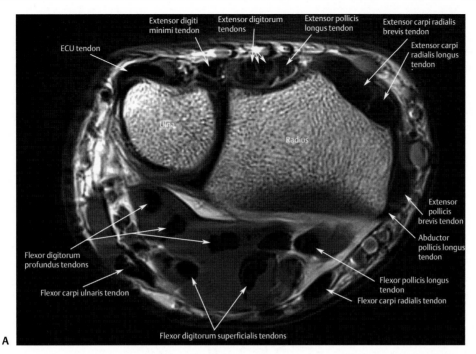

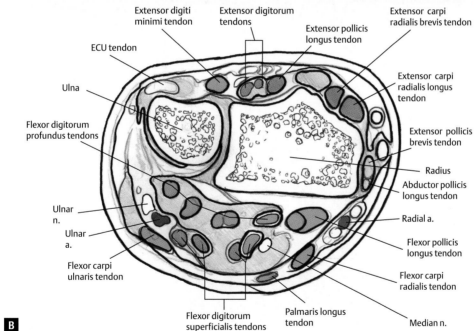

Fig. 2.19 An axial proton-density image **(A)** and artist's sketch **(B)** of the wrist, proximal to the carpal tunnel, showing the large, low signal intensity musculotendinous units along the volar and dorsal aspects of the left distal forearm.

force not only on the elbow but also on the wrist and hand. Muscles in the distal forearm can be classified by location (superficial or deep).

There are five superficial muscles in the dorsal aspect of the distal forearm:

- Extensor carpi radialis brevis
- Extensor carpi radialis longus
- Extensor digitorum
- Extensor digiti minimi
- ECU

Four superficial muscles are found in the distal forearm:

- Flexor carpi radialis
- Flexor carpi ulnaris
- Flexor digitorum superficialis
- Palmaris longus (not always present)

There are four deep muscles in the dorsal aspect of the distal forearm:

- Abductor pollicis longus
- Extensor pollicis brevis

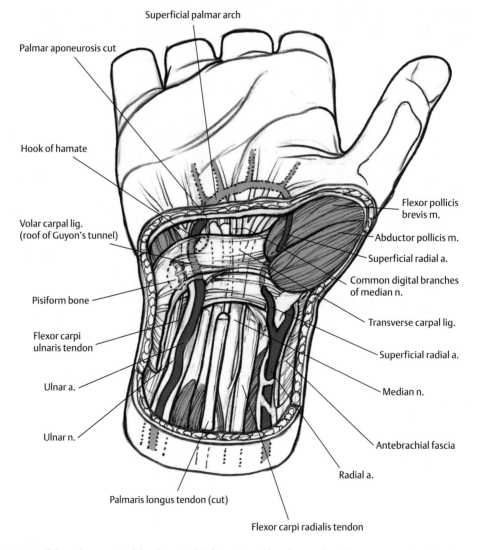

Fig. 2.20 A 3D illustration of the volar aspect of the dissected right wrist and hand, revealing the neurovascular structures, including the ulnar and median nerves and ulnar and radial arteries.

• Extensor pollicis longus
• Extensor indicis

Three deep muscles are found in the volar aspect of the distal forearm:

• Flexor digitorum profundus
• Flexor pollicis longus
• Pronator quadratus

The flexor carpi radialis originates from the common flexor tendon at the medial epicondyle and inserts on the base of the second and third metacarpals. The muscle belly of the flexor carpi radialis is intermediate in signal intensity, and its tendon should be low in signal intensity. The palmaris longus lies medial to the flexor carpi radialis, originating from the common flexor tendon at the medial epicondyle and inserting along the flexor retinaculum and palmar aponeurosis. Both the flexor retinaculum and palmar aponeurosis are seen as dark bands within the superficial palmar aspect of the wrist. The flexor carpi ulnaris originates from the common flexor tendon and the olecranon; inserts on the fifth metacarpal, hamate, and pisiform; and lies in close association with the ulnar nerve, which is seen as a thin, intermediate signal intensity structure running just deep and lateral to the flexor carpi ulnaris (**Fig. 2.20**).

The flexor digitorum superficialis originates at the medial epicondyle, coronoid process, and radial head. It inserts along the volar aspect of the middle phalanx of each finger (**Fig. 2.21**). Proximal to its insertions, the flexor digitorum superficialis divides into four musculotendinous units within the distal forearm, before entering the carpal tunnel. Within the carpal tunnel, the median nerve most often lies immediately superficial to the flexor digitorum superficialis tendons (**Figs. 2.18, 2.19,** and **2.20**), although it may have an intertendinous position. However, within the forearm, the median nerve lies immediately deep to the flexor digitorum superficialis muscle. The large, dark musculotendinous units of the flexor digitorum superficialis are easily identified as they converge within the forearm to enter the carpal tunnel. In contrast to the large, low signal intensity musculotendinous units of the flexor digitorum superficialis, the median nerve is a thinner structure with intermediate signal intensity, which can be more challenging to identify. Thus, the musculotendinous units of the flexor digitorum superficialis may be used as a landmark for the adjacent median nerve. The flexor digitorum profundus (**Fig. 2.22**) originates from the anteromedial aspect of the ulnar and interosseous membrane and inserts along the distal phalanges of each finger (**Fig. 2.21**). As does the flexor digitorum superficialis, the flexor digitorum profundus divides into four musculotendinous units within the forearm before entering the carpal tunnel. Within the carpal tunnel, the tendons of the flexor digitorum profundus lie immediately deep to the tendons of the flexor digitorum superficialis and are easy to identify based on this predictable relationship. The flexor pollicis longus originates from the coronoid process of the ulna, the mid-radius, and the interosseous membrane. It inserts along the volar aspect of the base of the distal phalanx of the thumb. The pronator quadratus originates from the volar aspect of the distal ulna and inserts along the volar aspect of the distal radius.

The extensor carpi radialis longus originates along the supracondylar ridge of the humerus and the lateral intermuscular septum. It inserts along the dorsal aspect of the second (index finger) metacarpal base. The extensor carpi radialis brevis originates from the common extensor tendon at the lateral epicondyle and inserts at the dorsal aspect of the third metacarpal base. The extensor digitorum (**Fig. 2.18**) originates from the common extensor tendon at the lateral epicondyle and inserts along the dorsal aspect of each finger (digits 2 through 5) (**Fig. 2.21**). The extensor digiti minimi (**Fig. 2.23**) originates from the common extensor tendon at the lateral epicondyle and inserts along the dorsal aspect of the fifth digit. The extensor digiti minimi runs immediately superficial to the radioulnar joint. The ECU originates from the dorsal aspect of the mid-ulna and from the lateral epicondyle. It inserts at the base of the fifth metacarpal. Proximal to its insertion, it can be seen coursing along the groove of the distal ulna. The pisiform is actually a sesamoid bone within the ECU. The TFCC is composed of the following:

• Fibrocartilaginous articular disc
• Dorsal and volar radioulnar ligaments
• Ulnolunate ligament
• Ulnotriquetral ligament
• UCL
• ECU subsheath
• A variable meniscus homologue

The abductor pollicis longus originates from the dorsal aspect of the proximal third of the radius and ulna and from the interosseous membrane. It inserts at the dorsal aspect of the first metacarpal base. The extensor pollicis brevis originates at the posterior aspect of the distal third of the radius and the interosseous membrane. It inserts at the dorsal aspect of the base of the proximal phalanx of the thumb, forms the lateral margin of the anatomic snuffbox, and runs in close association with the abductor pollicis longus. These tendons run deep to the extensor retinaculum at the level of the distal radial groove (**Fig. 2.23**). The extensor retinaculum is seen in the dorsal aspect of the wrist as a thin, dark band immediately deep to the subcutaneous tissues, which are very bright on non–fat-suppressed images. The extensor pollicis longus originates from the posterior aspect of the mid-ulna and the interosseous membrane, and it inserts at the dorsal aspect of the base of the distal phalanx of the thumb. The extensor indicis originates from the posterior aspect of the distal ulna and the interosseous membrane, and it inserts at the dorsal aspect of the second digit (index finger). The abductor pollicis brevis originates at the scaphoid, trapezius, and flexor retinaculum. It inserts at the base of the proximal

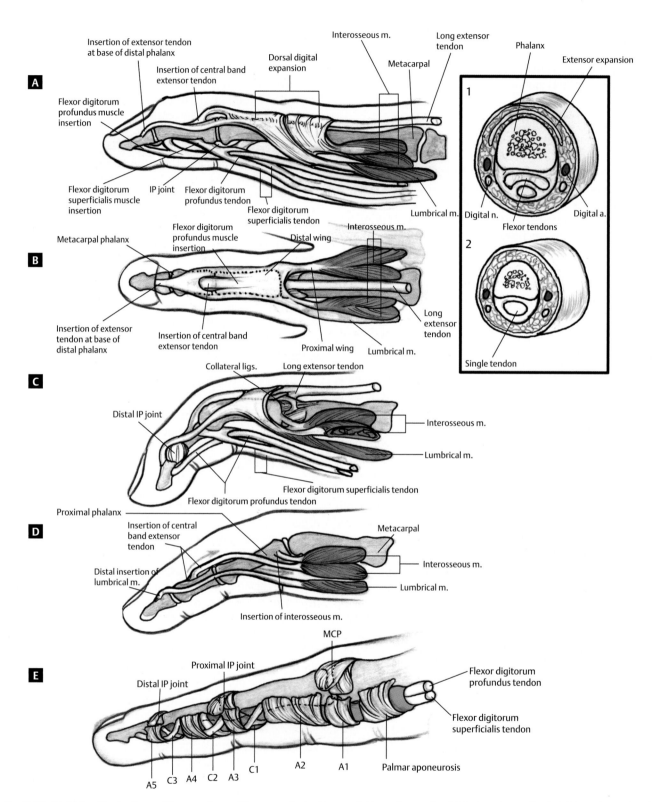

Fig. 2.21 Multiview illustrations of the muscles and ligaments in the fingers: **(A)** lateral superficial, **(B)** dorsal superficial, **(C)** lateral superficial in flexion, **(D)** lateral deep, and **(E)** pulley system (numbers and letters designate specific pulleys). *Inset*: axial cross-section through the middle (*1*) and distal (*2*) phalanxes.

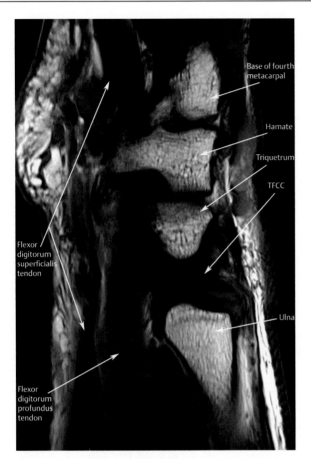

Fig. 2.22 A sagittal T1-weighted image of the wrist showing the normal appearance of the flexor digitorum profundus and flexor digitorum superficialis tendons, as well as the triangular fibrocartilage.

structures such as the scapholunate and lunotriquetral ligaments are usually best seen on coronal images, and with thin sections; these structures are routinely well delineated. The radiocarpal compartment is separated from the radioulnar joint by the triangular fibrocartilage. Most information about the triangular fibrocartilage is also gained from coronal images. The triangular fibrocartilage looks like a curvilinear bowtie, and it extends horizontally from the ulnar surface of the distal radius to the base of the ulnar styloid process. It is low in signal intensity. In the coronal plane, the triangular fibrocartilage and interosseous ligaments are often seen on the same sections as the ECU tendon. Within the hand, the ligaments of the IP and MCP joints (in particular, the UCL of the thumb) are most readily assessed in this plane. However, thumb imaging should be performed separately with

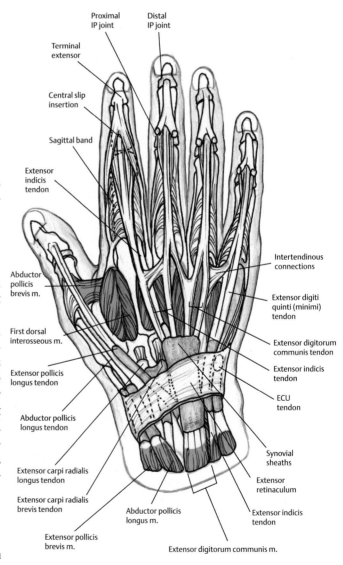

Fig. 2.23 Illustration of the dorsal aspect of the right hand showing the muscles and tendons.

phalanx of the thumb. Unlike the other muscles described in this section, the abductor pollicis brevis has no function at the wrist joint, and thus is considered a hand muscle.

In the axial plane, the distal radioulnar joint is examined at the sigmoid notch of the radius. Particular osseous structures, such as the hook of the hamate, and the articulations between carpal bones can be assessed on axial images. The extrinsic carpal ligaments (**Fig. 2.24**), seen as uniformly low intensity structures in close relationship with the wrist capsule, may be accentuated with intraarticular contrast. Axial images of the digits provide cross-sectional visualization of small anatomic structures such as the flexor tendons, extensor mechanism, volar plates, and neurovascular bundles (**Figs. 2.21** and **2.25**).

Coronal Images

Coronal plane images provide useful anatomic information about the wrist and hand, and show well the osseous structures and their respective relationships (**Fig. 2.26**). Small

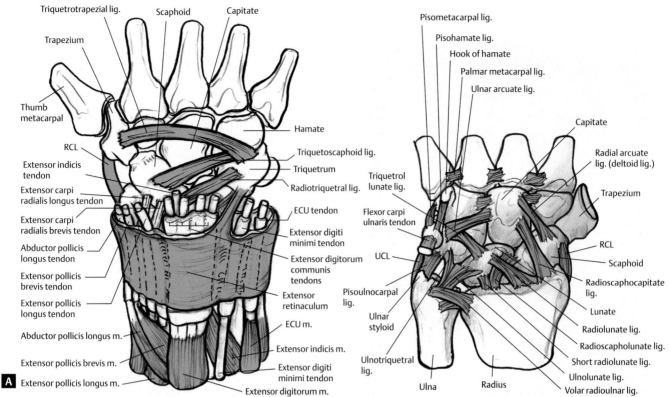

Fig. 2.24 Illustrations of the wrist showing the dorsal **(A)** and volar **(B)** aspects of the left distal radius and ulna, carpal bones, musculotendinous units, and intercarpal ligaments.

specialized planes. The abductor pollicis longus and extensor pollicis brevis tendons are seen within the medial/volar aspect of the wrist at the level of the volar aspect of the scaphoid and lunate. Also within the volar aspect of the wrist are the radioscaphocapitate ligament and the radiolunotriquetral ligament, which extend in the ulnar direction from the radial styloid. Located slightly ulnar to these ligaments is the radioscapholunate ligament (**Fig. 2.24**). These three carpal ligaments are low in signal intensity and are often seen on the same image in the coronal plane.

Despite the advantages of coronal images for evaluation of the TFCC and intercarpal ligaments, the variable courses of the tendons and neurovascular structures crossing the wrist and hand joints make evaluation of these structures difficult in the coronal plane, and therefore these structures are primarily assessed on axial images. On the dorsal coronal images, the extensor digiti minimi tendon is seen as it courses obliquely along the ulnar side of the triquetrum. The extensor pollicis longus and the extensor carpi radialis brevis are separated by Lister's tubercle, which shows fatty marrow signal intensity. On the volar coronal images, the flexor tendons are seen coursing deep to the flexor retinaculum, which appears as a dark, transverse band. The flexor tendons appear as hypointense bands and can be followed as they pass through the carpal tunnel between the trapezium and the hook of the hamate. The median nerve is intermediate in signal, slightly brighter than that of the adjacent tendons.

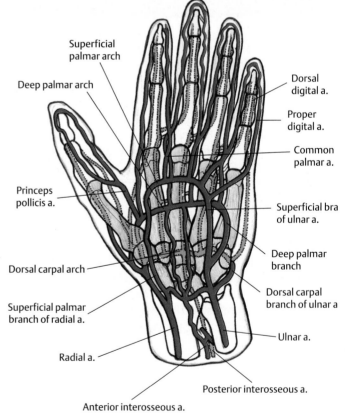

Fig. 2.25 A 3D illustration of the volar (red) and dorsal (pink) vasculature in the left wrist and hand.

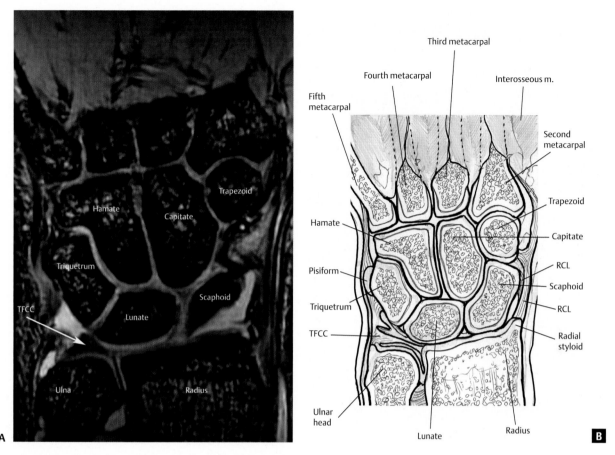

Fig. 2.26 A coronal T2*-weighted image **(A)** and artist's sketch **(B)** of the wrist at the level of the TFCC. The carpal bone architecture is well delineated on this image, which was acquired on a high field strength magnet with an eight-channel surface coil.

The radial and ulnar styloid may be evaluated for fractures on coronal images. The joints, including the distal radioulnar, radiocarpal, intercarpal, and carpometacarpal joints, can also be evaluated for degenerative or traumatic changes. The articular surfaces of the carpal bones show intermediate signal intensity.

Sagittal Images

The sagittal plane is useful for depicting the longitudinal course of structures and providing an orthogonal section for bones in the wrist and hand. Information from sagittal images can be used to evaluate the TFCC (**Fig. 2.22**) and overall carpal alignment, especially with regard to the scapholunate and capitolunate articulations (**Figs. 2.27** and **2.28**). Deformity of the scaphoid and abnormalities of the pisotriquetral joint are also examined in this plane. Fractures of the other carpal bones, including the hook of the hamate and the lu-

nate, are also well visualized. The course of the flexor and extensor tendons is well shown on sagittal images of the digits, as is the course of the median nerve in the wrist.

■ Hip

Axial Images

The hip (femoroacetabulum), a diarthrodial joint, is an articulation between the acetabulum and the head of the femur (**Fig. 2.29**). The acetabulum is formed by the union of the ilium, ischium, and pubis; is normally oriented approximately 45 degrees caudally; and has between 14 and 26.5 degrees of anteversion (averages: men, 18.5 ± 4.5 degrees; women, 21.5 ± 5.0 degrees).[8] The normal femoral neck–shaft angle ranges between 125 and 140 degrees.[8,9] Given the complex 3D geometry of the hip joint, MRI of the hip should use all

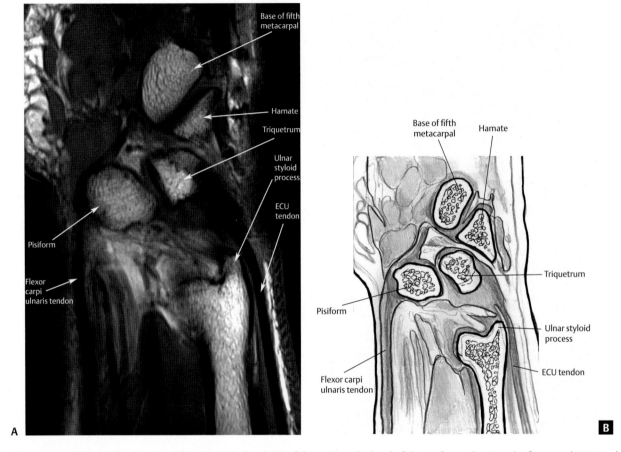

Fig. 2.27 A sagittal T1-weighted image (**A**) and artist's sketch (**B**) of the wrist at the level of the pisiform, showing the flexor and ECU tendons within the forearm and wrist.

three standard planes of imaging and a specialized plane along (parallel to) the femoral neck. The muscles of the hip can be grouped according to function or anatomic location (medial, anterior, lateral, and posterior). There is no single accepted grouping technique, but some form of a systematic review should be performed. Functional muscle grouping is a logical technique:

- Abductors: gluteus medius, gluteus minimus, and tensor fascia lata
- Adductors: pectineus, gracilis, adductor longus, adductor brevis, and adductor magnus
- Flexors: iliopsoas, rectus femoris, sartorius
- Extensors: gluteus maximus, hamstrings
- External rotators: piriformis, obturator externus, obturature internus, superior gemelli, inferior gemelli, and quadratus femoris

Although most of the musculature in the region of the hip is best evaluated on axial images (**Figs. 2.30** and **2.31**), the

hamstrings and gluteus medius and minimus are more easily evaluated in the coronal plane (**Fig. 2.32**).

Generally, in addition to the conventional axial images, oblique axial images oriented along the axis of the femoral neck are also obtained. These oblique images allow visualization of the head–neck junction and can aid in evaluating anatomy associated with femoroacetabular impingement. Axial images allow for good visualization of the anterior and posterior portions of the labrum (**Fig. 2.31**), which are seen as low signal intensity structures. Axial images are also useful for identifying the regional neurovascular bundles, specifically the sciatic nerve, obturator, and femoral neurovascular bundles; in these bundles, the nerves are seen in cross-section as intermediate signal structures, and often discrete fascicles can be discerned.

The gluteus maximus, gluteus medius, and gluteus minimus can be identified and differentiated by fascial divisions. The tensor fascia latae is located anterior to the gluteus medius (**Fig. 2.31**). At the level of the inferior pubic ramus, the

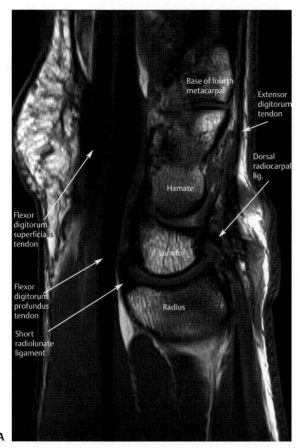

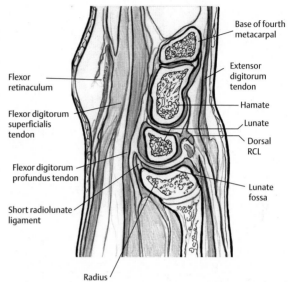

Fig. 2.28 A sagittal T1-weighted image **(A)** and artist's sketch **(B)** of the wrist at the radiolunate articulation showing the normal relationship of the radius, lunate, hamate, and fourth (ring finger) metacarpal. Long segments of the flexor digitorum superficialis and profundus tendons are seen as they pass through the carpal tunnel.

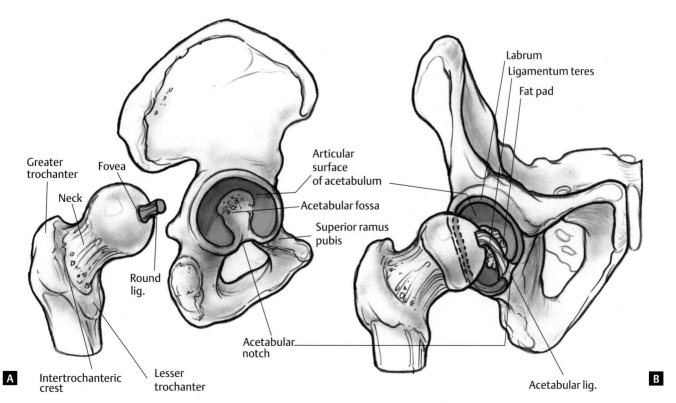

Fig. 2.29 Disarticulated lateral **(A)** and partially disarticulated anterior oblique **(B)** 3D illustrations of the femoroacetabular articular surfaces.

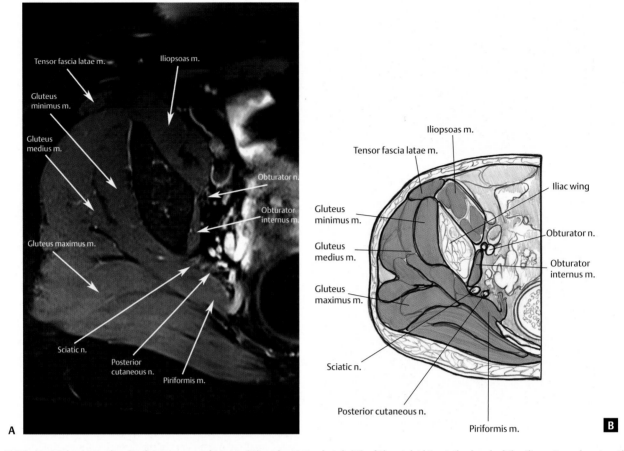

Fig. 2.30 An axial proton-density fat-suppressed image **(A)** and artist's sketch **(B)** of the right hip at the level of the iliac wing, showing the fascial layers separating the gluteus maximus, gluteus medius, and gluteus minimus musculature. The sciatic nerve is also seen.

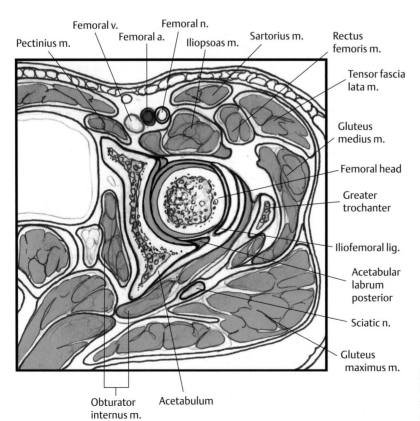

Fig. 2.31 An axial illustration of the left hip at the level of the femoroacetabular joint showing the anterior and posterior labrum, articular cartilage, and surrounding musculature.

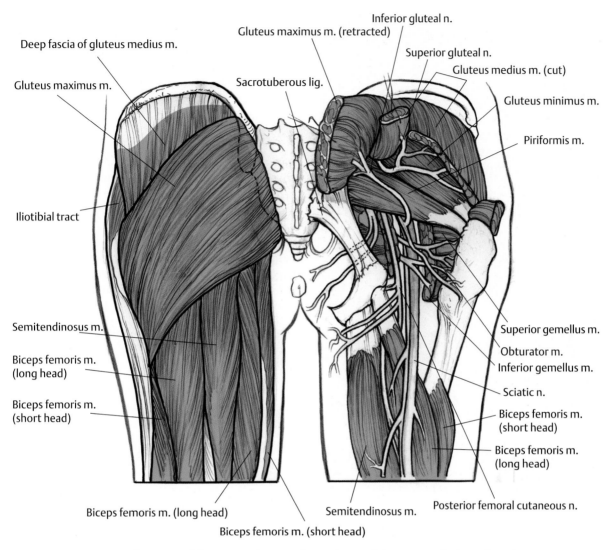

Fig. 2.32 A 3D posteroanterior illustration of the intact and removed musculature of the posterior thigh overlying the sciatic nerve and other neural structures.

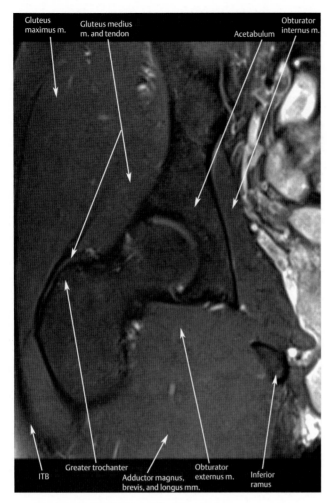

Gluteus maximus m.

Gluteus medius m. and tendon

Acetabulum

Obturator internus m.

ITB

Greater trochanter

Adductor magnus, brevis, and longus mm.

Obturator externus m.

Inferior ramus

Fig. 2.33 A coronal proton-density image of the right hip showing the suprafoveal aspect of the femoral head and acetabular dome.

iliopsoas inserts along the lesser trochanter. The ITB is identified laterally. The external iliac vessels are seen anterior to the anterior column of the acetabulum and medial to the iliopsoas muscle.

Coronal Images

The coronal plane is helpful for evaluating the weight-bearing, suprafoveal aspect of the femoral head and acetabular dome (**Fig. 2.33**), the trochanteric bursa, and the superior labrum (**Fig. 2.34**). The normal labrum appears as a triangular structure of low signal at the lateral (peripheral) margin of the acetabulum (**Fig. 2.35**). To view the anterior superior, superior, and posterior superior labrum, images should be examined successively from anterior to posterior. The inferior portion of the acetabulum is not covered by the labrum and contains the transverse ligament. The joint capsule and capsular ligaments surround the femoral neck and appear as a low signal intensity structure.

The trochanteric bursa, the iliopsoas tendon, and the distal insertions of the gluteus medius and minimus tendons onto the greater trochanter are well visualized in the coronal plane. The articular cartilage appears as an intermediate signal overlying the low signal cortical bone.

Sagittal Images

The sagittal images are helpful for evaluating the weight-bearing portion of the femoral head and acetabular dome, as well as the anterior superior labrum (**Fig. 2.36**). Articular cartilage is also well evaluated in the sagittal plane. The entire course of the labrum should be evaluated from medial to lateral. The hip adductors are visualized in cross-section in the sagittal plane, which is helpful in localizing pathologic changes to specific muscles in this group. The origin of the reflected tendon of the rectus femoris muscle can be visualized at the anterior inferior iliac spine.

Sagittal images also visualize the following:

- Iliopsoas muscle (which runs anterior to the hip joint as it courses toward its insertion on the lesser trochanter)
- Iliofemoral ligament (at its insertion on the anterior labrum)
- Ischiofemoral ligament (located posterior to the iliofemoral ligament)

■ Knee

Axial Images

Axial images are useful for examining the patellofemoral joint and the medial and lateral retinaculum, and for assessing tilt and subluxation (**Fig. 2.37**). The patellar cartilage surfaces also are well visualized in this plane, and plicae can be seen (**Fig. 2.38**). The suprapatellar bursa can be evaluated for knee effusions. The axial images can also be used to correlate quadriceps or patellar tendon anatomy seen on sagittal images, as well as collateral ligament anatomy seen on coronal images.

The ACL can be followed as it courses in an anteromedial direction through the intercondylar notch (**Fig. 2.37A**) to the surface of the tibia just lateral and slightly posterior to the anterior horn of the medial meniscus. The tibial insertion of the PCL is just medial to midline. This position can be verified on sagittal images because the PCL is in the same plane as the anterior and posterior horns of the medial meniscus.

The menisci can be visualized on axial images, although meniscal pathology is better evaluated in the sagittal and coronal planes. The transverse ligament usually can be seen running from the anterior horn of the medial meniscus to the lateral meniscus.

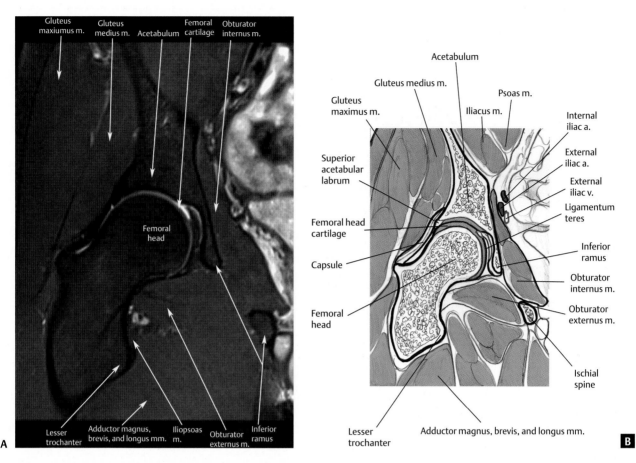

Fig. 2.34 A coronal proton-density image **(A)** and artist's sketch **(B)** of the right hip at the level of the lesser trochanter showing the articular cartilage of the femoral head and acetabulum.

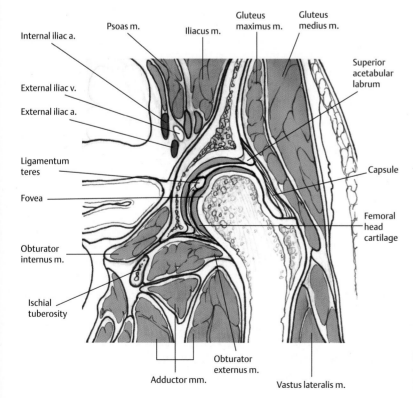

Fig. 2.35 A coronal illustration of the left hip showing the articular cartilage of the femoral head and acetabulum, the labrum, and the surrounding musculature.

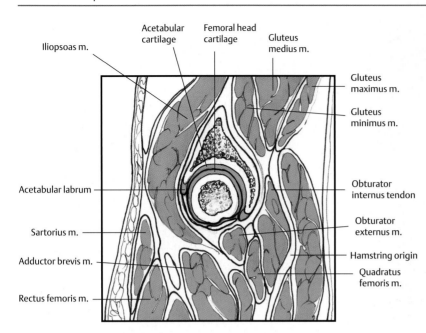

Iliopsoas m.

Acetabular cartilage

Femoral head cartilage

Gluteus medius m.

Gluteus maximus m.

Gluteus minimus m.

Acetabular labrum

Sartorius m.

Adductor brevis m.

Rectus femoris m.

Obturator internus tendon

Obturator externus m.

Hamstring origin

Quadratus femoris m.

Fig. 2.36 A sagittal illustration of the left hip showing the articular cartilage, labrum, and surrounding musculature.

The MCL and LCL complex components are seen as low signal intensity structures. The popliteal neurovascular structures can be seen just posterior to the joint capsule and are surrounded by fat. The popliteus tendon and posterolateral complex structures can also be seen in this plane.

Coronal Images

The coronal images are best for evaluating the collateral ligaments and the posterolateral and posteromedial corner complexes (**Fig. 2.39**), but they should be viewed in conjunction with the axial and sagittal sequences to better understand the location in all three dimensions.

Posterolateral and Posteromedial Corners

This complex layer of tissues lies deep to the popliteal neurovascular structures (**Fig. 2.40**). The posterolateral corner is composed of the arcuate ligament, fabellofibular ligament, popliteofibular ligament, popliteal tendon, fibular collateral ligament, and biceps femoris tendon. The posteromedial ligament corner is composed of the posterior oblique ligament and the insertion of the semimembranosus tendon with its five extensions, including the oblique popliteal ligament.[10] The fabella (variably present) can be seen as a circular structure superior to the most proximal aspect of the fibular head. The fabella frequently contains marrow and can be bright on T1-weighted sequences. Differentiating the individual components of these two complexes is difficult because they vary in consistency and are relatively thin. MR images acquired with thick sections may capture only

a small portion of the complexes. The intricacy of the posterolateral complex structures makes evaluation especially sensitive to artifact in this region, particularly from patient motion or limited technical quality of the scan.

Collateral Ligaments

The MCL, which runs from the medial femoral epicondyle to the proximal tibia, deep to the pes anserinus tendon, has deep and superficial components. The lateral side is composed of a multistructure tendon and ligament unit known as the LCL complex. It comprises the ITB, the fibular collateral ligament, and the biceps femoris tendon. The fibular collateral ligament (**Fig. 2.40**) extends from the lateral femoral epicondyle to the fibular head, anterior to the insertion of the biceps femoris tendon. The MCL and LCL are low signal intensity structures (**Fig. 2.41**). The ITB is seen on anterior coronal sections and inserts into Gerdy's tubercle on the anterolateral proximal tibia.

ACL and PCL

The ACL, which can be visualized running just anterior to the PCL, fills up the lateral aspect of the intercondylar notch, whereas the PCL is located in the medial aspect of the notch. The ACL can be seen almost in its entirety, whereas the PCL is captured by successive sections through its substance as it courses posteriorly and inferiorly. It should be noted that although the ACL and PCL are more easily evaluated on sagittal images, these structures are also well visualized in the coronal plane (**Fig. 2.41**).

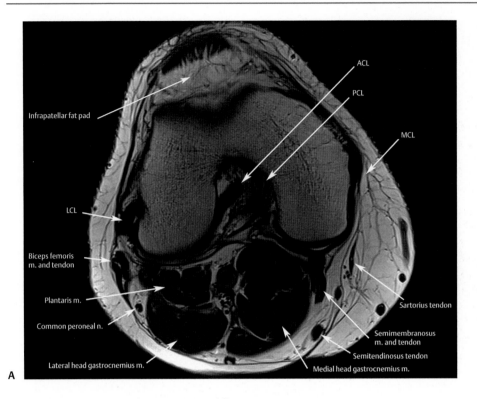

A

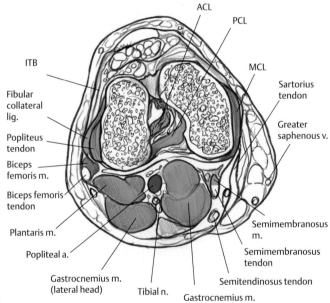

B

Fig. 2.37 An axial T2-weighted image **(A)** and artist's sketch **(B)** of the right knee at the level of the intercondylar notch showing the ACL and PCL.

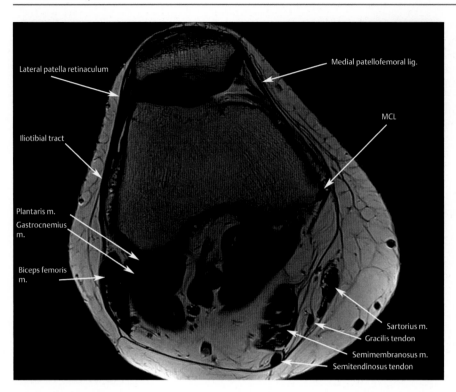

Lateral patella retinaculum

Iliotibial tract

Plantaris m.
Gastrocnemius m.

Biceps femoris m.

Medial patellofemoral lig.

MCL

Sartorius m.
Gracilis tendon

Semimembranosus m.
Semitendinosus tendon

Fig. 2.38 An axial T2-weighted image of the right knee showing the patellofemoral joint, including the articular cartilage.

Sagittal Images

Structures that are well visualized on sagittal images include the cruciate ligaments, menisci, articular cartilage, and extensor mechanism (**Figs. 2.42** and **2.43**). It is important to localize the images to the lateral or medial compartment. Medial or lateral compartment localization on sagittal images is guided by the presence of the fibular head and the convex lateral tibial condyle. Another clue to medial or lateral location is that the ACL is seen before the PCL when progressing from lateral to medial images. It may also be helpful to have a coronal image with localizer lines available as a reference guide while scrolling through the sagittal plane images.

ACL

The ACL is best evaluated on sagittal images but should be identified in all planes. The ligament runs obliquely from its origin on the posteromedial aspect of the lateral femoral condyle to its insertion site just lateral to the anterior horn of the medial meniscus. The ACL is composed of the anteromedial and posterolateral bundles. The ligament is intraarticular but extrasynovial. Because of this anatomic feature, the ACL may have fatty as well as fluid signal interspersed between the fibers.

On 5-mm sagittal sections, the ACL is usually visualized on at least one section. However, 3-mm sections for SE imaging and 1- to 2-mm sections for gradient-echo imaging are preferable because they allow for better visualization of the ACL. Normally, the ligament takes a straight course and has low signal intensity. However, the normal ACL does have some variation in its signal pattern, and subtle regions of increased T2-weighted signal may be seen in the uninjured ACL. Compared with the PCL, the ACL is less well defined and has higher signal intensity. Appreciating this normal appearance will help prevent inappropriate interpretations of a normal ACL as an ACL strain or partial tear. In a normal ACL, there should be at least one identifiable dark fiber bundle, and the ACL often appears as one thick dark band. There should be a clear anterior edge to the ligament. The ACL should not show marked increased signal on T2-weighted imaging, but it may have minimally increased signal on T1-weighted images because of the presence of fatty tissue. The normal ACL should follow the contour of the intercondylar roof, and attachments should be well delineated. Again, clinicians should be aware of these characteristics to avoid misdiagnosing ACL injuries.[11]

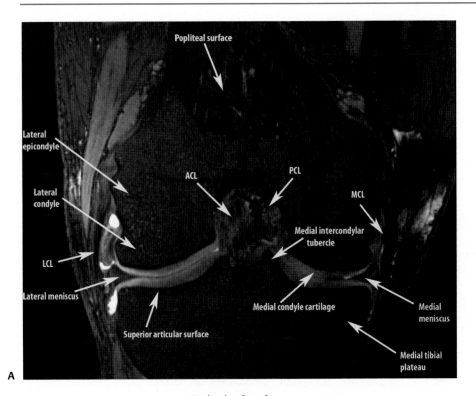

Popliteal surface

Lateral epicondyle

ACL

PCL

MCL

Lateral condyle

Medial intercondylar tubercle

LCL

Lateral meniscus

Superior articular surface

Medial condyle cartilage

Medial meniscus

Medial tibial plateau

A

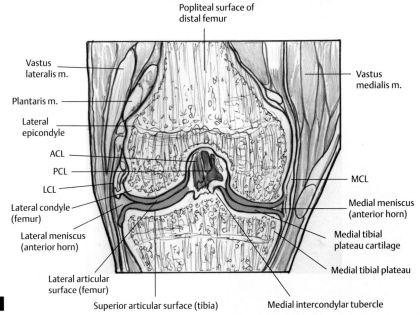

Popliteal surface of distal femur

Vastus lateralis m.

Plantaris m.

Lateral epicondyle

ACL

PCL

LCL

Lateral condyle (femur)

Lateral meniscus (anterior horn)

Lateral articular surface (femur)

Superior articular surface (tibia)

Vastus medialis m.

MCL

Medial meniscus (anterior horn)

Medial tibial plateau cartilage

Medial tibial plateau

Medial intercondylar tubercle

B

Fig. 2.39 A coronal T2-weighted image **(A)** and artist's sketch **(B)** of the right knee at the level of the intercondylar notch showing the MCL and LCL. The femoral and tibial articular cartilage is well shown.

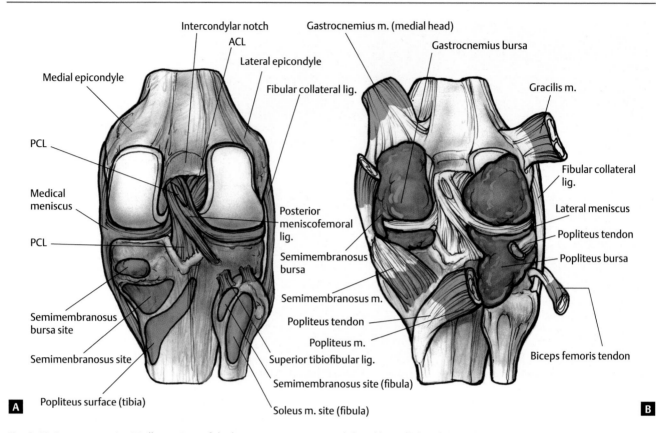

A

B

Fig. 2.40 Posteroanterior 3D illustrations of the ligamentous structures **(A)** and bursa **(B)** at the posterior aspect of the right knee.

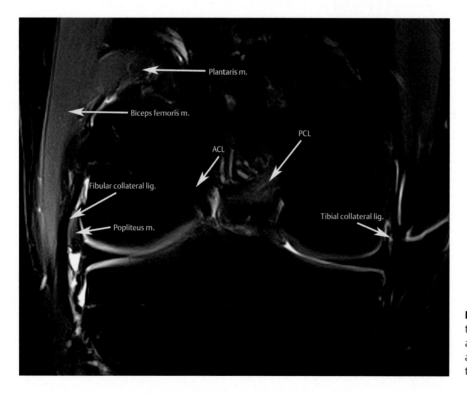

Fig. 2.41 A coronal T2-weighted image of the right knee showing the normal appearance of the collateral ligaments. The cruciate ligaments are shown coursing through the intercondylar notch.

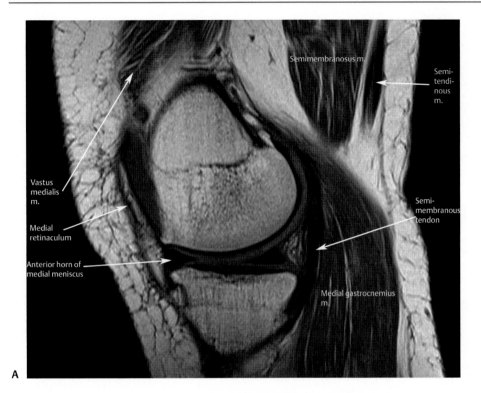

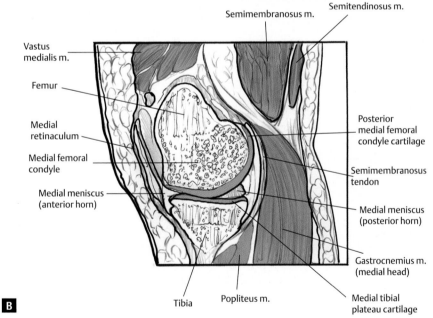

Fig. 2.42 A sagittal proton-density image **(A)** and artist's sketch **(B)** of the knee showing the articular cartilage and the anterior and posterior horns of the medial meniscus.

PCL

The PCL attaches on the posterior proximal tibia, inferior to the tibial joint surface. In contrast to the straight course of the ACL, the PCL curves anteriorly to insert on the anterolateral aspect of the medial femoral condyle (**Fig. 2.44**) because the knee is always imaged in extension. The PCL is usually seen on at least two images, even on examinations acquired with thick sections. The PCL usually appears as a thicker, darker, curved band compared with the ACL. When present, the ligaments of Humphry and Wrisberg (anterior and posterior meniscofemoral ligaments, which occur concurrently in 70% of knees[12]) can be seen adjacent to the PCL.

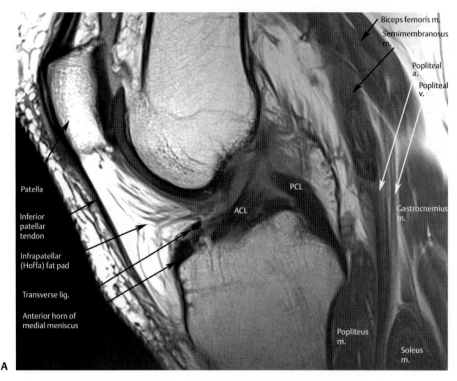

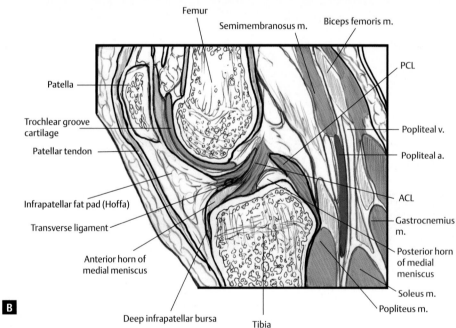

Fig. 2.43 A sagittal proton-density image **(A)** and artist's sketch **(B)** of the knee at the level of the intercondylar notch showing the ACL and PCL. The transverse ligament is seen in close association with the anterior horn of the medial meniscus. Also shown are the patellofemoral cartilage and the patellar and quadriceps tendons.

Menisci

The medial and lateral menisci are uniformly low signal intensity, triangle-shaped structures (when imaged in cross-section) under the femoral condyles. The menisci increase in thickness toward the periphery of the joint. At the edge of the joint, near the capsule, the menisci can be seen as thick, dark bands running parallel to the articular surface.

The transverse ligament can be seen as a tiny dark circle or triangle just superior to the anterior aspect of the tibial surface in midsagittal images. The transverse ligament also can be seen just superior to the anterior horns of the menisci, separated from the menisci in some images by a thin line of high signal intensity (**Fig. 2.44**). Clinicians unaware of this normal appearance may interpret the hyperintense line

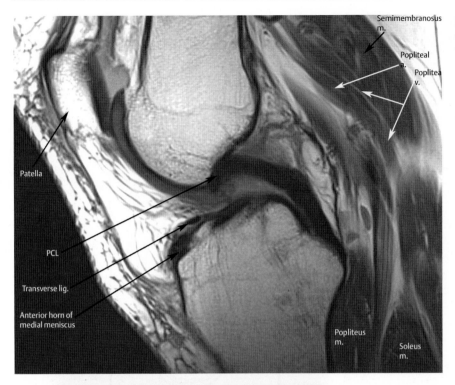

Fig. 2.44 A sagittal proton-density image of the knee showing the entire course of the PCL.

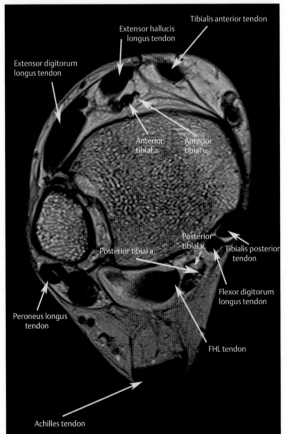

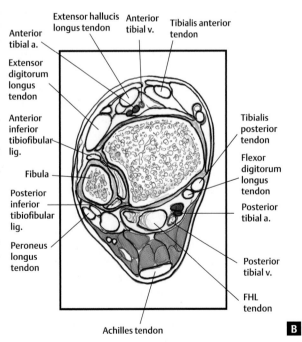

Fig. 2.45 An axial T2-weighted image **(A)** and artist's sketch **(B)** of the right ankle at the level of the tibial plafond. The tibialis posterior, flexor digitorum longus, and FHL tendons are seen posterior to the medial malleolus. The normal concave appearance of the Achilles tendon is seen in the midline posteriorly. The peroneus longus and brevis tendons are shown posterior to the lateral malleolus.

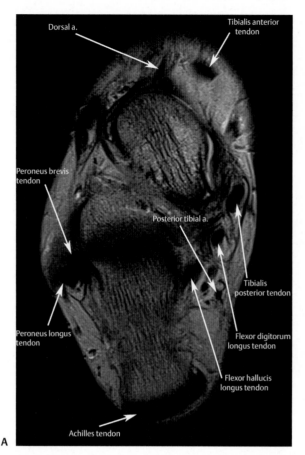

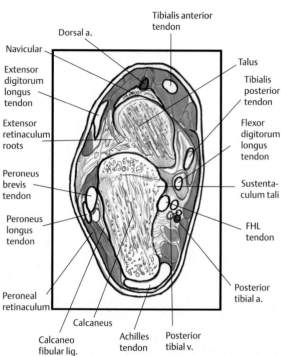

Fig. 2.46 An axial T2-weighted image **(A)** and artist's sketch **(B)** of the right ankle at the level of the calcaneus, showing the posterior tibialis, flexor digitorum longus, and FHL tendons in their expected locations from anteromedial to posterolateral, respectively. The peroneus longus and brevis tendons are seen coursing along the lateral aspect of the calcaneus.

between the menisci and the transverse ligament as pathologic, leading to a mistaken diagnosis of a meniscal tear.

The so called *magic-angle phenomenon* can cause the false diagnosis of a lateral meniscus tear. Specifically, the up-sloping portion of the posterior horn of the lateral meniscus may have increased signal on short-TE images secondary to this phenomenon.[13]

Extensor Mechanism

The structures of the extensor mechanism of the knee (the patella, patella tendon, quadriceps tendon, and medial and lateral retinaculum) are well seen on midsagittal images (**Fig. 2.43**). The fat pad is just posterior to the patellar tendon. The patellar and femoral bone marrow signal should be uniform without edema. The signal of the patellar tendon should be uniformly dark. The quadriceps tendon may have a laminated appearance reflecting its multiple tendon composition. There should be no areas of focal thickening of the tendons. The cartilage surfaces of the patella are particularly thick (up to 1 cm). There should be no areas of signal change, fibrillation, or thinning; the presence of these findings is indicative of chondromalacia.

Neurovascular Structures

The popliteal artery courses several millimeters posterior to the knee joint. The popliteal vein is just posterior and lateral to the artery (**Fig. 2.43**) and has a large cross-section. The tibial nerve runs just posterior and lateral to the vein. The common peroneal nerve arises from the tibial nerve above the joint line and may be seen coursing inferiorly and laterally toward the fibular head. The relationships between these structures are easily identified on coronal images.

■ Foot/Ankle

Axial Images

Axial images are extremely helpful in identifying normal and abnormal anatomy of the ankle (**Figs. 2.45** and **2.46**) and are usually evaluated from superior to inferior (proximal to distal). These images are acquired perpendicular to the plane of the tibia and fibula. The tibia and fibula expand distally to

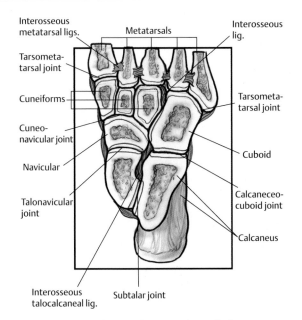

Fig. 2.47 Illustration of an axial section through the osseous structures of the right foot showing the tarsometatarsal and intertarsal joints and the interosseous ligaments.

form the tibial plafond, medial malleolus, and lateral malleolus. Axial images also show the distal tibiofibular joint and ankle syndesmosis, with the fibula located laterally and posteriorly in the syndesmotic notch. More inferiorly, the talar dome is visualized, followed sequentially by the calcaneus and the midfoot osseous structures (**Fig. 2.47**). The navicular bone can be seen on axial images and can be evaluated in this plane. More distally, the tarsometatarsal joints and metatarsals are seen. These structures are not all in the same axial plane because of the transverse arch of the foot. Therefore, they must be examined on sequential images, which is facilitated by correlation with the coronal and sagittal images. The forefoot structures (**Fig. 2.48**) are usually best evaluated with specialized planes for the hallux and separate planes for the lesser metatarsals.

On axial images, most tendon structures in the ankle are seen in cross-section. Therefore, it is important to identify and follow each tendon from image to image along its course. These tendons should be dark on all sequences. At the level of the ankle joint, the tibialis anterior and extensor hallucis longus tendons are the most anteromedial structures, anterior to the neurovascular bundle. The extensor digitorum longus tendon (**Fig. 2.49**) has a more muscular, broad appearance at the level of the ankle joint and lies more laterally than does the extensor hallucis longus. The most

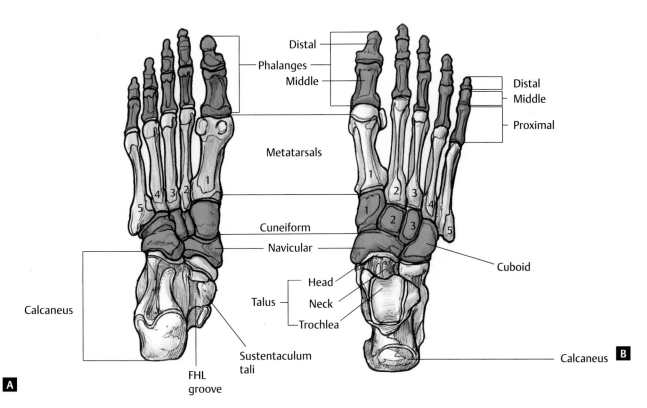

Fig. 2.48 Illustrations of the osseous structures of the plantar **(A)** and dorsal **(B)** surface views of the right foot.

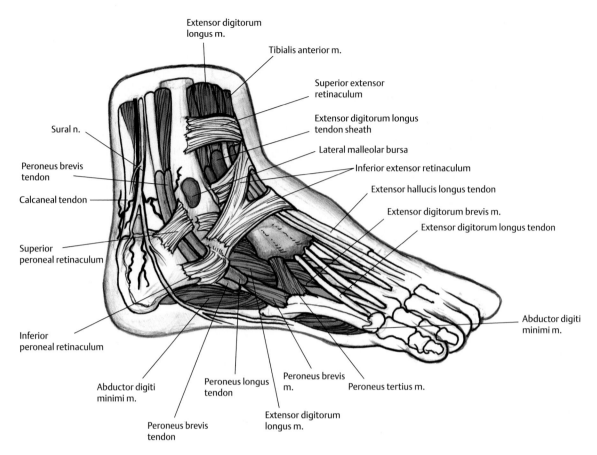

Extensor digitorum longus m.

Tibialis anterior m.

Superior extensor retinaculum

Extensor digitorum longus tendon sheath

Lateral malleolar bursa

Inferior extensor retinaculum

Extensor hallucis longus tendon

Extensor digitorum brevis m.

Extensor digitorum longus tendon

Abductor digiti minimi m.

Sural n.

Peroneus brevis tendon

Calcaneal tendon

Superior peroneal retinaculum

Inferior peroneal retinaculum

Abductor digiti minimi m.

Peroneus longus tendon

Peroneus brevis m.

Peroneus tertius m.

Extensor digitorum longus m.

Peroneus brevis tendon

Fig. 2.49 A 3D illustration of the ankle and foot from the lateral aspect showing the musculotendinous units passing deep to the superior and inferior extensor retinacula.

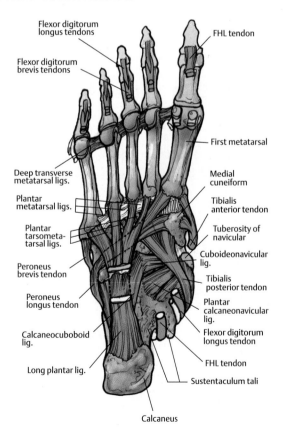

Flexor digitorum longus tendons

FHL tendon

Flexor digitorum brevis tendons

First metatarsal

Deep transverse metatarsal ligs.

Medial cuneiform

Plantar metatarsal ligs.

Tibialis anterior tendon

Plantar tarsometa-tarsal ligs.

Tuberosity of navicular

Cuboideonavicular lig.

Peroneus brevis tendon

Tibialis posterior tendon

Peroneus longus tendon

Plantar calcaneonavicular lig.

Calcaneocuboboid lig.

Flexor digitorum longus tendon

Long plantar lig.

FHL tendon

Sustentaculum tali

Calcaneus

Fig. 2.50 An axial 3D illustration of the plantar aspect of the right foot showing the tarsometatarsal and intertarsal ligaments, as well as the tendons crossing the ankle into the foot.

anterolateral structure is the peroneus tertius tendon (variably present), which can sometimes be difficult to visualize because of its small size.

The posterior tibialis tendon is the most obvious tendon structure just posterior to the medial malleolus. The flexor digitorum longus tendon is just posterior to the posterior tibialis tendon and medial to the posterior neurovascular bundle. It is approximately one third the diameter of the posterior tibialis tendon. Lateral and deep to the posterior neurovascular bundle is the FHL, which has a broad muscular cross-section at the level of the ankle joint. This tendon can be followed further distally in its sheath between the posteromedial and posterolateral processes of the talus. These three tendons can be identified not only by their appearance and insertions but also by their predictable relationships to each other as they pass posterior to the medial malleolus.

The peroneus brevis and longus (**Figs. 2.50** and **2.51**) are easily identified posterior to the fibula. The peroneus brevis lies directly against the fibula, and the longus is more superficial at the level of the ankle joint. The overlying superior peroneal retinaculum should be assessed for integrity.

The Achilles tendon is the most posterior tendinous structure in the ankle. At its insertion on the calcaneus, it has an oblong appearance on axial images and should appear concave more proximally on the anterior surface.

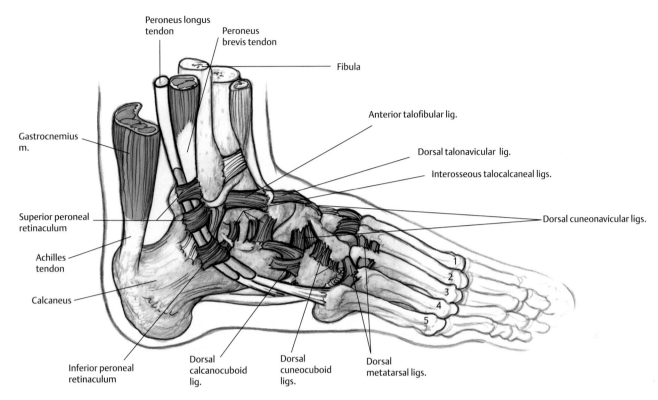

Fig. 2.51 A 3D illustration of the ankle and foot from the lateral aspect showing the deep ligaments and the peroneus longus and brevis tendons passing posterior to the lateral malleolus, deep to the peroneal retinaculum.

The anterior and posterior tibiofibular ligaments, along with the dense interosseous tibiofibular ligament, constitute the syndesmotic complex between the tibia and fibula. The anterior and posterior tibiofibular ligaments are identified easily as low signal intensity ligamentous connections between the distal tibia and fibula at the level of the ankle joint.

Of the lateral ligamentous complex structures, the anterior and posterior talofibular ligaments are best seen on axial images. They appear as dark, thin, ligamentous bands extending distally from the fibula anteriorly and posteriorly to insert on the talus. The anterior band attaches to the neck of the talus, and the posterior band attaches to the posterior lateral process of the talus. However, the structures of the lateral ligamentous complex do not all run in the same plane, and thus, the calcaneofibular ligament component of the lateral ligamentous complex is best seen on the coronal images, whereas the anterior and posterior talofibular ligaments are best seen on axial images.

The anterior neurovascular bundle (anterior tibial artery, anterior tibial vein, and deep peroneal nerve) is slightly lateral and deep to the extensor hallucis longus (**Fig. 2.52**). The posterior neurovascular bundle (posterior tibial artery, vein, and nerve) lies between the flexor digitorum longus and FHL and deep to the flexor retinaculum.

Coronal Images

Coronal images of the ankle are obtained in the plane of the tibia (**Figs. 2.53** and **2.54**). The tibial plafond, medial and lateral malleoli, and talar dome are well visualized on proton-density and T2-weighted coronal images. Such images are useful in diagnosing osseous pathology such as occult fractures, stress fractures, OCDs, degenerative arthritis, osseous infections, and neoplastic processes.

The ankle structures identified on coronal images are the medial and lateral ligament complexes. The deltoid ligament forms the MCL complex of the ankle and consists of superficial and deep layers. The tibionavicular and tibiocalcaneal ligaments constitute the superficial layer, and the tibiotalar ligament constitutes the deep layer (**Fig. 2.55**). The tibionavicular ligament originates from the medial malleolus and attaches to the tuberosity of the navicular. The tibiocalcaneal ligament is seen as a thick, dark band extending from the medial malleolus inferiorly to the sustentaculum tali of the calcaneus. The tibiotalar ligament extends from the medial malleolus to the entire nonarticular medial aspect of the talus.

The lateral ligamentous complex of the ankle consists of the calcaneofibular, anterior talofibular, and posterior talofibular ligaments. Of these three structures, the calcaneofibular ligament is best seen on coronal images, extending from

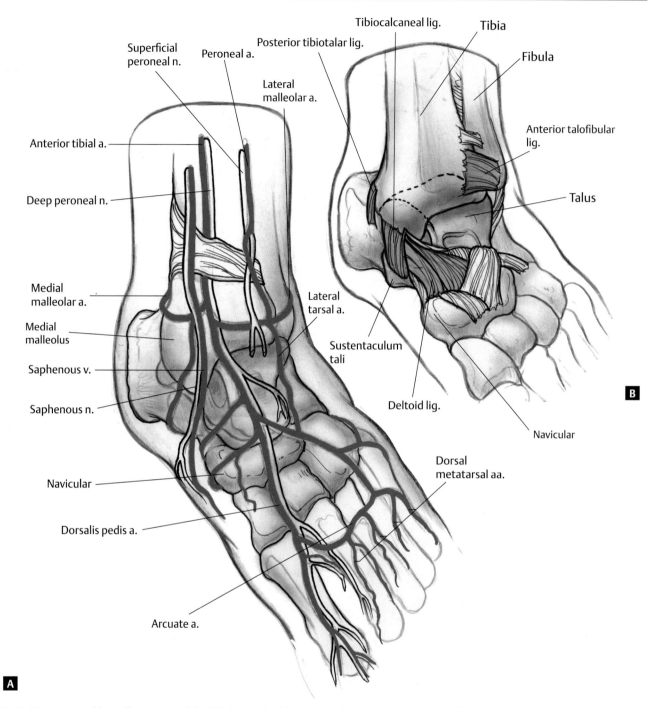

Fig. 2.52 Anterior oblique illustrations of the left foot and ankle showing the neurovascular **(A)** and ligamentous **(B)** structures.

the tip of the lateral malleolus to the lateral wall of the calcaneus. Despite the fact that many tendinous structures can be difficult to identify in the coronal plane, the posterior tibial tendon and the peroneus longus and brevis tendons can be identified inferior to the medial and lateral malleoli, respectively. The posterior tibial tendon should be seen as a longitudinal dark signal structure just posterior to the medial malleolus. The FHL can be identified at its broad origin from the posterior two thirds of the fibula. The peroneus longus and brevis tendons are seen as longitudinal dark signal structures on most coronal images, passing just posterior to the lateral malleolus.

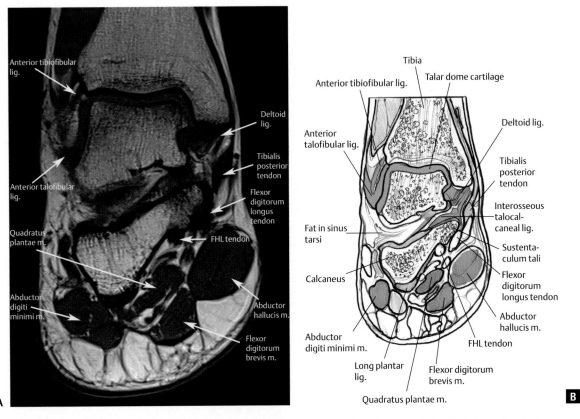

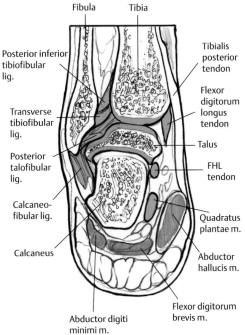

Fig. 2.53 A coronal T1-weighted image **(A)** and artist's sketch **(B)** of the right ankle at the level of the tibial plafond and talus.

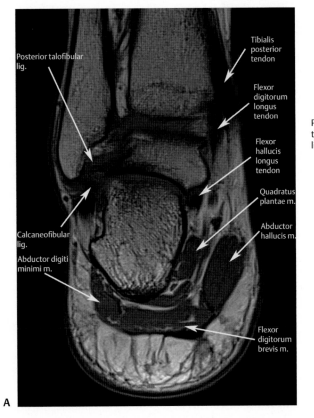

Fig. 2.54 A coronal T1-weighted image **(A)** and artist's sketch **(B)** of the right ankle through the posterior aspect of the joint showing the posterior tibialis, flexor digitorum longus, and FHL tendons coursing posterior to the medial malleolus in their expected locations from anteromedial to posterolateral, respectively.

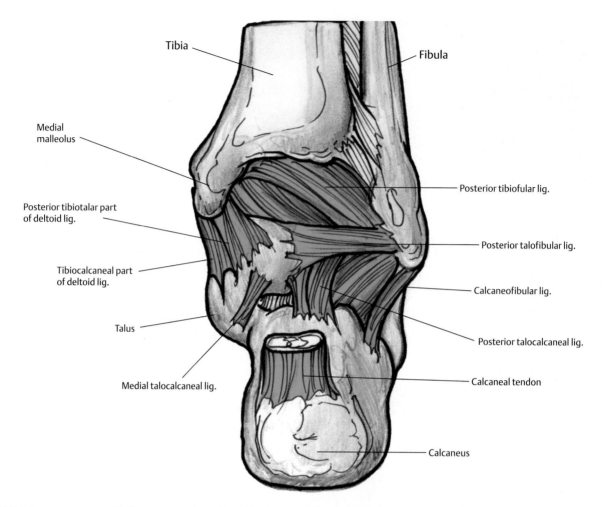

Fig. 2.55 A posteroanterior 3D illustration of the right ankle showing the posterior ligamentous structures, including the tibiocalcaneal and posterior tibiotalar parts of the deltoid ligament.

The osseous structures of the foot can also be evaluated on the coronal images. The hindfoot, including the talar body, calcaneus, and subtalar joint, can be examined for occult talocalcaneal coalitions or arthritic processes. The talocalcaneal ligaments and soft-tissue contents of the sinus tarsi can be examined on T2-weighted images or fat-suppressed proton-density images for evidence of increased signal secondary to ligament injury or soft-tissue impingement that supports a diagnosis of sinus tarsi syndrome. Coronal imaging of the midfoot also shows the talonavicular and calcaneocuboid joints, the navicular body and cuboid, and the tarsometatarsal joints. Coronal images through the midfoot are useful for diagnosing navicular or cuboid stress fractures, arthritis of the midfoot joints, or soft-tissue injuries of the tarsometatarsal (Lisfranc) complex. These images can show the plantar tarsometatarsal ligament complex and facilitate evaluation of tendinitis or tearing of the extensor and flexor tendons. Coronal imaging of the forefoot osseous structures includes the following:

- Metatarsals
- Phalanges
- MTP and IP joints
- Sesamoids

The flexor and extensor tendons can be visualized at the forefoot, particularly the extensor hallucis longus tendon and prominent flexor tendons at the first MTP level. The capsuloligamentous structures (plantar plate) of the MTP joints are also visualized in the coronal plane, allowing for diagnosis of MTP sprain injuries, such as the common turf-toe injury at the first MTP joint.

Sagittal Images

Like coronal images, sagittal images allow most structures to be visualized longitudinally along their courses (**Fig. 2.56**). The osseous structures of the ankle and foot can be visualized in sequence from medial to lateral (**Fig. 2.57**). The tibial plafond, talar dome, and lateral malleolus can be inspected for arthritic, degenerative, neoplastic, infectious, or traumatic conditions. Sagittal imaging shows the midfoot bones (particularly the talar head, navicular, and cuboid) and can permit sequential examination of the cuneiforms

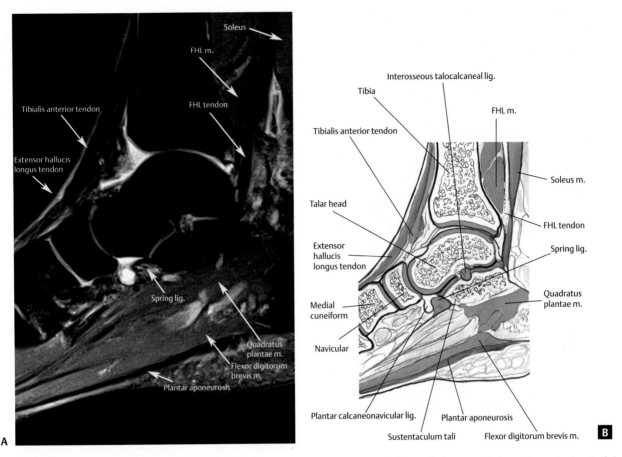

Fig. 2.56 A sagittal proton-density fat-suppressed image **(A)** and artist's sketch **(B)** of the medial aspect of the ankle at the level of the navicular.

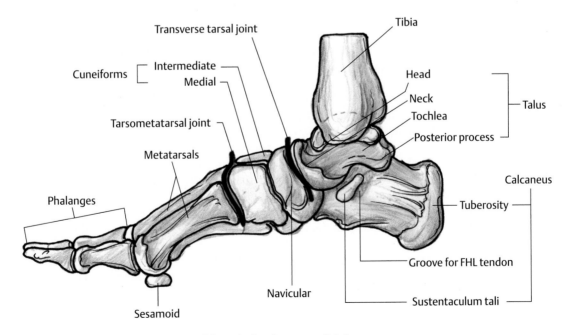

Fig. 2.57 An illustration of the osseous structures of the right foot from a medial view.

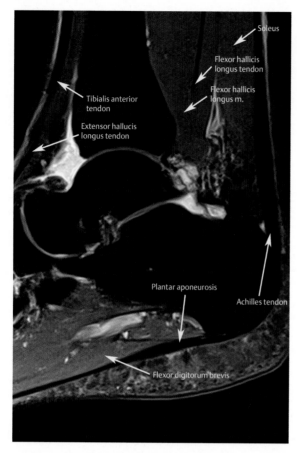

Fig. 2.58 A sagittal proton-density fat-suppressed image of the ankle showing the Achilles tendon and plantar aponeurosis. Flexor and extensor tendons crossing the ankle are also seen.

and metatarsals. Precise identification of the central osseous structures is facilitated by concurrent correlation with the axial and coronal images. The first MTP joint structures are visualized particularly well in the sagittal plane. Although coronal and axial images are better suited for identification of the ligamentous complexes of the ankle, the plantar plate and ligament structures of the MTP joints can be identified in the sagittal plane.

The Achilles tendon, easily identified as the most posterior tendon inserting onto the posterior calcaneal tuberosity, can be inspected for thickening, intratendinous signal heterogeneity, partial tearing, or complete rupture with retraction (**Fig. 2.58**). Immediately deep to this structure is the retrocalcaneal bursa, which can show increased signal intensity on T2-weighted images, suggestive of retrocalcaneal bursitis. The posterior tibial tendon is the first structure posterior to the medial malleolus. The course of this tendon can be appreciated as it curves around the medial malleolus to insert onto the tuberosity of the navicular bone. The next two medial tendons are the flexor digito-

rum longus and FHL (**Fig. 2.59**). The flexor digitorum longus tendon is located just posterior to the posterior tibialis tendon and medial to the posterior neurovascular bundle. The FHL, the deepest muscle in the posterior compartment, lies against the tibia. Lateral to the FHL are the peroneal tendons, which course posterior to the lateral malleolus and then toward the plantar midfoot. The anterior tibialis, extensor hallucis longus, and extensor digitorum longus tendons can be visualized anteriorly. In particular, the anterior tibialis tendon can be identified on sagittal imaging and should be evaluated for tenosynovitis, partial tear, or rupture.

General Spine Anatomy

Intervertebral Discs

The normal discovertebral complex has three components:

- Cartilaginous end plate
- Annulus fibrosus
- Nucleus pulposus

Overall, the intervertebral discs show intermediate signal intensity on T1-weighted images and high signal intensity on T2-weighted images. The outer annulus appears hypointense on T2-weighted images, whereas the inner annulus, which is composed of fibrocartilage and a high proportion of type II collagen, is indistinguishable from the hyperintense nucleus pulposus. Compared with normal vertebral marrow, the nucleus pulposus, which is composed of a proteoglycan matrix and type II collagen, appears hyperintense on T2-weighted images and hypointense on T1-weighted images.[14] As the disc degenerates and as patients age, the signal intensity of the nucleus pulposus decreases on T2-weighted images and becomes dark on all pulse sequences with advanced degenerative changes. Additional pulse sequences, such as fat-suppressed T2-weighted images, are useful for accentuating fluid and edema, which may help in delineating spine pathology. Special attention should be given to the posterior aspect of the disc on both sagittal and axial T2-weighted images to evaluate for disc protrusion, extrusion, sequestration, or other pathology that may be contributing to central canal or neural foraminal stenosis.

The end plate is a flat, osseous disc with a slightly elevated rim secondary to the attached ring apophysis, which produces a central depression in the end plate that is occupied by hyaline cartilage.[14] The annulus is composed of type I collagen fibers (Sharpey's fibers) that are attached to the ring apophysis periosteum. The annulus also blends with the anterior and posterior longitudinal ligaments. T1-weighted images provide optimal evaluation of anatomy, fracture lines, and other osseous detail. T1-weighted images also clearly

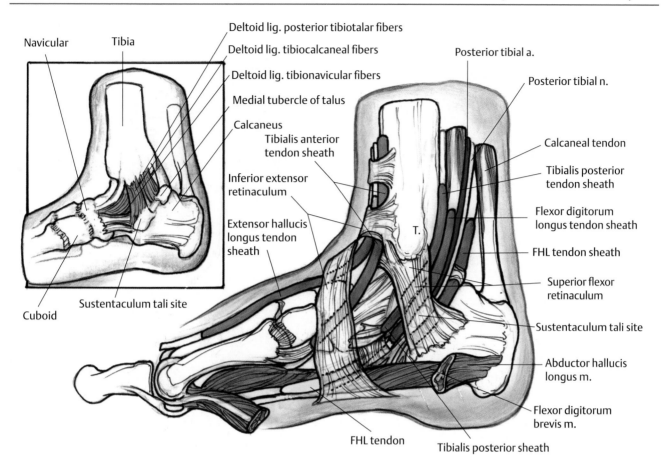

Fig. 2.59 Medial 3D illustrations of the right ankle showing the tibialis posterior tendon, flexor digitorum longus tendon, and the FHL tendon coursing posterior to the medial malleolus, deep to the flexor retinaculum. The inset shows the various components of the deltoid ligament.

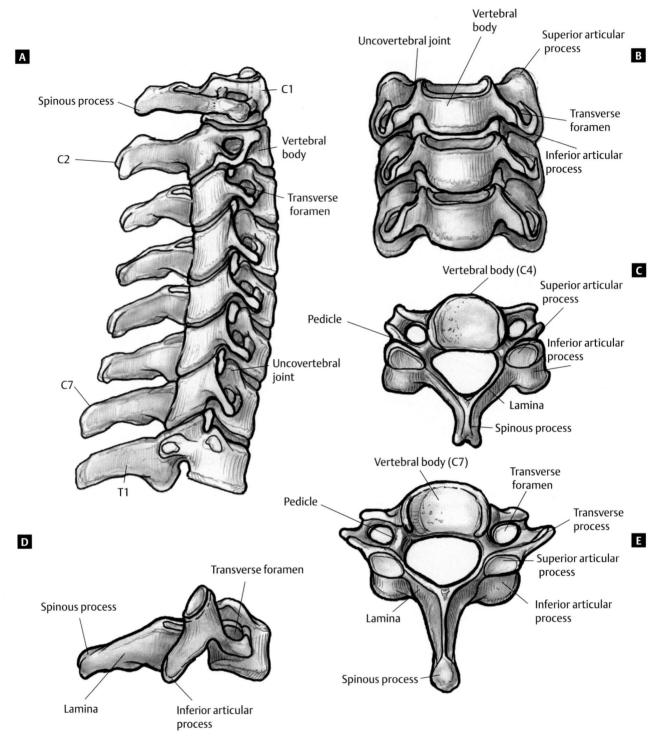

Fig. 2.60 Various views of the cervical vertebral bodies: **(A)** lateral vertebral body at C1-T1, **(B)** lateral AP vertebral body at C4-C7, **(C)** axial vertebral body at C4, **(D)** lateral vertebral body at C7, and **(E)** axial vertebral body at C7.

delineate the relationships of the vertebral bodies, intervertebral discs, central canal, and posterior elements.

Vertebral Bodies

Normal lordosis should be seen in the cervical and lumbar spine, and normal kyphosis should be present in the thoracic spine. The superior and inferior end plates should be intact and parallel to one another in the absence of vertebral compression fractures, other fractures, or infection. The subaxial cervical vertebral bodies all have a similar appearance (**Fig. 2.60**), whereas the atlas (C1) has no vertebral body and the axis (C2) has an odontoid process. Each of the lumbar vertebral bodies also has a similar appearance (**Fig. 2.61**), as do the

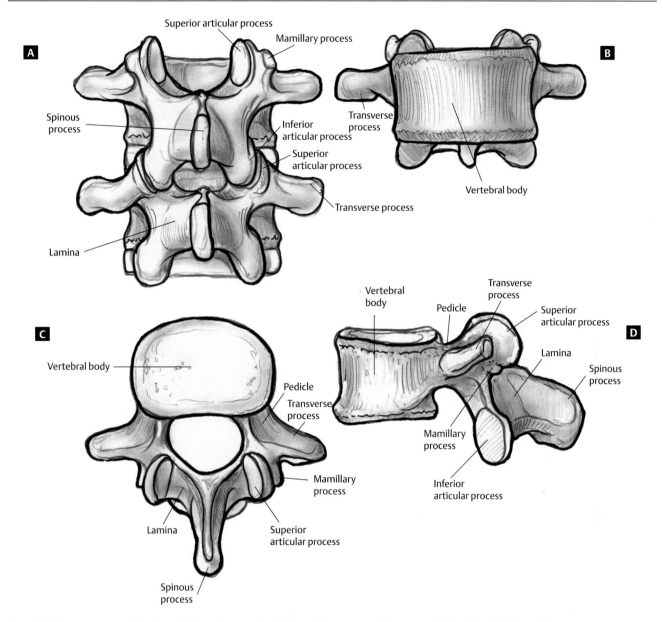

Fig. 2.61 Various views of the L3 and L4 lumbar vertebral bodies: **(A)** posterior, **(B)** anterior, **(C)** axial, and **(D)** lateral.

thoracic vertebral bodies (**Fig. 2.62**). The anterior and posterior longitudinal ligaments, seen along the vertebral bodies, have low signal intensity. The entry site of the basivertebral veins is seen at the midportion of the posterior vertebral bodies. The spinal and radicular arteries course around the cord's anterior, posterior, and lateral aspects within the vertebral canal (**Fig. 2.63**). Fat-suppression techniques can be used to nullify marrow signal and increase the sensitivity in the evaluation of neoplastic and infiltrative processes.

CSF

Like other fluids, CSF has low signal intensity on T1-weighted images and high signal intensity on T2-weighted images. On sagittal and axial images, CSF is seen surrounding the spinal cord in the cervical, thoracic, and lumbar spine and around the cauda equina in the lower lumbar spine. Thus, T2-weighted images provide a myelographic appearance that allows for the detection of spinal stenosis.

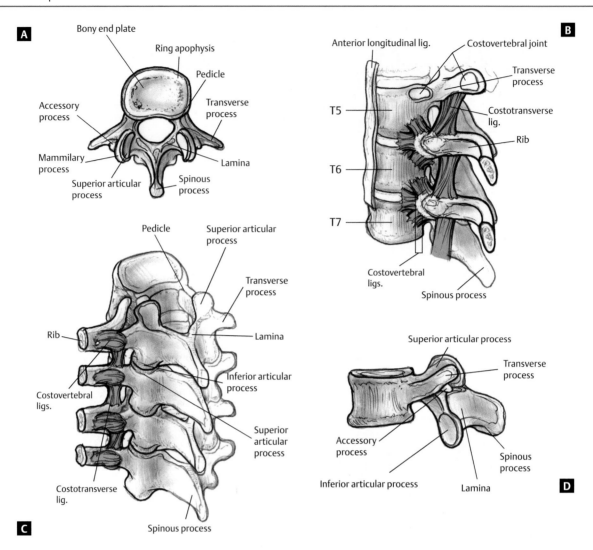

Fig. 2.62 Axial **(A)**, lateral **(B)**, posterior oblique **(C)**, and lateral **(D)** illustrations of the osseous structures of the thoracic spine, the costovertebral joints, and the costotransverse and costovertebral ligaments.

Spinal Cord

Sagittal T2-weighted images provide a myelographic effect that allows for the evaluation of spinal cord morphology and the presence of extrinsic compression. The cord should have homogeneous signal intensity in the absence of intrinsic pathology. On axial T2-weighted images, the central gray matter can be faintly identified. Specialized sequences obtained with high magnetic field magnets allow for detailed evaluation of central gray matter (**Fig. 2.64**). The spinal cord should terminate at or above the L1-L2 level in adults.

Ligaments

Normal ligaments should have low signal intensity on all pulse sequences. The transverse ligament can be seen posterior to the odontoid process (**Fig. 2.65**) and is best visualized on axial images. The ligamentum flavum connects the lamina of adjacent vertebrae and is seen as a hypointense band posterior to the dura. The anterior longitudinal ligament is broad, thick, and adherent to the anterior vertebral bodies. The posterior longitudinal ligament is thin, attached to the posterior vertebral cortex via the midline septum,

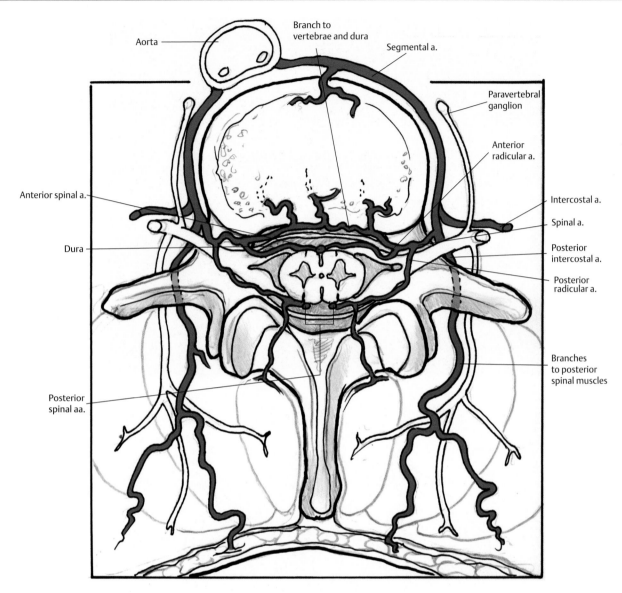

Fig. 2.63 A 3D illustration (axial view) of the spinal, intercostal, and other arteries that supply the thoracic spine.

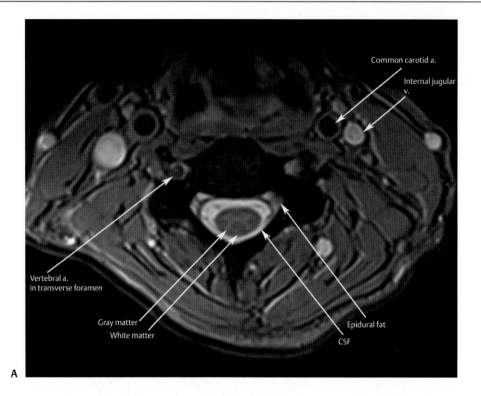

Common carotid a.

Internal jugular v.

Vertebral a. in transverse foramen

Gray matter

White matter

Epidural fat

CSF

A

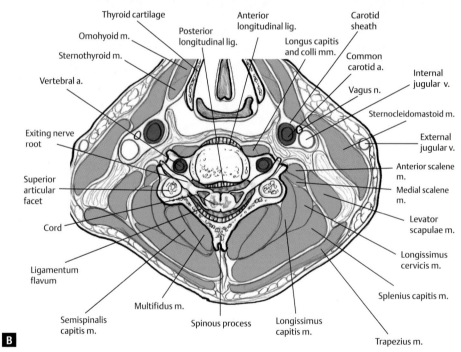

Thyroid cartilage

Omohyoid m.

Sternothyroid m.

Vertebral a.

Exiting nerve root

Superior articular facet

Cord

Ligamentum flavum

Semispinalis capitis m.

Posterior longitudinal lig.

Anterior longitudinal lig.

Longus capitis and colli mm.

Carotid sheath

Common carotid a.

Vagus n.

Internal jugular v.

Sternocleidomastoid m.

External jugular v.

Anterior scalene m.

Medial scalene m.

Levator scapulae m.

Longissimus cervicis m.

Splenius capitis m.

Multifidus m.

Spinous process

Longissimus capitis m.

Trapezius m.

B

Fig. 2.64 An axial T2-weighted image **(A)** and artist's sketch **(B)** clearly defining the gray and white matter of the cervical spinal cord, the CSF within the subarachnoid space, and epidural fat. Normal flow voids are seen within the carotid and vertebral arteries.

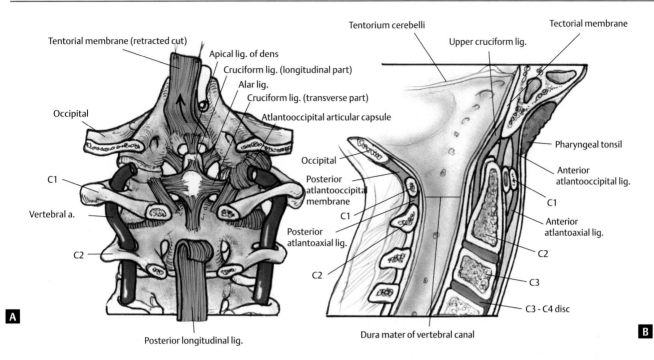

Fig. 2.65 Posteroanterior **(A)** and sagittal **(B)** illustrations showing the ligamentous structures of the skull base and cervical spine, including the alar ligament, cruciform ligament, and atlantooccipital ligaments.

and defines the posterior margin of the anterior epidural space at the midline (**Fig. 2.66**). The anterior epidural space is not apparent at the disc level because the posterior longitudinal ligament fuses to the discs. Visualization of these structures may be limited with MRI because of partial volume averaging with the adjacent vertebral body.[15]

Roots and Foramina

The dorsal and ventral nerve roots can be identified within the neural foramina on the parasagittal images and the axial images, and the exiting nerve root is located just posterior to the vertebral artery in the cervical spine (**Fig. 2.67**). Additional neural structures, including the sympathetic chain, are located in and around the cervical vertebral bodies (**Fig. 2.68**). Note that the C2 nerve root exits the spine above the C2 pedicle and runs parallel to the C1-C2 facet joint (**Fig. 2.69**). The nerve roots have intermediate signal intensity and are surrounded by high signal intensity fat on T1-weighted images and by high signal intensity CSF on T2-weighted images.

■ Cervical Spine

Sagittal Images

The T1-weighted and T2-weighted sagittal images should be reviewed first to evaluate the spinal anatomy (**Fig. 2.70**). The midsagittal image from the cervicomedullary to cervicothoracic junctions is a good anatomic screen of the cervical vertebral bodies, intervertebral discs, spinal cord, thecal sac, and posterior elements. To find the midsagittal image, the sagittal series should be reviewed for the image that best shows the entire cervical spinal cord and the odontoid process, basion, opisthion, midbrain, and fourth ventricle.

Sequential evaluation of the sagittal series away from the midsagittal image allows for assessment of facet joints and neural foramina (**Fig. 2.71**). The foramina have an oblique orientation to the sagittal plane, which can cause distortion and lead to artifactual narrowing. T1-weighted images are somewhat limited because they afford poor differentiation of the vertebral body, the annular-posterior longitudinal ligament complex, and the CSF in the adjacent thecal sac[16]; the posterior longitudinal ligament, a disc herniation, an osseous

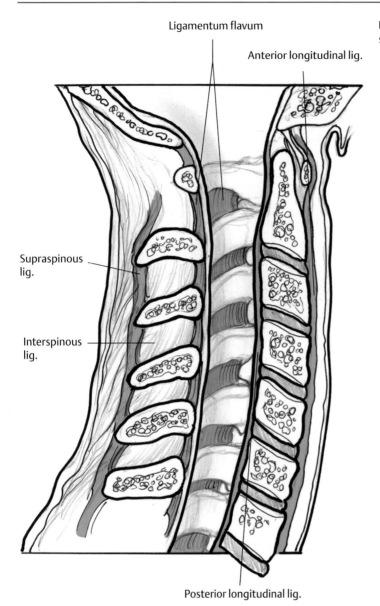

Ligamentum flavum

Anterior longitudinal lig.

Supraspinous lig.

Interspinous lig.

Posterior longitudinal lig.

Fig. 2.66 An illustration (lateral view) of the cervical spine showing the midsagittal ligaments.

spur, and CSF all appear as a low-intensity signal on T1-weighted sagittal images.[16] The CSF–extradural interface is well defined on T2-weighted images, and a myelographic appearance is produced on T2-weighted sagittal images because of the CSF's high signal. The intervertebral discs show intermediate signal intensity on T1-weighted images and high signal intensity on T2-weighted and gradient-echo images.

The cervical vertebral body has bright signal intensity on T1-weighted images because of the presence of normal fatty bone marrow. Normal cervical spine lordosis should be observed. The AP diameter of the canal tapers from the first to third cervical levels and then is relatively constant. Parasagittal images show the short cervical pedicles. The anterior and posterior longitudinal ligaments are depicted as low signal intensity linear structures along the vertebral bodies.[15,17,18] Often, a small cortical defect is seen in the midportion of the posterior vertebral body; this defect represents a vascular channel and is a normal finding.

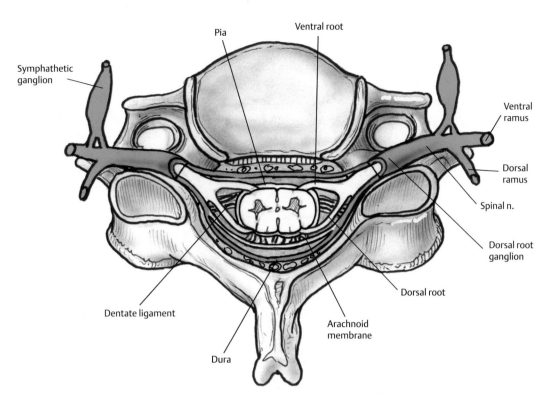

Fig. 2.67 An illustration (axial view) of the neural structures originating from the cervical spinal cord.

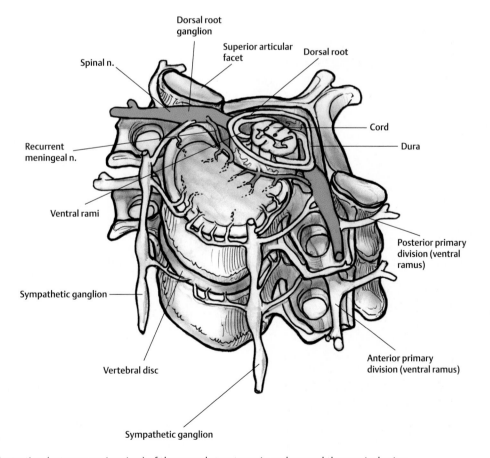

Fig. 2.68 A 3D illustration (anterosuperior view) of the neural structures in and around the cervical spine.

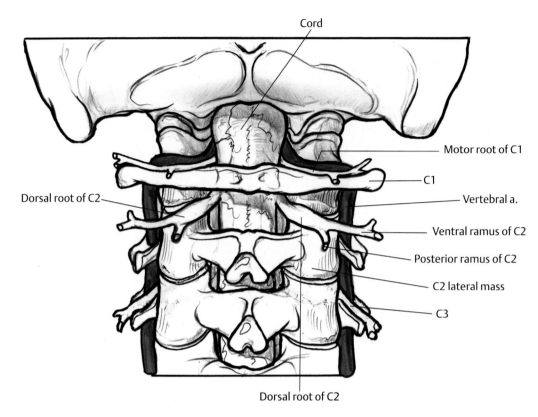

Fig. 2.69 A posterior 3D illustration of the upper cervical spine showing the location of the vertebral artery relative to the posterior arch of C1 and the exit of the C2 nerve root above the pedicle of C2.

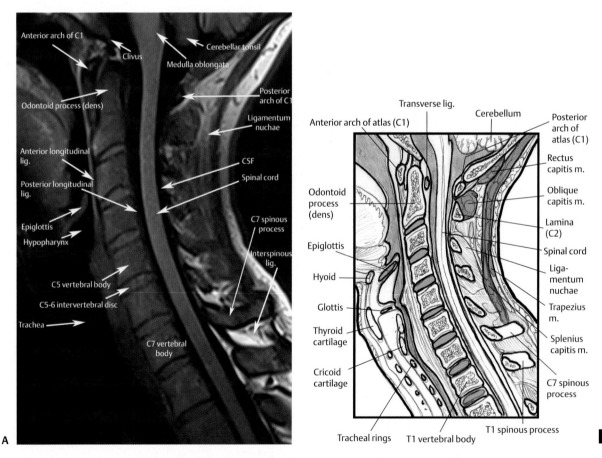

Fig. 2.70 A sagittal T1-weighted midline image **(A)** and artist's sketch **(B)** of the cervical spine depicting the cervical cord, CSF, and the anterior and posterior longitudinal ligaments, as well as the anterior and posterior elements of the cervical spine and the intervertebral discs.

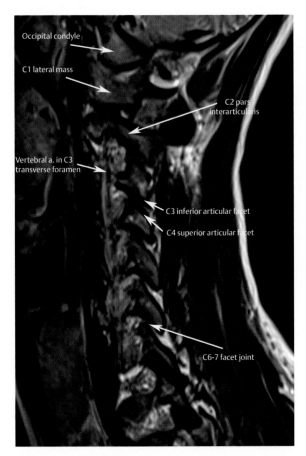

Fig. 2.71 A sagittal T2-weighted paramidline image of the cervical spine showing the vertebral artery in long axis coursing through the transverse foramina of the cervical spine. The facet joints are most easily evaluated in the parasagittal plane, as shown here.

Axial Images

Evaluation of the cervical spine on axial MRI initially requires the correct identification of the spinal level, which can be accomplished by using the localizing sagittal images or by evaluating signal intensity differences between the intervertebral discs and vertebral bodies and sequentially numbering the levels caudal to the odontoid process. Given the potential risk of wrong-level surgery, special care should be taken to identify the level by using a combination of these two labeling techniques (see Chapter 3). In addition, most imaging workstations have a tool that allows the vertebral bodies to be identified using the numbering techniques outlined above, which facilitates rapid localization on the midsagittal images while evaluating the associated axial images.

Cervical spine anatomy and anatomic pathology are well visualized on axial T1-weighted images; T2-weighted images have good CSF-to-cord contrast (**Fig. 2.64**), which allows evaluation of spinal cord or nerve root compression.[15,17,18] Knowledge of the location of the various spinal tracts can allow a clinician to correlate the clinical and radiographic findings in a patient with known or suspected spinal cord injury (**Fig. 2.72**). Compared with sagittal images, axial T2-weighted images can provide a higher resolution depiction of the cord (because of the smaller field of view), enabling a more sensitive assessment of its signal intensity. Sagittal images are also helpful in evaluating signal abnormalities in the spinal cord because one image can show a long segment of the spinal cord. Neural foramina are best depicted with gradient-echo and T2-weighted images and should be evaluated on axial and parasagittal images. Evaluation of the neural foramina in the axial and sagittal planes takes experience and training, especially with patients who have scoliosis or poor positioning

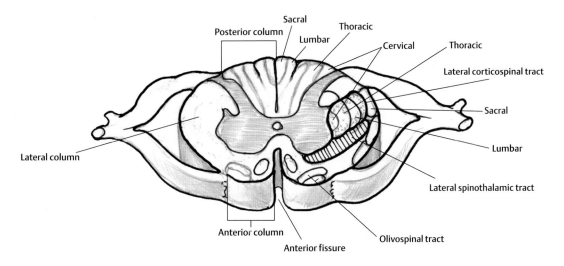

Fig. 2.72 An axial 3D illustration of cervical spinal cord anatomy with location of various spinal tracts.

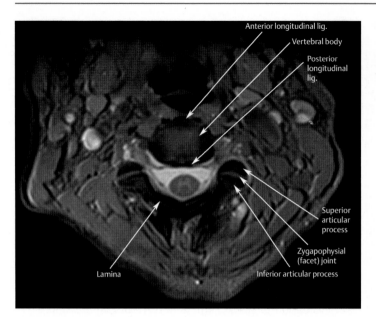

Anterior longitudinal lig.

Vertebral body

Posterior
longitudinal
lig.

Superior
articular
process

Zygapophysial
(facet) joint

Lamina

Inferior articular process

Fig. 2.73 An axial T2-weighted image of the cervical spine showing the anterior and posterior longitudinal ligaments and the superior and inferior articular processes of the facet joints.

in the scanner, which can cause each neural foramen to be visualized on individual parasagittal images. Care should be taken to evaluate the axial T2-weighted images and to recognize the normal shape and size of the central canal and the neural foramina. Specifically, the degree of contribution of the three primary contributors to cervical spinal stenosis (disc pathology, facet arthropathy, and ligamentum flavum hypertrophy) should be noted, and their combined contribution to the degree of central and foraminal stenosis should be assessed. The anterior border of the neural foramen is the disc, and the posterior border is the facet joint (**Fig. 2.73**). It is important to note the location and course of the vertebral arteries on the axial images. Aberrant vertebral arteries should be identified preoperatively, especially if a cervical corpectomy is being considered. Furthermore, the vertebral arteries should show normal hypointense pulsation signal. Incidentally imaged structures should also be evaluated. For instance, lymph nodes in the neck should be evaluated for size and the presence of a normal fatty hilum. The thyroid should also be evaluated for size and to exclude large nodules.

Coronal Images

Coronal images show the craniocervical spine articulations, intervertebral discs, uncinate processes, atlantooccipital joints, and lateral atlantoaxial joints.[15] Although the sagittal and axial images provide enough information for diagnosis in most cases, coronal images may be especially valuable for evaluating the craniocervical junction or assessing for spinal tumors. Coronal plane MR images, along with conventional radiographs, also facilitate evaluation of the rarely occurring cervical scoliosis because the entire scoliotic spine can be included within a single imaging plane.

■ Thoracic Spine

MRI of the thoracic spine is obtained relatively less frequently than that of the lumbar and cervical spine. The anatomic structures in the thoracic spine are unique in that the ribs form two additional articulations with the vertebrae:

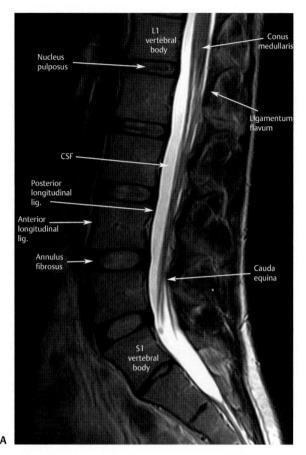

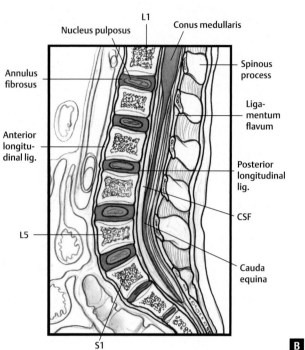

Fig. 2.74 A sagittal T2-weighted midline image **(A)** and artist's sketch **(B)** of the lumbar spine showing the conus medullaris. The posterior longitudinal ligament, intervertebral discs, and vertebral bodies are better differentiated on the T2-weighted images than on T1-weighted images (see Fig. 2.70).

the costocentral joint (between the vertebral body and the rib head) and the costotransverse joint (between the transverse process and proximal rib). The thoracic intervertebral discs are fairly uniform and monotonous. The facet joints are coronally oriented.

■ Lumbar Spine

Sagittal Images

Sagittal imaging of the lumbar spine is usually obtained with T1-weighted and T2-weighted pulse sequences (**Figs. 2.74** and **2.75**). The T1-weighted images are best used for evaluating the anatomic detail of the lumbar spine. The midsagittal image should be evaluated first. This image shows the full profile of the sacrum and most of the lumbar vertebral bodies, spinal cord, and cauda equina in patients without substantial scoliosis. After evaluating the midsagittal image, the sagittal images are sequentially evaluated toward each side to assess the facet joints and neural foramina.

The sagittal images can be concurrently evaluated with the axial sequence to confirm laterality. The bright signal from CSF on T2-weighted images provides a myelographic effect. T1-weighted gradient-echo images assist by providing improved evaluation of end plate and osteophyte anatomy and differentiation of the anterior and posterior longitudinal ligaments from the cortical bone.

Axial Images

When evaluating axial MR images, it is important to accurately identify the level at which the pathology exists, which can be achieved by using the localizing sagittal image. In addition, each level can be identified by starting at the sacrum and numbering each vertebral body from L5 to L1. In complex cases where severe pathology is present at multiple levels, it may also be helpful to use the spine labeling tool (see Cervical Spine, above). On axial images, the difference in signal intensity between the intervertebral discs and vertebral bodies allows for the distinction between vertebral levels.

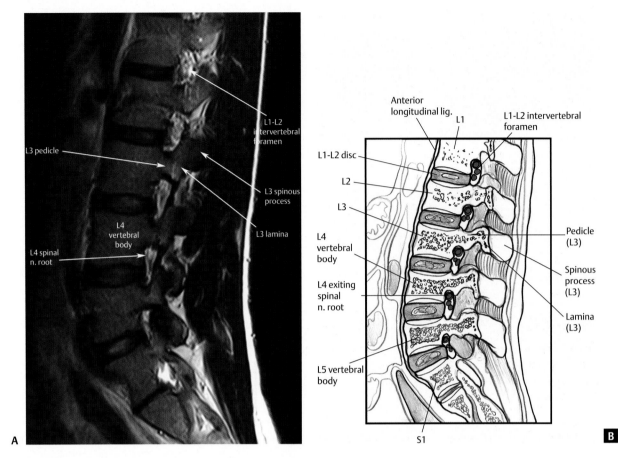

Fig. 2.75 A parasagittal T2-weighted image **(A)** and artist's sketch **(B)** of the lumbar spine showing the neural foramina and exiting nerve roots at multiple levels.

Evaluation of the axial images requires more experience and training than does the evaluation of the sagittal images. Care should be taken to evaluate the axial T2-weighted images and recognize the normal shape and size of the central canal and the neural foramina (**Fig. 2.76**). Specifically, the degree of contribution of the three primary contributors to spinal stenosis (disc pathology, facet arthropathy, and ligamentum flavum hypertrophy) should be noted, and their combined contribution to the degree of central and foraminal stenosis should be carefully assessed (**Fig. 2.77**). The relationship between the superior articular process from the caudal level and the exiting nerve root should be evaluated because hypertrophy of this structure leads to lateral recess and foraminal stenosis. The extraforaminal zone should also be studied at each level to rule out far lateral disc pathology. The psoas muscles are seen adjacent to the vertebral bodies in the lumbar spine (**Fig. 2.77**), and the major vessels (including the aorta and vena cava) are seen anterior to the vertebral bodies. Along with the spine, these structures should also be evaluated for pathologic processes such as aneurysm, thrombosis, and infection.

Coronal Images

Coronal images provide a clear evaluation of the general alignment and anatomy of the lumbar spine, allowing for the identification of the vertebrae and intervertebral discs. Because lordosis increases toward the caudal aspect of the lumbar spine, it is impossible to obtain one image that visualizes the entire spinal canal and its contents. The coronal plane images can be used to evaluate spinal alignment and transitional anatomy at the lumbosacral junction.

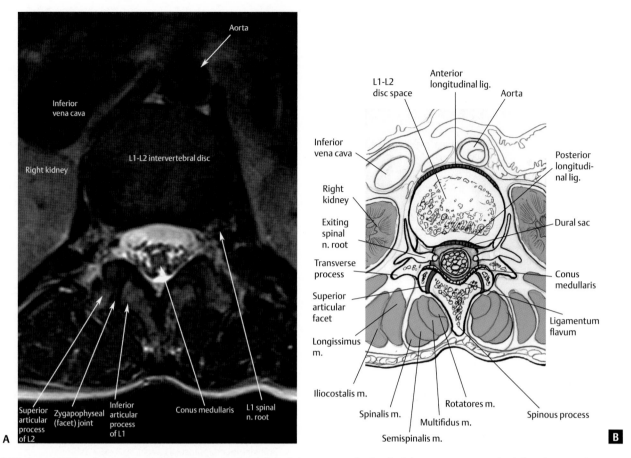

A

Aorta

Inferior
vena cava

Right kidney

L1-L2 intervertebral disc

Superior articular process of L2

Zygapophyseal (facet) joint

Inferior articular process of L1

Conus medullaris

L1 spinal n. root

L1-L2 disc space

Anterior longitudinal lig.

Aorta

Inferior vena cava

Right kidney

Exiting spinal n. root

Transverse process

Superior articular facet

Longissimus m.

Iliocostalis m.

Spinalis m.

Semispinalis m.

Multifidus m.

Rotatores m.

Spinous process

Posterior longitudinal lig.

Dural sac

Conus medullaris

Ligamentum flavum

B

Fig. 2.76 An axial T2-weighted image **(A)** and artist's sketch **(B)** of the spine at the level of the L1-L2 intervertebral disc showing the conus medullaris and the L1 spinal nerve root, as well as the superior and inferior articular processes of the L1-L2 facet joint.

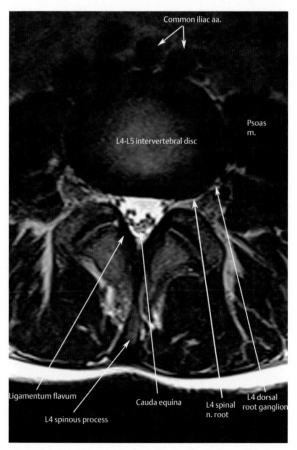

Common iliac aa.

L4-L5 intervertebral disc

Psoas m.

Ligamentum flavum

L4 spinous process

Cauda equina

L4 spinal n. root

L4 dorsal root ganglion

Fig. 2.77 An axial T2-weighted image at the level of the L4-L5 intervertebral disc showing the cauda equina, L4 spinal nerve root, and L4 dorsal root ganglion. Normal flow voids are seen within the common iliac arteries, just below the aortic bifurcation.

References

1. Stoller DW, ed. Stoller's Atlas of Orthopaedics and Sports Medicine. Baltimore: Lippincott Williams & Wilkins; 2008
2. El-Khoury GY, Montgomery WJ, Bergman RA, eds. Sectional Anatomy by MRI and CT. 3rd ed. Philadelphia: Churchill Livingstone (Elsevier); 2007
3. Uri DS. MR imaging of shoulder impingement and rotator cuff disease. Radiol Clin North Am 1997;35:77–96
4. Bredella MA, Tirman PFJ, Peterfy CG, et al. Accuracy of T2-weighted fast spin-echo MR imaging with fat saturation in detecting cartilage defects in the knee: comparison with arthroscopy in 130 patients. AJR Am J Roentgenol 1999;172:1073–1080
5. Disler DG, Recht MP, McCauley TR. MR imaging of articular cartilage. Skeletal Radiol 2000;29:367–377
6. Potter HG, Linklater JM, Allen AA, Hannafin JA, Haas SB. Magnetic resonance imaging of articular cartilage in the knee. An evaluation with use of fast-spin-echo imaging. J Bone Joint Surg Am 1998;80:1276–1284
7. Blease S, Stoller DW, Safran MR, Li AE, Fritz RC. The elbow. In: Stoller DW, ed. Magnetic Resonance Imaging in Orthopaedics and Sports Medicine. Philadelphia: Lippincott Williams & Wilkins; 2007:1463–1625
8. Werlen S, Leunig M, Ganz R. Magnetic resonance arthrography of the hip in femoracetabular impingement: technique and findings. Oper Tech Orthop 2005;15:191–203
9. Fitzgerald RH Jr. Acetabular labrum tears. Diagnosis and treatment. Clin Orthop Relat Res 1995;311:60–68
10. Loredo R, Hodler J, Pedowitz R, Yeh LR, Trudell D, Resnick D. Posteromedial corner of the knee: MR imaging with gross anatomic correlation. Skeletal Radiol 1999;28:305–311
11. Cone RO III. Knee. Section B. Imaging sports-related injuries of the knee. In: DeLee JC, Drez D Jr, Miller MD, eds. DeLee and Drez's Orthopaedic Sports Medicine: Principles and Practice. Philadelphia: WB Saunders; 2003:1595–1652
12. Stanitski CL. Knee. Section D. Meniscal injuries. Part 2. Meniscal injuries in the skeletally immature patient. In: DeLee JC, Drez D Jr, Miller MD, eds. DeLee and Drez's Orthopaedic Sports Medicine: Principles and Practice. Philadelphia: WB Saunders; 2003:1686–1696
13. Peterfy CG, Janzen DL, Tirman PFJ, van Dijke CF, Pollack M, Genant HK. "Magic-angle" phenomenon: a cause of increased signal in the normal lateral meniscus on short-TE MR images of the knee. AJR Am J Roentgenol 1994;163:149–154
14. Morgan S, Saifuddin A. MRI of the lumbar intervertebral disc. Clin Radiol 1999;54:703–723
15. White ML. Cervical spine: MR imaging techniques and anatomy. Magn Reson Imaging Clin N Am 2000;8:453–469
16. Kaiser JA, Holland BA. Imaging of the cervical spine. Spine (Phila Pa 1976) 1998;23:2701–2712
17. Khanna AJ, Carbone JJ, Kebaish KM, et al. Magnetic resonance imaging of the cervical spine. Current techniques and spectrum of disease. J Bone Joint Surg Am 2002;84(Suppl 2):70–80
18. Boden SD, Lee RR, Herzog RJ. Magnetic resonance imaging of the spine. In: Frymoyer JW, ed. The Adult Spine: Principles and Practice. Philadelphia: Lippincott-Raven; 1997:563–629

3 A Systematic Approach to the Review of Musculoskeletal MRI Studies

A. Jay Khanna

■ General Concepts

As with any new skill, learning the process for evaluating an MRI study begins with a systematic approach. Less experienced clinicians may have a tendency to review films without paying special attention to the type of imaging studies, the pulse sequences that are being evaluated, or the plane in which they are being evaluated. When reviewing films on a computer workstation, they also may tend to review only one pulse sequence or one or two imaging planes. These shortcuts, especially early in a clinician's experience in evaluating MRI studies, may lead to less accurate and less reliable MR study interpretation.

Chapter 1 provided a summary of the technical foundation that radiologists often use to select the appropriate pulse sequences and imaging techniques for the study of a given region or pathologic process. The purpose of this more clinically oriented chapter is to provide the clinician or radiologist with a method for evaluating MRI studies in an organized and systematic fashion. The adoption of such a system early in a clinician's experience is believed to lead to improved accuracy and reliability in the interpretation of MRI studies. Over time, clinicians may be able to incorporate a more informal method of evaluating the MRI studies and rely more on their own experience and personalized method of study evaluation.

The evaluation of an MRI study can be divided into the following five steps:

1. Determination of which conventional and specialized MRI pulse sequences are available for review
2. Evaluation of T2-weighted images for recognition of areas of increased T2-weighted signal that are not expected or physiologic
3. Evaluation of T1-weighted images for improved detection of anatomic detail and correlation of the alteration in local and regional anatomy on the T1-weighted images with areas of increased signal intensity on the T2-weighted images
4. Evaluation of specialized MRI pulse sequences that may be specific to the region or disease process that is being evaluated
5. Correlation of the above imaging information with the patient's history, physical examination, and laboratory study results to identify the most likely differential diagnostic considerations

The use of a general technique of MRI study evaluation described in this chapter in conjunction with the more region- and concept-specific information provided in subsequent chapters will help improve a clinician's ability to accurately interpret an MRI study of the musculoskeletal system.

■ Step 1: Determination of Pulse Sequences Available for Review

The first step in the evaluation of an MRI study is to determine which pulse sequences are available for review. For

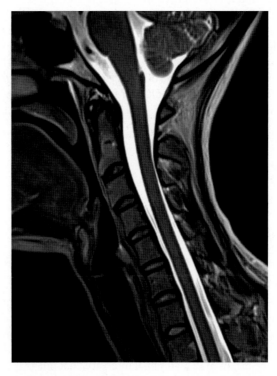

Fig. 3.1 A sagittal T2-weighted image of the cervical spine. Note that the CSF is of high signal intensity.

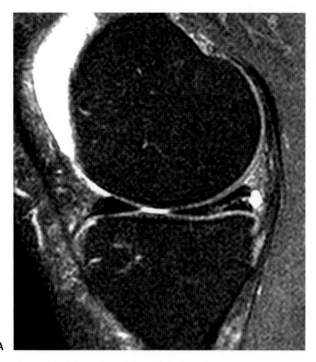

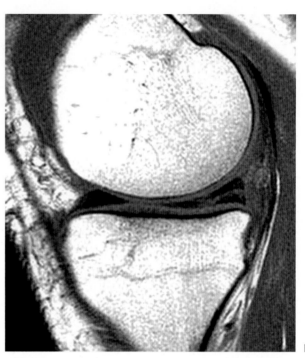

A   B

Fig. 3.2 Sagittal fat-suppressed T2-weighted **(A)** and T1-weighted **(B)** images of the knee. Note that the joint fluid is high signal on the former and low signal on the latter. Note also that there is a horizontal tear of the posterior horn of the medial meniscus with an associated meniscal cyst, which is best seen on the T2-weighted image **(A)**.

most cases, such sequences include at least T1-weighted and conventional T2-weighted images, acquired in the sagittal, axial, and (frequently) coronal planes. MR images of the spine (cervical, thoracic, and lumbar) are often acquired only in the sagittal and axial planes.

In addition to conventional T1-weighted and T2-weighted pulse sequences, there are other pulse sequences that are often acquired and that should be recognizable, including the following:

- Fat-suppressed T2-weighted images or STIR images
- Postgadolinium T1-weighted images
- Gradient-echo images
- MR arthrography images
- MR angiography images

T1-Weighted and T2-Weighted Images

One should be able to determine whether an image is T1-weighted or T2-weighted using the following techniques:

- Recognition of an area within an image that is known to contain fluid, such as the spine (CSF) (**Fig. 3.1**), the region of the hip (bladder), and the knee or other joints (intraarticular fluid) (**Fig. 3.2**). If this fluid is noted to be bright or of high signal intensity, that image is likely T2-weighted. If the region of the fluid is noted to be dark, that image is likely T1-weighted.

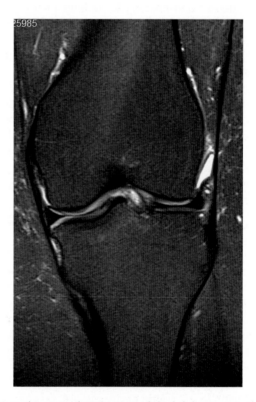

Fig. 3.3 In this coronal STIR image of the left knee, note that this image is relatively dark. Thus, if an area of increased signal is noted in the tibial plateau, for example, it would be relatively conspicuous and difficult to miss.

• Recognition of the TR and TE values, which are often printed on the film or are visible on the workstation screen. Recognizing these values may allow the clinician to determine whether an image is T1-weighted or T2-weighted. In most institutions and in most cases, images are acquired using an SE technique (for additional details, see Chapter 1). When this technique or similar techniques are used, the TR value is usually 300 to 800 ms for T1-weighted images and 2000 to 5000 ms for T2-weighted images. If the clinician evaluates the image and is unable to use the technique in which fluid recognition allows the differentiation of T1-weighted and T2-weighted images, this technique is a good second option. If the TR number is found on the film and is noted to be in the 100s range, it likely is a T1-weighted image. If the TR number is found to be in the 1000s range, it likely is a T2-weighted image. With newer and more variable pulse sequences, this method may be less reliable.

Fat-Suppressed T2-Weighted Images or STIR Images

Fat-suppressed T2-weighted images are acquired using techniques similar to those for conventional T2-weighted images, and then various computer algorithms and processes are used to "suppress" the signal that is coming from fat. A more "pure" way of achieving this goal is to acquire a STIR image, in which case the signal from fat is not acquired. Because of the suppression of signal from fat in either of these techniques, the images tend to appear quite a bit "darker" than images obtained via other techniques (such as conventional T2-weighted images) and thus help accentuate the increase in T2-weighted signal (relative to the adjacent tissues), which may otherwise be missed (**Fig. 3.3**). Specifically, this technique facilitates the evaluation of bone marrow edema and edema secondary to other pathologic processes. Fat-suppressed T2-weighted images or STIR images show areas of edema with markedly greater conspicuity than that seen on conventional T2-weighted images (see individual chapters for applications of these techniques for region-specific pathology).

As an example, in the evaluation of a nondisplaced femoral neck fracture, coronal T1-weighted or T2-weighted images may not show edema along the fracture line, whereas a fat-suppressed T2-weighted image or a STIR image would make such a finding quite obvious (**Fig. 3.4**). These latter images are also useful for determining whether a vertebral compression fracture represents a chronic fracture or an acute or subacute fracture (**Fig. 3.5**).

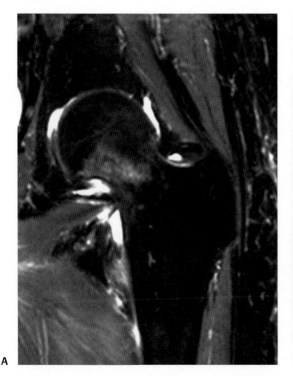

A

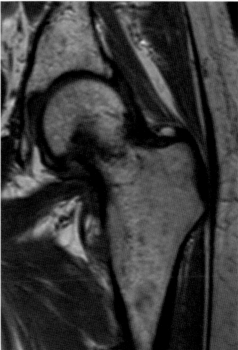

B

Fig. 3.4 Nondisplaced femoral neck fracture in the left hip. **(A)** A coronal STIR image shows a region of increased signal intensity in the femoral neck, suggestive of an acute or subacute nondisplaced fracture. **(B)** A T1-weighted image shows a linear pattern of low signal within the femoral neck, which helps confirm the diagnosis of an acute, nondisplaced femoral neck fracture.

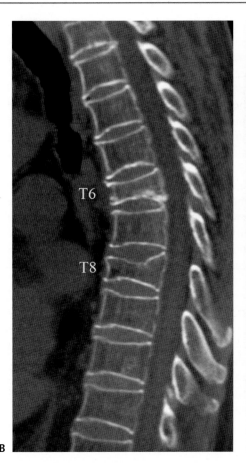 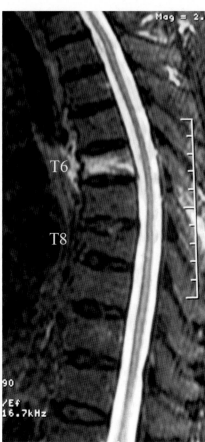

A, B

Fig. 3.5 Vertebral compression fracture. **(A)** A sagittal reconstructed CT image shows vertebral compression fractures at the T6 and T8 levels. **(B)** A sagittal STIR image shows that the T6 vertebral compression fracture has increased signal compatible with edema within it, which is representative of an acute or subacute fracture. The T8 vertebral compression fracture shows no increase in signal within it, which is compatible with a chronic vertebral compression fracture.

Postgadolinium T1-Weighted Images

Postgadolinium T1-weighted images and fat-suppressed postgadolinium T1-weighted images are typically obtained for the evaluation of infection, tumor, and postsurgical changes or scar. These images can sometimes be confused with T2-weighted images because they may show areas of increased signal in the presence of pathology (**Fig. 3.6**); the distinction can be made using the techniques outlined above. Specifically, the clinician should evaluate the areas in which one may expect to find physiologic fluid, such as fluid within a joint or CSF in the spine. If this fluid is bright, then the images are T2-weighted. If this fluid seems to be dark, and the pathology seems to be bright, then the image is likely a postgadolinium T1-weighted image. In addition, the technique of TR evaluation described above can also be used to differentiate a postgadolinium T1-weighted image (TR is in the 100s range) from a T2-weighted image (TR is in the 1000s range).

Gradient-Echo Images

Gradient-echo images, which appear to be somewhat grayer in their general appearance than other images (including T1-weighted and T2-weighted images), are especially useful for the evaluation of articular cartilage (**Fig. 3.7**). In addition, it is important to note that the gradient-echo images are especially susceptible to ferromagnetic materials, such as metallic implants or hemosiderin, and therefore show "signal dropout" in the presence of these substances.

MR Arthrography Images

MR arthrography images are obtained after the joint of interest is injected with gadolinium or normal saline (see Chapter 16) (**Fig. 3.8**). They may be difficult to differentiate from T2-weighted images, which also contain bright fluid within the joint. MR arthrography images are often marked by the radiologist or the radiology technician so that it is relatively obvious that gadolinium has been injected into the joint.

MR Angiography Images

MR angiography images highlight the blood vessels and allow for evaluation of the arterial and venous vascular structures (see Chapter 16) (**Fig. 3.9**). These images are obviously different in appearance from the images acquired using the more conventional pulse sequences and MRI techniques.

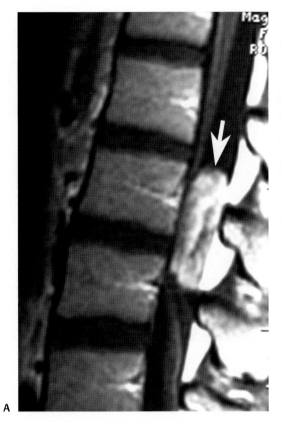

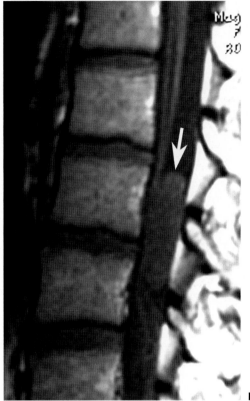

Fig. 3.6 Lumbar spine intradural-extramedullary mass. **(A)** A post-gadolinium sagittal T1-weighted image shows a high-signal intensity mass (*arrow*) just dorsal to the filum terminal. **(B)** The associated pregadolinium T1-weighted image shows the mass (*arrow*) to be less conspicuous. Note that if specific attention is not given to the fact that the CSF is dark, one may mistakenly identify the first image as a T2-weighted image and the second image as the associated T1-weighted image.

■ Step 2: Evaluation of T2-Weighted Images

After the clinician has identified all of the T2-weighted images, they should be systematically evaluated, plane by plane. In almost all instances, the clinician should begin with sagittal T2-weighted images, views especially useful for the spine, knee, elbow, and ankle. In some instances, such as for the hip and shoulder, it may be best to begin with the coronal or coronal oblique images.

If the images are being evaluated as films on a light box, they should be hung in sequential order, starting with all sagittal images, then all coronal images, and then all axial images. The same process should be used when evaluating an imaging study on a computer workstation.

Cervical Spine Example

A description of the evaluation of the cervical spine serves as an illustrative example.

- First, evaluate the sagittal T2-weighted images. Ensure that all of the sagittal T2-weighted images are being visualized in order from one side to the other (in this case, from left to right) (**Fig. 3.10**).
- Next, look for the midline image (**Fig. 3.11**).

  o For the cervical spine, recognize the midline image by noting that the spinal cord is seen in its entirety (in the patient without scoliosis), extending from the midbrain to the upper thoracic spine.

  o Visualize the CSF anterior and posterior to the cervical spinal cord.

  o Confirm that the midline image is being evaluated by noting the basion and opisthion at the foramen magnum. In addition, the fourth ventricle is visualized, the vertebral bodies are seen as rectangular or square structures, and the odontoid process is seen in profile with its domed tip.

- After evaluating all of the structures at the midline, continue the review to the left or right side to evaluate for foraminal or lateral recess stenosis.

  o Each institution has its own convention as to whether the images for sagittal images are acquired from left to right or right to left.

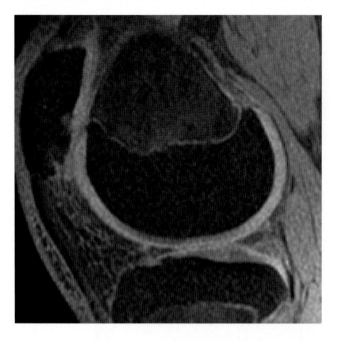

Fig. 3.7 A sagittal 3D fat-suppressed T1-weighted gradient-echo image of the knee shows high contrast between hyperintense articular cartilage and hypointense bone. (From Shindle MK, Foo LF, Kelly BT, Khanna AJ, Domb BG, Farber A, Wanich T, Potter HG: Magnetic resonance imaging of cartilage in the athlete: current techniques and spectrum of disease. J Bone Joint Surg Am 2006;88(suppl 4):27–46. Reprinted by permission.)

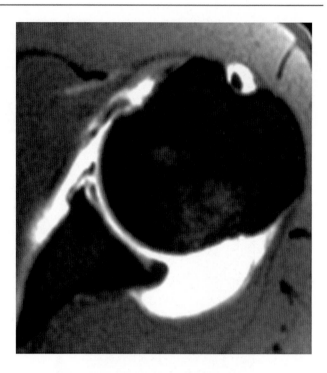

Fig. 3.8 An axial postgadolinium MR arthrogram of the left shoulder shows a Bankart lesion.

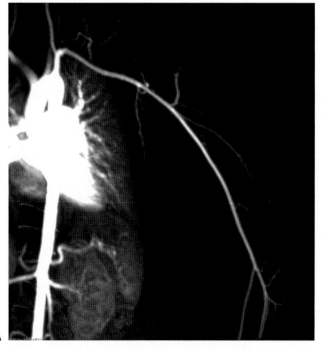

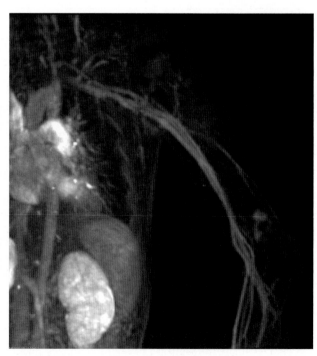

A   B

Fig. 3.9 MR arteriogram **(A)** and venogram **(B)** of the left shoulder obtained for the evaluation of a vascular malformation.

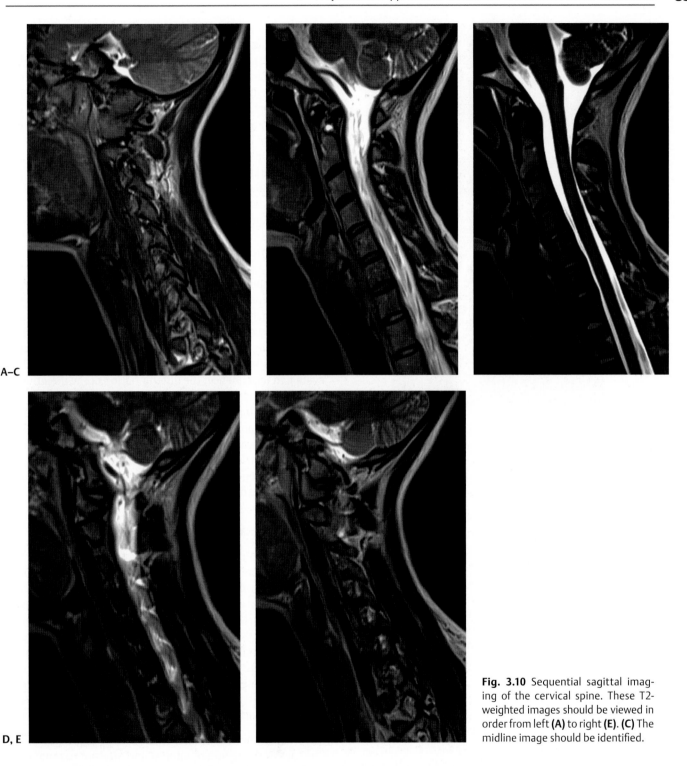

A–C

D, E

Fig. 3.10 Sequential sagittal imaging of the cervical spine. These T2-weighted images should be viewed in order from left **(A)** to right **(E)**. **(C)** The midline image should be identified.

○ The only way to be 100% positive about which side of the cervical spine is being visualized is to evaluate the coronal localizing pulse sequence, which often displays numbers that correspond to the numbers seen on the sagittal images. The other way to see whether a specific pathologic finding (for example, a disc herniation) is right or left or paracentral is to correlate the sagittal images with the findings seen on the axial images.

• Next, evaluate all of the axial T2-weighted images from the occipitocervical junction to the lower cervical spine (**Fig. 3.12**).

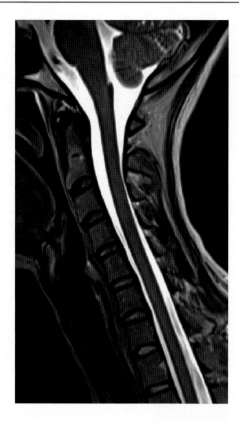

Fig. 3.11 A midline sagittal T2-weighted image of the cervical spine. Note that the spinal cord is seen in its entirety; CSF is seen anterior and posterior to the spinal cord; and the vertebral bodies, odontoid process, and fourth ventricle are seen in profile.

o The only way to ensure that all of the images are seen in sequence and that none is missed is to look at the image numbers on the printed film or on the screen and to confirm that the image number at the beginning of one sheet is the next sequential number after that on the previous sheet.

o Confirm the location at the occipitocervical junction by noting that the odontoid process appears different than the remaining cervical vertebral bodies in the subaxial cervical spine.

• Finally, evaluate all of the images in sequence to view the cervical spinal cord and note that there is CSF (bright signal) around it and adequate space available for the nerve roots at the neural foramina; correlating the axial image number with the sagittal localizing image, which contains lines corresponding with numbers that indicate the level of the axial image, will ensure accurate identification of the level being evaluated.

Knee Example

The same technique can be used for evaluating knee MR images. Again, all of the sagittal T2-weighted images are hung (or viewed on a work station) in sequence from the lateral to the medial side or vice versa. Looking for differences in the lateral-side knee anatomy (such as the presence of the fibular head or the shape of the lateral tibial plateau compared with that of the medial tibial plateau) or correlating the sagittal image numbers with the number seen on the coronal or axial localizing pulse sequence (**Fig. 3.13**) will ensure that the lateral side is being evaluated. These images are then evaluated from the lateral to the medial side, beginning with the lateral femoral condyle, and then in sequence the ACL or PCL and the medial femoral condyle (see Chapter 2 for additional details regarding knee anatomy) (**Fig. 3.14**).

After evaluation of the sagittal T2-weighted images, the next step is to evaluate the coronal T2-weighted images in sequence, from anterior to posterior or vice versa. Using the sagittal- or axial-localizing pulse sequence and matching the image numbers will ensure that an image is relatively anterior or relatively posterior. In addition, it is obvious that the anterior images begin with the patella, whereas the posterior images contain the popliteal artery and vein (**Fig. 3.15**).

Next, the axial T2-weighted images can be evaluated from proximal to distal or vice versa. The images should be evaluated in sequence; the differentiation of the direction of film progression can be made based on whether the femur or the tibia/fibula is visualized (**Fig. 3.16**). However, if there is any uncertainty in the region of the femoral condyles or the tibial plateau, the image number seen on the sagittal- or coronal-localizing pulse sequence can be correlated with the image number seen on the axial images to determine the exact location of the axial cut.

Pattern Recognition

The next step is to evaluate for any areas of increased T2-weighted signal that should not have increased T2-weighted signal. This evaluation may be relatively easy for a clinician with extensive experience in evaluating MRI studies of a particular region. Most clinicians would agree that in determining these areas of increased T2-weighted signal, they tend to use the gestalt method. However, for the less experienced clinician or the clinician in training, several techniques can be used to determine whether or not an area should show increased T2-weighted signal. These techniques rely on the concepts of pattern recognition and experience:

• Recall the evaluations of the last 20 to 50 MRI studies of the region of interest and attempt to remember exactly where the increase in T2-weighted signal was seen.

o Increased T2-weighted signal outside of that pattern on the current study may represent an area of pathology.

o This technique of pattern recognition is commonly used by experienced radiologists to read

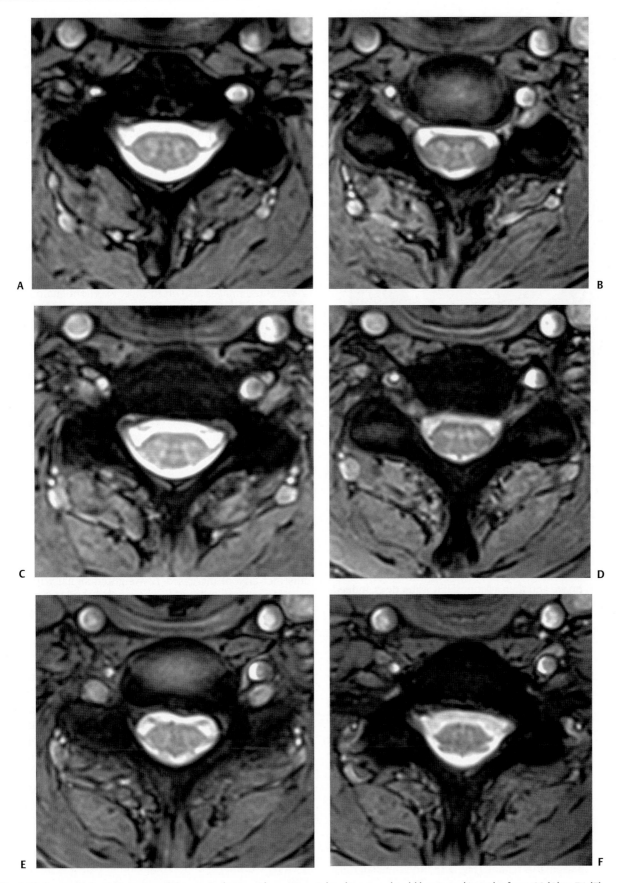

Fig. 3.12 Sequential axial imaging of the cervical spine. These T2-weighted images should be viewed in order from C6 **(A)** to T1 **(F)**.

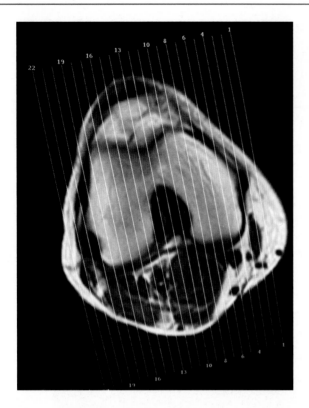

Fig. 3.13 Axial localizing pulse sequence of the right knee with numbers of prescribed sagittal images from medial (*number 1*) to most lateral (*number 22*).

films. Although clinicians tend to use this technique for in-office patient evaluation, it may or may not be a safe and effective technique.[1]

- The other method with which one can evaluate for areas of abnormal increased T2-weighted signal is to note all areas of increased T2-weighted signal within a given image and then ask oneself if water does, indeed, "belong" in that area.

    o For example, if the shoulder is being evaluated on a T2-weighted coronal oblique image and a thin sliver of high signal is seen between the humeral head and the glenoid (anatomic structures that are obvious, even to the least-experienced clinician), then one may assume that it represents fluid within the joint (**Fig. 3.17**). The question, then, is whether it is a normal (physiologic) or an excessive (pathologic) amount of fluid. The ability to make this determination comes from experience or from comparison to a normal contralateral joint.

    o In the same coronal oblique image, if increased T2-weighted signal is seen superior and lateral to the humeral head in the expected location of the supraspinatus tendon (**Fig. 3.18**), the clinician must

ask this question: Does water or edema belong in the tendons? If the answer is no, the clinician may assume that there is edema within the tendon and then may be able to deduce that the signal may represent a partial or complete tear of the supraspinatus tendon. Additional findings such as retraction of the tendon and other morphologic changes may help make this determination.

■ Step 3: Evaluation of T1-Weighted Images

T1-weighted images allow for optimal evaluation of anatomic detail. With current improvements in MRI techniques and equipment, including dedicated surface and other coils, T2-weighted images also often show excellent anatomic detail. This improvement may be the reason that the author believes the routine use of T1-weighted images by clinicians and radiologists is declining. Nevertheless, the most appropriate way to evaluate an MRI study fully and most effectively is to review all of the images and pulse sequences.

Therefore, after identification of the pulse sequences obtained (step 1) and evaluation of the T2-weighted images (step 2), the next step is to review the T1-weighted images for improved evaluation of anatomic detail. This author's routine is to correlate the areas of increased T2-weighted signal seen during the very detailed and systematic evaluation of the T2-weighted images outlined above with the same region on the T1-weighted images. The improved spatial resolution of the T1-weighted images facilitates the evaluation of regional and local disturbances in anatomic detail. For example, a coronal fat-suppressed T2-weighted image of a nondisplaced femoral neck fracture shows a somewhat indistinct area of increased T2-weighted signal within the femoral neck (**Fig. 3.4A**). The clinician may decide that it represents a nondisplaced femoral neck fracture but may also consider the possibility of other diagnoses. However, a relatively sharp and crisp fracture line seen within the femoral neck on the coronal T1-weighted image (**Fig. 3.4B**) would likely leave no doubt in the clinician's mind that it represents a fracture and not some other process such as a bone bruise, infection, or tumor.

In addition, the T1-weighted images may help the clinician determine the type of tissue that is present in a lesion. Central to this concept is the fact that T1-weighted images tend to show fat as bright signal and fluid as dark signal. Therefore, lesions such as a lipoma (see Chapter 15) are noted to be bright on T1-weighted images, and, in fact, follow the signal of subcutaneous fat on all pulse sequences, including fat-suppressed or STIR pulse sequences. As another example, one of the few lesions that is bright on both T2-weighted and T1-weighted images is a hemangioma, which is often seen

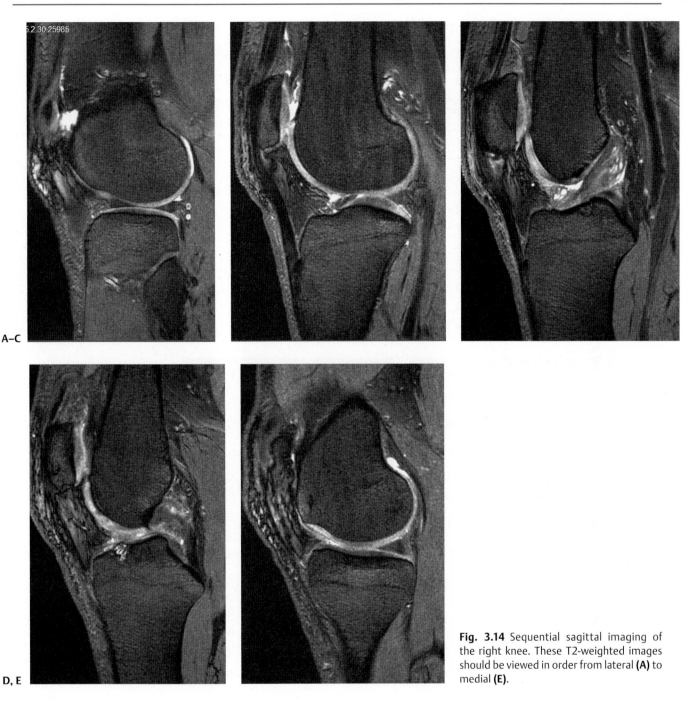

A–C

D, E

Fig. 3.14 Sequential sagittal imaging of the right knee. These T2-weighted images should be viewed in order from lateral **(A)** to medial **(E)**.

in the vertebral body (**Fig. 3.19**). Thus, if the lesion is seen to be bright on both of these images and displays the typical pattern of striations, the diagnosis of vertebral body hemangioma can be made with relative certainty.

As with T2-weighted images, T1-weighted images should be evaluated in all planes and in the same sequence as described in Step 2.

■ Step 4: Evaluation of Specialized Pulse Sequences

Fat-Suppressed T2-Weighted or STIR Images

The fat-suppressed T2-weighted or STIR pulse sequences are used to accentuate the increase in signal and edema seen

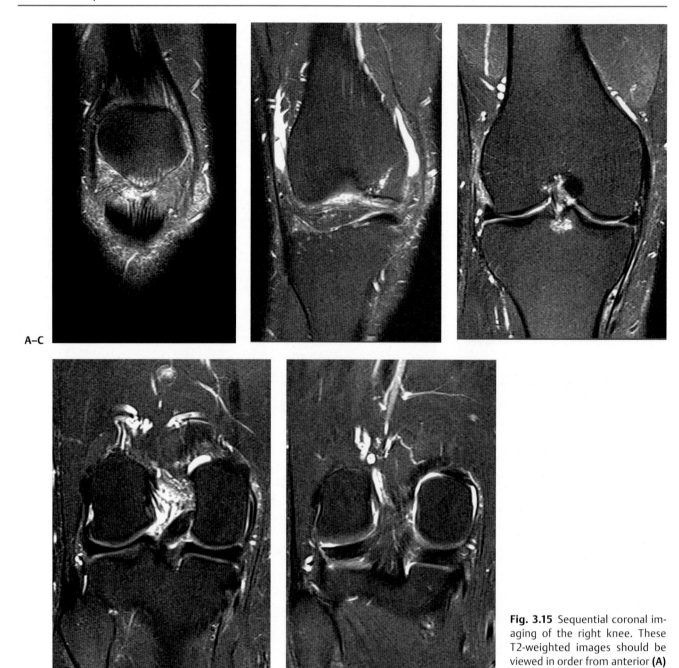

A–C

D, E

Fig. 3.15 Sequential coronal imaging of the right knee. These T2-weighted images should be viewed in order from anterior **(A)** to posterior **(E)**.

in pathologic processes such as fracture, infection, and tumor. On conventional T2-weighted images, the signal from bone marrow fat is maintained, and one attempts to recognize edema by noting the presence or absence of a very bright region (marrow pathology or edema) within a bright background (fatty marrow) (**Fig. 3.20A**). On fat-suppressed T2-weighted images, all of the subcutaneous, bone marrow, and other fat is suppressed, and one can more easily recognize an area of edema as a bright region within a dark background (**Fig. 3.20B**). This author considers fat-suppressed T2-weighted and STIR images to be somewhat like a three-

phase nuclear scintigraphy (bone scan) study (see Chapter 17), which is relatively sensitive to increased bone turnover but not very specific. Similarly, if a region is evaluated with fat-suppressed T2-weighted imaging or STIR imaging and there is no area of increased signal, one can be somewhat reassured that a pathologic process is not present in that region. Conversely, if an area of increased signal is noted, it may represent pathologic change or a normal region of increased signal such as physiologic fluid within the joint or CSF. Other pulse sequences, such as T2-weighted and T1-weighted images, provide better anatomic detail for evaluation and help

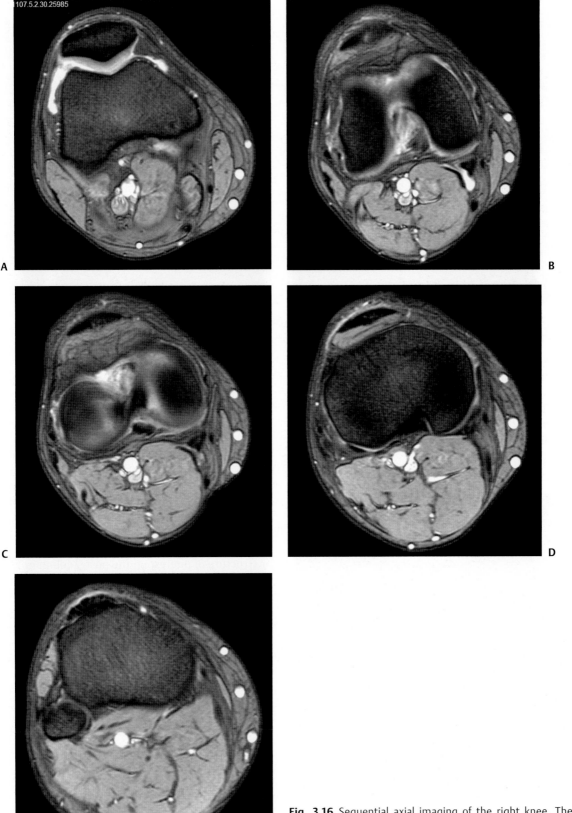

Fig. 3.16 Sequential axial imaging of the right knee. These T2-weighted images should be viewed in order from proximal **(A)** to distal **(E)**.

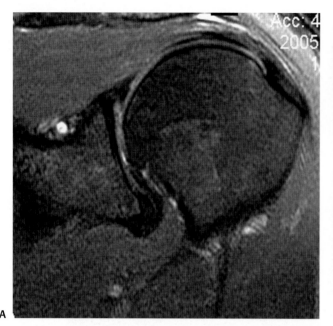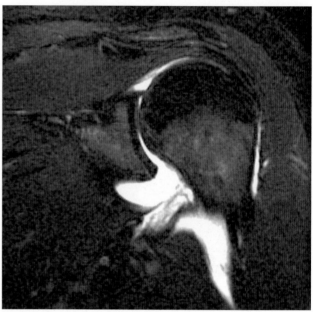

A   B

Fig. 3.17 Coronal oblique STIR images show minimal, if any, fluid within the left shoulder joint of a patient with no pathology **(A)** and a pathologically increased amount of joint fluid in the left shoulder joint of a patient with a HAGHL lesion **(B)**.

the clinician identify a more specific diagnosis. As discussed above and in region-specific chapters, fat-suppressed T2-weighted images can be used to evaluate for nondisplaced fractures and to determine the approximate age or chronicity of fractures, including vertebral compression fractures.

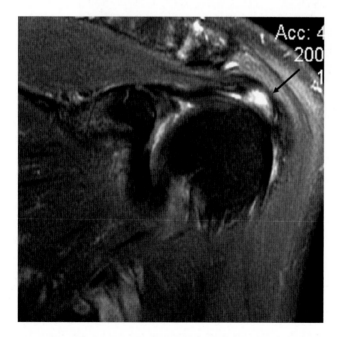

Fig. 3.18 A coronal oblique T2-weighted image of the left shoulder shows increased signal within the supraspinatus tendon (*arrow*), compatible with a high-grade partial-thickness tear.

Postgadolinium T1-Weighted Images

Postgadolinium T1-weighted images are often acquired to evaluate for the presence or absence of infection and tumor and to assess the postoperative joint or spine. For example, in the spine, postgadolinium T1-weighted images can help differentiate recurrent disc herniation from epidural fibrosis and scar. The recommended method for evaluating these images is to place the postgadolinium T1-weighted images side by side with the pregadolinium T1-weighted images. The region of interest is then compared in the same planes and on matching images. Higher signal intensity in the region or structure of interest on the postgadolinium T1-weighted images is termed postgadolinium or contrast enhancement. An evaluation can then be made with regard to the degree and pattern of enhancement. For example, peripheral rim enhancement with a central region of nonenhancement in a relatively well-circumscribed lesion is considered, in the appropriate clinical setting, to be a finding suggestive of an abscess (**Fig. 3.21**).

■ Step 5: Correlation of Imaging Findings with Patient History and Examination Findings to Determine the Most Likely Diagnosis

Clinicians and radiologists have distinct advantages and disadvantages in terms of evaluating an MRI study. The radiologist has the advantage of often being trained with a process

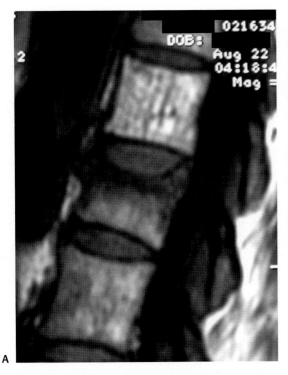

Fig. 3.19 Sagittal T1-weighted **(A)** and T2-weighted **(B)** images show a lesion at the T12 level with high signal intensity on both images and with the typical striations compatible with a vertebral body hemangioma. An incidentally noted vertebral compression fracture is seen at the L1 level.

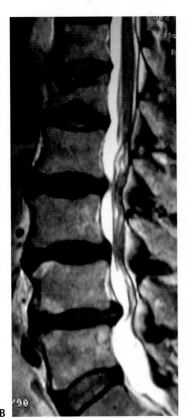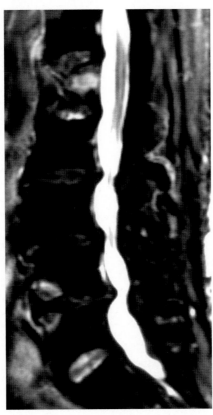

Fig. 3.20 Vertebral compression fracture. **(A)** A sagittal T2-weighted image of the lumbar spine showing an L1 vertebral body compression fracture of an indeterminate age, given that edema is not definitely seen. **(B)** A sagittal STIR image of the same patient shows edema within the L1 vertebral body, which is compatible with an acute or subacute vertebral compression fracture.

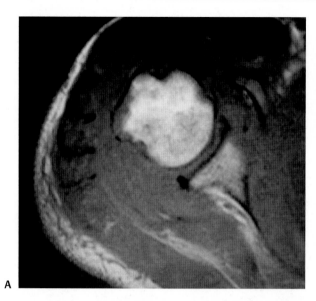
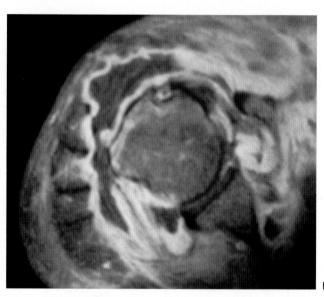

A   B

Fig. 3.21 Pregadolinium **(A)** and postgadolinium **(B)** T1-weighted images of the right shoulder showing a fluid collection around the glenohumeral joint with peripheral rim enhancement on the postga- dolinium image **(B)** in a patient with infectious symptoms and find- ings. The imaging characteristics are compatible with an abscess and associated septic joint.

similar to the one described above and often has, and takes, the time to evaluate the images in a systematic fashion. However, the clinician has the advantage of knowing the patient's history and physical examination findings, labora- tory results, and other parameters. It is essential that clini- cians use this advantage to help maximize the accuracy and reliability of their MRI interpretations. An accurate diagno- sis, or differential diagnosis, occurs at the "intersection" of a patient's history, physical examination results, radiographic findings, and laboratory study results (**Fig. 3.22**). With an

understanding of the clinical scenario, clinicians can arrive at an accurate diagnosis, especially when they are armed with the appropriate techniques for evaluating the MRI studies. One way to leverage the advantages of both clinicians and radiologists is to use a collaborative team approach to the evaluation of patients with complex pathology.

For example, if a patient presents with knee pain after trauma and is point-tender at the proximal anterior tibia and if the MR image shows an area of increased T2-weighted sig- nal within the tibial plateau, the diagnosis of a bone bruise

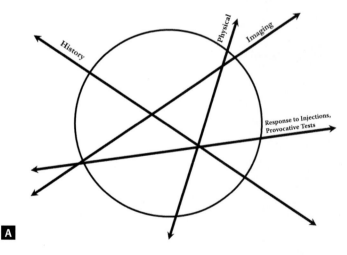
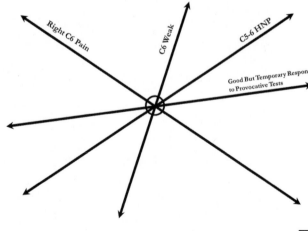

A   B

Fig. 3.22 The concept of intersecting lines for diagnosis and surgi- cal decision-making. **(A)** In a patient for whom the history, physical examination, imaging findings, and response to provocative tests do not "intersect" within a small circle, it is difficult to identify a diag- nosis or to narrow a differential diagnosis. **(B)** Conversely, for a pa- tient with a smaller region of intersection, such as one with a right C6 radiculopathy, one may expect to see a C5-C6 disc protrusion on MRI.

or a nondisplaced tibial plateau fracture can be suggested. However, if a patient with the same imaging findings presents with no history of trauma, is elderly, has a history of insidious onset of knee pain (particularly at night), and has a history of a primary malignancy, another diagnosis (e.g., metastatic disease) might be higher on the differential diagnosis. To determine the correct diagnosis, the clinician would likely obtain a CT scan to evaluate further the osseous anatomy in both patients. The second patient might also benefit from a primary malignancy survey and a three-phase bone scan.

In summary, the above-described five-step technique will help guide the clinician in systematically evaluating MRI studies of various regions of the musculoskeletal system. This author strongly believes that such a systematic technique should be used for the evaluation of all MRI studies and that the tendency to become less meticulous and systematic over time should be avoided. One additional concept taught to the residents in the author's institution is always to attempt to read the MRI study using the above-described technique and then to evaluate the "official" radiologist's reading to determine the degree of correlation between the two readings. Occasionally, findings are noted by the clinicians that were not reported by the radiologist, and vice versa. Over time, this method of checking one's own evaluation against that of another trained specialist will serve as method of quality control and assurance and will likely result in a continuously improving ability to evaluate MRI studies accurately.

Reference

1. Groopman J. How Doctors Think. Boston: Houghton Mifflin; 2007.

II Upper Extremity

4 The Shoulder

Adam J. Farber, A. Jay Khanna, Laura M. Fayad, Timothy S. Johnson, and Edward G. McFarland

■ Specialized Pulse Sequences and Imaging Protocols

MRI of the shoulder has improved with the development of high-field systems and enhanced surface coil technology.[1] The patient is imaged in the supine position and the arm is held at the side, rather than across the chest, to minimize transmission of respiratory motion to the shoulder. To optimally visualize the supraspinatus tendon and its insertion and to prevent confusing overlap with the infraspinatus tendon on coronal oblique images, the arm is placed in slight external rotation. Axial, coronal oblique, and sagittal oblique images are obtained routinely.

Most centers use a standard screening examination, consisting of an array of specified imaging planes and pulse sequences.[1] In addition to standard intermediate-weighted (proton-density) images, fat-suppressed proton-density, fat-suppressed T2-weighted, and STIR sequences are sensitive to the presence of fluid. The latter sequences allow the detection of soft-tissue pathology by accentuating the increased signal of edema relative to the surrounding structures. In some centers, non–fat-suppressed T2-weighted imaging is preferred for the evaluation of the rotator cuff tendons because it aids in the distinction of tendinosis and partial tears. In general, these sequences are acquired with an FSE technique that produces the desired contrast in a fraction of the time needed for conventional SE sequences. In addition, gradient-echo sequences may be used to evaluate the articular cartilage (see Chapter 14) and to delineate the presence of intraarticular bodies or accentuate calcification seen with calcium hydroxyapatite deposition. However, gradient-echo sequences should be avoided after shoulder surgery (especially in the presence of metal hardware) because of the increased artifact inherent to the gradient-echo technique (see Chapter 1).

MR arthrography can be performed via direct or indirect methods. Direct MR arthrography is performed by injecting approximately 10 to 15 mL of diluted gadolinium contrast agent into the glenohumeral joint from an anterior or posterior approach and acquiring fat-suppressed T1-weighted and T2-weighted images. Indirect MR arthrography is performed by injecting gadolinium intravenously and imaging the joint after contrast has been taken up by the synovium and then diffused into the joint. Direct MR arthrography of the shoulder has been shown to improve visualization of the labrum, the articular cartilage, and the rotator cuff tendons. Indirect MR arthrography has limited use for evaluation of the labrum, but it aids in the detection of rotator cuff pathology and in the assessment of arthritis, neoplasm, and infection. However, with the advent of high-field, high-resolution imaging and novel noncontrast MR techniques, direct and indirect MR arthrography techniques may be rendered obsolete in the future.[2]

■ Traumatic Conditions

Traumatic conditions affecting the shoulder that are commonly evaluated by MRI include the following:

- Glenohumeral instability
- Labral pathology
- Occult fractures
- Rotator cuff tears

Many rotator cuff tears occur in the setting of long-standing tendinosis (see Degenerative Conditions, below).

Glenohumeral Instability

Because of the shoulder's extensive range of motion, it is the most commonly dislocated joint in the body.[3,4] Instability encompasses a spectrum of disorders of varying direction, degree, and etiology. Shoulder instability is classified based on the direction of dislocation (i.e., anterior [most common], posterior, or multidirectional) and by degree (dislocation, subluxation, and microinstability), force (traumatic versus atraumatic), and patient contribution (voluntary versus involuntary). Instability episodes range from subluxation to complete dislocation and are associated with a spectrum of injury to the shoulder stabilizers.

Patients with recurrent anterior shoulder instability typically have a history of a traumatic (direct or indirect) anterior shoulder dislocation, report recurrent episodes of subluxation or dislocation, and describe symptoms such as pain or apprehension during arm abduction and external rotation. Patients with recurrent posterior instability pose more complex diagnostic challenges and can present

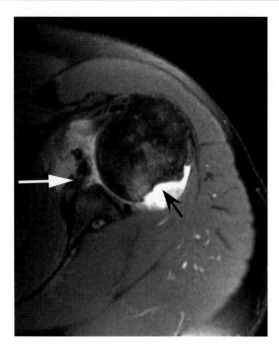

Fig. 4.1 An axial fat-suppressed proton-density image of the left shoulder showing an osseous Bankart lesion (*white arrow*) and a Hill-Sachs lesion (*black arrow*).

with traumatic posterior instability or with atraumatic subluxations not associated with trauma. Trauma, direct or indirect, also may be the mechanism of injury of a posterior shoulder instability or dislocation. Seizures and electrocution are common causes of posterior shoulder dislocation.

Although conventional radiographs often are sufficient for diagnosing shoulder dislocation, MRI is valuable in evaluating patients with presumed instability but no history of a dislocation, or to evaluate the status of the rotator cuff in patients preoperatively.

The MRI findings of anterior instability vary depending on the degree of instability and the chronicity of instability. The most common pathologies associated with traumatic anterior shoulder instability are detachment of the anterior-inferior labrum (known as a Perthes-Bankart lesion) and tears of the anterior capsule.[5] The Bankart lesion (**Figs. 4.1** and **4.2**) represents an avulsion of the anterior-inferior glenoid labrum from the glenoid rim (soft-tissue Bankart lesion). When this lesion is associated with an intact anterior scapular periosteum, it is called an anterior labrum periosteal sleeve avulsion lesion. There may be an associated fracture of the anterior inferior glenoid rim (osseous Bankart lesion)[6] or a contusion of the posterior aspect of the humeral head (Hill-Sachs lesion).[6]

The MRI appearance of a Bankart lesion includes the following[7]:

- A linear high signal intensity coursing through the normally homogeneously low signal intensity labral substance,

- An abnormally small or absent anterior labrum, or
- A displaced anterior glenoid labrum with the presence of fluid signal intensity between the anterior rim of the osseous glenoid and the displaced labrum.

In addition, a low signal intensity fracture line surrounded by edema (intermediate T1-weighted signal intensity and high T2-weighted signal intensity) is seen in the presence of a fracture.[8] These findings are best appreciated on the axial images (**Figs. 4.1** and **4.2**). As with most traumatic conditions, the pattern of MRI signal intensity often can be used to estimate the approximate age of a given injury. High signal intensity on T2-weighted or fat-suppressed T2-weighted images (along with low signal intensity on T1-weighted images) suggests the presence of an acute, or at least subacute, injury because it indicates the presence of edema at the site of injury. Conversely, the absence of increased signal intensity on T2-weighted or fat-suppressed T2-weighted images suggests the presence of a chronic injury with no substantial edema present. A finding known as the double axillary pouch sign is assessed with coronal oblique images and is very specific for anterior labral tears.[9]

A lesion known as the anterior labroligamentous periosteal sleeve avulsion injury is a variation of the Bankart lesion; unlike a Bankart lesion, the anterior labroligamentous periosteal sleeve avulsion lesion has an intact anterior scapular periosteum, allowing the labroligamentous structures to displace medially and to rotate inferiorly on the scapular neck.[10] This lesion is visualized on axial MR images as medial

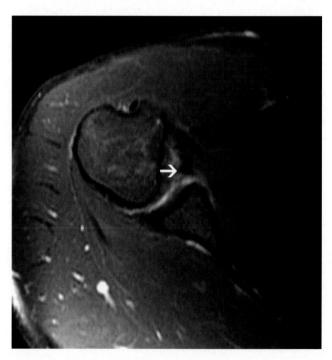

Fig. 4.2 An axial fat-suppressed proton-density image of the right shoulder showing the labral tear of a Bankart lesion (*arrow*).

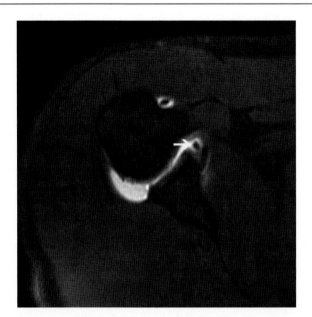

Fig. 4.3 An axial fat-suppressed T2-weighted image of an anterior labroligamentous periosteal sleeve avulsion lesion in the right shoulder showing the medially displaced anterior labrum (*arrow*).

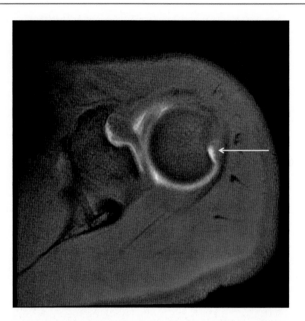

Fig. 4.4 An axial fat-suppressed T1-weighted image showing a Hill-Sachs impression fracture (*arrow*) on the posterolateral aspect of the humeral head in a left shoulder.

displacement and inferior rotation of a torn anterior labrum (**Fig. 4.3**).[10]

Anterior shoulder dislocations may also produce a posterolateral impression fracture in the humeral head, known as a Hill-Sachs lesion.[11] This lesion is seen on MRI as a flattening or concavity of the posterolateral humeral head detected on the two most superior axial images through the level of the humeral head; on those superior images, the humeral head is normally round above the bicipital groove and tuberosities (**Fig. 4.4**).[12,13]

Finally, an anterior shoulder dislocation may tear the IGHL without injuring the anterior labrum. This injury, known as a HAGHL, is defined as an avulsion of the IGHL from the anatomic neck of the humerus.[14,15] On MRI, a HAGHL shows morphologic disruption of the normally low signal intensity IGHL on axial images.[14] In addition, fluid signal intensity often is seen within the soft tissues anterior and inferior to the shoulder joint, which likely represents edema, hematoma, or extravasated joint fluid (**Fig. 4.5**).[14] The HAGHL is frequently associated with tears of the subscapularis tendon.[14]

Posterior instability of the shoulder is much less common than anterior instability. MRI findings of posterior instability are analogous to the findings seen with anterior instability, but the word *reverse* is used to describe lesions that convey a posterior direction to the instability. Therefore, in a patient who has sustained posterior shoulder instability in which the humeral head has subluxated or dislocated posterior to the glenoid, a reverse Bankart lesion represents an avulsion of the posterior-inferior capsulolabral structures from the glenoid rim (**Fig. 4.6**); similarly, a reverse Hill-Sachs lesion represents edema or an impaction fracture of the anterome-

dial humeral head[16] (**Fig. 4.7**). In addition to these findings, MRI typically reveals posterior capsular disruption, which is evident as a disruption or marked irregularity of the normally low signal intensity line representing the posterior capsule.[16]

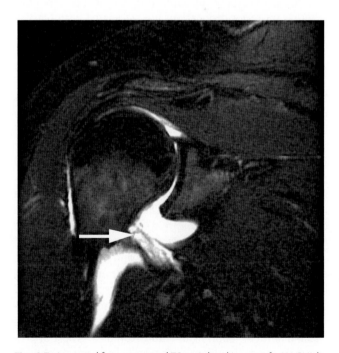

Fig. 4.5 A coronal fat-suppressed T2-weighted image of a HAGHL lesion in the right shoulder showing fluid signal passage through the anterior band of the IGHL (*arrow*).

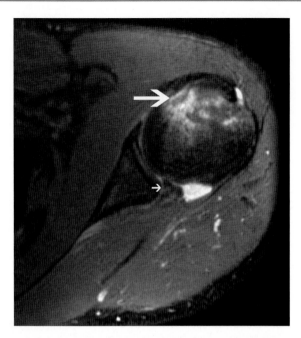

Fig. 4.6 An axial fat-suppressed proton-density image of a reverse soft-tissue Bankart lesion in the left shoulder showing an avulsion of the posterior-inferior labrum from the glenoid rim (*small arrow*) and a reverse Hill-Sachs impaction fracture on the anteromedial aspect of the humeral head (*large arrow*).

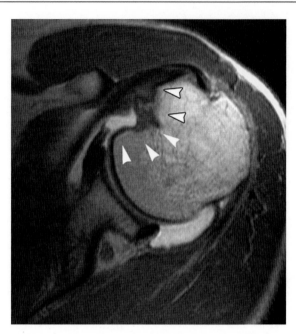

Fig. 4.7 An axial intermediate weighted MR arthrographic image of the left shoulder showing a medium-sized reverse Hill-Sachs defect (*arrowheads*) involving 25% to 50% of the articular surface of the humeral head. Reprinted by permission from Saupe N, White LM, Bleakney R, et al.: Acute traumatic posterior shoulder dislocation: MR findings. Radiology 2008;248:185–193.

Other MRI findings associated with episodes of shoulder instability include injuries to the rotator cuff, especially in patients more than 40 years old. Anterior dislocations are associated with tears of the supraspinatus and subscapularis, whereas posterior dislocations are associated with tears of the subscapularis or fractures of the lesser tuberosity.

Labral Pathology and SLAP Lesions

MRI has proved to be a sensitive, specific, and accurate modality for evaluating the glenoid labrum,[7,17,18] which routinely is assessed in all three imaging planes.[19] Coronal oblique and axial plane images, however, provide the most diagnostic information.[20] The axial plane best shows the anterior and posterior labrum, whereas the coronal oblique plane visualizes the superior and inferior portions.[21] The normal labrum is approximately 3 mm in craniocaudal dimension from base to apex and is 4 mm in width at its base of insertion into the glenoid cartilage.[22] The classic morphology is described as smooth, with triangular anterior and posterior wedges, as seen on axial images.[21] The intact fibrous labrum shows low signal intensity on all pulse sequences. The peripheral attachment of the labrum joins the capsule and glenohumeral ligaments, creating the capsulolabral complex. This capsulolabral or labral ligamentous complex is best appreciated on sagittal oblique MR images. The sagittal oblique plane also is useful for evaluating displaced bucket-handle tears of the labrum.[22] Labral tears and SLAP lesions (superior labrum from anterior to posterior, relative to the bi-

ceps tendon anchor) are best appreciated on fluid-sensitive sequences.[17]

There is considerable variation in the attachment and morphology of the glenoid labrum. Labral anatomy anteriorly and posteriorly is best evaluated with axial images. Above the equator of the glenoid, the labrum may not be attached to the glenoid, but inferior to the middle of the glenoid, the labrum often is confluent with the articular cartilage. The greatest variation in labrum anatomy occurs in the anterosuperior glenoid.[23] To detect true abnormalities, knowledge of these normal variants of labral anatomy as visualized on MRI is very important. Specifically, the absence of a labral attachment in the anterosuperior quadrant is a normal variant and should be differentiated from pathologic labral tears. Therefore, one must be cautious about interpreting an isolated labral tear in the anterosuperior quadrant.

A normal sublabral foramen, or hole, between the labrum and the glenoid rim is often misinterpreted as an anterior labral disruption or tear. When present, the sublabral foramen is located in the 1 o'clock to 3 o'clock positions, anterior to the biceps-labral complex, and represents space between the anterosuperior labrum and the adjacent glenoid cartilage.[22] A sublabral foramen can vary in size from a few millimeters to the entire anterosuperior quadrant above the level of the subscapularis tendon.[24]

Another normal anatomic variant, known as the Buford complex (**Fig. 4.8**), consists of three elements[25]:

- A cord-like MGHL
- An MGHL that attaches directly to the superior labrum anterior to the biceps (at the base of the biceps anchor)
- The absence of anterosuperior labral tissue

The sagittal oblique plane shows the course of the cord-like MGHL attaching directly to the superior labrum at the anterior base of the biceps tendon.

The sublabral recess, or sublabral sulcus, is an additional anatomic variant that should be recognized. In this variant, the superior labrum (from the 11 o'clock to 1 o'clock positions) is meniscoid in morphology.[22,26] On coronal oblique views, a recess appears as an area of high signal intensity on T2-weighted images between the labrum and the superior glenoid. The recess curves medially and follows the contour between the superior labrum and adjacent hyaline cartilage of the superior glenoid.[22,26] The caudal meniscoid portion of the labrum is not attached to the superior portion of the glenoid, but the base of the superior labrum remains attached near the insertion of the long head of the biceps tendon.[22,26]

In 1990, Snyder and associates[27] were the first to describe SLAP lesions. Patients with SLAP lesions usually present with

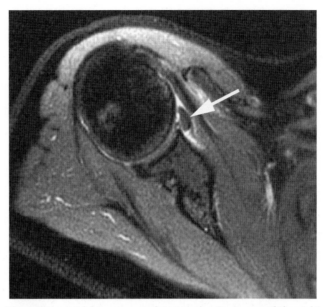

Fig. 4.8 An axial fat-suppressed proton-density image of the right shoulder showing the Buford complex, which consists of three elements: a cord-like MGHL (*arrow*), an MGHL that attaches directly to the superior labrum anterior to the biceps (at the base of the biceps anchor), and an absence of anterosuperior labral tissue.

SLAP LESIONS

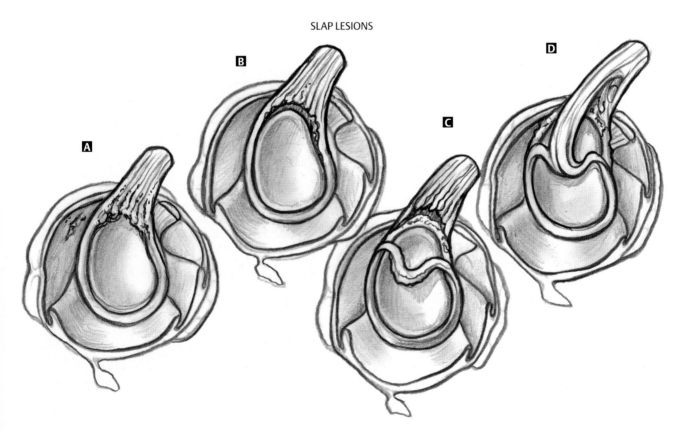

Fig. 4.9 Types of SLAP lesions. **(A)** Type I, a frayed and degenerative superior labrum with a normal (stable) biceps tendon anchor. **(B)** Type II, detachment of the superior labrum and biceps anchor. **(C)** Type III, a bucket-handle tear of a meniscoid superior labrum without extension into the biceps tendon. The biceps anchor is stable and the remaining labrum is intact. **(D)** Type IV, a bucket-handle tear of a meniscoid superior labrum with extension into the biceps tendon. (Based on Powell SE, Nord KD, Ryu RKN: The diagnosis, classification, and treatment of SLAP lesions. Oper Tech Sports Med 2004;12:99–110.)

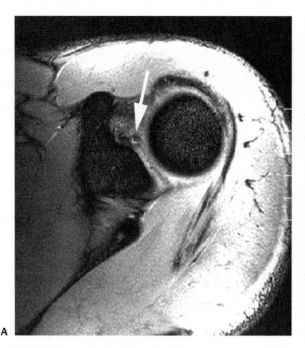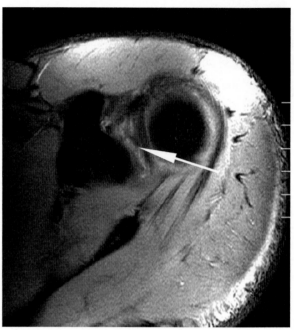

Fig. 4.10 Type II SLAP lesion. **(A,B)** Axial fat-suppressed gradient-echo images of the left shoulder showing increased signal intensity within the superior glenoid labrum (arrow) in a patient with a type II SLAP lesion verified by arthroscopy.

complaints of deep pain (typically with overhead activities) and/or mechanical symptoms of catching, locking, popping, or grinding.[28] Frequently, there is a history of overhead activities or sports. The mechanism of injury often is traction or compression.[28]

The most common classification of SLAP tears includes four distinct lesions, although recently new lesions and sub-classifications have been added (**Fig. 4.9**).[27,29]

In type I lesions, there is a frayed and degenerative superior labrum with a normal (stable) biceps tendon anchor. On MRI, the labral contour appears blunted or irregular with a slight increase in signal intensity on T2-weighted images.[30,31]

Type II lesions have similar labral fraying but have detachment of the superior labrum and biceps anchor, making them unstable. MRI findings of type II SLAP lesions include a line of high-intensity signal coursing across the base of the hyperintense labrum to the periphery (**Figs. 4.10** and **4.11**). The long head of the biceps tendon has normal signal and shape and is attached to the avulsed labrum.[31] The sublabral recess can be differentiated from a type II SLAP lesion by two MRI signs on T2-weighted images present in these SLAP lesions, but not in sublabral recesses[26]:

- High signal intensity in the labrum posterior to the biceps anchor, which extends to the articular surface
- An area of high signal intensity irregular or curved laterally and distinct from the medial curvilinear area of signal intensity at the labral–glenoid junction seen in a sublabral recess

In type III lesions, there is a bucket-handle tear of a meniscoid superior labrum without extension into the biceps tendon. The biceps anchor is stable and the remaining

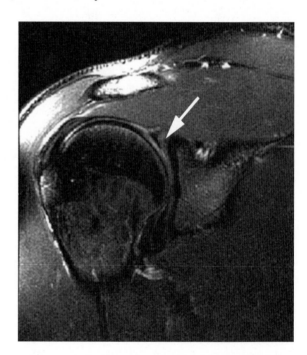

Fig. 4.11 A coronal oblique fat-suppressed T2-weighted image of the right shoulder showing increased signal intensity within the superior glenoid labrum (*arrow*) posterior to the long head of the biceps tendon origin in a patient with a type II SLAP lesion verified by arthroscopy.

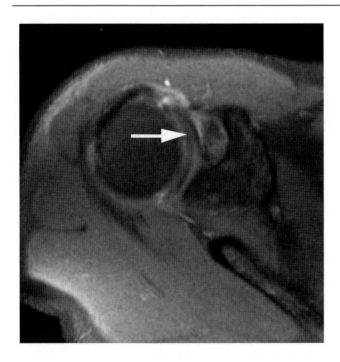

Fig. 4.12 An axial fat-suppressed proton-density image of a type IV SLAP lesion in the right shoulder showing increased signal intensity within the superior glenoid labrum with extension into the biceps anchor (*arrow*).

labrum is intact. On MRI, type III SLAP lesions are characterized by a line of high signal intensity coursing across the base of the hyperintense labrum but extending beyond the equator in the case of a nondisplaced bucket-handle tear. In the case of a displaced bucket-handle tear, a discrete piece of fibrocartilage is identified within the joint capsule. On MRI, the displaced piece of fibrocartilage appears as a low signal intensity intraarticular fragment surrounded by high signal intensity joint fluid.[32] In type III SLAP lesions, the superior labrum also is deficient, yet the biceps tendon can be followed to the supraglenoid tubercle.[31]

In type IV SLAP lesions, there is a bucket-handle tear of a meniscoid superior labrum with extension into the biceps tendon. On MRI, a type IV SLAP lesion is characterized by a line of high signal intensity coursing across the base of the normally hypointense labrum to the periphery and extending beyond the equator with a deficient labrum (**Fig. 4.12**).[30] In addition, there is hyperintensity and splitting of fibers of the biceps tendon.[31]

SLAP lesions frequently are associated with other shoulder pathology that can be visualized on MRI. The presence of paralabral cysts, almost invariably associated with labral tears,[21,33,34] should incite the search for a labral tear. The imaging features include a cystic-appearing mass adjacent to the labrum or capsule with increased signal on T2-weighted sequences.[21] Rotator cuff tears (both partial thickness and full thickness) and Bankart lesions are commonly associated with SLAP lesions.[35,36]

■ Degenerative Conditions

The shoulder is affected by numerous degenerative conditions, including the following:

- Subacromial impingement syndrome
- Rotator cuff tears
- Glenohumeral osteoarthritis
- AC osteoarthritis
- Pathologic conditions affecting the biceps tendon

Subacromial Impingement Syndrome

Subacromial impingement syndrome is a continuum of abnormalities and clinical symptoms; in its final stages, it may be associated with full-thickness rotator cuff tears. Impingement syndrome is secondary to compression of the rotator cuff by abnormal morphology of structures within the supraspinatus outlet. Patients with chronic impingement syndrome typically present with the insidious onset of diffuse shoulder pain in the area of the deltoid muscle; the pain is activity related, worse with overhead activities, and often worse at night.[37] However, it must be stated that there is often no correlation between clinical symptoms and rotator cuff pathology found on MRI or during autopsy.

Osseous factors that contribute to subacromial impingement syndrome include the following[38,39]:

- Anterior acromial spurs
- The shape of the acromion
- The slope of the acromion
- The morphology of the AC joint (e.g., hypertrophic bone, calcification of the coracoacromial ligament, callus formation)

The shape of the acromion (acromial morphology) is best evaluated with sagittal oblique MR images. Bigliani and associates[38] classified acromial morphology into three types:

- Type I, a flat undersurface (**Fig. 4.13**)
- Type II, a smooth curved inferior surface (**Fig. 4.14**)
- Type III, an anteroinferior hook or beak (**Fig. 4.15**)

The type II and type III acromions that create narrowing of the supraspinatus outlet are associated with a predisposition to rotator cuff disease.[40,41]

In addition to acromial morphology in the sagittal plane, the slope of the acromion in the coronal plane may predispose patients to impingement syndrome and subsequent rotator cuff tears. Normally, the anterior acromion should be nearly horizontal when viewed in the oblique coronal plane. Lateral downsloping of the acromion narrows the supraspinatus outlet and may predispose to impingement syndrome.[42] Sagittal oblique MR images can be used to assess the morphology of the acromion from posterior to anterior,

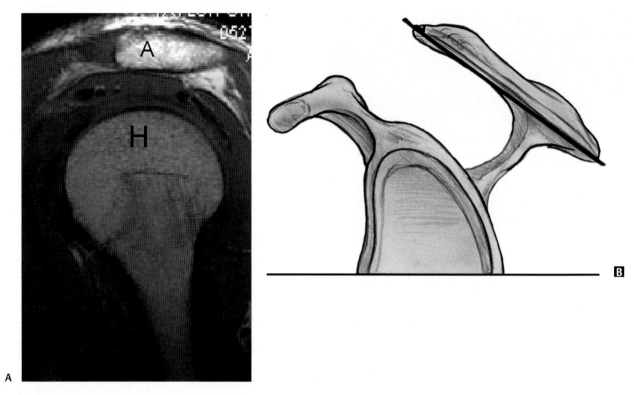

Fig. 4.13 Type I acromion. **(A)** A sagittal oblique T1-weighted image. *A*, acromion; *H*, humeral head. **(B)** Artist's sketch. Straight line indicates flat inferior surface.

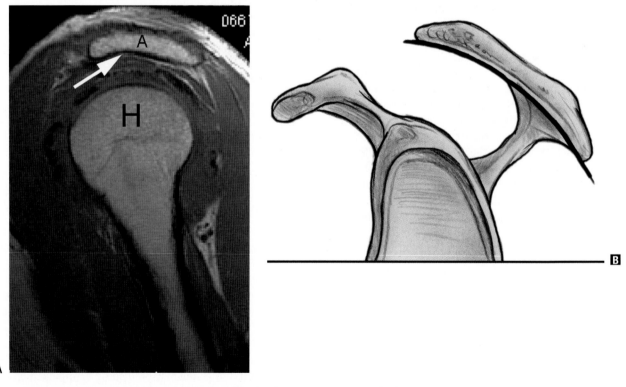

Fig. 4.14 Type II acromion. **(A)** A sagittal oblique T1-weighted image (*arrow*, curved inferior surface). *A*, acromion; *H*, humeral head. **(B)** Artist's sketch. Curved line indicates curved inferior surface.

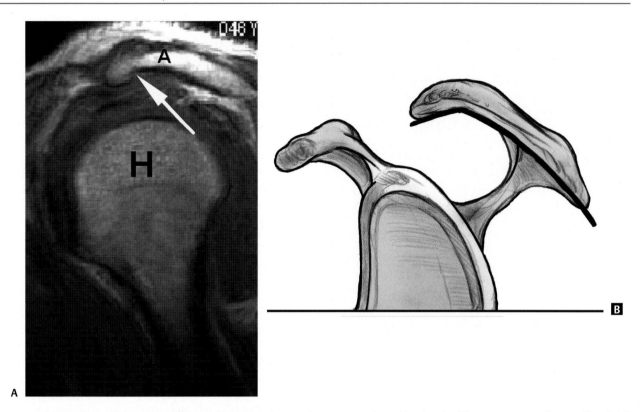

Fig. 4.15 Type III acromion. **(A)** A sagittal oblique T1-weighted image (*arrow*, anterolateral hook or beak). *A*, acromion; *H*, humeral head. **(B)** Artist's sketch. Bent line indicates an anteroinferior hook or beak.

whereas coronal oblique MR images can be used to evaluate the lateral acromial slope.

The spectrum of MRI changes in subacromial impingement syndrome have been characterized and documented.[43,44] Rotator cuff disease is evaluated on the basis of tendon morphology and changes in the observed signal intensity within the specific cuff tendons. In addition, pathologic processes within the supraspinatus outlet, including abnormalities of the acromion, AC joint, and the subacromial-subdeltoid bursa, may be identified in the spectrum of findings in patients with impingement symptoms.

Changes in the subacromial bursa often are seen on MRI in association with impingement syndrome.[45,46] Bursal inflammation is seen as decreased signal intensity, or loss of peribursal fat, on T1-weighted images and as increased signal intensity (from associated fluid, inflammation, or bursal proliferative disease) on T2-weighted or fat-suppressed T2-weighted sequences.[42,47] Low signal intensity within a thickened subacromial bursa on T1-weighted and T2-weighted images indicates a proliferative process in chronic bursitis, which also is associated with rotator cuff disease.[48]

Capsular hypertrophy of the AC joint has also been identified on coronal oblique MR images in patients with impingement syndrome.[44] Other MRI findings associated with impingement syndrome include inferior acromial and AC spurs, which are visualized as alterations in the normal smooth contour of the inferior acromion and AC joint. However, recent studies have suggested that small acromial spurs may be a normal finding associated with advancing age, whereas spurs larger than 5 mm are strongly associated with the presence of rotator cuff pathology.[41,49]

Normal rotator cuff tendons display uniformly low signal intensity on all pulse sequences. In cuff tendon degeneration (tendinosis), there is intermediate signal intensity on T1-weighted or proton-density images, with no evidence of fluid signal intensity on T2-weighted images (**Fig. 4.16**). Fat-suppressed T2-weighted sequences are sensitive to changes of degeneration, and, in the absence of a partial or complete rotator cuff tear, they display areas or regions of hyperintensity.[50] These areas of increased signal intensity often occur adjacent to acromial or AC spurs (as described above) or a low-lying acromion.[44] More severe changes or degeneration may be characterized by intermediate to increased signal intensity on T1-weighted and proton-density images, which persist without additional increase in signal intensity on T2-weighted images. Other findings of rotator cuff tendinosis include areas of thickening and irregularity within the tendon.[42]

Caution must be used to avoid confusing rotator cuff abnormalities with the *magic angle phenomenon*. This phenomenon, which results in spuriously increased signal intensity on sequences with a short TE (including T1-weighted and proton-density sequences), occurs in tissues containing highly

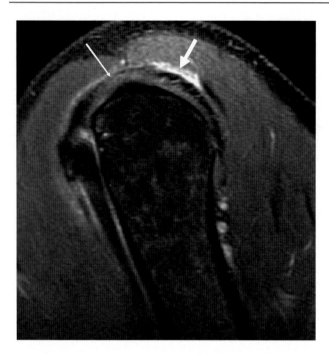

Fig. 4.16 A sagittal oblique T2-weighted image showing hyperintense signal in the tendon (*thin arrow*) without a discrete defect, consistent with supraspinatus tendinosis. Compare this finding with the fluid signal intensity in the subacromial bursa (*thick arrow*), consistent with subacromial bursitis.

structured collagen fibers that lie at an angle of 55 degrees to the main magnetic field.[51] In the shoulder, this phenomenon is common just proximal to the insertion of the supraspinatus tendon on the greater tuberosity. The increased signal intensity associated with the magic angle phenomenon disappears on T2-weighted images, making it possible to differentiate this phenomenon from true pathology.[51]

Rotator Cuff Tears

Rotator cuff tears represent the end of the spectrum of abnormalities associated with chronic subacromial impingement syndrome. Therefore, the clinical presentation often is similar to that described for impingement syndrome. Some patients may present with acute pain and weakness after traumatic rotator cuff rupture, whereas other patients with rotator cuff tears may have minimal to no symptoms. Patients also may report weakness and limited active range of motion despite normal passive motion.[37] The supraspinatus and infraspinatus tendons are the most common tendons torn.[52] MR images, particularly in the coronal oblique and sagittal oblique planes, are most useful in showing tears of these two tendons.[40] These tears are best shown with fat-suppressed T2-weighted images.[53] Rotator cuff tears can be characterized as partial thickness or full thickness.[54] Partial-thickness tears may involve the articular or bursal surface or, less commonly, they may be completely intratendinous.

Intratendinous lesions are defined as tears that do not communicate with the bursal or articular surface.

Coronal oblique and sagittal oblique images are ideal for the evaluation of partial-thickness tears of the supraspinatus and infraspinatus tendons. Similarly, axial and sagittal oblique images are best for evaluating the subscapularis and teres minor tendons. The diagnosis of this type of tear is suggested by increased signal in the rotator cuff that only partially traverses the rotator cuff substance.[55] Typically, there is abnormal morphology of the tendon insertion onto bone with evidence of partial tendon discontinuity on T1-weighted images. Partial-thickness tears show low to intermediate signal intensity on T1-weighted images, intermediate to high signal intensity on proton-density images, and fluid signal intensity on T2-weighted sequences (**Figs. 4.17** and **4.18**). Increased signal intensity is the result of tracking of fluid within the bursal or articular surface of the cuff.

The diagnosis of a partial-thickness rotator cuff tear is most difficult at either end of the spectrum: low-grade partial-thickness tears tend to be mistaken for tendinosis and high-grade partial-thickness tears may be mistaken for full-thickness rotator cuff tears (**Fig. 4.19**).[42] MRI findings in degeneration and partial-thickness rotator cuff tears may overlap, and tendon abnormalities must be evaluated on the basis of bursal, intrasubstance, and articular surface morphology and on signal intensity changes on T1-weighted, proton-density, and T2-weighted sequences.[8]

Full-thickness tears of the supraspinatus and infraspinatus are best visualized with the coronal oblique and sagittal

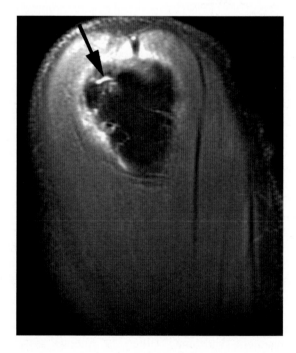

Fig. 4.17 A sagittal oblique T2-weighted image showing a partial-thickness rotator cuff tear (*arrow*) on a background of tendinosis.

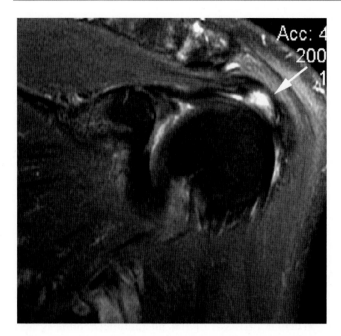

Fig. 4.18 A coronal oblique T2-weighted image of the left shoulder showing a high-grade partial-thickness rotator cuff tear (*arrow*).

oblique images. Full-thickness tears of the subscapularis and teres minor are best visualized using the axial and sagittal oblique images. The direct signs of a full-thickness rotator cuff tear consist of a complete tendon defect or complete discontinuity of the tendon with retraction, and abnormal increased signal intensity within the tendon defect (**Table 4.1**).[53,56–60] A complete tear cannot be diagnosed unequivo-

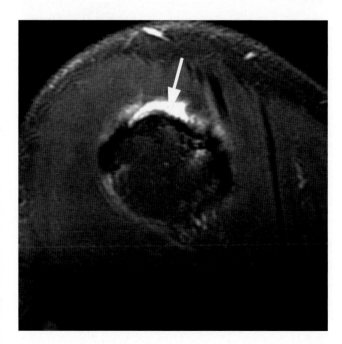

Fig. 4.19 A sagittal oblique T2-weighted image showing a full-thickness rotator cuff tear (*arrow*).

cally without visualization of a complete tendon defect or a direct communication between the glenohumeral joint and the subacromial-subdeltoid bursa. The defect, or tendinous gap, is seen as an interruption or loss of continuity of the normally low signal intensity tendon. This gap appears as a continuous band of increased signal intensity that traverses the full thickness of the rotator cuff, extending from the glenohumeral joint to the subacromial bursa.[56] The signal intensity is increased on T1-weighted and proton-density images and increased additionally on T2-weighted and fat-suppressed T2-weighted sequences.[42] The increased signal intensity is secondary to interposed joint fluid or granulation tissue at the cuff tear site. Large cuff tears may fill in with fibrous or granulation tissue that may have low-signal intensity on T2-weighted images.[47]

Indirect signs of rotator cuff tears can be used in conjunction with the primary assessment of changes in tendon signal intensity and morphology to help in the diagnosis of full-thickness rotator cuff tears. Indirect signs of rotator cuff abnormality include the following (**Table 4.1**)[61,62]:

- Fluid within the subacromial-subdeltoid bursa
- Obliteration of the peribursal fat stripe
- The presence of a glenohumeral effusion
- Atrophy of the involved muscle

Subacromial-subdeltoid bursal fluid is associated with a full-thickness rotator cuff tear, but it is not specific for this condition. This fluid is manifested on MRI as high signal intensity changes in the subacromial-subdeltoid bursa that equal the intensity of fluid on T2-weighted images. Changes in subacromial and subdeltoid peribursal fat also may be considered indirect signs of cuff abnormality. Because peribursal fat may be replaced by low signal intensity granulation tissue or scar or high signal intensity fluid, which is often limited to the site of the cuff tear, this abnormality is considered a secondary sign when a cuff tear is not clearly visualized.

Most rotator cuff tears can be identified by a good history and physical examination. MRI is most useful in planning and predicting the prognosis for successful rotator cuff repair. Identification of tendon retraction and cuff muscle atrophy on MRI is imperative in the evaluation of a full-thickness tear. Large, retracted cuff tears with atrophy of the

Table 4.1 Characteristics of Rotator Cuff Tears on MRI

Direct Signs	Indirect Signs
Visualization of tendon defect	Subacromial-subdeltoid fluid
Indication of direct communication between glenohumeral joint and subacromial bursa	Retraction of supraspinatus musculotendinous junction
Retraction of supraspinatus or infraspinatus tendon	Changes in subacromial and subdeltoid peribursal fat Fatty atrophy of rotator cuff muscles

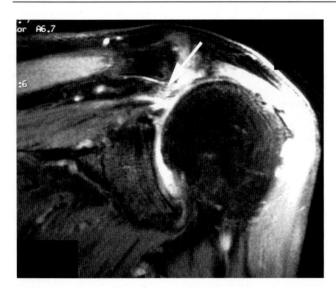

Fig. 4.20 A coronal oblique proton-density MR image showing a full-thickness supraspinatus tear with tendon retraction (*arrow*). Note the slightly increased signal intensity of the muscle, consistent with early atrophy.

muscle may not be repairable. Retraction of the torn rotator cuff tendon is assessed by medial displacement of the musculotendinous junction from its normal position, which lies in a 45-degree arc lateral to the highest point of the humeral head.[47] Other authors consider the supraspinatus tendon retracted if the musculotendinous junction is located more medial than the middle third of the humeral head (**Fig. 4.20**).[56] Retraction of the supraspinatus or infraspinatus tendons is best seen on coronal oblique images that show the medial and lateral extension of the cuff tear. Similarly, axial images are best for identifying subscapularis and teres minor retraction. T2-weighted sagittal oblique images provide additional information, allowing identification of articular and bursal surface extension and the quantification of the size of the tear in the AP direction.[42]

Large or chronic rotator cuff tears frequently are accompanied by atrophy of the rotator cuff muscle. Muscle atrophy can be identified in two forms, which often are present simultaneously: fatty replacement and decreased muscle bulk. T1-weighted or proton-density images are best suited for this assessment. Fatty replacement is best shown on T1-weighted images, which display high signal intensity (equal to fat) horizontal streaks parallel to the long axis of the involved muscle (**Fig. 4.20**).[44] In addition, MRI can visualize the diminution in cross-sectional size of the involved muscle, which is best seen on the sagittal oblique images.[56]

Glenohumeral Osteoarthritis

Osteoarthritis in the glenohumeral joint is similar to that in other joints, such as the hip and knee. Patients with this condition, who tend to be older than those with rotator cuff

injuries and glenohumeral instability, present with complaints of shoulder pain and stiffness. In osteoarthritis of the shoulder, the glenoid articular cartilage and subchondral bone typically are worn posteriorly, the humeral head may be subluxed posteriorly, and the articular cartilage of the humeral head is eroded centrally, with a surrounding rim of remaining articular cartilage and osteophytes.[63] Although glenohumeral osteoarthritis usually is diagnosed with conventional radiographs, early arthritis frequently is missed with this modality because conventional radiographs do not directly image the cartilage and therefore cannot detect early chondral damage. Rather, conventional radiographs rely on signs such as joint space narrowing and secondary changes such as the presence of subchondral cysts and osteophyte formation, but these findings often are not seen until the disease process is more advanced. MRI, the optimal imaging modality for assessing articular cartilage, can provide morphologic information, such as fissuring and the presence of partial- or full-thickness cartilage defects.[64,65]

Articular cartilage of the glenohumeral joint is best evaluated on gradient-echo or fat-suppressed T2-weighted sequences with images in the coronal oblique and axial planes.[64,66,67] Normal articular cartilage has a uniform thickness and homogeneous intermediate signal intensity on T1-weighted, fat-suppressed T2-weighted, and gradient-echo sequences.[66,67] Osteoarthritis is associated with multiple defects and erosions in the articular cartilage; in glenohumeral osteoarthritis, these changes typically occur centrally

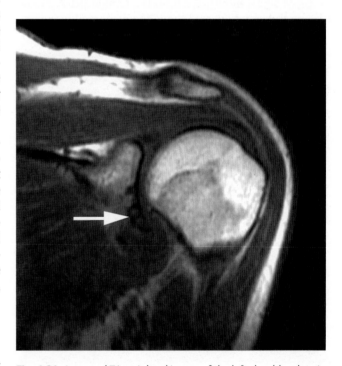

Fig. 4.21 A coronal T1-weighted image of the left shoulder showing subchondral cyst formation (*arrow*) in a patient with glenohumeral osteoarthrosis.

in the humeral head and posteriorly on the glenoid.[63] This altered morphology of the articular cartilage can be seen on MRI as surface irregularities, partial-thickness focal defects, and full-thickness focal defects because the normally intermediate signal intensity cartilage is occupied by fluid signal intensity joint fluid.[66] With osteoarthritis, there usually are multiple defects of variable size and depth or diffuse cartilage thinning.[64] Other MRI findings of osteoarthritis include bone marrow edema, osteophytes, subchondral cysts, and subchondral sclerosis (**Fig. 4.21**).[64] Less commonly, signal intensity abnormalities, such as foci of high signal intensity in morphologically normal cartilage, may suggest early osteoarthritis.[66]

AC Osteoarthritis

AC joint osteoarthritis is a common condition associated with the normal aging process.[68] Patients with AC joint osteoarthritis who manifest symptoms typically present with anterior shoulder pain that is exacerbated by activities such as bench presses and shoulder elevation or adduction. Physical examination reveals focal tenderness over the AC joint, pain with passive cross-body adduction, and pain with resisted AC extension. Although degenerative changes of the AC joint are extremely common, most patients with this condition are asymptomatic.

MRI findings of AC joint arthritis include the following (**Fig. 4.22**)[68–70]:

- Subacromial fat effacement
- Joint space narrowing
- Osseous irregularity of the joint
- Capsular distention
- Osteophyte formation

These AC joint arthritic changes are seen on MRI in more than 80% of asymptomatic patients and in approximately 95% of asymptomatic patients more than 30 years old.[68,70] A study has suggested that the presence of reactive bone marrow edema on fat-suppressed T2-weighted MR images in the distal clavicle or acromion, or both sides of the AC joint, is a reliable predictor of symptomatic AC joint pathology, and is not seen in asymptomatic patients.[70] AC joint degenerative changes commonly are associated with other shoulder pathology, such as impingement syndrome, rotator cuff tears, and glenohumeral osteoarthritis.[68]

Abnormalities of the Long Head of the Biceps Tendon

The biceps tendon may be followed on multiple sequences from its origin at the supraglenoid tubercle through the bicipital groove.[21] The long head of the biceps tendon should be inspected on coronal oblique, axial, and sagittal oblique images. The origin of the biceps tendon and its proximal

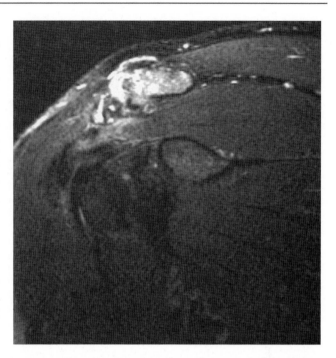

Fig. 4.22 A coronal oblique fat-suppressed T2-weighted image of the right shoulder shows hypertrophy of the AC joint, joint effusion, and subchondral bone marrow edema related to AC joint osteoarthrosis.

intraarticular portion are best visualized on sagittal oblique and coronal oblique images, but more distally, as it courses within the bicipital groove, it is best visualized on axial images. The normal MRI appearance of the long head of the biceps tendon includes low signal intensity on all pulse sequences and identification in its normal anatomic location (**Figs. 4.23** and **4.24**).[21] On axial images at the level of the bicipital groove, the tendon appears as an oval-shaped low signal intensity structure surrounded by a thin moderate signal intensity synovial sheath.[47] Pathologic conditions involving the long head of the biceps tendon include tendinosis, partial-thickness tears, complete tears (rupture), subluxation, and dislocation.

The clinical presentation of patients with disorders of the long head of the biceps tendon varies with the underlying abnormality; such patients often have concomitant chronic impingement syndrome or rotator cuff tears. Patients with biceps tendinosis, partial tears, and subluxation may have pain and tenderness in the bicipital groove.[71] This pain may radiate down the arm anteriorly to the biceps muscle belly, but it is often difficult to distinguish from that of impingement syndrome.[71] When long-standing, the pain often will resolve spontaneously after rupture, and complete tears are often asymptomatic.[71]

The MRI findings in tendinosis include high signal intensity within the tendon on all pulse sequences, and thickening and inhomogeneity of the tendon (**Fig. 4.25**).[21,72] This finding

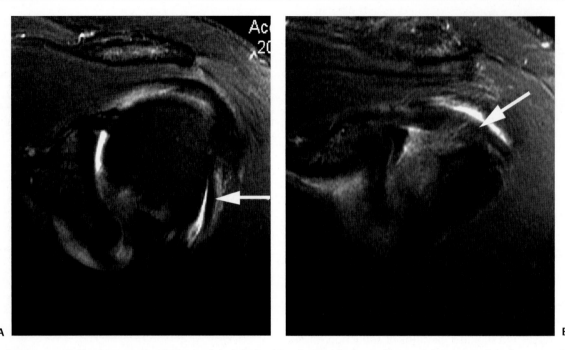

A   B

Fig. 4.23 (A,B) Coronal oblique T2-weighted images of the left shoulder showing the normal low signal intensity of the biceps tendon (*arrow on each*).

is particularly evident on sagittal oblique images obtained at the level of the intracapsular portion of the long head of the biceps tendon.[21] Biceps tendinosis frequently is associated with impingement syndrome and rotator cuff tears. There-

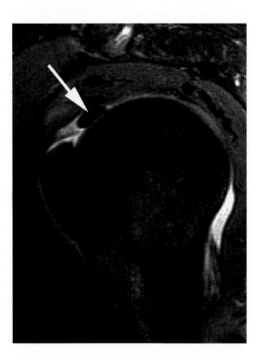

Fig. 4.24 A sagittal oblique T2-weighted image showing the normal low signal intensity of the biceps tendon (*arrow*) as it courses through the glenohumeral joint.

fore, MRI often visualizes the associated pathologic findings, including joint effusion and increased fluid in the bicipital synovial sheath, which is nonspecific for inflammation of the long head of the biceps tendon.[72,73] However, fluid in the tendon sheath of the long head of the biceps is abnormal if it completely surrounds the tendon in the absence of a glenohumeral joint effusion.[61,62]

Biceps tendinosis is the earliest stage of biceps tendon disease, but it can progress to partial or complete tears of the tendon. Transverse partial tears are difficult to diagnose and usually are shown by a sudden change in the cross-sectional diameter of the tendon.[72] However, a longitudinal tear is easier to identify because the tendon surrounds the high signal intensity tear on T2-weighted images (**Fig. 4.26**).[72] More often, complete rupture occurs proximally, at the level of the proximal portion of the extracapsular segment, within the bicipital groove.[74] Any axial image that definitively shows no tendon in the bicipital groove and no medial dislocation is diagnostic of rupture of the long head of the biceps tendon (**Fig. 4.27**).[72] Additional MRI findings include atrophy and distal retraction of the tendon and fluid within the tendon sheath.[21,72,73] These findings are best shown on axial sections. Intraarticular tears of the biceps tendon frequently are associated with rotator cuff tears, and are visualized on MRI as the absence of the intraarticular portion of the tendon and the associated rotator cuff lesion.[21]

Biceps subluxations, although rare, can be seen in disease processes in which loss of the integrity of the rotator cuff has occurred or in which the biceps tendon loses the supporting structures that contain it in within the bicipital

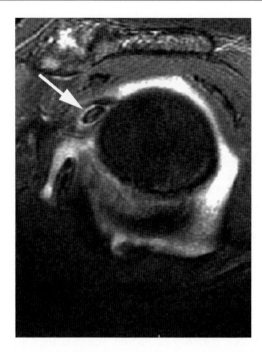

Fig. 4.25 A sagittal oblique T2-weighted image showing a thickened biceps tendon (biceps tendinosis) with increased T2 signal (*arrow*). Note also the glenohumeral joint effusion.

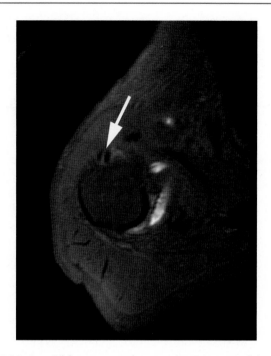

Fig. 4.26 An axial fat-suppressed proton-density image of the right shoulder showing a longitudinal tear of the biceps tendon (*arrow*).

groove (i.e., the transverse humeral ligament).[72] Because of the forces acting on the biceps tendon, displacement always occurs in the medial direction.[72] The subluxation is best visualized on axial sections (**Fig. 4.28**). In addition to subluxation, frank dislocation of the biceps tendon can occur. The

MRI findings of a dislocated biceps tendon include visualization of the dislocated tendon medial to an empty bicipital groove (**Fig. 4.29**).[72] This condition also is best visualized on axial images.[72,73,75,76] On sagittal oblique images, dislocation of the biceps tendon is identified as a more medial position

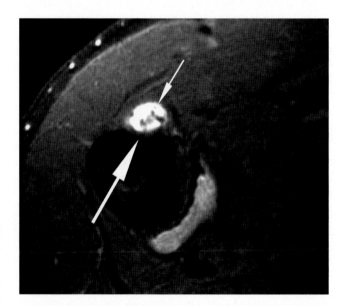

Fig. 4.27 An axial fat-suppressed T2-weighted image of the right shoulder showing absence of the biceps tendon within the bicipital groove (*thin arrow*) and complex fluid in the biceps tendon sheath (*thick arrow*), which represents hemorrhage related to complete rupture.

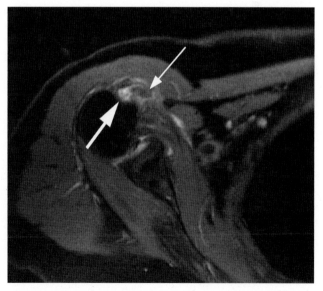

Fig. 4.28 An axial fat-suppressed proton-density image of the right shoulder showing subluxation of the biceps tendon (*thin arrow*) and the bicipital groove (*thick arrow*). Note also the subscapularis tear.

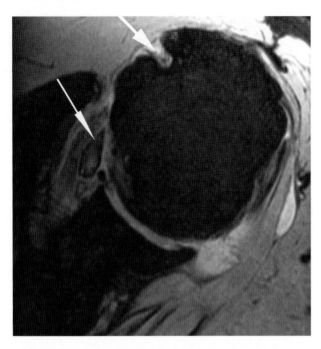

Fig. 4.29 An axial fat-suppressed T2-weighted image of the left shoulder showing the dislocated biceps tendon (*thin arrow*) medial to an empty bicipital groove (*thick arrow*). Note the ruptured subscapularis tendon and the resulting intraarticular entrapment of the biceps tendon.

of the descending tendon and as an abnormal course of the intraarticular portion of the tendon.[72] Associated findings may include a shallow bicipital groove and tears of the coracohumeral ligament, subscapularis tendon, and supraspinatus tendon. The biceps tendon is located medial and anterior to the subscapularis tendon, with disruption of the transverse ligament and an intact subscapularis. If the subscapularis tendon is detached from its insertion on the lesser tuberosity, however, the biceps tendon becomes entrapped in an intraarticular position.[21,73]

■ Infectious Conditions: Septic Arthritis

The glenohumeral joint is the third most common site for septic arthritis, after the hip and knee.[77] As do patients with septic arthritis in other joints, patients with septic arthritis in the glenohumeral joint present with a combination of findings, including the following:

- Pain
- Decreased range of motion
- Fevers
- Focal swelling
- Warmth
- Tenderness
- Erythema

This condition usually occurs in patients older than those with septic knees and hips. Patients with glenohumeral septic arthritis often have substantial comorbidities, including the following[77]:

- Coronary artery disease
- Congestive heart failure
- Cancer
- RA
- Alcoholism
- Cirrhosis
- Diabetes mellitus
- End-stage renal disease
- Intravenous drug abuse
- HIV

Frequently, there is a history of recent shoulder surgery, intraarticular cortisone injections, or another infectious source, such as endocarditis, urinary tract infections, or pneumonia.[77,78]

The diagnosis usually is made on the basis of physical examination, laboratory evaluation, and joint fluid aspiration with subsequent microbiologic analysis. Conventional radiographs usually are not useful in establishing the diagnosis, especially early in the course of the infection[77,78]; MRI may be useful in ambiguous cases of septic arthritis or to determine the extent of the bone and soft-tissue infection.[78,79] The joint effusion and synovitis associated with septic arthritis are shown on T2-weighted and fat-suppressed T2-weighted MRI sequences.[78] In the acute stage of the infection, bone marrow edema also may be visualized with MRI.[78] If gadolinium contrast is administered intravenously, a prominent rim enhancement of the thickened synovium can be seen on the postgadolinium T1-weighted images.[78,80] If untreated, cartilage destruction, marginal erosions, joint space narrowing, and subchondral cyst formation are eventually seen on both MR images and conventional radiographs.[78]

■ Other Pathologic Conditions

Certain pathologic conditions that affect the shoulder, such as adhesive capsulitis and calcific tendinitis, cannot be classified as traumatic, degenerative, or infectious.

Adhesive Capsulitis

Adhesive capsulitis occurs when inflammation, thickening, and contracture of the joint capsule and synovium result in capsular fibrosis that causes pain and a global limitation of glenohumeral motion.[81,82] Patients with diabetes mellitus are at increased risk for this condition.[83] Patients present with a history of shoulder pain and stiffness. Physical examination reveals a global loss of active and passive range of motion. Although this condition is primarily a clinical diagnosis, MRI can be useful in confirming clinical suspicions and ruling out concomitant abnormalities. Studies have found that a combined thickness of more than 4 mm for the joint capsule and synovium, as assessed on the coronal oblique images at the level of the axillary recess, is a useful MRI criterion for the diagnosis of adhesive capsulitis.[81,84] Furthermore, a thickened region of soft-tissue signal intensity in the rotator interval that encases the middle and superior glenohumeral ligaments and extends to the biceps anchor is another common finding in patients with adhesive capsulitis; this soft tissue enhances with gadolinium and is best assessed on sagittal oblique images (**Fig. 4.30**).[84,85]

Calcific Tendinitis

Calcific tendinitis of the shoulder is an acute or chronically painful and self-limiting condition of unknown cause that is associated with inflammation around calcium deposits located in or around the rotator cuff tendons.[86,87] This condition predominantly affects middle-aged women.[86,87] The most common site of occurrence is within the supraspinatus tendon and at a location 1.5 to 2.0 cm proximal to its insertion on the greater tuberosity.[87] Patients usually exhibit specific tenderness over the greater tuberosity and symptoms similar to those of subacromial impingement syndrome. The diagnosis is made by history, physical examination, and radiographic workup. Calcium deposits usually are visualized on conventional radiographs, and therefore MRI evaluation

is not indicated routinely. If MRI is obtained, the calcifications appear as areas of decreased signal intensity on T1-weighted and T2-weighted images; T2-weighted images frequently show a perifocal band of increased signal intensity surrounding the lesion, compatible with edema.[86,87]

■ Postoperative MRI Findings

The accuracy of MRI of the postoperative shoulder is limited by several factors, including the following[80]:

- Surgical distortions of native anatomy
- Changes in the signal intensity of tissues secondary to surgical trauma
- Image degradation caused by metallic artifacts associated with surgical implants

The key questions to consider with MRI evaluation of the postoperative shoulder are the following:

- What imaging sequences limit the effects of artifact?
- What are the expected MRI findings in the postoperative shoulder?
- What MRI findings suggest new/recurrent pathology?

Furthermore, it is optimal that the person interpreting the MR images, whether a radiologist or an orthopaedic surgeon, be familiar with the details of the shoulder's operative procedure. Finally, during image interpretation, preoperative and postoperative images should be correlated closely.[80]

MR images of the postoperative shoulder are often affected by metallic artifacts because of the presence of ferromagnetic surgical implants such as anchors, screws, tacks, or shoulder arthroplasty prostheses.[88,89] These artifacts are most pronounced on images obtained with a long TE, on gradient-echo images, and on fat-suppression sequences.[80,90] Certain pulse sequences can minimize the effects of these artifacts and thus maximize the accuracy of MRI. To avoid magnetic susceptibility artifacts, inversion recovery may be used instead of fat suppression, and FSE sequences may be used instead of conventional SE sequences; gradient-echo sequences may be avoided.[80,91,92] These specialized pulse sequences usually are prescribed by a radiologist with expertise in musculoskeletal MRI, which highlights the need for good communication between the orthopaedic surgeon and the radiologist during MRI evaluation of patients with complex processes affecting the shoulder joint.

The most frequently performed surgical procedures that are evaluated postoperatively with MRI of the shoulder include the following[93]:

- Subacromial decompression (impingement syndrome)
- Rotator cuff repair
- Glenohumeral instability treatment
- Arthroplasty

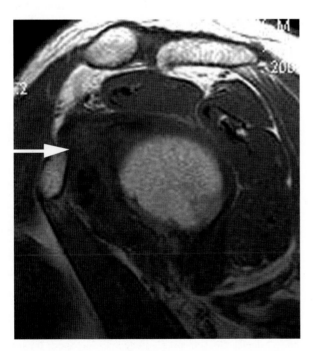

Fig. 4.30 A sagittal T1-weighted image showing decreased signal in the subcoracoid triangle (*arrow*).

Expected MRI findings after arthroscopic subacromial decompression include morphologic changes in the acromion and coracoacromial ligament and widening of the AC distance. The acromion, as viewed on the sagittal images, usually changes from a hook or curve to a more flat and slightly tapered configuration.[80] Decreased signal intensity in the distal acromion on T1-weighted, T2-weighted, and proton-density sequences usually is present and represents fibrosis in the acromial bone marrow.[93,94] After resection, the coracoacromial ligament often is replaced by fatty tissue; this site also may have abnormal signal intensity and an irregular morphology caused by scar tissue and metallic artifacts.[80] In addition, bursitis-like signal abnormalities at the bursal surface of the rotator cuff are common.[95] Finally, if a Mumford procedure (distal clavicle excision) is performed, widening of the AC joint by 1 to 2 cm may be visualized.[93]

Expected MRI findings after rotator cuff repair include signal intensity changes in the repaired tendon and regular or irregular tendon morphology, depending on the procedure performed and the quality of the remaining tendon.[92,93] The signal intensity changes include intermediate signal intensity (representing granulation tissue) or low signal intensity (representing fibrosis).[92,93] Irregularities of the tendon surfaces do not have the same relevance as those in preoperative assessments because even perfect tendon repairs are associated with tendon distortion and variable diameters.[91] In one study, only 10% of repaired rotator cuff tendons in asymptomatic patients had a normal appearance on MRI.[96] Fluid in the subacromial space is another nonspecific, postoperative finding that may be associated with a functional but not watertight repair, a recurrent tear in the rotator cuff, or an otherwise normal postoperative rotator cuff.[96] Nonvisualization of the subacromial fat and the presence of a joint effusion are other common findings.[96] Granulation tissue may also be seen around the sutures, resulting in a high-signal abnormality on T2-weighted images, which may mimic a recurrent tear.[91] After rotator cuff repair, susceptibility artifacts are common on MRI, especially in the presence of bone anchors.[91] The criteria for MRI diagnosis of a recurrent full-thickness rotator cuff tear are nonvisualization of a portion of the rotator cuff tendon and the presence of a fluid-like signal in the tendinous gap on T2-weighted sequences.[91,93] Recurrent partial-thickness rotator cuff tears are difficult to distinguish from granulation tissue, fluid trapped in sutures, and recurrent full-thickness tears of the rotator cuff.[80] MR arthrography would help distinguish these possibilities.

Expected MRI findings after a procedure for glenohumeral instability, such as a Bankart repair, include the presence of paramagnetic artifacts from anchors and the restoration of normal anatomy, including the reattachment of the capsulolabral complex to the glenoid rim.[80] The labrum-like structure found after Bankart repair usually is rounded and may have an inhomogeneous signal.[91] In addition, thickening of the anterior capsule often is visualized on MRI images after surgical repair of instability and labral tears.[91,97] MR arthrography is useful for optimal evaluation of the rotator cuff, capsulolabral structures, and tendon defects in the postoperative shoulder.[80]

MRI evaluation of the painful shoulder arthroplasty (total arthroplasty or hemiarthroplasty) is limited by the signal loss associated with imaging adjacent to the metallic prosthesis. Despite this limitation, MRI may be useful in evaluating the integrity of the rotator cuff tendons and residual glenoid articular cartilage (in the presence of hemiarthroplasty).[98] To optimize the value of MRI, pulse sequences should be manipulated to reduce the susceptibility artifact from the shoulder prosthesis.[98]

References

1. Kassarjian A, Bencardino JT, Palmer WE. MR imaging of the rotator cuff. Radiol Clin North Am 2006;44:503–523
2. Chung CB, Lektrakul N, Gigena L, Resnick D. Magnetic resonance imaging of the upper extremity: advances in technique and application. Clin Orthop Relat Res 2001;383:162–174
3. Kazár B, Relovszky E. Prognosis of primary dislocation of the shoulder. Acta Orthop Scand 1969;40:216–224
4. McFarland EG, Torpey BM, Curl LA. Evaluation of shoulder laxity. Sports Med 1996;22:264–272
5. Baker CL, Uribe JW, Whitman C. Arthroscopic evaluation of acute initial anterior shoulder dislocations. Am J Sports Med 1990;18:25–28
6. Bankart ASB. The pathology and treatment of recurrent dislocation of the shoulder-joint. Br J Surg 1938;26:23–29
7. Chandnani VP, Yeager TD, DeBerardino T, et al. Glenoid labral tears: prospective evaluation with MRI imaging, MR arthrography, and CT arthrography. AJR Am J Roentgenol 1993;161:1229–1235
8. Stoller DW, Wolf EM. The shoulder. In: Stoller DW, ed. Magnetic Resonance Imaging in Orthopaedics and Sports Medicine. 2nd ed. Philadelphia: Lippincott-Raven; 1997:597–742
9. Sanders TG, Miller MD. A systematic approach to magnetic resonance imaging interpretation of sports medicine injuries of the shoulder. Am J Sports Med 2005;33:1088–1105
10. Neviaser TJ. The anterior labroligamentous periosteal sleeve avulsion lesion: a cause of anterior instability of the shoulder. Arthroscopy 1993;9:17–21
11. Hill HA, Sachs MD. The grooved defect of the humeral head. A frequently unrecognized complication of dislocations of the shoulder. Radiology 1940;35:690–700
12. Denti M, Monteleone M, Trevisan C, De Romedis B, Barmettler F. Magnetic resonance imaging versus arthroscopy for the investigation of the osteochondral humeral defect in anterior shoulder instability. A double-blind prospective study. Knee Surg Sports Traumatol Arthrosc 1995;3:184–186

13. Richards RD, Sartoris DJ, Pathria MN, Resnick D. Hill-Sachs lesion and normal humeral groove: MR imaging features allowing their differentiation. Radiology 1994;190:665–668

14. Tirman PFJ, Steinbach LS, Feller JF, Stauffer AE. Humeral avulsion of the anterior shoulder stabilizing structures after anterior shoulder dislocation: demonstration by MRI and MR arthrography. Skeletal Radiol 1996;25:743–748

15. Wolf EM, Cheng JC, Dickson K. Humeral avulsion of glenohumeral ligaments as a cause of anterior shoulder instability. Arthroscopy 1995;11:600–607

16. Hottya GA, Tirman PFJ, Bost FW, Montgomery WH, Wolf EM, Genant HK. Tear of the posterior shoulder stabilizers after posterior dislocation: MR imaging and MR arthrographic findings with arthroscopic correlation. AJR Am J Roentgenol 1998;171:763–768

17. Gusmer PB, Potter HG, Schatz JA, et al. Labral injuries: accuracy of detection with unenhanced MR imaging of the shoulder. Radiology 1996;200:519–524

18. Loredo R, Longo C, Salonen D, et al. Glenoid labrum: MR imaging with histologic correlation. Radiology 1995;196:33–41

19. Monu JUV, Pope TL Jr, Chabon SJ, Vanarthos WJ. MR diagnosis of superior labral anterior posterior (SLAP) injuries of the glenoid labrum: value of routine imaging without intraarticular injection of contrast material. AJR Am J Roentgenol 1994;163:1425–1429

20. Jee WH, McCauley TR, Katz LD, Matheny JM, Ruwe PA, Daigneault JP. Superior labral anterior posterior (SLAP) lesions of the glenoid labrum: reliability and accuracy of MR arthrography for diagnosis. Radiology 2001;218:127–132

21. Beltran J, Jbara M, Maimon R. Shoulder: labrum and bicipital tendon. Top Magn Reson Imaging 2003;14:35–49

22. Mohana-Borges AVR, Chung CB, Resnick D. Superior labral anteroposterior tear: classification and diagnosis on MRI and MR arthrography. AJR Am J Roentgenol 2003;181:1449–1462

23. Rao AG, Kim TK, Chronopoulos E, McFarland EG. Anatomical variants in the anterosuperior aspect of the glenoid labrum: a statistical analysis of seventy-three cases. J Bone Joint Surg Am 2003;85:653–659

24. Wall MS, O'Brien SJ. Arthroscopic evaluation of the unstable shoulder. Clin Sports Med 1995;14:817–839

25. Williams MM, Snyder SJ, Buford D Jr. The Buford complex—the "cordlike" middle glenohumeral ligament and absent anterosuperior labrum complex: a normal anatomic capsulolabral variant. Arthroscopy 1994;10:241–247

26. Tuite MJ, Cirillo RL, De Smet AA, Orwin JF. Superior labrum anterior-posterior (SLAP) tears: evaluation of three MR signs on T2-weighted images. Radiology 2000;215:841–845

27. Snyder SJ, Karzel RP, Del Pizzo W, Ferkel RD, Friedman MJ. SLAP lesions of the shoulder. Arthroscopy 1990;6:274–279

28. Mileski RA, Snyder SJ. Superior labral lesions in the shoulder: pathoanatomy and surgical management. J Am Acad Orthop Surg 1998;6:121–131

29. Maffet MW, Gartsman GM, Moseley B. Superior labrum-biceps tendon complex lesions of the shoulder. Am J Sports Med 1995;23:93–98

30. Cartland JP, Crues JV III, Stauffer A, Nottage W, Ryu RKN. MR imaging in the evaluation of SLAP injuries of the shoulder: findings in 10 patients. AJR Am J Roentgenol 1992;159:787–792

31. Connell DA, Potter HG, Wickiewicz TL, Altchek DW, Warren RF. Noncontrast magnetic resonance imaging of superior labral lesions. 102 cases confirmed at arthroscopic surgery. Am J Sports Med 1999;27:208–213

32. Hunter JC, Blatz DJ, Escobedo EM. SLAP lesions of the glenoid labrum: CT arthrographic and arthroscopic correlation. Radiology 1992;184:513–518

33. Nam EK, Snyder SJ. The diagnosis and treatment of superior labrum, anterior and posterior (SLAP) lesions. Am J Sports Med 2003;31:798–810

34. Tirman PFJ, Feller JF, Janzen DL, Peterfy CG, Bergman AG. Association of glenoid labral cysts with labral tears and glenohumeral instability: radiologic findings and clinical significance. Radiology 1994;190:653–658

35. Snyder SJ, Banas MP, Karzel RP. An analysis of 140 injuries to the superior glenoid labrum. J Shoulder Elbow Surg 1995;4:243–248

36. Kim TK, Queale WS, Cosgarea AJ, McFarland EG. Clinical features of the different types of SLAP lesions: an analysis of one hundred and thirty-nine cases. J Bone Joint Surg Am 2003;85:66–71

37. Almekinders LC. Impingement syndrome. Clin Sports Med 2001;20:491–504

38. Bigliani LU, Morrison DS, April EW. The morphology of the acromion and its relationship to rotator cuff tears. [Abstr] Orthop Trans. 1986;10:216

39. Ozaki J, Fujimoto S, Nakagawa Y, Masuhara K, Tamai S. Tears of the rotator cuff of the shoulder associated with pathological changes in the acromion. A study in cadavera. J Bone Joint Surg Am 1988;70:1224–1230

40. Morrison DS, Ofstein R. The use of magnetic resonance imaging in the diagnosis of rotator cuff tears. Orthopedics 1990;13:633–637

41. Panni AS, Milano G, Lucania L, Fabbriciani C, Logroscino CA. Histological analysis of the coracoacromial arch: correlation between age-related changes and rotator cuff tears. Arthroscopy 1996;12:531–540

42. Uri DS. MR imaging of shoulder impingement and rotator cuff disease. Radiol Clin North Am 1997;35:77–96

43. Kieft GJ, Bloem JL, Rozing PM, Obermann WR. Rotator cuff impingement syndrome: MR imaging. Radiology 1988;166(1 Pt 1):211–214

44. Seeger LL, Gold RH, Bassett LW, Ellman H. Shoulder impingement syndrome: MR findings in 53 shoulders. AJR Am J Roentgenol 1988;150:343–347

45. Hawkins RJ, Kennedy JC. Impingement syndrome in athletes. Am J Sports Med 1980;8:151–158

46. Neer CS II, Welsh RP. The shoulder in sports. Orthop Clin North Am 1977;8:583–591

47. Miniaci A, Salonen D. Rotator cuff evaluation: imaging and diagnosis. Orthop Clin North Am 1997;28:43–58

48. Rafii M. Shoulder. In: Firooznia H, Golimbu CN, Rafii M, Rauschning W, Weinreb JC, eds. MRI and CT of the Musculoskeletal System. St. Louis: Mosby-Year Book; 1992:465–549

49. Ogawa K, Yoshida A, Inokuchi W, Naniwa T. Acromial spur: relationship to aging and morphologic changes in the rotator cuff. J Shoulder Elbow Surg 2005;14:591–598

50. Mirowitz SA. Normal rotator cuff: MR imaging with conventional and fat-suppression techniques. Radiology 1991;180:735–740

51. Erickson SJ, Cox IH, Hyde JS, Carrera GF, Strandt JA, Estkowski LD. Effect of tendon orientation on MR imaging signal intensity: a manifestation of the "magic angle" phenomenon. Radiology 1991;181:389–392

52. Jerosch J, Müller T, Castro WHM. The incidence of rotator cuff rupture. An anatomic study. Acta Orthop Belg 1991;57:124–129

53. Quinn SF, Sheley RC, Demlow TA, Szumowski J. Rotator cuff tendon tears: evaluation with fat-suppressed MR imaging with arthroscopic correlation in 100 patients. Radiology 1995;195:497–500

54. Ellman H. Shoulder arthroscopy: current indications and techniques. Orthopedics 1988;11:45–51

55. McConville OR, Iannotti JP. Partial-thickness tears of the rotator cuff: evaluation and management. J Am Acad Orthop Surg 1999;7:32–43

56. Farley TE, Neumann CH, Steinbach LS, Jahnke AJ, Petersen SS. Full-thickness tears of the rotator cuff of the shoulder: diagnosis with MR imaging. AJR Am J Roentgenol 1992;158:347–351

57. Hodler J, Kursunoglu-Brahme S, Snyder SJ, et al. Rotator cuff disease: assessment with MR arthrography versus standard MR imaging in 36 patients with arthroscopic confirmation. Radiology 1992;182:431–436

58. Hodler J, Kursunoglu-Brahme S, Flannigan B, Snyder SJ, Karzel RP, Resnick D. Injuries of the superior portion of the glenoid labrum involving the insertion of the biceps tendon: MR imaging findings in nine cases. AJR Am J Roentgenol 1992;159:565–568

59. Patten RM. Tears of the anterior portion of the rotator cuff (the subscapularis tendon): MR imaging findings. AJR Am J Roentgenol 1994;162:351–354

60. Reinus WR, Shady KL, Mirowitz SA, Totty WG. MR diagnosis of rotator cuff tears of the shoulder: value of using T2-weighted fat-saturated images. AJR Am J Roentgenol 1995;164:1451–1455

61. Kaplan PA, Bryans KC, Davick JP, Otte M, Stinson WW, Dussault RG. MR imaging of the normal shoulder: variants and pitfalls. Radiology 1992;184:519–524

62. Kaplan PA, Helms CA, Dussault R, Anderson MW, Major NM. Shoulder. In: Kaplan PA, et al., eds. Musculoskeletal MRI. Philadelphia: WB Saunders; 2001:175–223

63. Matsen FA III, Rockwood CA Jr, Wirth MA, Lippitt SB. Glenohumeral arthritis and its management. In: Rockwood CA Jr, Matsen FA III, eds. The Shoulder. 2nd ed. Philadelphia: WB Saunders; 1998:840–964

64. Disler DG, Recht MP, McCauley TR. MR imaging of articular cartilage. Skeletal Radiol 2000;29:367–377

65. Gold GE, Reeder SB, Beaulieu CF. Advanced MR imaging of the shoulder: dedicated cartilage techniques. Magn Reson Imaging Clin N Am 2004;12:143–159

66. Bredella MA, Tirman PFJ, Peterfy CG, et al. Accuracy of T2-weighted fast spin-echo MR imaging with fat saturation in detecting cartilage defects in the knee: comparison with arthroscopy in 130 patients. AJR Am J Roentgenol 1999;172:1073–1080

67. Potter HG, Linklater JM, Allen AA, Hannafin JA, Haas SB. Magnetic resonance imaging of articular cartilage in the knee. An evaluation with use of fast-spin-echo imaging. J Bone Joint Surg Am 1998;80:1276–1284

68. Needell SD, Zlatkin MB, Sher JS, Murphy BJ, Uribe JW. MR imaging of the rotator cuff: peritendinous and bone abnormalities in an asymptomatic population. AJR Am J Roentgenol 1996;166:863–867

69. de Abreu MR, Chung CB, Wesselly M, Jin-Kim H, Resnick D. Acromioclavicular joint osteoarthritis: comparison of findings derived from MR imaging and conventional radiography. Clin Imaging 2005;29:273–277

70. Stein BES, Wiater JM, Pfaff HC, Bigliani LU, Levine WN. Detection of acromioclavicular joint pathology in asymptomatic shoulders with magnetic resonance imaging. J Shoulder Elbow Surg 2001;10:204–208

71. Sethi N, Wright R, Yamaguchi K. Disorders of the long head of the biceps tendon. J Shoulder Elbow Surg 1999;8:644–654

72. Tuckman GA. Abnormalities of the long head of the biceps tendon of the shoulder: MR imaging findings. AJR Am J Roentgenol 1994;163:1183–1188

73. Erickson SJ, Fitzgerald SW, Quinn SF, Carrera GF, Black KP, Lawson TL. Long bicipital tendon of the shoulder: normal anatomy and pathologic findings on MR imaging. AJR Am J Roentgenol 1992;158:1091–1096

74. Van Leersum M, Schweitzer ME. Magnetic resonance imaging of the biceps complex. Magn Reson Imaging Clin N Am 1993;1:77–86

75. Cervilla V, Schweitzer ME, Ho C, Motta A, Kerr R, Resnick D. Medial dislocation of the biceps brachii tendon: appearance at MR imaging. Radiology 1991;180:523–526

76. Chan TW, Dalinka MK, Kneeland JB, Chervrot A. Biceps tendon dislocation: evaluation with MR imaging. Radiology 1991;179:649–652

77. Cleeman E, Auerbach JD, Klingenstein GG, Flatow EL. Septic arthritis of the glenohumeral joint: a review of 23 cases. J Surg Orthop Adv 2005;14:102–107

78. Weishaupt D, Schweitzer ME. MR imaging of septic arthritis and rheumatoid arthritis of the shoulder. Magn Reson Imaging Clin N Am 2004;12:111–124

79. Learch TJ, Farooki S. Magnetic resonance imaging of septic arthritis. Clin Imaging 2000;24:236–242

80. Mohana-Borges AVR, Chung CB, Resnick D. MR imaging and MR arthrography of the postoperative shoulder: spectrum of normal and abnormal findings. Radiographics 2004;24:69–85

81. Emig EW, Schweitzer ME, Karasick D, Lubowitz J. Adhesive capsulitis of the shoulder: MR diagnosis. AJR Am J Roentgenol 1995;164:1457–1459

82. Warner JJP. Frozen shoulder: diagnosis and management. J Am Acad Orthop Surg 1997;5:130–140

83. Kordella T. Frozen shoulder & diabetes. Frozen shoulder affects 20 percent of people with diabetes. Proper treatment can help you work through it. Diabetes Forecast 2002;55:60–64

84. Connell D, Padmanabhan R, Buchbinder R. Adhesive capsulitis: role of MR imaging in differential diagnosis. Eur Radiol 2002;12:2100–2106

85. Lefevre-Colau MM, Drapé JL, Fayad F, et al. Magnetic resonance imaging of shoulders with idiopathic adhesive capsulitis: reliability of measures. Eur Radiol 2005;15:2415–2422

86. Hurt G, Baker CL Jr. Calcific tendinitis of the shoulder. Orthop Clin North Am 2003;34:567–575

87. Uhthoff HK, Loehr JW. Calcific tendinopathy of the rotator cuff: pathogenesis, diagnosis, and management. J Am Acad Orthop Surg 1997;5:183–191

88. McMenamin D, Koulouris G, Morrison WB. Imaging of the shoulder after surgery. Eur J Radiol 2008;68:106–119

89. Potter HG, Jawetz ST, Foo LF. Imaging of the rotator cuff following repair: human and animal models. J Shoulder Elbow Surg 2007;16(5, Suppl):S134–S139

90. Guermazi A, Miaux Y, Zaim S, Peterfy CG, White D, Genant HK. Metallic artefacts in MR imaging: effects of main field orientation and strength. Clin Radiol 2003;58:322–328

91. Zanetti M, Hodler J. MR imaging of the shoulder after surgery. Magn Reson Imaging Clin N Am 2004;12:169–183

92. Zlatkin MB. MRI of the postoperative shoulder. Skeletal Radiol 2002;31:63–80

93. Resnick D, Kang HS. Shoulder. In: Resnick D, Kang HS, eds. Internal Derangement of Joints. Emphasis on MR Imaging. Philadelphia: WB Saunders; 1997:163–333

94. Owen RS, Iannotti JP, Kneeland JB, Dalinka MK, Deren JA, Oleaga L. Shoulder after surgery: MR imaging with surgical validation. Radiology 1993;186:443–447

95. Zanetti M, Jost B, Hodler J, Gerber C. MR imaging after rotator cuff repair: full-thickness defects and bursitis-like subacromial abnormalities in asymptomatic subjects. Skeletal Radiol 2000;29:314–319

96. Spielmann AL, Forster BB, Kokan P, Hawkins RH, Janzen DL. Shoulder after rotator cuff repair: MR imaging findings in asymptomatic individuals—initial experience. Radiology 1999;213:705–708

97. Vahlensieck M, Lang P, Wagner U, et al. Shoulder MRI after surgical treatment of instability. Eur J Radiol 1999;30:2–4

98. Sperling JW, Potter HG, Craig EV, Flatow E, Warren RF. Magnetic resonance imaging of painful shoulder arthroplasty. J Shoulder Elbow Surg 2002;11:315–321

5 The Elbow

Lance M. Brunton, Mark W. Anderson, and A. Bobby Chhabra

■ Specialized Pulse Sequences and Imaging Protocols

MRI of the elbow has improved with the development of high-field systems and enhanced surface coil technology.[1] Most centers image the elbow with the patient in the supine position and the arm comfortably positioned at the patient's side, with the elbow in full extension. This position limits rotation of the proximal radioulnar joint with respect to the distal humerus and minimizes motion artifact compared with imaging the patient prone with the arm overhead. Axial, coronal, and sagittal images are obtained routinely.[2]

Most centers use a standard screening examination, consisting of an array of specified imaging planes and pulse sequences.[3] In addition to standard T1-weighted and T2-weighted images, fat-suppressed T2-weighted and STIR sequences are extremely sensitive for detecting marrow and soft-tissue pathology by accentuating the increased signal of fluid and edema relative to the surrounding structures. These sequences are acquired with an FSE technique that produces the desired contrast in a fraction of the time needed for conventional T2-weighted sequences. Gradient-echo sequences are often used to evaluate ligaments and articular cartilage (see Chapter 14) and to delineate loose bodies in the elbow joint. However, these sequences should be avoided after elbow surgery (especially in the presence of metal hardware) because of the increased artifact inherent to the gradient-echo technique (see Chapter 1). A proton-density pulse sequence is occasionally used, often with fat suppression, and combines characteristics of T1-weighted and T2-weighted images. FSE pulse sequences have substantially reduced the length of examination, a great benefit for claustrophobic patients. Imaging parameters can be refined additionally for optimal cartilage visualization when indicated (see Chapter 14).[4]

MR arthrography is performed by injecting approximately 5 to 10 mL of diluted gadolinium contrast agent into the radiocapitellar joint from a lateral approach and acquiring fat-suppressed T1-weighted and T2-weighted images.[5] Although somewhat controversial, MR arthrography of the elbow may help evaluate undersurface collateral ligament tears, capsular disruption, OCD, and intraarticular loose bodies. When investigating infectious, neoplastic, or synovial disorders involving the elbow, intravenous gadolinium is often used to evaluate for synovial hypertrophy or enhancement of pathologic tissues. Intravenous contrast is also useful for detecting soft-tissue abscesses, which show a thick enhancing wall surrounding the nonenhancing central fluid. Additional refinement of conventional MRI pulse sequences may eventually render these invasive techniques obsolete.[6]

■ Traumatic Conditions

Most patients with elbow trauma may be evaluated and treated adequately without the use of advanced imaging. However, for select patients, MRI may facilitate the diagnosis of suspected occult fractures, loose bodies, ligamentous injuries, and tendinous pathology.

Occult Fractures

Conventional radiographs often are unrevealing in a patient presenting with elbow pain after acute trauma. In this setting, a joint effusion is often detected clinically, and an elevated posterior fat pad sign may be evident on conventional radiographs. Prospective studies in adults and children have shown that the presence of a posterior fat pad sign correlates with an occult fracture in more than 75% of patients.[7,8] However, localizing the injury is a challenging endeavor, and patients often may be overtreated with immobilization in the absence of advanced imaging.

MRI may be used in the setting of elbow trauma to localize and characterize osseous injury when conventional radiographs are unrevealing or equivocal. Fat-suppressed T2-weighted (or STIR) pulse sequences are the most sensitive images for detecting radiographically occult traumatic or stress fractures. Fractures show a linear pattern of signal change on T1-weighted (decreased signal) or T2-weighted (increased signal) images, whereas an osseous contusion often has a more nonspecific appearance (**Fig. 5.1A**). The most frequent site of occult fracture is the radial head; other sites, such as the lateral epicondyle or olecranon, are much less common.[7] Radial head fractures may be accompanied by associated injuries that are most effectively detected by MRI, such as ligament or capsular disruptions, OCD, loose bodies, or capitellar bone contusions.[9]

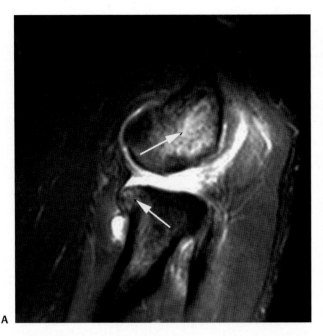

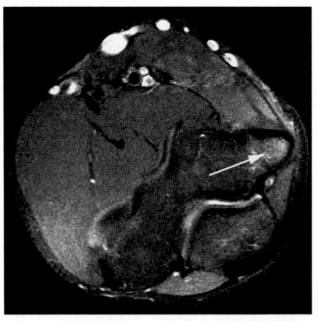

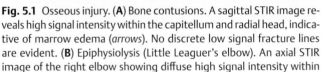

Fig. 5.1 Osseous injury. (**A**) Bone contusions. A sagittal STIR image reveals high signal intensity within the capitellum and radial head, indicative of marrow edema (*arrows*). No discrete low signal fracture lines are evident. (**B**) Epiphysiolysis (Little Leaguer's elbow). An axial STIR image of the right elbow showing diffuse high signal intensity within the medial epicondyle consistent with epiphysiolysis from repetitive valgus stress to the elbow (*arrow*). Part A is adapted with permission from Brunton LM, Anderson MW, Pannunzio ME, Khanna AJ, Chhabra AB: Magnetic resonance imaging of the elbow: update on current techniques and indications. J Hand Surg Am 2006;31:1001–1011.

In children with a traumatic injury to the elbow and radiographic evidence of only a joint effusion, MRI is a sensitive and accurate modality for identifying or excluding an occult fracture.[10] MRI reveals a broad spectrum of elbow pathology in this setting, including the following[11]:

- Bone bruises
- Ligamentous disruptions
- Muscle injury

MRI also may be effective in evaluating pediatric physeal injuries, especially in young children with poorly visualized ossification centers.[12] Finally, MRI has a role in the detection of Little Leaguer's elbow, a valgus stress injury in skeletally immature throwing athletes in which epiphysiolysis occurs at the medial epicondylar apophysis (**Fig. 5.1B**).[13]

Loose Bodies

The clinical manifestation of loose bodies within the elbow joint is typically pain with motion, often accompanied by mechanical symptoms, such as catching or locking. Loose bodies may originate from a traumatic shear injury to the osteochondral surface, synovial disorders, or OCD. The definitive treatment of symptomatic loose bodies is arthroscopic or open removal, but accurate diagnosis is imperative to prevent unnecessary surgery.

Although conventional radiographs or CT may detect the presence of osseous loose bodies in the elbow joint, MRI is especially useful for detecting intraarticular cartilaginous or osteocartilaginous loose bodies. Loose bodies are found most commonly in the olecranon or coronoid fossae on T2-weighted images (**Fig. 5.2**). Osteophytes and synovial hypertrophy may mimic loose bodies on MRI images.[3] The use of MRI for detecting loose bodies in the elbow has been disputed, and an overall low specificity and sensitivity, similar to that of conventional radiography, when compared with arthroscopic findings have been reported.[14] MR arthrography may be effective in this setting, but it has not been studied adequately.

MCL Injury

The MCL is composed of the anterior, posterior, and transverse bundles. The anterior bundle is the most important stabilizer against valgus stress, and it can be divided into anterior and posterior bands. The anterior band is the primary restraint with the elbow in extension, and the posterior band is the primary restraint with the elbow in increasing amounts of flexion. MCL injuries have received tremendous attention because of their prevalence in throwing athletes of all ages and at all levels of competition.[15] Accurate diagnosis of a full-thickness or partial-thickness tear of the MCL has important implications for treatment, as does the differentiation between MCL pathology and other causes of medial-side elbow pain, such as ulnar neuropathy, stress fracture, and flexor-pronator mass injury.

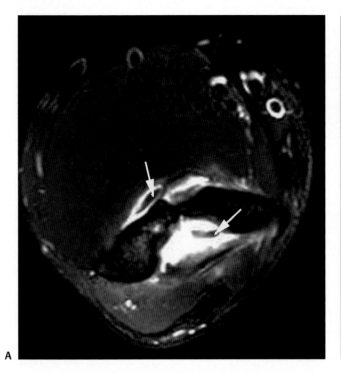

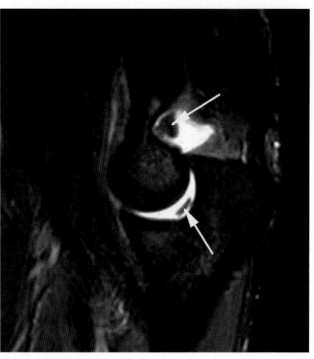

Fig. 5.2 Axial (**A**) and sagittal (**B**) T2-weighted images showing loose bodies in the coronoid and olecranon fossae and in the trochlear ulnar joint (*arrows on each*). Adapted with permission from Brunton LM, Anderson MW, Pannunzio ME, Khanna AJ, Chhabra AB: Magnetic resonance imaging of the elbow: update on current techniques and indications. J Hand Surg Am 2006;31: 1001–1011.

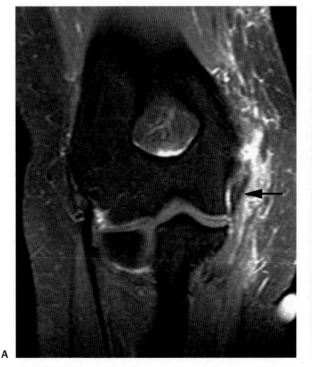

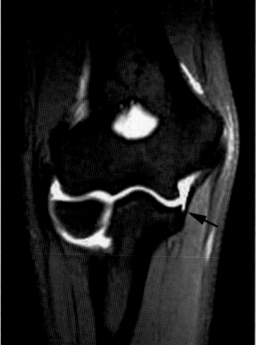

Fig. 5.3 MCL injury of the right elbow. (**A**) A coronal fat-suppressed T2-weighted image showing discontinuity (complete tear) of the MCL with surrounding edema and hemorrhage (*arrow*). (**B**) A coronal fat-suppressed T1-weighted arthrogram showing a partial tear of the MCL as a "T-sign" with leakage of intraarticular contrast at the undersurface of the MCL at its distal insertion on the sublime tubercle (*arrow*). Part A is adapted with permission from Brunton LM, Anderson MW, Pannunzio ME, Khanna AJ, Chhabra AB: Magnetic resonance imaging of the elbow: update on current techniques and indications. J Hand Surg Am 2006;31:1001–1011.

Full-thickness tears of the anterior bundle of the MCL can be detected accurately by MRI. The MCL is seen on MRI as a vertically oriented, uniformly low signal intensity structure coursing between the medial epicondyle and the sublime tubercle on coronal images. The abnormalities detectable by MRI include ligament attenuation, redundancy, or discontinuity. Increased signal intensity often is found within and adjacent to the ligament on fat-suppressed T2-weighted images, indicating edema or hemorrhage (**Fig. 5.3A**).[16] Concomitant findings, such as adjacent muscle edema and ulnar neuritis, are not unusual. MRI is less reliable for detecting partial-thickness tears, but the addition of intraarticular contrast may improve the sensitivity in this regard (**Fig. 5.3B**).[17,18]

LCL Complex Injury

The LCL complex of the elbow consists of four separate components:

- RCL
- LUCL
- Annular ligament
- Variable accessory LCL

Injury to this complex from an acute elbow dislocation may lead to chronic mechanical symptoms or recurrent instability when early treatment is inadequate. Tears of the LUCL and RCL are common in acute elbow dislocations. Chronic insufficiency of the LUCL is believed to lead to posterolateral rotatory instability, which is often difficult to diagnose clinically.[19]

The ability of MRI to visualize tears of the LCL complex historically has been less dependable, especially in patients with chronic instability.[20] One study of asymptomatic individuals revealed inconsistent MRI signal characteristics within the LUCL.[21] Other investigators, however, have found MRI to be effective in detecting abnormalities of the LUCL in the setting of posterolateral rotatory instability when 3D gradient-echo and FSE sequences were used.[22] Findings are similar to those seen in MCL injuries, with combinations of ligament attenuation, redundancy, and/or discontinuity evident on coronal or axial images (**Fig. 5.4**).[12,16] MR arthrography in this setting has not been studied sufficiently to date.

Biceps Tendon Injury

Injury to the distal biceps tendon is relatively common. Complete rupture occurs almost exclusively in men after forced extension of the flexed elbow against an eccentric load. However, symptoms arising from a partial tear may have an insidious onset, and such tears usually occur from repetitive microtrauma in an already degenerative tendon. Although MRI is not always necessary to diagnose a complete distal biceps tendon rupture, it can distinguish between tendino-

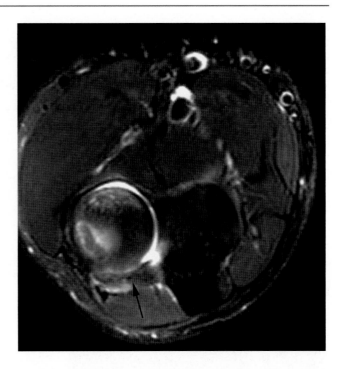

Fig. 5.4 An axial T2-weighted image of the right elbow showing thickening and abnormal signal (sprain vs. partial tear) of the LUCL with adjacent high signal intensity edema posterior to the radial head (*arrow*). Adapted with permission from Brunton LM, Anderson MW, Pannunzio ME, Khanna AJ, Chhabra AB: Magnetic resonance imaging of the elbow: update on current techniques and indications. J Hand Surg Am 2006;31:1001–1011.

sis, partial tears, and complete tears. MRI may also allow for the diagnosis of concomitant injuries. A complete rupture is characterized by the absence of the low signal intensity tendon tissue at the radial tuberosity insertion on axial images. The less experienced clinician may have difficulty localizing the biceps tendon insertion on the axial images and may find it easier to make or confirm the diagnosis on the sagittal T2-weighted images. A large amount of high signal intensity fluid and/or hemorrhage in the antecubital fossa usually accompanies an acute distal biceps tendon injury. The extent of tendon retraction is assessed on sagittal images, although the course of the tendon often is oriented obliquely to this plane (**Fig. 5.5**). An abnormally thickened or attenuated distal biceps tendon with increased signal intensity may represent tendinopathy or a partial tear. Associated bone marrow edema within the radial tuberosity is likely related to microavulsive injury. Increased fluid within the bicipitoradial bursa may accompany a partial tear in some patients.[12,23]

Triceps Tendon Injury

Ruptures of the triceps tendon are far less common than are injuries to the distal biceps tendon. Complete tears result from a traumatic event and are manifested clinically by the inability to extend the elbow against gravity. Extensive

Fig. 5.5 Distal biceps tendon injury. (**A**) An axial T2-weighted image of the right elbow showing rupture of the distal biceps tendon (*short arrow*) from its insertion (*long arrow*) at the radial tuberosity, accompanied by surrounding edema. (**B**) A sagittal T2-weighted image showing a complete tear of the biceps tendon with prominent edema and hemorrhage surrounding the thickened, retracted tendon (*arrow*). (**C**) Artist's sketch. Part B is adapted with permission from Brunton LM, Anderson MW, Pannunzio ME, Khanna AJ, Chhabra AB: Magnetic resonance imaging of the elbow: update on current techniques and indications. J Hand Surg Am 2006;31:1001–1011.

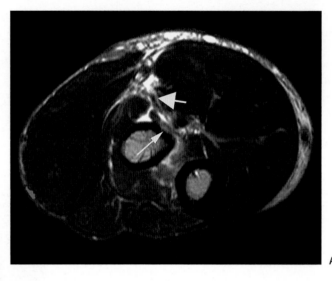

A

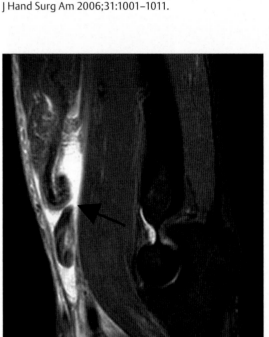

B

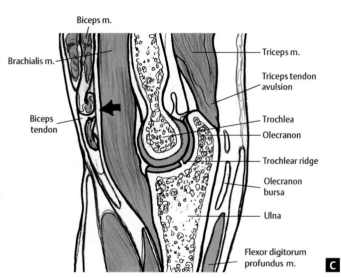

C

posterior elbow swelling, ecchymosis, and a palpable tendon defect are also common findings. The tendon typically is detached from its insertion on the olecranon process of the proximal ulna, and a small osseous avulsion may be seen on conventional radiographs.

MRI has a role in diagnosing triceps tendon injury in patients with equivocal clinical findings. A complete rupture is accompanied by extensive adjacent soft-tissue edema, and the retracted tendon margin is seen on sagittal images (**Fig. 5.6**).[12,16] Partial injury or tendinopathy may result only in thickening or thinning of the tendon, usually without related abnormal signal intensity. Findings of olecranon bursitis may accompany triceps tendon injury in some patients.

■ Degenerative Conditions: Lateral and Medial Epicondylitis

The term *epicondylitis* may be a misnomer because mucoid degeneration and tearing of the extensor carpi radialis brevis tendon (in the case of lateral epicondylitis), rather than inflammation, are the key histologic features of the disorder.[24]

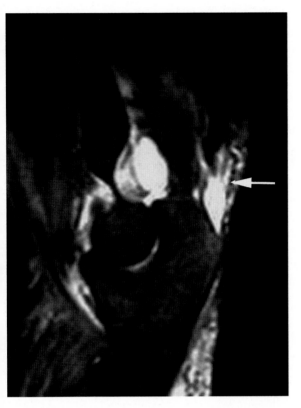

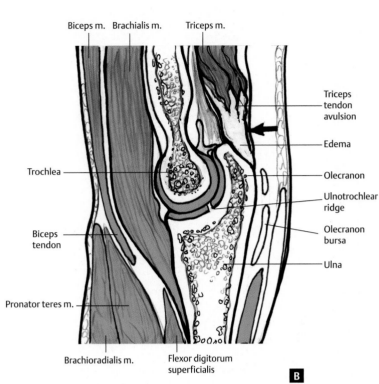

Fig. 5.6 A sagittal T2-weighted image (**A**) and artist's sketch (**B**) revealing a torn, retracted triceps tendon with a large amount of high signal intensity edema between the olecranon process and the tendon end (*arrows on each*). Part A is adapted with permission from Brunton LM, Anderson MW, Pannunzio ME, Khanna AJ, Chhabra AB: Magnetic resonance imaging of the elbow: update on current techniques and indications. J Hand Surg Am 2006;31:1001–1011.

Nevertheless, in the absence of a more accurate term, lateral epicondylitis (also known as tennis elbow) is the most common overuse disorder of the elbow, occurring most frequently in individuals who participate in racquet sports and in middle-aged persons who perform repetitive wrist extension in their daily activities. Patients complain of lateral elbow pain that increases with the offending activity. Examination reveals tenderness over the insertion of the common extensor tendon at the lateral epicondyle, and the pain is exacerbated by resisted wrist extension with the elbow fully extended. Although the diagnosis usually is obvious by history and physical examination, concurrent underlying pathology cannot be ruled out easily. The differential diagnosis for lateral elbow pain includes the following:

- Degenerative joint disease
- OCD
- Radial tunnel syndrome
- Posterolateral rotatory instability
- Occult fracture
- Loose bodies

It is important to consider these other etiologies when nonoperative treatment of lateral epicondylitis for more than 6 to 12 months has failed.

Usually, MRI is used to rule out concomitant causes of refractory elbow pain rather than to diagnose lateral epicondylitis.[25] Abnormalities of the LCL complex are not unusual in patients with severe lateral epicondylitis (**Fig. 5.7**).[26] The typical finding of isolated lateral epicondylitis is increased signal intensity in a thickened common extensor tendon. If the common extensor tendon appears normal, adjacent soft-tissue edema usually predominates (**Fig. 5.8**).[12,16] Although asymptomatic individuals may have abnormal MRI findings, these findings are usually limited to tendon thickening and intermediate signal intensity on T1-weighted or T2-weighted images without adjacent soft-tissue edema.[27]

Despite the relatively low prevalence of medial epicondylitis, MRI has an additional role in excluding other causes of medial elbow pain, such as MCL injury or ulnar neuritis, in patients for whom nonoperative treatment fails. A thickened common flexor tendon and local soft-tissue edema are the typical MRI features.

■ Infectious Conditions

Depending on the acuity of presentation, various imaging modalities are used in the evaluation of patients with signs

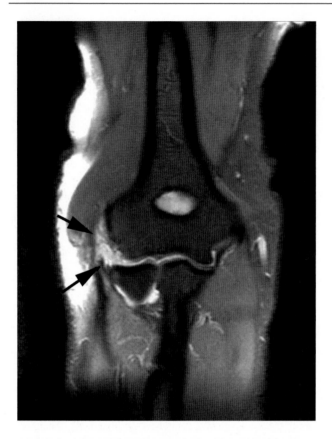

Fig. 5.7 A coronal T2-weighted image of the right elbow showing concurrent severe lateral epicondylitis (*upper arrow*) with high signal intensity within a thickened common extensor tendon and discontinuity of the underlying RCL (*lower arrow*).

fluid as normal, bloody, or purulent is less reliable. MRI often is used to determine the extent of involvement in patients with severe cellulitis, septic bursitis, or other superficial infections that are unresponsive to nonoperative measures. MRI also is an excellent method for diagnosing a suspected deep abscess about the elbow that may require surgical incision and drainage.[29]

The MRI findings in septic and nonseptic olecranon bursitis may be markedly similar. Abnormalities may include the following:

- Marginal lobulation
- Bursal septation
- Heterogeneous internal signal
- Poorly defined margins
- Adjacent soft-tissue edema
- Thickening or edema of the triceps tendon
- Localized bone marrow edema

The most consistent finding in septic olecranon bursitis is rim and soft-tissue enhancement on postgadolinium T1-weighted images.[30]

and symptoms of musculoskeletal infection. Conventional radiographs, CT, and radioisotope studies all have roles in the diagnosis of an infectious process, although MRI is the single most useful study for determining the precise anatomic location and extent of infection.

Acute osteomyelitis causes inflammation of medullary bone, which can be detected by MRI well before findings are evident on conventional radiographs. On T1-weighted images, areas of marrow involvement show a low signal intensity that contrasts with the surrounding bright normal marrow. STIR images, or other fat-suppressed T2-weighted images, are the most sensitive for infection, showing affected areas as high signal intensity. Sometimes these regions of high T2-weighted signal are accompanied by a well-defined low-intensity margin. Because these findings may be similar in patients with tumor or early osteonecrosis, correlation with the history and physical examination is critical.[28]

The role of MRI in patients with presumed septic arthritis is less clear. Although the presence of an elbow joint effusion can be well depicted by MRI, characterizing the synovial

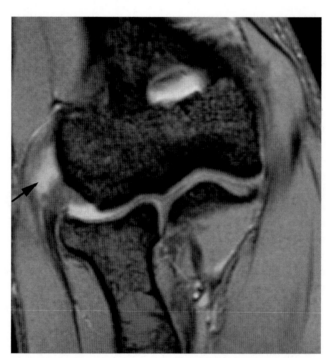

Fig. 5.8 A coronal STIR image of the right elbow showing isolated lateral epicondylitis, indicated by the thickened common extensor tendon with amorphous features and high signal intensity (*arrow*). Adapted with permission from Brunton LM, Anderson MW, Pannunzio ME, Khanna AJ, Chhabra AB: Magnetic resonance imaging of the elbow: update on current techniques and indications. J Hand Surg Am 2006;31:1001–1011.

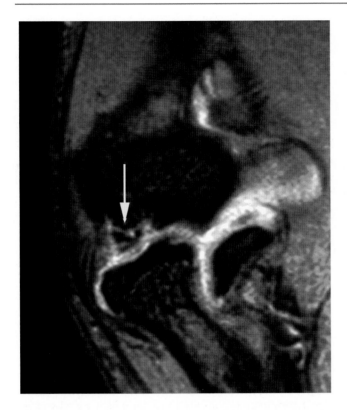

Fig. 5.9 A coronal oblique STIR image of the right elbow showing an unstable OCD fragment of the capitellum with joint fluid tracking behind the fragment (*arrow*). Adapted with permission from Brunton LM, Anderson MW, Pannunzio ME, Khanna AJ, Chhabra AB: Magnetic resonance imaging of the elbow: update on current techniques and indications. J Hand Surg Am 2006;31:1001–1011.

■ Other Pathologic Conditions

OCD

OCD of the humeral capitellum is an idiopathic disorder affecting adolescents with a history of repetitive overuse of the elbow. Affected individuals commonly present with pain and swelling of the lateral aspect of the elbow. Mechanical symptoms and/or limitations of motion may be indicative of an associated loose body. Conventional radiographs taken in the early stages of OCD may show only subtle changes within the capitellum.

In contrast, MRI can be helpful in the early detection of OCD. Focal areas of subchondral low signal intensity on T1-weighted images are characteristic. Fat-suppressed T2-weighted images provide the most sensitive evaluation for a potential OCD lesion at the capitellar articular surface; however, these images are the least specific. With a patient in whom the clinical suspicion is relatively high, the fat-suppressed T2-weighted image can be used as a "screening" examination and then correlated with the T1-weighted image where anatomic detail may be better seen. MRI can also help to evaluate the stability and viability of the OCD

fragment. Fluid surrounding the fragment on fat-suppressed T2-weighted images or surrounding contrast material on MR arthrography are signs of an unstable fragment (**Fig. 5.9**). Enhancement of a fragment after intravenous gadolinium contrast has been administered suggests adequate blood supply and fragment viability.[31]

Compression Neuropathies

The most commonly occurring compression neuropathies about the elbow include the following:

- Cubital tunnel syndrome (ulnar nerve)
- Radial tunnel syndrome (posterior interosseous nerve—pain)
- Posterior interosseous nerve syndrome (posterior interosseous nerve—motor deficits)
- Pronator syndrome (median nerve)

Each syndrome has key historical and physical examination findings that have been addressed elsewhere.[32] Electromyography and nerve conduction studies are the most frequently used adjunctive diagnostic tests. Advanced imaging may have a role in evaluating patients for whom nonoperative treatment fails or those with recurrence after surgical intervention.

MRI is most useful for assessing cubital tunnel syndrome, especially when electrodiagnostic testing is equivocal, or for excluding accompanying pathology in patients in whom this syndrome recurs. MRI may be more sensitive than nerve conduction studies in the diagnosis of ulnar neurop-

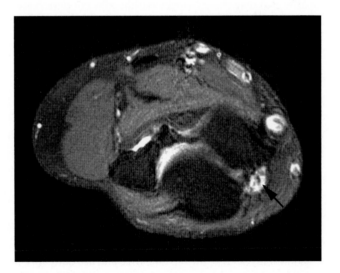

Fig. 5.10 An axial STIR image of the right elbow showing a thickened ulnar nerve with a mottled appearance and surrounding increased signal intensity consistent with edema from inflammation (ulnar neuritis) (*arrow*). Adapted with permission from Brunton LM, Anderson MW, Pannunzio ME, Khanna AJ, Chhabra AB: Magnetic resonance imaging of the elbow: update on current techniques and indications. J Hand Surg Am 2006;31:1001–1011.

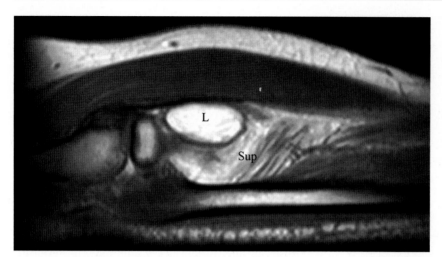

Fig. 5.11 A sagittal T1-weighted image revealing a lipoma (*L*) within the supinator muscle (*Sup*). The supinator shows diffuse high signal intensity, which matches that of the lipoma and subcutaneous fat, indicating fatty atrophy of the denervated muscle from long-standing compression of the posterior interosseous nerve by the lipoma. Adapted with permission from Brunton LM, Anderson MW, Pannunzio ME, Khanna AJ, Chhabra AB: Magnetic resonance imaging of the elbow: update on current techniques and indications. J Hand Surg Am 2006;31:1001–1011.

athy at the elbow.[33] Prolonged compression of peripheral nerves leads to a spectrum of MRI findings, including the following:

- Thickening of the nerve
- Increased signal intensity within the nerve
- A mottled appearance of the nerve
- A surrounding fluid collection, which may represent varying degrees of inflammatory changes (**Fig. 5.10**)

The median and radial nerves are more difficult to evaluate; however, MRI can detect adjacent space-occupying lesions that may produce compression. Patients with chronic neuropathy also may show changes within adjacent denervated muscles, such as fatty atrophy on T1-weighted images (**Fig. 5.11**) or muscle edema on T2-weighted images.[5]

Synovial Disorders

MRI can depict numerous abnormal synovial-based processes, such as RA, crystal deposition disorders, PVNS, and idiopathic synovial osteochondromatosis.[13] When synovial fluid analysis is equivocal, MRI may aid in differentiating conditions that produce a joint effusion. With the use of intravenous gadolinium, MRI has become a powerful tool for detecting the early stages of inflammatory arthritides, such as RA, because of the striking enhancement of the proliferative synovium (see Chapter 6 for specific MRI findings in patients with RA). Although PVNS and synovial chondromatosis are commonly seen in the hip and knee and are quite rare in the elbow, these syndromes should be considered in the differential diagnosis of the patient with multiple loose bodies in the elbow. Gradient-echo imaging shows accentuated "signal dropout" in areas of PVNS, relating to the presence of hemosiderin in this disease process. Other nonspecific MRI findings of PVNS include variable synovial proliferation, bone erosion, and joint effusion.[34,35]

Soft-Tissue Masses

Although soft-tissue masses are less common around the elbow than in the lower extremity, MRI is essential for evaluating such lesions. The primary role of MRI is differentiating determinate from indeterminate lesions (see Chapter 15). Determinate lesions are those for which a well-trained

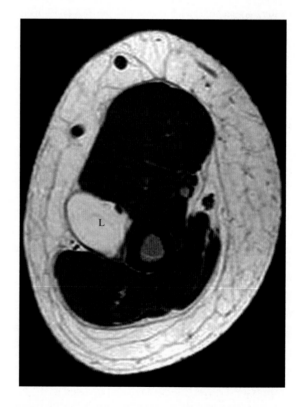

Fig. 5.12 An axial T1-weighted image showing the similarity in signal intensity between the well-circumscribed lipoma (*L*) and the adjacent subcutaneous fat.

musculoskeletal radiologist or clinician can provide a single diagnosis after MRI evaluation with a high degree of certainty based on the imaging appearance. Such lesions include the following[12,36,37]:

- Lipomas
- Ganglions
- Hemangiomas
- Neurofibromas
- Muscle tears

- Myositis ossificans (chronic stage)
- PVNS

A lipoma matches the signal intensity of subcutaneous fat on all pulse sequences, including fat-suppressed sequences (**Fig. 5.12**). Indeterminate lesions are those lesions in which the radiologist or clinician is unable to provide a definitive diagnosis and therefore warrant a needle or open biopsy (see Chapter 15 for additional information on MRI of soft-tissue masses).[36]

References

1. Fritz RC, Breidahl WH. Radiographic and special studies: recent advances in imaging of the elbow. Clin Sports Med 2004;23:567–580
2. Kijowski R, Tuite M, Sanford M. Magnetic resonance imaging of the elbow. Part I: normal anatomy, imaging technique, and osseous abnormalities. Skeletal Radiol 2004;33:685–697
3. Potter HG. Imaging of posttraumatic and soft tissue dysfunction of the elbow. Clin Orthop Relat Res 2000;370:9–18
4. Burstein D, Gray M. New MRI techniques for imaging cartilage. J Bone Joint Surg Am 2003;85(suppl 2):70–77
5. Kijowski R, Tuite M, Sanford M. Magnetic resonance imaging of the elbow. Part II: abnormalities of the ligaments, tendons, and nerves. Skeletal Radiol 2005;34:1–18
6. Chung CB, Lektrakul N, Gigena L, Resnick D. Magnetic resonance imaging of the upper extremity: advances in technique and application. Clin Orthop Relat Res 2001;383:162–174
7. O'Dwyer H, O'Sullivan P, Fitzgerald D, Lee MJ, McGrath F, Logan PM. The fat pad sign following elbow trauma in adults: its usefulness and reliability in suspecting occult fracture. J Comput Assist Tomogr 2004;28:562–565
8. Skaggs DL, Mirzayan R. The posterior fat pad sign in association with occult fracture of the elbow in children. J Bone Joint Surg Am 1999;81:1429–1433
9. Itamura J, Roidis N, Mirzayan R, Vaishnav S, Learch T, Shean C. Radial head fractures: MRI evaluation of associated injuries. J Shoulder Elbow Surg 2005;14:421–424
10. Pudas T, Hurme T, Mattila K, Svedström E. Magnetic resonance imaging in pediatric elbow fractures. Acta Radiol 2005;46:636–644
11. Griffith JF, Roebuck DJ, Cheng JCY, et al. Acute elbow trauma in children: spectrum of injury revealed by MR imaging not apparent on radiographs. AJR Am J Roentgenol 2001;176:53–60
12. Melloni P, Valls R. The use of MRI scanning for investigating soft-tissue abnormalities in the elbow. Eur J Radiol 2005;54:303–313
13. Chen FS, Diaz VA, Loebenberg M, Rosen JE. Shoulder and elbow injuries in the skeletally immature athlete. J Am Acad Orthop Surg 2005;13:172–185
14. Dubberley JH, Faber KJ, Patterson SD, et al. The detection of loose bodies in the elbow: the value of MRI and CT arthrography. J Bone Joint Surg Br 2005;87:684–686
15. Cain EL Jr, Dugas JR, Wolf RS, Andrews JR. Elbow injuries in throwing athletes: a current concepts review. Am J Sports Med 2003;31:621–635
16. Fritz RC, Steinbach LS. Magnetic resonance imaging of the musculoskeletal system: Part 3. The elbow. Clin Orthop Relat Res 1996;324:321–339

17. Hill NB Jr, Bucchieri JS, Shon F, Miller TT, Rosenwasser MP. Magnetic resonance imaging of injury to the medial collateral ligament of the elbow: a cadaver model. J Shoulder Elbow Surg 2000;9:418–422
18. Schwartz ML, Al-Zahrani S, Morwessel RM, Andrews JR. Ulnar collateral ligament injury in the throwing athlete: evaluation with saline-enhanced MR arthrography. Radiology 1995;197:297–299
19. O'Driscoll SW, Bell DF, Morrey BF. Posterolateral rotatory instability of the elbow. J Bone Joint Surg Am 1991;73:440–446
20. Grafe MW, McAdams TR, Beaulieu CF, Ladd AL. Magnetic resonance imaging in diagnosis of chronic posterolateral rotatory instability of the elbow. Am J Orthop 2003;32:501–503, discussion 504
21. Terada N, Yamada H, Toyama Y. The appearance of the lateral ulnar collateral ligament on magnetic resonance imaging. J Shoulder Elbow Surg 2004;13:214–216
22. Potter HG, Weiland AJ, Schatz JA, Paletta GA, Hotchkiss RN. Posterolateral rotatory instability of the elbow: usefulness of MR imaging in diagnosis. Radiology 1997;204:185–189
23. Williams BD, Schweitzer ME, Weishaupt D, et al. Partial tears of the distal biceps tendon: MR appearance and associated clinical findings. Skeletal Radiol 2001;30:560–564
24. Kraushaar BS, Nirschl RP. Tendinosis of the elbow (tennis elbow). Clinical features and findings of histological, immunohistochemical, and electron microscopy studies. J Bone Joint Surg Am 1999;81:259–278
25. Aoki M, Wada T, Isogai S, Kanaya K, Aiki H, Yamashita T. Magnetic resonance imaging findings of refractory tennis elbows and their relationship to surgical treatment. J Shoulder Elbow Surg 2005;14:172–177
26. Bredella MA, Tirman PFJ, Fritz RC, Feller JF, Wischer TK, Genant HK. MR imaging findings of lateral ulnar collateral ligament abnormalities in patients with lateral epicondylitis. AJR Am J Roentgenol 1999;173:1379–1382
27. Kijowski R, De Smet AA. Magnetic resonance imaging findings in patients with medial epicondylitis. Skeletal Radiol 2005;34:196–202
28. Boutin RD, Brossmann J, Sartoris DJ, Reilly D, Resnick D. Update on imaging of orthopedic infections. Orthop Clin North Am 1998;29:41–66
29. Berquist TH, Broderick DF. Musculoskeletal infection. In: Berquist TH, ed. MRI of the Musculoskeletal System. 5th ed. Philadelphia: Lippincott Williams & Wilkins; 2006:916–947
30. Floemer F, Morrison WB, Bongartz G, Ledermann HP. MRI characteristics of olecranon bursitis. AJR Am J Roentgenol 2004;183:29–34
31. Kijowski R, De Smet AA. MRI findings of osteochondritis dissecans of the capitellum with surgical correlation. AJR Am J Roentgenol 2005;185:1453–1459

32. Lubahn JD, Cermak MB. Uncommon nerve compression syndromes of the upper extremity. J Am Acad Orthop Surg 1998;6:378–386

33. Vucic S, Cordato DJ, Yiannikas C, Schwartz RS, Shnier RC. Utility of magnetic resonance imaging in diagnosing ulnar neuropathy at the elbow. Clin Neurophysiol 2006;117:590–595

34. Khanna AJ, Cosgarea AJ, Mont MA, et al. Magnetic resonance imaging of the knee. Current techniques and spectrum of disease. J Bone Joint Surg Am 2001;83(suppl 2 Pt 2):128–141

35. Cheng XG, You YH, Liu W, Zhao T, Qu H. MRI features of pigmented villonodular synovitis (PVNS). Clin Rheumatol 2004;23:31–34

36. Frassica FJ, Khanna JA, McCarthy EF. The role of MR imaging in soft tissue tumor evaluation: perspective of the orthopedic oncologist and musculoskeletal pathologist. Magn Reson Imaging Clin N Am 2000;8:915–927

37. Chen AL, Youm T, Ong BC, Rafii M, Rokito AS. Imaging of the elbow in the overhead throwing athlete. Am J Sports Med 2003;31:466–473

6 The Wrist and Hand

Lance M. Brunton, Mark W. Anderson, and A. Bobby Chhabra

■ Six Specialized Pulse Sequences and Imaging Protocols

The routine use of MRI for the distal upper extremity, compared with its use for larger joints, has been hindered by the technical challenges of imaging small anatomic structures. MRI of the wrist and hand typically is performed at a magnetic field strength of 0.2 to 3.0 T, using systems with dedicated surface coils. Recent advances in high field strength magnets and extremity surface coil design, however, have resulted in additional improvement in image quality. One prospective study revealed significantly higher contrast-to-noise ratios between muscle and bone and between bone and cartilage for all sequences with a 3-T system than with a 1.5-T system.[1] 3-T systems are now becoming available for clinical use, but most hand and wrist examinations are still performed with 1.5-T magnets.

The hand or wrist is best imaged with the patient prone and the affected extremity placed above the head with the forearm pronated. Typically, the closer the body part being imaged is to the isocenter of the magnet, the better the image quality that is obtained. Because this position is uncomfortable for many patients, scanning may also be performed with the patient supine, the arm positioned at the patient's side, and the forearm in neutral, with the attendant risk of some degradation of image quality. A small field of view and 1- to 3-mm-thick sections are preferable.

Scanning is routinely performed in the axial, coronal, and sagittal planes. Most centers use a standard screening examination, consisting of an array of specified imaging planes and their corresponding pulse sequences. Based on the indication, additional pulse sequences may be added. Standard pulse sequences include the following:

- T1-weighted
- T2-weighted FSE with fat suppression
- STIR
- Gradient-echo

T1-weighted images provide good anatomic detail and are especially useful for identifying fat (given its high signal intensity on these images) in lipomatous masses or atrophied muscles. Fat- suppressed, T2-weighted sequences are the most sensitive for detecting many pathologic conditions by accentuating the presence of abnormal fluid, edema, or hemorrhage related to traumatic injury or an inflammatory process. Gradient-echo sequences, especially with a 3D, thin-section technique, are useful for evaluating the carpal ligaments and articular cartilage (see Chapter 14).

MR arthrography of the wrist can be performed with single-, double-, or triple-compartment (radiocarpal, intercarpal, or distal radioulnar compartments) injection of contrast material. Approximately 2 to 5 mL of contrast are administered under sterile technique and fluoroscopic guidance. A single-compartment radiocarpal technique is used most often, with normal dissemination of contrast material between the proximal carpal row and the distal radius. Fat-suppressed, T1-weighted images are typically obtained in all three planes, in addition to other sequences. MR arthrography of the wrist has proven useful in the evaluation of the scapholunate ligament, the lunotriquetral ligament, and the TFCC.[2]

Intravenous contrast provides valuable information for the evaluation of a soft-tissue mass or possible synovial process involving the wrist and hand, especially when combined with fat-suppressed T1-weighted images. It is useful for differentiating solid and cystic lesions, showing rim-enhancing soft-tissue abscesses, and determining bone vascularity in cases of suspected osteonecrosis. Intravenous contrast may also be used to perform indirect arthrography, in which the contrast may migrate into the joint over time. This effect is most notable in an inflamed joint. The potential information gained from these procedures must always be weighed against the additional cost and risk associated with an invasive procedure.

■ Traumatic Conditions

Traumatic conditions affecting the wrist and hand that are commonly evaluated by MRI include occult fractures, tears of the TFCC, and injuries to the interosseous carpal ligaments and small joint ligaments and tendons.

Occult Fractures of the Scaphoid and Other Bones

At initial presentation, a patient with wrist pain after a traumatic injury to the outstretched hand may not have radiographic evidence of a fractured scaphoid. However, when a patient continues to have tenderness in the anatomic snuff-box or over the scaphoid tubercle at follow-up examination, other advanced imaging modalities often are used for the detection of a radiographically occult scaphoid fracture. Recent comparative studies have sought to determine the superior modality for confirming the diagnosis: bone scintigraphy, CT, MRI, or ultrasound.[3–6] MRI has consistently outperformed other methods in the accurate early detection of scaphoid fracture and other radiographically indeterminate carpal injuries.[7–9] In addition, the use of early MRI in the management of clinically suspected scaphoid fractures may prove to be more cost-effective than follow-up conventional radiography.[10,11]

A fracture may be identified on T1-weighted images as a distinct line of low signal intensity that contrasts with the surrounding high-signal marrow (**Fig. 6.1A**). Fat-suppressed, T2-weighted images typically show high-signal marrow edema surrounding the fracture line (**Fig. 6.1B**). A scaphoid humpback deformity may also be shown on sagittal images (**Fig. 6.1C**).

MRI has proven to be sensitive in the detection of occult fractures in the distal radius, distal ulna, and other carpal bones (**Fig. 6.2**)[12,13] and can also differentiate fractures from

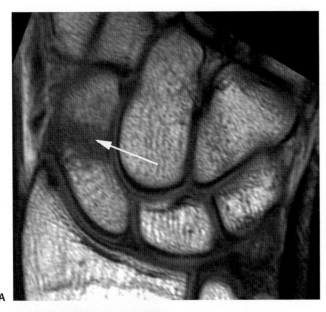

A

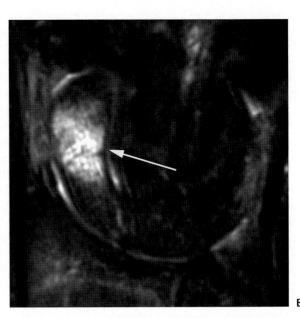

B

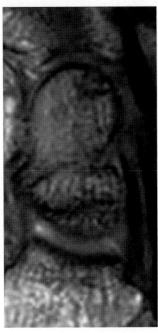

C

Fig. 6.1 Scaphoid fracture/deformity. **(A)** A coronal T1-weighted image of the wrist showing a fracture through the scaphoid waist (*arrow*), seen as a discrete line of low signal intensity. **(B)** A coronal fat-suppressed T2-weighted image showing the same fracture as in (A), with focal marrow edema in the scaphoid waist consistent with fracture (*arrow*). **(C)** A sagittal gradient-echo image showing a humpback deformity of the scaphoid.

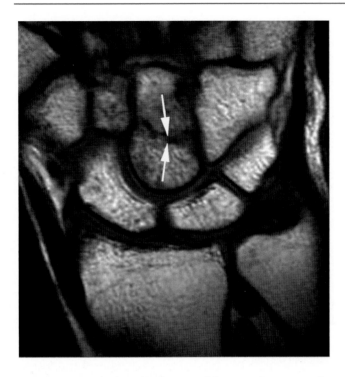

Fig. 6.2 A coronal T1-weighted image of the wrist showing a radiographically occult capitate fracture (*arrows*).

bone bruises (contusions), which show marrow edema without a discrete fracture line. MRI is also sensitive for diagnosing subtle physeal injuries in children (**Fig. 6.3**) and for evaluating physeal bars and growth arrest.[14] Radiographically occult fractures of the metacarpals and phalanges are uncommon.

TFCC Injury

The TFCC encompasses the major stabilizing structures of the ulnar aspect of the wrist, spanning the distal radioulnar joint and consisting of the following components[15]:

- Fibrocartilaginous articular disc
- Dorsal and volar radioulnar ligaments
- Ulnolunate ligament
- Ulnotriquetral ligament
- UCL
- ECU subsheath
- A variable meniscus homologue

In general, tears of the TFCC are classified as degenerative or traumatic.[16] Degenerative central perforations of the TFCC are common and often asymptomatic. On the other hand, acute injuries to the TFCC frequently lead to ulnar-side wrist pain and dysfunction. It is difficult to distinguish this condition from other causes of ulnar-side wrist pain (such as occult fractures, lunotriquetral ligament injury, ECU tendinopathy or subluxation, distal radioulnar joint injury, or

pisotriquetral joint injury) by history and physical examination. Historically, three-compartment wrist arthrography was the imaging test of choice for evaluation of the TFCC. However, this modality suffers from unacceptably low sensitivity and specificity and lacks the ability to determine lesion size, location, and acuity.[17,18] Although wrist arthroscopy remains the standard for the diagnosis of TFCC pathology, advances in MRI and MR arthrography are increasing the reliability in accurate diagnosis of the size, location, and character of TFCC tears before wrist arthroscopy. In the most specialized centers, the sensitivity and accuracy of MRI for detecting TFCC tears approaches 100%, using arthroscopy as the standard diagnostic modality.[19]

The normal TFCC is a low signal intensity structure shaped like a bowtie in the coronal plane. The articular disc is readily apparent on coronal and sagittal images. Advances in imaging techniques have enabled MRI to visualize some other individual components of the TFCC, such as the radioulnar ligaments and the ECU subsheath. T2-weighted images may help to differentiate between degenerative and traumatic tears of the TFCC, with traumatic tears showing increased signal intensity in adjacent tissues. The excellent anatomic

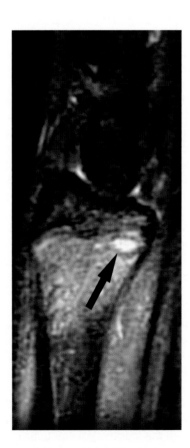

Fig. 6.3 A sagittal STIR image of the wrist showing diffuse marrow edema in the distal radius metaphysis adjacent to the growth plate, which is widened along its volar aspect (*arrow*).

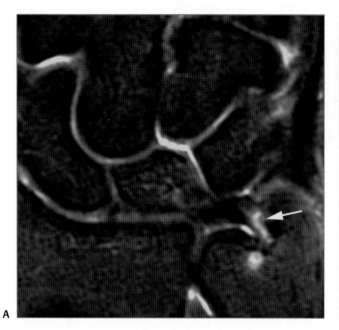
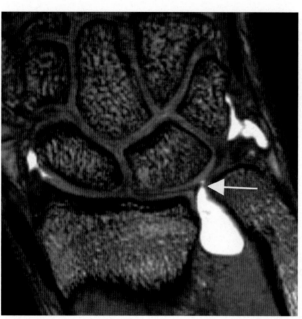

A   B

Fig. 6.4 Peripheral TFCC tear. **(A)** A coronal fat-suppressed T2-weighted image showing a tear of the peripheral portion of the TFCC near its ulnar attachment (*arrow*). **(B)** A coronal STIR image showing a perforation of the peripheral portion of the TFCC near its radial attachment (*arrow*).

detail afforded by MRI also helps in determining specific lesion location, with degenerative tears typically occurring in the thinner central portion and traumatic tears most often found in the periphery of the TFCC (**Fig. 6.4**). Nonetheless, all TFCC attachments must be carefully evaluated in all three planes. Ulnar attachment tears have been consistently more difficult to diagnose.[20] Concomitant pathology of the ECU tendon, lunotriquetral ligament, and surrounding osseous structures must be pursued. MR arthrography may prove superior to MRI in detecting TFCC lesions.[2,21] A TFCC tear is often shown by the presence of gadolinium contrast within the tear itself and/or in the distal radioulnar joint. Strong evidence exists that observer experience is critical for the accurate detection of TFCC pathology.[22]

Interosseous Ligament Injury

The scapholunate and lunotriquetral ligaments are the most commonly injured wrist ligaments secondary to acute trauma. These C-shaped ligaments vary in thickness throughout their courses. MRI has supplanted stress radiography and conventional wrist arthrography as the study of choice for suspected carpal ligament injury. Compared with arthroscopic findings, conventional MRI is highly specific but still has an overall low sensitivity for the detection of tears of the scapholunate ligament,[23] although the sensitivity seems to be improving with technologic advances in imaging techniques. Disruption of the interosseous ligaments is best evaluated on coronal gradient-echo (**Fig. 6.5**) and fat-suppressed T2-weighted images.

Carpal ligaments show low signal intensity on most MR images. However, the scapholunate ligament normally shows a more heterogeneous appearance on coronal images, which may lead to the misdiagnosis of a tear. Distinct linear areas of high signal intensity equal to that of fluid, especially in the thick dorsal portion of the ligament, usually indicate clinically significant tears, which may lead to carpal instability if not treated adequately. Alternative findings in ligament tears include nonvisualization of the ligament or morphologic distortion.[24] MR arthrography may be more accurate than conventional MRI for the detection of tears of the scapholunate ligament when compared with arthroscopic findings.[25] MR arthrography is most useful for the detection of tears of the lunotriquetral ligament, which although rarely an isolated injury, often accompanies an injury to the TFCC. The assessment of lunotriquetral ligament pathology by MRI techniques is still met with skepticism in the literature.[26,27]

Extrinsic Carpal Ligament Injury

The extrinsic carpal ligaments are a complex assortment of dorsal and volar structures that lie in close relation to the wrist joint capsule. The volar extrinsic ligaments are stronger and more robust than their dorsal counterparts. Isolated acute injuries to the extrinsic ligaments are rare. Typically, disruptions of these ligaments are part of a constellation of acute bone and soft-tissue injury about the wrist joint. Although MRI can distinguish the extrinsic ligament complexes with multiple image planes or 3D reconstructions

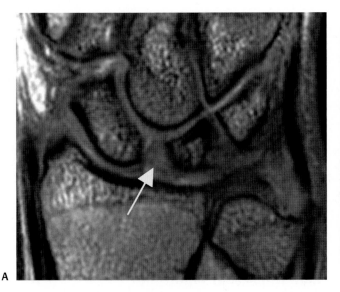 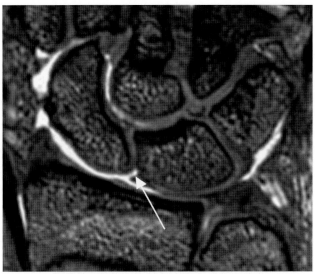

A B

Fig. 6.5 Scapholunate ligament tear. **(A)** A coronal gradient-echo image of the wrist showing partial stretching of the scapholunate ligament with concurrent widening of the scapholunate interval (*arrow*). **(B)** A coronal gradient-echo image of the wrist showing a small perforation in the membranous portion of the scapholunate ligament (*arrow*).

(**Fig. 6.6**), the role of MRI in this clinical setting is more often to exclude occult fracture, disruption of the intrinsic carpal ligaments, or injury to the TFCC. If diagnosed, these conditions may require a change in treatment algorithm.

Thumb UCL Injury

The UCL of the MCP joint is the primary stabilizer of the ulnar aspect of the thumb. Rupture of this ligament is common in skiers and results from forced abduction of the thumb. A

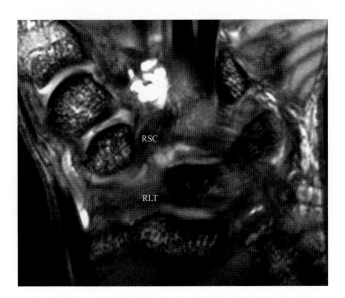

Fig. 6.6 A coronal STIR image of the wrist showing the extrinsic ligaments comprising part of the volar wrist capsule, including the radioscaphocapitate (*RSC*) and radiolunotriquetral (*RLT*) ligaments.

Stener lesion describes displacement of the torn ligament to a position superficial to the aponeurosis of the adductor pollicis muscle, a conformation that inhibits adequate ligament healing. Although clinical presentation and stress radiography may be enough for the diagnosis of a torn UCL, MRI may detect a Stener lesion and help guide the surgical treatment of acute injuries (**Fig. 6.7**).[28,29]

Tendon Injuries

Tendon pathology may occur as a result of acute trauma, chronic overuse, or inflammatory arthropathies such as RA. The spectrum of pathology ranges from tendon thickening and various degrees of tendon or tendon sheath inflammation to frank tears. In patients with traumatic injury, partial or complete rupture of a hand or wrist tendon may be difficult to diagnose clinically. Although tenderness and localized swelling are often present, the degree of flexion or extension loss may be equivocal. The use of MRI and ultrasound in this setting is evolving. Occasionally, ruptures of the extensor wrist tendons can be detected by MRI (**Fig. 6.8**). On T2-weighted sequences, partial tendon tears typically show increased intrasubstance signal intensity (**Fig. 6.9**), whereas complete tears show separation of the tendon ends with fluid tracking between its margins. Timely and accurate diagnosis has important clinical implications because early surgical repair provides the best outcome for zone II flexor tendon tears comprising >50% of their width.[30] Similarly, identifying the location of the retracted tendon end after a zone I flexor digitorum profundus avulsion injury (Jersey finger) is important for determining the appropriate treatment. Advances in image quality with sophisticated systems and MR

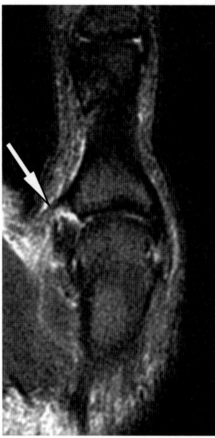

Fig. 6.7 A coronal oblique T2-weighted image of the thumb showing a complete rupture of the UCL at the MCP joint with increased fluid emanating from the joint (*arrow*).

tenography, in which contrast material is injected within the tendon sheath, have led to the detection of flexor pulley system injuries (see **Fig. 2.21**) and concomitant bowstringing deformities of the flexor tendons.[31]

■ Degenerative Conditions

The wrist and hand are affected by various degenerative conditions, although the usefulness of MRI may be limited to the evaluation of ulnar impaction syndrome, tendon disorders, and carpal instability in select patients. Other common degenerative conditions in the hand and wrist, such as first carpometacarpal joint and radiocarpal joint osteoarthritis, are adequately imaged with conventional radiography.

Ulnar Impaction Syndrome

Ulnar variance relates to the relative lengths of the radius and ulna. In patients with ulnar positive variance, the relatively long ulna may abut the proximal carpal row when the wrist is ulnarly deviated, leading to ulnar-side wrist pain from excessive loading across the ulnar aspect of the wrist. Chronic impaction may lead to subchondral sclerosis or cyst formation of the proximal and ulnar portions of the lunate, the radial portion of the triquetrum, and/or the distal and radial portions of the ulnar head. Focal defects of the articular cartilage or increased marrow signal on T2-weighted images may be visualized (**Fig. 6.10**). These findings can be differen-

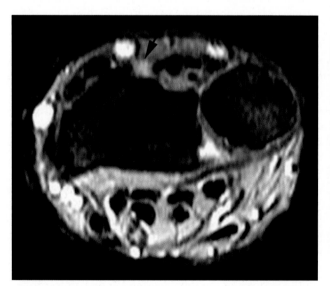

Fig. 6.8 An axial STIR image of the wrist showing absence of the extensor pollicis longus tendon in the third extensor compartment, indicative of complete rupture (*arrow*).

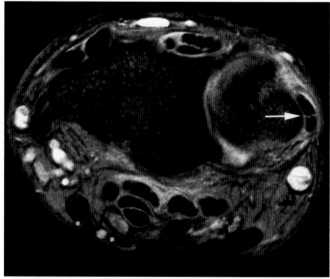

Fig. 6.9 An axial fat-suppressed T2-weighted image at the level of the distal radioulnar joint, showing thickening of the ECU tendon and a high signal intensity split within the tendon, indicating a partial tear (*arrow*).

tiated from Kienböck disease because the signal changes are focal rather than diffuse, and the ulnar variance is usually positive rather than negative or neutral. MRI may also detect accompanying degenerative TFCC or lunotriquetral ligament tears.[32]

Tendon Disorders

Pain and diminished function of the wrist and hand may be caused by various forms of tendon pathology, ranging from tendinosis to tenosynovitis to partial or complete tears. Although these conditions may result from simple overuse, other etiologies include inflammatory arthropathies, indolent infections, PVNS, gout, sarcoidosis, or amyloidosis.[33] Although tendon pathology is often self-limiting, MRI is excellent for assessing the spectrum of tendon pathology. MRI may reveal tendon thickening or thinning in patients with tendinosis or tendinitis. T2-weighted images may reveal distended tendon sheaths filled with high signal intensity fluid in patients with tenosynovitis (**Fig. 6.10**). Occasionally, tiny foci of low signal intensity, called *rice bodies*, are seen within the fluid in patients with chronic tenosynovitis.

As an example, de Quervain tenosynovitis is a common inflammatory disorder of the first dorsal compartment. A spectrum of MRI findings may be seen, including thickening of the abductor pollicis longus and extensor pollicis brevis tendons, adjacent fluid collections, and increased intraten-dinous T2-weighted signal intensity (**Fig. 6.11**). Similar findings are described for other commonly affected tendons, including the ECU, extensor carpi radialis longus, extensor pollicis longus, flexor carpi radialis, and flexor carpi ulnaris (**Fig. 6.12**). Tendon subluxation or dislocation from chronic overuse may be detected on axial images. MRI may help to differentiate chronic tenosynovitis and soft-tissue masses such as giant cell tumor of the tendon sheath.

The clinician should keep in mind that when a tendon lies at approximately 55 degrees relative to the direction of the external magnetic field during scanning, artifactual increased intratendinous signal intensity may be observed on some imaging sequences secondary to the *magic angle phenomenon*, not to true pathology.[34,35] This phenomenon is recognized easily because the signal disappears and the tendon appears normal on heavily T2-weighted images. This phenomenon also is seen in the shoulder where the presence of the magic angle effect may be mistaken for rotator cuff tendinopathy (see chapter 4).

Given that the clinical findings are typically diagnostic, MRI is not necessary for the diagnosis of stenosing tenosynovitis of the digits (trigger finger), although it may have a role in evaluating patients with postoperative recurrence or in ruling out other causes of symptoms, such as tendon sheath tumor, rheumatoid synovitis, or volar plate pathology.

Carpal Instability

The most common pattern of carpal instability is dorsal intercalated segment instability, often associated with disruption of the scapholunate and volar extrinsic carpal ligaments. Volar intercalated segment instability from lunotriquetral ligament deficiency is far less common. Clinically, carpal instabilities usually present as chronic wrist pain months to years after traumatic injury or secondary to inflammatory arthropathy. Physical examination findings are often equivocal, and standard lateral wrist radiographs may not always show abnormal carpal alignment. In patients with static carpal instability, the malalignment will be evident on sagittal images, and MRI may also detect associated abnormalities of the stabilizing carpal ligaments, such as laxity, thickening, retraction, edema, or absence. MR arthrography and thin-section coronal gradient-echo images are the most useful for identifying the pathology of these structures. Perforations of the central portions of the interosseous ligaments may be asymptomatic and consistent with normal aging.[36]

■ Infectious Conditions

Soft-tissue abscesses within the hand or wrist typically show intermediate to low signal intensity on T1-weighted images and high signal intensity on T2-weighted images. A thick, enhancing wall is usually seen after the administra-

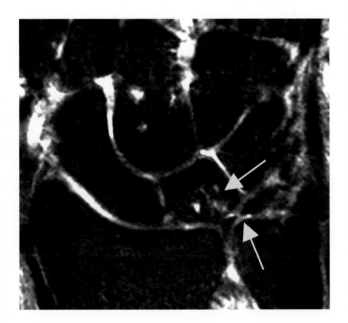

Fig. 6.10 A coronal STIR image of the wrist showing focal edema and cystic changes at the proximal ulnar aspect of the lunate consistent with ulnar impaction syndrome (*top arrow*). A small perforation of the central portion of the TFCC is also shown (*bottom arrow*).

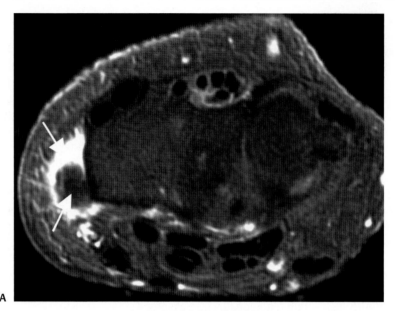

Fig. 6.11 De Quervain tenosynovitis. An axial fat-suppressed T2-weighted image **(A)** and artist's sketch **(B)** showing thickening of the first compartment tendons and surrounding edema (*arrows on* **A**).

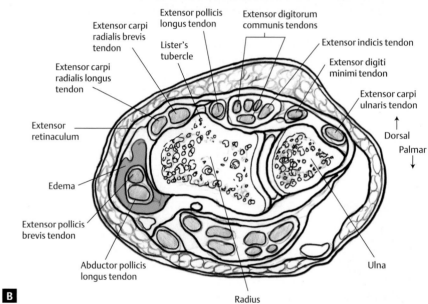

tion of intravenous contrast. MRI can evaluate the extent of soft-tissue involvement and the presence or absence of accompanying osteomyelitis. An emergent MRI may be necessary in select patients with suspected necrotizing fasciitis, where T2-weighted images may help confirm the diagnosis with increased signal intensity seen in the deep fascia, although this imaging finding is nonspecific. Given the need for urgent treatment of this diagnosis, the clinician should also carefully evaluate for the presence of crepitus within the soft tissues and rapidly spreading erythema and induration. Prompt treatment of infectious processes in critically ill patients should never be delayed while awaiting an MRI study.

■ Other Pathologic Conditions

MRI has proven useful in the evaluation of other pathologic conditions affecting the wrist and hand, such as osteonecrosis, RA, compression neuropathies, and soft-tissue masses.

Kienböck Disease

Idiopathic osteonecrosis of the lunate is known as Kienböck disease. This diagnosis must be considered in patients with subacute or chronic dorsal wrist pain of unknown etiology. A strong association with negative ulnar variance exists, and the etiology of the disorder may stem from chronic micro-

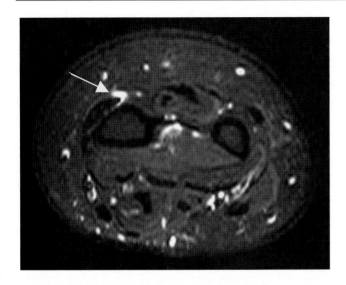

Fig. 6.12 Axial fat-suppressed T2-weighted image showing fluid between the first and second extensor compartments consistent with intersection syndrome from chronic overuse (*arrow*).

trauma secondary to increased shear stress on the lunate. Lichtman et al[37] defined four stages of Kienböck disease:

- Stage I: normal conventional radiographs, changes in the lunate on MRI
- Stage II: lunate sclerosis on conventional radiographs
- Stage III: lunate collapse
- Stage IV: pancarpal arthritis

Early diagnosis by MRI is critical because both nonoperative measures and surgical intervention are most successful in the initial stages of the disease, long before progression to lunate collapse or pancarpal arthritis.

In the first stage of Kienböck disease, MRI shows distinct changes in the lunate. On T1-weighted images, decreased lunate vascularity leads to diffuse low signal intensity of the bone marrow compared with the surrounding carpal bones (**Fig. 6.13**). This diffuse involvement distinguishes Kienböck disease from focal T1-weighted signal loss secondary to ulnar impaction syndrome, fracture, or tumor. The findings on T2-weighted images have been correlated with prognosis, showing low signal intensity with complete marrow fibrosis and increased signal intensity with lunate revascularization. When stage I Kienböck disease is diagnosed, patients are typically immobilized for up to 3 months, and follow-up MRI examinations are used to monitor the success of nonoperative treatment.

MRI findings are similar in idiopathic osteonecrosis of the scaphoid, also known as Preiser disease, and other carpal bones. One study supports the possibility of two patterns of Preiser disease based on disparate MRI patterns of vascular impairment[38]:

- Type 1 variant, diffuse involvement of the scaphoid
- Type 2 variant, only partial necrosis

The recognition of two distinct patterns has implications for treatment, and the clinical outcome may be more favorable for patients with type 2 involvement.[38]

Posttraumatic Scaphoid Osteonecrosis

The tenuous retrograde blood supply of the scaphoid often results in delayed union, nonunion, and/or osteonecrosis of the proximal pole. These complications are minimized with the early diagnosis of a scaphoid fracture and the implementation of appropriate treatment. In patients with scaphoid nonunion, determination of bone viability is critical to subsequent management. Vascularity of the proximal fragment has been shown to be an important determinant of outcome after surgical reconstruction of a scaphoid nonunion.[39] Patients with proximal pole osteonecrosis may require vascularized bone grafting. Visual inspection of intraoperative punctate bleeding typically corresponds with viability of the proximal pole. Because conventional radiographs are unreliable for detecting bone vascularity, MRI with intravenous gadolinium contrast can be used to assess the degree of osteonecrosis preoperatively. Osteonecrosis is indicated by low signal intensity on T1-weighted images, in stark contrast to the high signal intensity of the marrow of the normal surrounding carpal bones (**Fig. 6.14**). T2-weighted images also show low signal intensity.

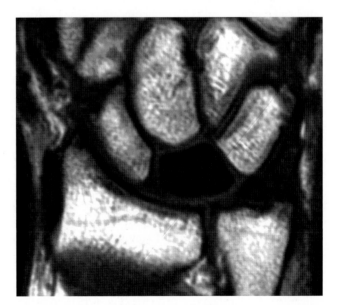

Fig. 6.13 Coronal T1-weighted image showing complete loss of normal marrow signal within the lunate, indicating necrosis (Kienböck disease).

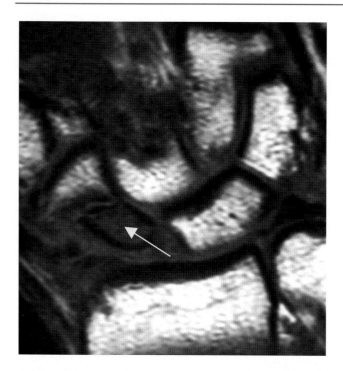

Fig. 6.14 A coronal T1-weighted image showing loss of normal marrow signal in the proximal pole of the scaphoid (*arrow*), indicative of posttraumatic osteonecrosis.

ture so that other diagnoses (systemic lupus erythematosus, scleroderma, polymyositis, dermatomyositis, Behçet disease, or mixed connective disease) are excluded.[43] Advanced techniques have been developed to quantify the volume of affected synovium and bone erosion with MRI. These methods may prove useful in predicting disease progression and monitoring the response to treatment.[44]

Compression Neuropathies

The nerve branches in the hand and wrist most frequently affected by compression syndromes are the median nerve in the carpal tunnel and the ulnar nerve in Guyon's canal. The superficial sensory branch of the radial nerve is affected much less commonly. Compression neuropathies may be triggered by intrinsic or extrinsic sources. Most patients are diagnosed by history and physical examination findings, which are then corroborated by electrodiagnostic testing. MRI can serve as a useful adjunctive diagnostic modality in the evaluation of compression neuropathies. Some patients present with atypical or equivocal clinical features or nerve conduction study results, and an MRI examination may be indicated for the investigation of unusual etiologies, such as nerve sheath tumors or extrinsic space-occupying lesions. Another indication for MRI is patients with recurrent symptoms after surgical intervention, in whom incomplete

RA

RA, the most common form of inflammatory arthritis, is characterized by inflammation of the synovial lining of joints and tendon sheaths. It frequently affects the hand and wrist early in the disease process. Although RA may become a severely disabling condition, recent clinical trials unequivocally support early intervention with aggressive pharmacologic therapy for the prevention of rapid joint erosion and the improvement of long-term outcomes.[40] The importance of timely and accurate diagnosis is implicit within this strategy. For many patients, this diagnosis is achieved only by history, physical examination, laboratory data, and conventional radiographic findings; a more expeditious diagnosis of early RA, however, may be provided with MRI.

Several reports have shown the value of MRI in detecting bone erosion and active synovitis before changes are visible on conventional radiographs.[41,42] To investigate a possible diagnosis of RA via MRI, contrast-enhanced images are obtained after an intravenous injection of contrast material. Intense bilateral contrast enhancement in the wrist, MCP, or proximal IP joints suggests active synovitis and is indicative of inflammatory arthritis (**Fig. 6.15**). Additionally, adjacent bone edema or frank erosions can be detected (**Fig. 6.16**). Because these imaging findings are nonspecific, the clinician must take into account the entire clinical pic-

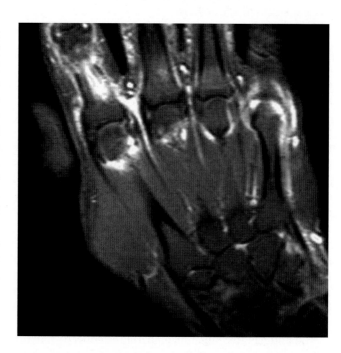

Fig. 6.15 A coronal fat-suppressed postgadolinium T1-weighted image showing diffuse high signal enhancement surrounding the MCP joints, consistent with synovitis from early RA. Conventional radiographs were normal.

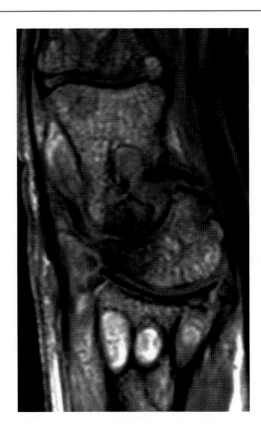

Fig. 6.16 A sagittal gradient-echo image of the wrist showing multiple subchondral cysts and periarticular erosions in the setting of advanced RA.

masses (**Fig. 6.18**). Again, axial images are best for evaluating the ulnar nerve in Guyon's canal. The information gained from MRI may help guide treatment decisions, with surgical decompression reserved for those patients in whom an extrinsic source of compression is found.

In chronic cases of any nerve compression syndrome, MRI may reveal patterns of muscle atrophy consistent with denervation of the affected nerve. Denervated muscles typically show increased signal intensity on T1-weighted images, representing fatty replacement in the more chronic setting, or on fat-suppressed T2-weighted sequences, representing muscle edema in the more acute to subacute phases.

Soft-Tissue Masses

Soft-tissue masses occur commonly in the wrist and hand. Many of these lesions, such as ganglia, can be managed reliably without the use of advanced imaging. Nevertheless, MRI remains the standard for evaluating soft-tissue masses of unclear clinical diagnoses. The primary role of MRI is in differentiating determinate from indeterminate lesions (see Chapter 15).[46] Determinate lesions are lesions that may be diagnosed on MRI by a radiologist or clinician with a high degree of certainty based on the imaging characteristics. Indeterminate lesions are lesions for which the radiologist or clinician is unable to provide a definitive diagnosis and which therefore warrant a needle or open biopsy. Intravenous contrast may help in distinguishing solid and cystic lesions.

Benign solid lesions of the wrist and hand with characteristic MRI features include hemangioma, giant cell tumor of

decompression, excessive scarring, hematoma formation, or another space-occupying lesion may be detected and for whom additional treatment can be initiated accordingly (**Fig. 6.17**).

In the evaluation of the median nerve at the carpal tunnel, T1-weighted and T2-weighted axial images are obtained to screen for obvious anatomic anomalies or pathologic findings. The median nerve is examined for changes in size, shape, or signal intensity. A predominant finding in patients with carpal tunnel syndrome is increased signal within the median nerve on T2-weighted images, which is related to chronic compression or ischemia. Other detectable abnormalities include bowing of the flexor retinaculum, deep palmar bursitis, tenosynovitis, or the presence of a space-occupying soft-tissue mass. Intraneural lesions usually are well delineated. Although dynamic and motion studies of the median nerve in the carpal tunnel have been described, they are rarely used.[45]

In the presence of ulnar nerve compression at the wrist, MRI may elucidate the cause when other diagnostic methods are unrevealing. Several etiologies include posttraumatic neuritis, occult fractures, pisotriquetral arthropathy, anatomic variants or ganglion cysts, and other soft-tissue

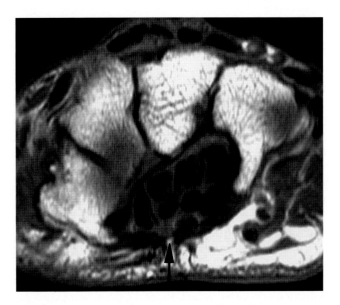

Fig. 6.17 A postoperative axial T1-weighted image at the level of the carpal tunnel showing incomplete release of the transverse carpal ligament (*arrow*).

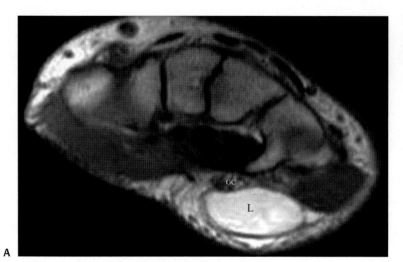

Fig. 6.18 Ulnar tunnel syndrome. An axial T1-weighted image (**A**) and artist's sketch (**B**) showing a large well-circumscribed lipoma (*L*) compressing Guyon's canal (*GC*).

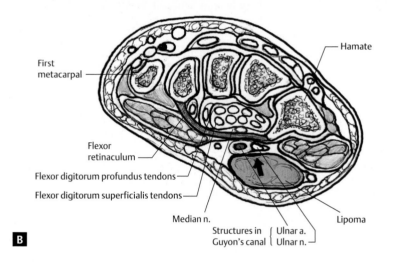

B

the tendon sheath, lipoma, Dupuytren disease, hamartoma, peripheral nerve sheath tumor, and glomus tumor (**Fig. 6.19**). Although malignant soft-tissue masses are rare in the hand and wrist, MRI may show irregular features or tissue necrosis that suggest a malignant process and require additional evaluation before excision.[47] Many malignant lesions, however, have a nonaggressive appearance on MR images. The value of MRI in the assessment of bone malignancies is to identify and characterize the extent of soft-tissue involvement.

Ganglion cysts can usually be diagnosed clinically with palpation and visualization. However, occult ganglions can be a cause of chronic dorsal wrist pain. Conventional radiography is usually normal. MRI may help in differentiating ganglion cysts from synovitis in the chronically painful wrist. In a recent study, significant differences were found between the two entities with regard to margins, shape, specific site of involvement, dimensions, internal structure, and contrast enhancement.[48] Ganglia have defined margins, a spherical shape, a septated, multilocular appearance, and wall enhancement (**Fig. 6.20**), whereas synovitis shows diffuse margins, a crescentic shape, lack of septa, and diffuse enhancement.[48] Distinguishing these two diagnoses in the setting of chronic wrist pain has obvious implications for treatment because patients with findings of chronic synovitis typically undergo a more prolonged course of nonoperative treatment than do patients with ganglia. Approximately 30% of patients with radial-side ganglia may have associated pathology, such as interosseous ligament tears, that are detectable by MRI.[49]

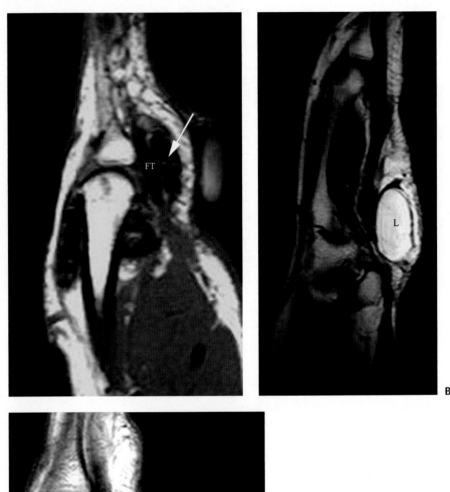

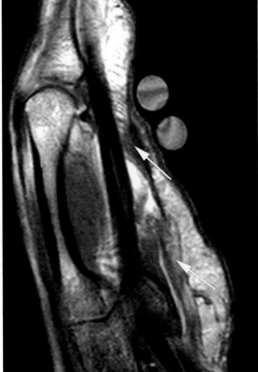

Fig. 6.19 Benign soft-tissue tumors of the hand. **(A)** Giant cell tumor of tendon sheath. A sagittal T1-weighted image of the hand and digit depicting a solid mass (*arrow*) of mixed signal intensity originating from the underlying flexor tendon (*FT*). **(B)** Lipoma. A sagittal T1-weighted image showing a well-circumscribed lipoma (*L*) in the distal palm. Note how the signal characteristics of the lipoma match those of surrounding subcutaneous fat. **(C)** Dupuytren contracture. A sagittal T1-weighted image showing thickened palmar fascial bands (*bottom arrow*) and a fibrotic nodule just proximal to the MCP joint (*top arrow*) in a patient with Dupuytren disease. The circular structures are fiduciary markers that delineate the site of the patient's symptoms.

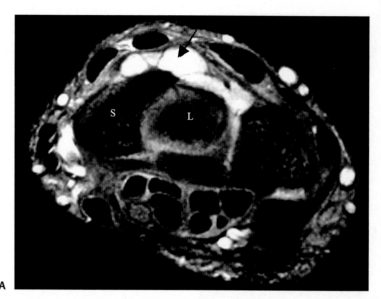
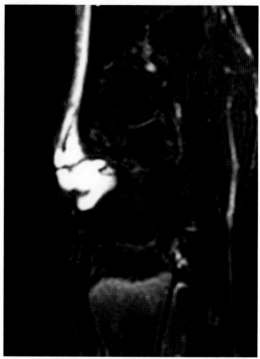

A B

Fig. 6.20 Ganglion cyst. **(A)** An axial STIR image of the wrist showing a multiloculated ganglion cyst (*arrow*) adjacent to the dorsal margin of the scapholunate articulation. *S*, scaphoid; *L*, lunate. **(B)** A sagittal STIR image depicting a dorsal ganglion cyst.

References

1. Saupe N, Prüssmann KP, Luechinger R, Bösiger P, Marincek B, Weishaupt D. MR imaging of the wrist: comparison between 1.5- and 3-T MR imaging—preliminary experience. Radiology 2005;234:256–264

2. Steinbach LS, Palmer WE, Schweitzer ME. Special focus session. MR arthrography. Radiographics 2002;22:1223–1246

3. Adey L, Souer JS, Lozano-Calderon S, Palmer W, Lee SG, Ring D. Computed tomography of suspected scaphoid fractures. J Hand Surg Am 2007;32:61–66

4. Fowler C, Sullivan B, Williams LA, McCarthy G, Savage R, Palmer A. A comparison of bone scintigraphy and MRI in the early diagnosis of the occult scaphoid waist fracture. Skeletal Radiol 1998;27:683–687

5. Memarsadeghi M, Breitenseher MJ, Schaefer-Prokop C, et al. Occult scaphoid fractures: comparison of multidetector CT and MR imaging—initial experience. Radiology 2006;240:169–176

6. Senall JA, Failla JM, Bouffard JA, van Holsbeeck M. Ultrasound for the early diagnosis of clinically suspected scaphoid fracture. J Hand Surg Am 2004;29:400–405

7. Brydie A, Raby N. Early MRI in the management of clinical scaphoid fracture. Br J Radiol 2003;76:296–300

8. Hunter JC, Escobedo EM, Wilson AJ, Hanel DP, Zink-Brody GC, Mann FA. MR imaging of clinically suspected scaphoid fractures. AJR Am J Roentgenol 1997;168:1287–1293

9. Low G, Raby N. Can follow-up radiography for acute scaphoid fracture still be considered a valid investigation? Clin Radiol 2005;60:1106–1110

10. Brooks S, Cicuttini FM, Lim S, Taylor D, Stuckey SL, Wluka AE. Cost effectiveness of adding magnetic resonance imaging to the usual management of suspected scaphoid fractures. Br J Sports Med 2005;39:75–79

11. Saxena P, McDonald R, Gull S, Hyder N. Diagnostic scanning for suspected scaphoid fractures: an economic evaluation based on cost-minimisation models. Injury 2003;34:503–511

12. Lohman M, Kivisaari A, Vehmas T, et al. MR imaging in suspected acute trauma of wrist bones. Acta Radiol 1999;40:615–618

13. Spence LD, Savenor A, Nwachuku I, Tilsley J, Eustace S. MRI of fractures of the distal radius: comparison with conventional radiographs. Skeletal Radiol 1998;27:244–249

14. Futami T, Foster BK, Morris LL, LeQuesne GW. Magnetic resonance imaging of growth plate injuries: the efficacy and indications for surgical procedures. Arch Orthop Trauma Surg 2000;120:390–396

15. Palmer AK, Werner FW. The triangular fibrocartilage complex of the wrist—anatomy and function. J Hand Surg Am 1981;6:153–162

16. Palmer AK. Triangular fibrocartilage complex lesions: a classification. J Hand Surg Am 1989;14:594–606

17. Cooney WP. Evaluation of chronic wrist pain by arthrography, arthroscopy, and arthrotomy. J Hand Surg Am 1993;18:815–822

18. Reinus WR, Hardy DC, Totty WG, Gilula LA. Arthrographic evaluation of the carpal triangular fibrocartilage complex. J Hand Surg Am 1987;12:495–503

19. Potter HG, Asnis-Ernberg L, Weiland AJ, Hotchkiss RN, Peterson MGE, McCormack RR Jr. The utility of high-resolution magnetic resonance imaging in the evaluation of the triangular fibrocartilage complex of the wrist. J Bone Joint Surg Am 1997;79:1675–1684

20. Haims AH, Schweitzer ME, Morrison WB, et al. Limitations of MR imaging in the diagnosis of peripheral tears of the triangular fibrocartilage of the wrist. AJR Am J Roentgenol 2002;178:419–422

21. Zanetti M, Bräm J, Hodler J. Triangular fibrocartilage and intercarpal ligaments of the wrist: does MR arthrography improve standard MRI? J Magn Reson Imaging 1997;7:590–594

22. Blazar PE, Chan PSH, Kneeland JB, Leatherwood D, Bozentka DJ, Kowalchick R. The effect of observer experience on magnetic resonance imaging interpretation and localization of triangular fibrocartilage complex lesions. J Hand Surg Am 2001;26:742–748

23. Daunt N. Magnetic resonance imaging of the wrist: anatomy and pathology of interosseous ligaments and the triangular fibrocartilage complex. Curr Probl Diagn Radiol 2002;31:158–176

24. Zlatkin MB, Chao PC, Osterman AL, Schnall MD, Dalinka MK, Kressel HY. Chronic wrist pain: evaluation with high-resolution MR imaging. Radiology 1989;173:723–729

25. Scheck RJ, Kubitzek C, Hierner R, et al. The scapholunate interosseous ligament in MR arthrography of the wrist: correlation with non-enhanced MRI and wrist arthroscopy. Skeletal Radiol 1997;26:263–271

26. Miller RJ. Information that orthopedists still need to know and what is missing from the MR images of the wrist. Semin Musculoskelet Radiol 2001;5:211–216

27. Shin AY, Battaglia MJ, Bishop AT. Lunotriquetral instability: diagnosis and treatment. J Am Acad Orthop Surg 2000;8:170–179

28. Ahn JM, Sartoris DJ, Kang HS, et al. Gamekeeper thumb: comparison of MR arthrography with conventional arthrography and MR imaging in cadavers. Radiology 1998;206:737–744

29. Harper MT, Chandnani VP, Spaeth J, Santangelo JR, Providence BC, Bagg MA. Gamekeeper thumb: diagnosis of ulnar collateral ligament injury using magnetic resonance imaging, magnetic resonance arthrography and stress radiography. J Magn Reson Imaging 1996;6:322–328

30. Verdan CE. Half a century of flexor-tendon surgery. Current status and changing philosophies. J Bone Joint Surg Am 1972;54:472–491

31. Hauger O, Chung CB, Lektrakul N, et al. Pulley system in the fingers: normal anatomy and simulated lesions in cadavers at MR imaging, CT, and US with and without contrast material distention of the tendon sheath. Radiology 2000;217:201–212

32. Cerezal L, del Piñal F, Abascal F, García-Valtuille R, Pereda T, Canga A. Imaging findings in ulnar-sided wrist impaction syndromes. Radiographics 2002;22:105–121

33. Berquist TH. Infection. In: Berquist TH, ed. MRI of the Hand and Wrist. Philadelphia: Lippincott Williams & Wilkins; 2003:142–152

34. Erickson SJ, Cox IH, Hyde JS, Carrera GF, Strandt JA, Estkowski LD. Effect of tendon orientation on MR imaging signal intensity: a manifestation of the "magic angle" phenomenon. Radiology 1991;181:389–392

35. Peh WCG, Chan JHM. The magic angle phenomenon in tendons: effect of varying the MR echo time. Br J Radiol 1998;71:31–36

36. Totterman SMS, Seo GS. MRI findings of scapholunate instabilities in coronal images: a short communication. Semin Musculoskelet Radiol 2001;5:251–255

37. Lichtman DM, Mack GR, MacDonald RI, Gunther SF, Wilson JN. Kienböck's disease: the role of silicone replacement arthroplasty. J Bone Joint Surg Am 1977;59:899–908

38. Kalainov DM, Cohen MS, Hendrix RW, Sweet S, Culp RW, Osterman AL. Preiser's disease: identification of two patterns. J Hand Surg Am 2003;28:767–778

39. Cerezal L, Abascal F, Canga A, García-Valtuille R, Bustamante M, del Piñal F. Usefulness of gadolinium-enhanced MR imaging in the evaluation of the vascularity of scaphoid nonunions. AJR Am J Roentgenol 2000;174:141–149

40. Quinn MA, Emery P. Potential for altering rheumatoid arthritis outcome. Rheum Dis Clin North Am 2005;31:763–772

41. Rominger MB, Bernreuter WK, Kenney PJ, Morgan SL, Blackburn WD, Alarcon GS. MR imaging of the hands in early rheumatoid arthritis: preliminary results. Radiographics 1993;13:37–46

42. Sugimoto H, Takeda A, Masuyama J, Furuse M. Early-stage rheumatoid arthritis: diagnostic accuracy of MR imaging. Radiology 1996;198:185–192

43. Sugimoto H, Takeda A, Hyodoh K. Early-stage rheumatoid arthritis: prospective study of the effectiveness of MR imaging for diagnosis. Radiology 2000;216:569–575

44. Taouli B, Guermazi A, Sack KE, Genant HK. Imaging of the hand and wrist in RA. Ann Rheum Dis 2002;61:867–869

45. Brahme SK, Hodler J, Braun RM, Sebrechts C, Jackson W, Resnick D. Dynamic MR imaging of carpal tunnel syndrome. Skeletal Radiol 1997;26:482–487

46. Frassica FJ, Khanna JA, McCarthy EF. The role of MR imaging in soft tissue tumor evaluation: perspective of the orthopedic oncologist and musculoskeletal pathologist. Magn Reson Imaging Clin North Am 2000;8:915–927

47. Teh J, Whiteley G. MRI of soft tissue masses of the hand and wrist. Br J Radiol 2007;80:47–63

48. Anderson SE, Steinbach LS, Stauffer E, Voegelin E. MRI for differentiating ganglion and synovitis in the chronic painful wrist. AJR Am J Roentgenol 2006;186:812–818

49. el-Noueam KI, Schweitzer ME, Blasbalg R, et al. Is a subset of wrist ganglia the sequela of internal derangements of the wrist joint? MR imaging findings. Radiology 1999;212:537–540

III Lower Extremity

7 The Hip

Michael K. Shindle, Bryan T. Kelly, Luis E. Moya, and Douglas N. Mintz

■ Specialized Pulse Sequences and Imaging Protocols

As with MRI of any anatomic region, accurate MRI assessment of the hip requires attention to technical detail. Traditionally, MRI of the hip performed for suspicion of osteonecrosis or an occult fracture used a large body coil within the magnet bore, which provided very poor in-plane resolution and little to no detail of the articular cartilage or labrum. More recently, surface coils have been used to evaluate the hip, providing much higher spatial resolution. However, initial body coil sequences of the entire pelvis are still helpful for screening for other etiologies of pain, such as the following:

- Muscle strains
- Pelvic masses
- Hernias
- Spine and sacroiliac joint pathology
- Occult fractures

At the authors' institution, coronal inversion recovery and axial proton-density sequences are obtained using a body coil, followed by the use of a surface coil with cartilage-sensitive, intermediate TE, FSE pulse sequences in the coronal, sagittal, and axial planes, with high in-plane and segment resolution. The authors' institution also prefers to use an intermediate TE sequence rather than T1-weighted and T2-weighted images for several reasons. First, T1 is not good for evaluating cartilage because there is no contrast between fluid and cartilage. Second, it is also not good for evaluating subtle muscle abnormalities, so another sequence in each plane would be required for a thorough evaluation, and yet a third for cartilage. The intermediate TE sequence eliminates that redundancy by allowing enough signal for excellent resolution and enough contrast to evaluate all the structures (bone, ligament, tendon, muscle, and articular cartilage) and the quality of synovitis, if present. One can obtain this sequence in each plane and then add one fat-suppressed sequence to evaluate for subtle findings and assess acuity.

Many authors advocate using MR arthrography of the hip for the evaluation of labral pathology and articular cartilage (see Chapter 14),[1–3] but this modality increases the cost and imaging time, and makes MRI an invasive procedure.[4] Mintz et al.[5] evaluated 92 patients before hip arthroscopy via an optimized protocol similar to that outlined above

and concluded that noncontrast imaging can identify labral and chondral pathology. However, many institutions in the United States and abroad continue to use MR arthrography to improve the visualization of intraarticular hip pathology, especially labral pathology.[6]

■ Traumatic Conditions and the Athletic Hip

Acetabular Labral Tears

The fibrocartilaginous labrum (type I collagen) appears as a triangular, low signal intensity structure attached to the rim of the acetabulum[7] (**Fig. 7.1**). Labral pathology can be a cause of substantial hip pain (**Table 7.1**) and is associated

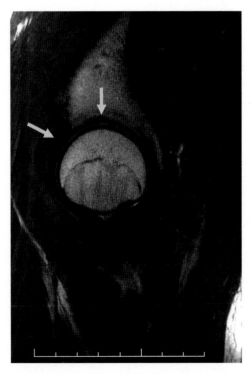

Fig. 7.1 A sagittal FSE image of the hip showing a normal anterior labrum (*left arrow*) as a triangular focus of low signal and normal articular cartilage of the acetabulum (*top arrow*). (© 2009 Hospital for Special Surgery, New York, NY.)

147

Table 7.1   Differential Diagnosis of Hip Pain

Primary labral pathology	Nonmusculoskeletal causes
Femoroacetabular impingement	Genitourinary
Laxity	Spine
Trauma	Psoas muscle abscess
Dysplasia	Hernia
Degenerative	Endometriosis
	Ovarian cyst
	Peripheral vascular disease
Primary chondral	**Unknown etiology**
Lateral impact	Transient osteoporosis of the hip
Subluxation/dislocation	Bone marrow edema syndrome
Osteonecrosis	
Loose bodies	
Degeneration	
Primary capsule	**Synovial proliferative disorders**
Laxity	PVNS
Adhesive capsulitis	Synovial chondromatosis
Synovitis/inflammation	Chondrocalcinosis
Extraarticular	**Infectious/tumor/metabolic**
Snapping hip (internal/external)	Septic arthritis
Trochanteric bursitis	Osteomyelitis
Ischial bursitis	
Psoas bursitis	Neoplasms
Osteitis pubis	Benign bone and soft tissue
Sports hernia	Malignant bone and soft tissue
Piriformis syndrome	Paget disease
Sacroiliac joint	Primary hyperparathyroidism
Tendinitis	Metastatic bone disease
Hip flexor	
Adductor	
Abductor	
Gluteus medius tear	
Inflammatory	**Systemic**
RA	Polyarticular
Reiter syndrome	Reflex sympathetic dystrophy
Psoriatic arthritis	Complex regional pain syndrome
Bursitis	Hormonal

Source: From Shindle MK, Ranawat AS, Kelly BT. Diagnosis and management of traumatic and atraumatic hip instability in the athletic patient. Clin Sports Med 2006;25:309–326. Reprinted by permission.

with the development of osteoarthritis.[8] The labrum surrounds the rim of the acetabulum nearly circumferentially and is contiguous with the transverse acetabular ligament across the acetabular notch. The labrum is thickest superiorly and posteriorly and widest anteriorly and superiorly. The joint capsule attaches to the acetabular rim adjacent to the labrum; however, at the superior aspect of the joint, the capsule inserts a few millimeters above the labrum, which creates a sublabral recess or sulcus.[9] Neuroreceptors that provide proprioception have been identified, and there is a limited blood supply to the periphery of the labrum.[10,11]

Labral tears are diagnosed by the presence of increased signal intensity (often equivalent to that of synovial fluid) on fat-suppressed images through the substance of the labrum, with or without displacement (**Fig. 7.2**). Partial or complete detachment is characterized by fluid-matching signal undermining the attachment between the labrum and acetabulum. The presence of paralabral cysts should prompt careful inspection of the labrum to discern the often subtle splits that serve as the origin for these cysts (**Fig. 7.3**). Lecouvet et al.[12] performed MRI of the hip in 200 asymptomatic individuals and showed that intralabral areas of high signal intensity communicating with the free surface increased with age.

To optimize outcomes, the underlying etiology of the injury must be identified. In addition to degenerative labral tears associated with arthritis, there are at least five causes of labral tears[13]:

- Femoroacetabular impingement
- Traumatic labral injury (dislocation/subluxation)
- Atraumatic capsular laxity (hypermobility)

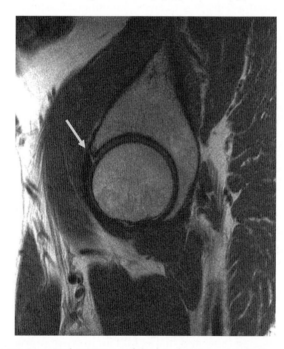

Fig. 7.2 A sagittal FSE image of the hip showing a nondisplaced anterior labral tear (*arrow*). (© 2009 Hospital for Special Surgery, New York, NY.)

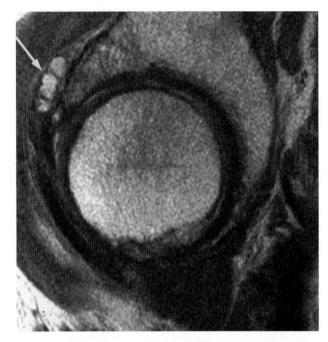

Fig. 7.3 A sagittal FSE image of the hip showing paralabral cysts associated with an anterior labral tear (*arrow*) and full-thickness cartilage loss of the anterior acetabulum. (© 2009 Hospital for Special Surgery, New York, NY)

- Psoas impingement
- Dysplastic labral tears

Several classification systems have been used for labral tears, two of which are described here. In a cadaveric study, Seldes et al.[14] determined histologically that there were two distinct types of tears (**Fig. 7.4**):

- Detachment of the labrum from the hyaline cartilage at the transitional zone (type 1)
- Cleavage of variable depth within the substance of the labrum (type 2)

In another study, Lage et al.[15] developed an arthroscopic classification based on morphology:

- Radial flap tear
- Radial fibrillated tear
- Longitudinal peripheral tear
- Unstable tear

A recent article by Ilizaliturri et al.[16] described a zone method with which to classify intraarticular pathology at hip arthroscopy (**Fig. 7.5**). Among a group of expert hip arthroscopists, the zone method was found to be more reproducible than the clock-face method.[16]

Two potential pitfalls may occur when interpreting noncontrast MRI and MR arthrography studies, potentially leading to an inaccurate diagnosis of a labral tear. First, there is a normal variant of the posteroinferior sublabral groove, which is a relatively common occurrence and typically seen on axial images.[9] The clinician should recognize that this location is distinct from that of most labral tears. The second variant is a superior sublabral recess at the anterosuperior margin of the acetabulum, which has been described in the presence of mild acetabular dysplasia.[17]

The prevalence of labral tears in the anterosuperior labrum reportedly is high, and several authors have speculated that this tear may be secondary to decreased vascularity in this zone.[13,14] In an evaluation of 12 hips from six cadavers, Kelly et al.[13] used a modified Spalteholz technique to map the

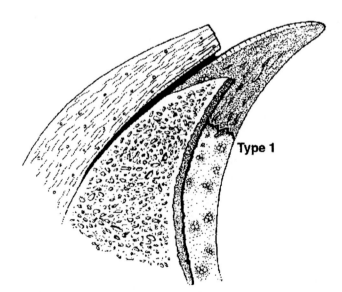

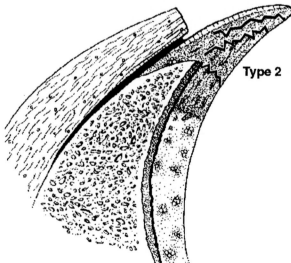

Fig. 7.4 Seldes type 1 and type 2 labral tears: detachment of the labrum from the hyaline cartilage at the transitional zone and cleavage of variable depth within the substance of the labrum, respectively. (From Seldes RM, Tan V, Hunt J, Katz M, Winiarsky R, Fitzgerald RH Jr. Anatomy, histologic features, and vascularity of the adult acetabular labrum. Clin Orthop Relat Res 2001;382:232–240. Reprinted by permission.)

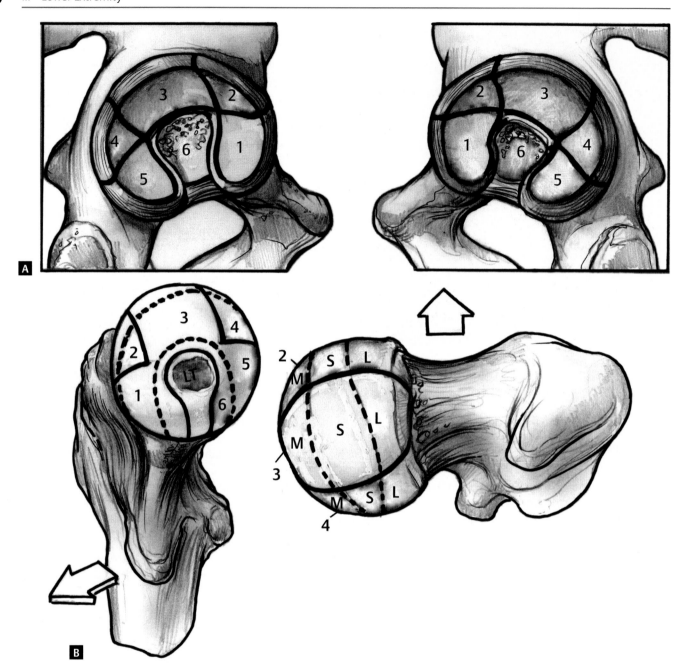

Fig. 7.5 Zone classification. **(A)** An artist's depiction of the left and right hemipelves. The acetabulum has been subdivided into six zones: 1, anterior-inferior; 2, anterior-superior; 3, central superior; 4, posterior-superior; 5, posterior-inferior; and 6, acetabular notch. **(B)** An artist's depiction of the left and right proximal femurs. (*Left*) The frontal view of the femoral head is divided into six zones around the acetabular fossa (there is a dotted line around the ligamentum teres [*LT*]): 1, anterior-inferior; 2, anterior-superior; 3, central superior; 4, posterior-superior; 5, posterior-inferior; and 6, area around the ligamentum teres. (*Right*) The superior view shows the three subdivisions of zones 2, 3, and 4: medial (*M*), superior (*S*), and lateral (*L*). (From Ilizaliturri VM Jr, Byrd JWT, Sampson TG, et al. A geographic zone method to describe intra-articular pathology in hip arthroscopy: cadaveric study and preliminary report. Arthroscopy 2008;24:534–539. Reprinted by permission.)

anatomic zones of labral vascularity. They reported that cadaveric specimens have relatively avascular hip labra, with no statistically significant ($p > .05$) differences among the anterior, superior, posterior, or inferior labral lesions, or in torn versus intact specimens. However, slightly increased vascularity was seen on the capsular compared with the articular side, suggesting that the vascularity usually is supplied by the capsule. Those authors also noted that all labral tears were associated with increased microvascularity at the labral base, adjacent to the attachment of bone. Such studies have important future implications for labral surgery in terms of determining the type and location of tears that would be amenable to successful repair, as opposed to arthroscopic debridement.

MRI evaluation of the postoperative labrum is similar to that of the postoperative meniscus in the knee. Because labral debridement causes a persistent intralabral signal secondary to abnormally mobile water in the degenerative fibrocartilage, the presence of abnormal signal alone should not serve as a primary indicator of a re-tear. The most reliable indicator of a re-tear of a labral remnant is the presence of a displaced fragment.

Stress Fractures

Stress fractures, which result from cyclic mechanical stress, can be subdivided into one of two groups: fatigue or insufficiency. Military recruits and athletes are more susceptible than the general population to fatigue fractures, given that they occur in normal bone that is exposed to a repetitive mechanical overload that overwhelms the normal remodeling process.[18] Insufficiency fractures occur more commonly in the elderly secondary to osteoporosis, osteomalacia, or other processes that weaken the bone, permitting osseous failure to occur after fewer loading cycles than in normal bone. Insufficiency fractures in the athletic population have also been described in female athletes, in association with the female athletic triad.[19] Stress fractures can occur on the compression or the tension side of the femoral neck.[20] Compression stress fractures are more common and begin at the inferior cortex of the femoral neck. Tension stress fractures begin in the superior cortex, have a greater propensity to displace, and thus require more aggressive treatment. A fracture line with a benign periosteal reaction may be visualized on conventional radiography or CT, and bone scintigraphy may be sensitive but not specific for the diagnosis of femoral neck stress fracture. However, MRI is sensitive and specific to the presence of underlying bone marrow lesions, and a linear fracture line associated with the preservation of fatty marrow should be sought to confirm the diagnosis of a stress fracture.[20,21] Fat-suppressed or STIR coronal images show a linear pattern of increased signal intensity, which is compatible with an acute or subacute fracture (**Fig. 7.6**). MRI is also useful for excluding underlying lesions, such as a tumor, or marrow disorders that may be the cause of a pathologic stress fracture.

Traumatic Posterior Subluxation/ Dislocation/Lateral Impaction

A traumatic posterior hip dislocation most commonly occurs as a result of a motor vehicle accident when the hip and knee are flexed and the knee impacts on the dashboard, producing

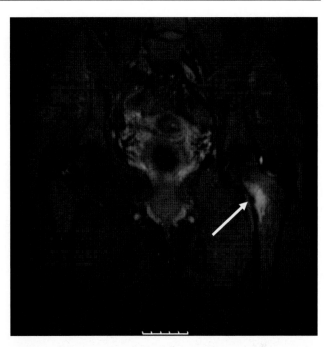

Fig. 7.6 A coronal fat-suppressed image obtained with a body coil technique, showing increased signal intensity (*arrow*) surrounding a stress fracture at the medial aspect of the left femoral neck. (© 2009 Hospital for Special Surgery, New York, NY.)

a posteriorly directed force on the hip. In the acute setting, MRI may aid in the diagnosis of the following[22,23]:

- Femoral head contusions
- Labral disruptions
- Sciatic nerve injury
- Intraarticular fragments

Hip subluxation usually has a more subtle presentation than does hip dislocation because of its lower energy mechanism of injury, such as a fall on a flexed hip and knee; however, subluxation is a potentially devastating injury that may be misdiagnosed as a simple hip strain or sprain. Traumatic posterior subluxation events in football or other high-level athletic activities may cause symptomatic cartilage-shearing injuries and labral tears, but they are not associated with radiographic documentation of a dislocation.[24] Depending on the degree of force applied to the hip at the time of translation, the posterior labrum or wall may be displaced and/or combined with anterior labral tears, disruption of the iliofemoral ligament, and parafoveal cartilage shearing injuries; the latter two typically are sustained at the time of reduction (**Fig. 7.7**). MRI is also a useful tool for detecting the complication of osteonecrosis and for assisting in the determination of when athletes may return safely to sports activity[24,25] (see Osteonecrosis, below). Byrd[26] described a lateral impaction injury as a direct blow to the greater trochanter, resulting in isolated traumatic chondral injuries in young, physically fit individuals as a consequence of sports

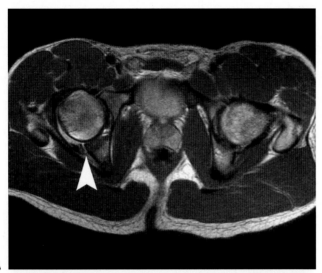

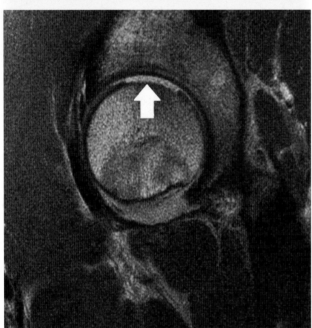

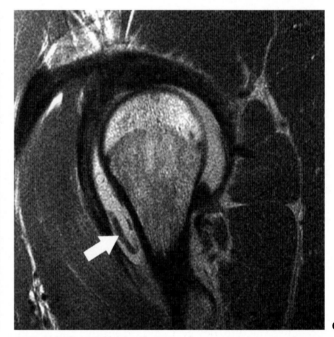

Fig. 7.7 Posterior hip subluxation. Axial body coil **(A)** and sagittal surface coil **(B,C)** FSE images of the hip in an 18-year-old patient with sequelae of posterior hip subluxation. An intact right posterior hip capsule is seen, attached to a posterior wall fracture (**A**, arrowhead), and associated with a large full-thickness chondral shear injury of the femoral head (**B**, arrow). Cartilaginous debris (**C**, arrow) is seen within the anteroinferior dependent recess of the joint. (From Shindle MK, Foo LF, Kelly BT, et al. Magnetic resonance imaging of cartilage in the athlete: current techniques and spectrum of disease. J Bone Joint Surg Am 2006;88:27–46. Reprinted by permission. © 2009 Hospital for Special Surgery, New York, NY.)

or activity. MRI is useful in this scenario for determining the extent of chondral damage and for evaluating the presence of osteochondral loose bodies.

Greater Trochanteric Pain Syndrome

Greater trochanteric pain syndrome is a common regional pain syndrome that encompasses greater trochanteric bursitis and tears/tendinosis of the gluteus medius and minimus. The major clinical findings are nonspecific, usually with tenderness localized to the lateral aspect of the hip or thigh. Clinically, distinguishing isolated bursal pathologic changes from tendon abnormalities or other soft-tissue lesions is difficult; therefore, the differential diagnosis is quite broad and

requires consideration of articular, periarticular, and distant processes as a source of lateral hip pain.[27]

Trochanteric Bursitis

The surface of the greater trochanter has four distinct facets:

- Anterior
- Posterior
- Lateral
- Superoposterior

The overlying trochanteric bursa is composed of three discrete components[27]:

- Subgluteus maximus bursa
- Subgluteus medius bursa
- Subgluteus minimus bursa

Excessive friction from the overlying ITB is the most likely etiology, but trochanteric bursitis often is a manifestation of underlying abductor tendon pathology. Thus, the presence of trochanteric bursitis should prompt careful attention to the underlying abductor tendons. Fat-suppressed MR sequences, particularly coronal and axial images, should be evaluated for bursal distention with high signal intensity.

Abductor Tears

The gluteus medius inserts onto the superoposterior and lateral facets, and the gluteus minimus inserts onto the anterior facet of the greater trochanter. MRI evaluation of the hip in patients more than 40 years old usually reveals several pathologic processes, including some degree of the following[28,29]:

- Cartilage degeneration
- Degenerative labral lesions
- Extracapsular abnormalities (including abductor or iliopsoas tendinosis)

Abductor tears have been termed the "rotator cuff tears of the hip" and are highly prevalent in patients with osteoarthritis.[30,31] Again, the coronal and axial sequences should be evaluated for the presence or absence of such tears. Greater trochanteric bursitis is usually indicated by increased signal on fat-suppressed images (**Fig. 7.8A**). Partial-thickness tears

show hyperintensity with abnormal morphology of the torn tendon fibers, and full-thickness tears show a fluid-filled gap with a retracted tendon (**Fig. 7.8B**). Some patients have "intractable" complaints of trochanteric bursitis despite multiple injections and nonoperative treatment. For such patients, MRI may be diagnostic for a gluteus medius or minimus rupture.[32] The MRI appearance of abductor tendinosis or tears, which includes alterations in tendon caliber and signal, is the same as that in other locations.

Snapping Hip Syndrome (Coxa Saltans)

The snapping hip syndrome, or coxa saltans, is characterized by an audible or palpable snapping of the hip with flexion and extension of the hip, occasionally resulting in pain. The etiology of coxa saltans has been divided into three categories[33]:

- Intraarticular
- Internal (snapping of iliopsoas tendon against an osseous ridge)
- External (snapping of the ITB or gluteus maximus muscle over the greater trochanter)

It is important to accurately determine the source of the snapping so that the appropriate treatment can be given. MRI is useful for excluding other intra- or extraarticular hip abnormalities, but its role in diagnosing coxa saltans is limited because of its lack of dynamic capabilities. With internal coxa saltans, fat-suppressed images may display a hyperintense iliopsoas bursa fluid. With external coxa saltans,

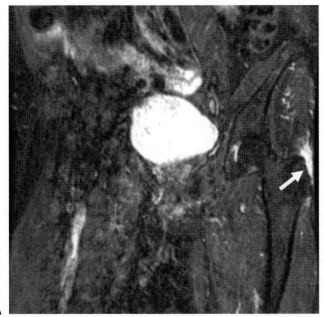

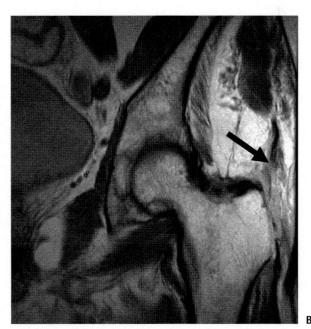

A   B

Fig. 7.8 Hip abductor tear. **(A)** A coronal fat-suppressed image of the hip showing a fluid-filled space that should be occupied by the left hip abductors, indicating a tear (*arrow*). **(B)** An FSE image showing tendinosis of the gluteus medius tendon (*arrow*) with dehiscence of its insertion from the greater trochanter. (© 2009 Hospital for Special Surgery, New York, NY.)

fat-suppressed images may show a hyperintense ITB, trochanteric bursa, and anterior border of the gluteus maximus. Because of MRI's lack of dynamic capabilities, dynamic sonography of the hip is beneficial as an adjuvant to confirm the diagnosis.

Piriformis Syndrome

The sciatic nerve exits the pelvis through the greater sciatic notch, which is formed, in part, by the piriformis tendon. Although variations exist, the nerve usually is located immediately anterior to the piriformis muscle. Irritation of the piriformis musculotendinous unit can cause compression of the sciatic nerve, which in turn may cause pain and dysesthesias in the gluteal region or radicular-type symptoms.[34] MRI may show an abnormal hypertrophic piriformis muscle and/or hyperintensity of the sciatic nerve on fat-suppressed images or a variant course of the nerve through the piriformis muscle. There is usually a mass effect, resulting in displacement of the muscle from anterior to posterior with a loss of normal muscle striations. There may be effacement of fat in the greater sciatic foramen, and gluteal atrophy may be present.[35] Neurophysiologic testing may be required to confirm the diagnosis.[34]

Muscle Strains

The most frequent injuries about the groin and hip are muscle strains and tears. These injuries usually affect the myotendinous junction, which is the weakest point of the musculotendinous unit, but they may also occur via avulsion at the osseous insertion or origin.[36] Apophyseal avulsion injuries usually occur in the adolescent population and

are equivalent to muscle strains in the adult. During running and jumping activities, the hamstring origins at the ischial tuberosity may be avulsed; these injuries have been referred to as hurdler's fractures.[37] Apophyseal injuries of the pelvis may also involve the rectus femoris or sartorius muscles at the anteroinferior or anterosuperior iliac spines, respectively. In competitive sports that require kicking motions with extreme hip flexion, avulsions of the iliopsoas tendon off the lesser trochanter may be seen.

The most commonly strained muscles around the hip joint are the following:

- Hamstrings (biceps femoris, semimembranosus, and semitendinosus)
- Rectus femoris
- Adductors

The adductor group is frequently involved, especially in hockey, soccer, and football players; in those athletes, medial thigh or groin pain is the presenting complaint.[36] The MRI classification is based on the extent of disruption present: in general, on fat-suppressed images, muscle avulsions and tears have high signal intensity in areas of hemorrhage or edema. First-degree strains have a minor degree of fiber disruption and a "feathery" pattern of increased signal intensity on fat-suppressed T2-weighted images secondary to interstitial edema and hemorrhage that extends into the adjacent muscle fascicles. Second-degree strains have a partial tear without retraction and often also have a hematoma at the myotendinous junction. Third-degree strains have a complete rupture of the myotendinous unit.[38] Acute tendinous avulsion injuries of the rectus femoris tendon at its origin at the anterior inferior iliac spine can be seen. This injury occurs most commonly after forceful extension of the hip[35] (**Fig. 7.9**). Hamstring tears are usually partial-thickness, and the proximal long head of the biceps femoris is the most frequently injured structure, followed by the semitendinosus and semimembranosus muscles. Injuries usually occur at the musculotendinous junction with the characteristic feather-like edema pattern described above.

■ Bone Marrow Abnormalities

Osteonecrosis

Osteonecrosis (also termed avascular necrosis or aseptic necrosis) of the femoral head is the cellular necrosis of the bone and bone marrow elements that compromise a part of or the entire femoral head. Osteonecrosis is the preferred term because it makes no reference to the pathophysiology of the disease. There are numerous predisposing causes, including the following[39]:

- Corticosteroid usage
- Collagen vascular disease

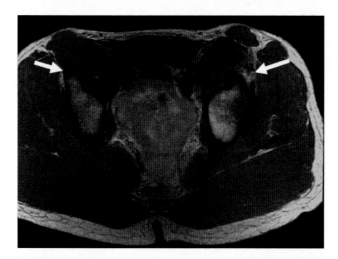

Fig. 7.9 An axial FSE image obtained with a body coil technique, showing avulsion of the proximal portion of the rectus femoris from the left anterior inferior iliac spine (*left arrow*). A normal low signal tendinous insertion is seen on the right (*right arrow*). (© 2009 Hospital for Special Surgery, New York, NY)

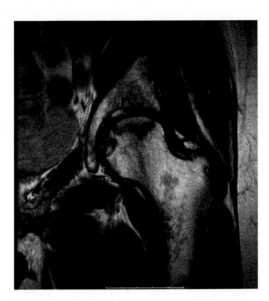

Fig. 7.10 A coronal FSE image of the left hip showing a region of osteonecrosis at the weight-bearing surface of the femoral head with a classic serpentine line of demarcation from the adjacent normal bone. (© 2009 Hospital for Special Surgery, New York, NY.)

- Dislocation of the hip
- Femoral neck fracture
- Hemoglobinopathies

MRI has been shown to be more sensitive than conventional radiography, nuclear scintigraphy, or CT for the early detection of osteonecrosis.[40–43] Besides aiding in this early detection, MRI is useful for differentiating osteonecrosis from other pathologic processes and for predicting the likelihood of femoral head collapse.[44,45] Osteonecrosis of the femoral head has a characteristic MRI appearance: a low-signal, crescent-shaped rim in a subchondral location that corresponds to the interface between normal and ischemic bone (**Fig. 7.10**). A second rim of increased signal that is pathognomonic of osteonecrosis usually is present on fat-suppressed images.[42,44] The presence of a band of low signal intensity on T1-weighted images or of the "double-line" sign on T2-weighted or fat-suppressed proton-density images are each reported to be an early specific sign of nontraumatic osteonecrosis of the femoral head.[42,43] The double-line sign, which appears as a low signal intensity peripheral line and a parallel inner line of high signal intensity, can be observed in up to 80% of lesions.[46] These MRI abnormalities represent the reactive interface between necrotic and viable bone.[42,47] MRI may also show a joint effusion on fat-suppressed sequences.

In the presence of a posterior hip subluxation, MRI is a useful tool for detecting osteonecrosis. In the acute setting, MRI is not an accurate predictor of osteonecrosis, and a repeat study is usually obtained at 6 weeks. If there is no evidence of osteonecrosis, patients may safely return to sports activity. However, if there is evidence of osteonecrosis, patients are at increased risk for subsequent collapse and joint degeneration.[24]

A limited MRI examination may be obtained for the detection of femoral head osteonecrosis and quantification of the size of the lesion in selected patients.[48] Several methods have been proposed to measure the extent of osteonecrosis for prognosis and treatment planning. Lafforgue et al[49] measured the α angle on the coronal T1-weighted images, selecting the largest area of necrosis and determining the angle formed at the center of the femoral head. An angle of more than 75 degrees was considered to have a poor prognosis, and an angle of less than 46 degrees corresponded to a satisfactory clinical response. Koo and Kim[50] measured the angle formed from the center of the femoral head on midcoronal and midsagittal MR images to quantify the size of the lesion objectively. Cherian et al[51] modified this method for quantifying the extent of osteonecrosis of the femoral head by using the coronal and sagittal MR images with maximal femoral head involvement. They concluded that that method was a reproducible and reliable way of determining the extent of osteonecrosis.

A low percentage of involvement of the femoral head weight-bearing surface has been well correlated with a favorable outcome in patients with early stages of the disease[49] and the unlikelihood of femoral head collapse after core decompressive surgery.[52] In one study, femoral head collapse did not occur when the MRI showed that less than 25% of the weight-bearing surface was involved.[52] However, when more than 50% of the surface was involved, 87% of hips had femoral head collapse.[52]

MRI is also useful for identifying and localizing the necrotic lesion before performing a core decompression procedure. It is also not infrequent to see cartilage loss and geode formation on the acetabular side as a result of osteonecrosis of the femoral head.[49] This finding is important because it may change the treatment approach—for example, total hip replacement rather than femoral head resurfacing or core decompression.

Idiopathic Transient Osteoporosis

Idiopathic transient osteoporosis is a rare and often unrecognized cause of hip pain that is usually seen healthy young adults. The condition most commonly affects women in the third trimester of pregnancy and middle-aged men. Symptoms often present insidiously, with pain in the affected hip, and then progress to gait disturbance and functional disability. Transient osteoporosis of the hip should be considered after more common causes of hip pain (such as infection, stress fractures, or malignancy) are ruled out. Conventional radiographs usually show focal osteopenia of the femoral head and neck with loss of cortical continuity, although this finding may be subtle and is frequently missed. Fat-suppressed MR images show diffuse high signal intensity compatible with edema in the femoral head and proximal femoral neck and a small hip joint effusion, which are the classic findings of transient osteoporosis of the hip. However, this diffuse edema pattern may be related to a subtle subchondral fracture[53,54] (**Fig. 7.11**). This entity can be differentiated from osteonecrosis of the hip, which shows signal changes at the weight-bearing surface of the femoral head and is not as diffuse as that seen with transient osteoporosis of the hip. Most cases resolve spontaneously within 6 to 12 months.

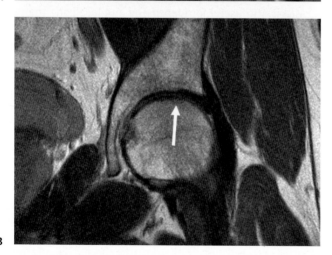

Fig. 7.11 Transient osteoporosis of the hip. **(A)** A coronal FSE image with fat suppression showing diffuse and extensive high signal of the left femoral head without a demarcated focus (*arrow*). Because there is no evidence of demarcation defining osteonecrosis, the diagnosis is consistent with transient osteoporosis of the hip. **(B)** Most cases of transient osteoporosis actually represent subchondral femoral head stress fractures, which can be appreciated on this coronal FSE image (*arrow*). (© 2009 Hospital for Special Surgery, New York, NY)

However, subchondral fractures leading to femoral head collapse have been reported.[46] Therefore, patients should be treated with protected weight bearing and monitored carefully with repeat MRI until the edema is resolved and the clinical symptoms subside.

■ Degenerative Conditions

Femoroacetabular Impingement

Femoroacetabular impingement is a well-described pathologic condition that has been associated with predisposing factors such as the following[55–59]:

- Slipped capital femoral epiphysis
- Abnormal extension of the femoral head epiphysis
- Acetabular retroversion

Repetitive microtrauma from impingement during hip flexion and internal rotation leads to degeneration of the acetabular labrum and articular cartilage. This progressive degeneration and tearing of the labrum, as well as damage to the articular cartilage, predisposes patients to osteoarthritis.[46,57,58,60,61] Femoroacetabular impingement is caused by two main types of mechanisms: "cam" and "pincer." Most femoroacetabular impingement cases represent a combination of both mechanisms[62] (see Chapter 14) (**Fig. 7.12**). MRI is an excellent modality for femoroacetabular impingement because it permits early detection of the disease process and can identify labral tears, cartilage damage, subchondral cysts, and underlying subtle anatomic variations of the femoral head–neck junction or acetabulum associated with cam or pincer impingement.

The cam type involves shear forces created by the nonspherical portion of the femoral head impinging on the acetabulum, resulting in a characteristic pattern of cartilage loss over the anterosuperior weight-bearing portion of the acetabulum and, eventually, possible tear or detachment of the principally uninvolved labrum[56,58] (**Fig. 7.13**). MRI is an excellent modality for assessment of femoroacetabular impingement because it can detect subtle anatomic variations of the femoral head–neck junction, labral pathology, adjacent cartilage damage, and subchondral cysts. Typical findings on fat-suppressed images may include any of the following:

- Intermediate-signal labral degeneration
- Labral tears with a hyperintense linear or diffuse signal intensity
- Defects or fissures in the articular cartilage
- Hyperintense femoral head/neck cysts

Typical findings on FSE sequences may include abnormal contour of the acetabular labrum and a cam lesion. Decreased offset of the femoral head–neck junction can be detected on conventional radiographs or MRI as a prominent lateral extension of the femoral head at the step-off to the adjacent femoral neck.[46] Other features that can be present on MR images are the following:

- Congruent but nonspherical head
- Small head-to-neck ratio
- Short neck

As part of the multiplanar assessment of femoroacetabular impingement, oblique axial MRI sequences can be helpful in defining the abnormal osseous neck-shaft offset. In those images, the segment prescription is parallel to the neck-shaft angle of a coronal image, passing directly through the center of the femoral head. The α angle, measured according to the method of Nötzli et al,[63] can help define the anterior margin of the waist of the femoral neck (**Fig. 7.14**).

The pincer type involves contact between a normal femoral neck and an abnormal anterior acetabular rim secondary to acetabular retroversion or protrusion. In this setting, the acetabular labrum fails first, which leads to degeneration and eventual ossification, worsening the over-coverage (retroversion). In patients with a retroverted acetabulum, axial MR images show increased coverage of the anterior femoral head.[64] During flexion and internal rotation, the prominent anterolateral edge of the acetabulum leads to impingement and subsequent labral degeneration. Synovial fluid may penetrate into the subchondral bone and lead to subchondral cyst formation.[56,64,65] In addition, persistent anterior abutment can result in contre-coup cartilage lesions of the posteroinferior acetabulum. Overall, the pincer type has limited chondral lesions compared with the deep chondral lesions associated with cam impingement.[59,66]

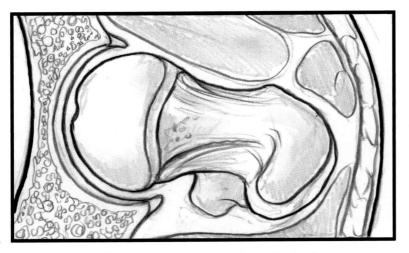

A

Acetabular over-coverage   Femoral head-neck convexity

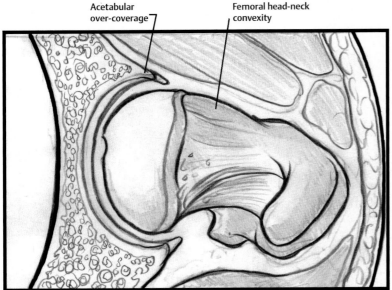

B

Fig. 7.12 Diagrammatic representation of **(A)** normal acetabulum and femur morphology and **(B)** combined femoroacetabular impingement with reduced head-neck offset (cam mechanism) and excessive anterior over-coverage (pincer mechanism).

Osteoarthritis

Osteoarthritis is characterized by articular cartilage degenerative change with hip joint space narrowing; the incidence of this process increases with age. There are several conditions that lead to osteoarthritis, including the following[46]:

- Femoroacetabular impingement
- Previous slipped capital femoral epiphysis
- Developmental dysplasia of the hip
- Legg-Calvé-Perthes disease
- Trauma
- Other anatomic variants

The appearance of osteoarthritis on MR images is similar to that on conventional radiographs, including the following:

- Hypointense subchondral sclerosis of the femoral head and acetabulum
- Joint space narrowing
- Osteophyte formation
- Subchondral cysts

Osteoarthritis may also be associated with labral tears, paralabral cysts, synovitis, or osteonecrosis of the femoral head.[67]

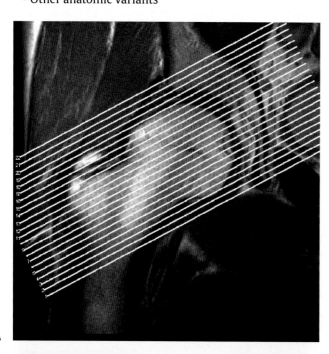

A

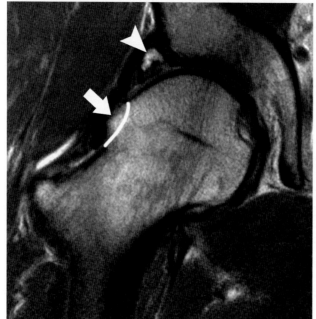

B

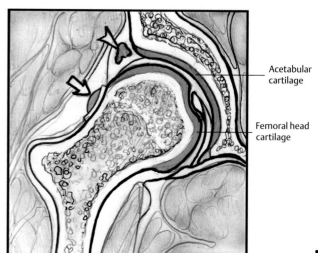

Acetabular cartilage

Femoral head cartilage

C

Fig. 7.13 FSE images and sketches of a 41-year-old patient with combined femoroacetabular impingement of the right hip. **(A)** The segment prescription (© 2009 Hospital for Special Surgery, New York, NY). The coronal image (© 2009 Hospital for Special Surgery, New York, NY) **(B)** and associated artist's sketch **(C)** show a torn superior labrum (*arrowhead on each*) and a cam lesion at the neck–shaft junction (*arrow on each*). (Adapted from Shindle MK, Foo LF, Kelly BT, et al. Magnetic resonance imaging of cartilage in the athlete: current techniques and spectrum of disease. J Bone Joint Surg Am 2006;88:27–46. Adapted by permission.) (Continued on page 159)

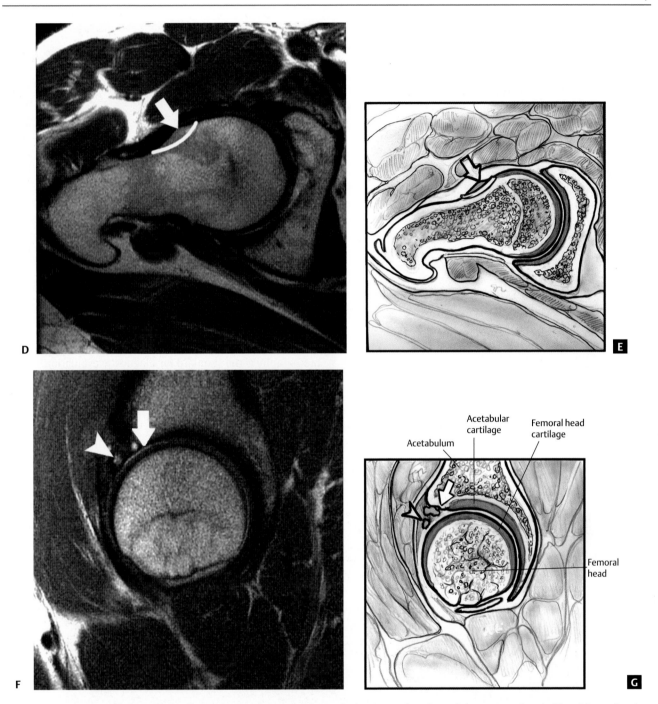

Fig. 7.13 (*Continued*) The oblique axial view (© 2009 Hospital for Special Surgery, New York, NY) **(D)** and associated artist's sketch **(E)** *(arrow on each)* accentuate the osseous defect (cam lesion). The sagittal image (© 2009 Hospital for Special Surgery, New York, NY) **(F)** and associated artist's sketch **(G)** show full-thickness cartilage loss over the anterior acetabular dome (*arrow on each*) and partial-thickness cartilage loss of the anterior femoral head (*arrowhead on each*). (Adapted from Shindle MK, Foo LF, Kelly BT, et al. Magnetic resonance imaging of cartilage in the athlete: current techniques and spectrum of disease. J Bone Joint Surg Am 2006;88:27–46. Adapted by permission.)

Inflammatory Disorders

RA is a systemic autoimmune inflammatory disorder that primarily affects the small joints of the hands and feet but may involve the hip joints late in the disease process. MRI is useful for evaluating erosions, effusion, and synovial pannus formation.[68] The synovial proliferation is typically a mass-like prominence of tissue within the joint that is hyperintense on fat-suppressed sequences.[46] The pannus may be heterogeneous or homogeneous in appearance, and pannus hemorrhages can form with areas of low signal hemosiderin.[68] As with osteoarthritis, the MR findings of inflammatory arthritis correlate with the radiographic appearance, including any of the following[68]:

- Symmetric joint space narrowing
- Periarticular erosions
- Juxtaarticular osteoporosis
- Protrusion acetabulae

Other findings may include the following[46]:

- Hyperintense joint effusion
- Joint capsule distention
- Hyperintense marrow edema

Ankylosing spondylitis is another form of inflammatory arthritis. It usually involves the spine and larger joints, so the hip is frequently affected and may be so early in the disease process.[46] The hip may be involved in 17 to 35% of patients, but

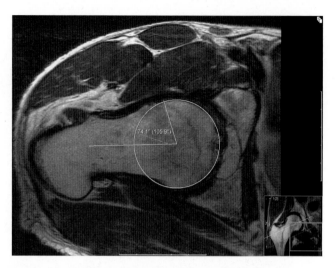

Fig. 7.14 An oblique axial FSE image of the left hip showing an increased α angle in a nonspherical femoral head with a cam lesion. (© 2009 Hospital for Special Surgery, New York, NY.)

the role of MRI has not been well defined, and conventional radiography is the standard for diagnostic evaluation.[69]

■ Synovial Disorders

A systematic examination of a hip MRI must include careful scrutiny of the synovium because synovial proliferative

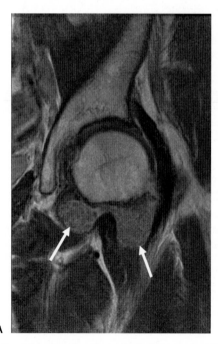

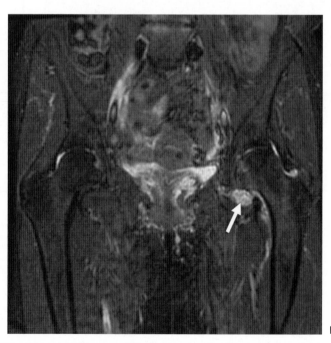

Fig. 7.15 Synovial osteochondromatosis. **(A)** A coronal FSE image of the left hip showing synovial osteochondromatosis with cartilaginous bodies in the inferior capsule (*arrows*). **(B)** A coronal fat-suppressed FSE image of the pelvis also showing large detached cartilaginous bodies (*arrow*). (© 2009 Hospital for Special Surgery, New York, NY.)

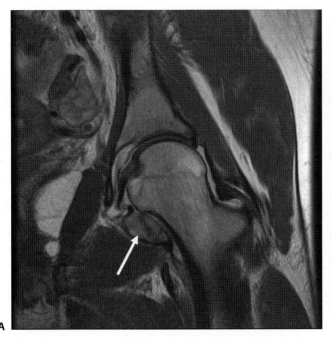 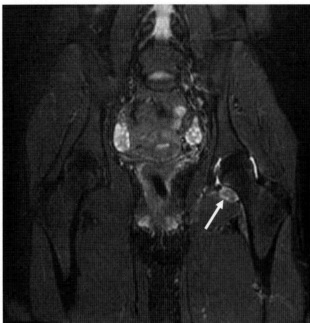

A   B

Fig. 7.16 PVNS. **(A)** A coronal FSE image of the left hip showing PVNS with hemosiderin-laden synovium (*arrow*). **(B)** A coronal fat-suppressed FSE image of the pelvis also showing the hemosiderin-laden synovium (*arrow*). (© 2009 Hospital for Special Surgery, New York, NY.)

disorders are not uncommon. In the hip, negative intraarticular pressure and the tight capsule may result in more prominent erosions than those associated with synovial proliferative disorders in other joints such as the knee, which has several patulous synovial recesses.[46] Asymmetric fluid is seen on body coil fat-suppressed images, and fine synovial debris is present on the surface coil images in the setting of synovial osteochondromatosis, which is a monoarticular synovium-based cartilage metaplasia that commonly involves the hip joint (**Fig. 7.15**).[46,70] The development of intraarticular loose bodies may converge to create large pressure erosions of the femoral neck and head or result in destruction of the hyaline cartilage. Typical MRI characteristics include multiple ossified loose bodies (low to intermediate signal intensity) surrounded by a high signal intensity joint effusion.[46]

PVNS may create a similar appearance, but the presence of hemosiderin degradation products creates a low signal intensity that can be quite helpful in confirming the diagnosis (**Fig. 7.16**).[71] PVNS has two forms: nodular and diffuse.[71] In its nodular form, it is seen as a focus of solitary, bulky synovial debris within the anteromedial recess or bare area.[46] If left untreated, synovial proliferative disorders may lead to a rapid degradation of articular cartilage with resultant osteoarthritis in a short period of time. (For a complete discussion of synovial proliferative disorders, see Chapter 15.)

References

1. Schmid MR, Nötzli HP, Zanetti M, Wyss TF, Hodler J. Cartilage lesions in the hip: diagnostic effectiveness of MR arthrography. Radiology 2003;226:382–386

2. Kassarjian A, Yoon LS, Belzile E, Connolly SA, Millis MB, Palmer WE. Triad of MR arthrographic findings in patients with cam-type femoroacetabular impingement. Radiology 2005;236:588–592

3. Kramer J, Recht MP. MR arthrography of the lower extremity. Radiol Clin North Am 2002;40:1121–1132

4. Potter HG, Foo LF. Magnetic resonance imaging of articular cartilage: trauma, degeneration, and repair. Am J Sports Med 2006;34:661–677

5. Mintz DN, Hooper T, Connell D, Buly R, Padgett DE, Potter HG. Magnetic resonance imaging of the hip: detection of labral and chondral abnormalities using noncontrast imaging. Arthroscopy 2005;21:385–393

6. Toomayan GA, Holman WR, Major NM, Kozlowicz SM, Vail TP. Sensitivity of MR arthrography in the evaluation of acetabular labral tears. AJR Am J Roentgenol 2006;186:449–453

7. Kelly BT, Williams RJ III, Philippon MJ. Hip arthroscopy: current indications, treatment options, and management issues. Am J Sports Med 2003;31:1020–1037

8. McCarthy JC, Noble PC, Schuck MR, Wright J, Lee J. The Otto E. Aufranc Award: the role of labral lesions to development of early degenerative hip disease. Clin Orthop Relat Res 2001;393:25–37

9. Dinauer PA, Murphy KP, Carroll JF. Sublabral sulcus at the posteroinferior acetabulum: a potential pitfall in MR arthrography diagnosis of acetabular labral tears. AJR Am J Roentgenol 2004;183:1745–1753

10. Kelly BT, Shapiro GS, Digiovanni CW, Buly RL, Potter HG, Hannafin JA. Vascularity of the hip labrum: a cadaveric investigation. Arthroscopy 2005;21:3–11

11. Kim YT, Azuma H. The nerve endings of the acetabular labrum. Clin Orthop Relat Res 1995;320:176–181

12. Lecouvet FE, Vande Berg BC, Malghem J, et al. MR imaging of the acetabular labrum: variations in 200 asymptomatic hips. AJR Am J Roentgenol 1996;167:1025–1028

13. Kelly BT, Weiland DE, Schenker ML, Philippon MJ. Arthroscopic labral repair in the hip: surgical technique and review of the literature. Arthroscopy 2005;21:1496–1504

14. Seldes RM, Tan V, Hunt J, Katz M, Winiarsky R, Fitzgerald RH Jr. Anatomy, histologic features, and vascularity of the adult acetabular labrum. Clin Orthop Relat Res 2001;382:232–240

15. Lage LA, Patel JV, Villar RN. The acetabular labral tear: an arthroscopic classification. Arthroscopy 1996;12:269–272

16. Ilizaliturri VM Jr, Byrd JWT, Sampson TG, et al. A geographic zone method to describe intra-articular pathology in hip arthroscopy: cadaveric study and preliminary report. Arthroscopy 2008;24:534–539

17. Byrd JWT. Labral lesions: an elusive source of hip pain case reports and literature review. Arthroscopy 1996;12:603–612

18. Armstrong DW III, Rue JPH, Wilckens JH, Frassica FJ. Stress fracture injury in young military men and women. Bone 2004;35:806–816

19. Anderson K, Strickland SM, Warren R. Hip and groin injuries in athletes. Am J Sports Med 2001;29:521–533

20. Boden BP, Osbahr DC. High-risk stress fractures: evaluation and treatment. J Am Acad Orthop Surg 2000;8:344–353

21. Fredericson M. Diagnosing tibial stress injuries in athletes. West J Med 1995;162:150

22. Potter HG, Montgomery KD, Heise CW, Helfet DL. MR imaging of acetabular fractures: value in detecting femoral head injury, intraarticular fragments, and sciatic nerve injury. AJR Am J Roentgenol 1994;163:881–886

23. Laorr A, Greenspan A, Anderson MW, Moehring HD, McKinley T. Traumatic hip dislocation: early MRI findings. Skeletal Radiol 1995;24:239–245

24. Moorman CT III, Warren RF, Hershman EB, et al. Traumatic posterior hip subluxation in American football. J Bone Joint Surg Am 2003;85:1190–1196

25. Shindle MK, Ranawat AS, Kelly BT. Diagnosis and management of traumatic and atraumatic hip instability in the athletic patient. Clin Sports Med 2006;25:309–326

26. Byrd JWT. Lateral impact injury. A source of occult hip pathology. Clin Sports Med 2001;20:801–815

27. Dwek J, Pfirrmann C, Stanley A, Pathria M, Chung CB. MR imaging of the hip abductors: normal anatomy and commonly encountered pathology at the greater trochanter. Magn Reson Imaging Clin N Am 2005;13:691–704

28. Kingzett-Taylor A, Tirman PF, Feller J, et al. Tendinosis and tears of gluteus medius and minimus muscles as a cause of hip pain: MR imaging findings. AJR Am J Roentgenol 1999;173:1123–1126

29. Chung CB, Robertson JE, Cho GJ, Vaughan LM, Copp SN, Resnick D. Gluteus medius tendon tears and avulsive injuries in elderly women: imaging findings in six patients. AJR Am J Roentgenol 1999;173:351–353

30. Bunker TD, Esler CNA, Leach WJ. Rotator-cuff tear of the hip. J Bone Joint Surg Br 1997;79:618–620

31. Howell GED, Biggs RE, Bourne RB. Prevalence of abductor mechanism tears of the hips in patients with osteoarthritis. J Arthroplasty 2001;16:121–123

32. LaBan MM, Weir SK, Taylor RS. "Bald trochanter" spontaneous rupture of the conjoined tendons of the gluteus medius and minimus presenting as a trochanteric bursitis. Am J Phys Med Rehabil 2004;83:806–809

33. Jacobson T, Allen WC. Surgical correction of the snapping iliopsoas tendon. Am J Sports Med 1990;18:470–474

34. Papadopoulos EC, Korres DS, Papachristou G, Efstathopoulos N. Piriformis syndrome. Orthopedics 2004;27:797, 799, author reply 799

35. Meislin R, Abeles A. Role of hip MR imaging in the management of sports-related injuries. Magn Reson Imaging Clin N Am 2005;13:635–640

36. Palmer WE, Kuong SJ, Elmadbouh HM. MR imaging of myotendinous strain. AJR Am J Roentgenol 1999;173:703–709

37. Pavlov H. Roentgen examination of groin and hip pain in the athlete. Clin Sports Med 1987;6:829–843

38. Bencardino JT, Kassarjian A, Palmer WE. Magnetic resonance imaging of the hip: sports-related injuries. Top Magn Reson Imaging 2003;14:145–160

39. Lavernia CJ, Sierra RJ, Grieco FR. Osteonecrosis of the femoral head. J Am Acad Orthop Surg 1999;7:250–261

40. Coleman BG, Kressel HY, Dalinka MK, Scheibler ML, Burk DL, Cohen EK. Radiographically negative avascular necrosis: detection with MR imaging. Radiology 1988;168:525–528

41. Hauzeur JP, Pasteels JL, Schoutens A, et al. The diagnostic value of magnetic resonance imaging in non-traumatic osteonecrosis of the femoral head. J Bone Joint Surg Am 1989;71:641–649

42. Mitchell DG, Steinberg ME, Dalinka MK, Rao VM, Fallon M, Kressel HY. Magnetic resonance imaging of the ischemic hip. Alterations within the osteonecrotic, viable, and reactive zones. Clin Orthop Relat Res 1989;244:60–77

43. Totty WG, Murphy WA, Ganz WI, Kumar B, Daum WJ, Siegel BA. Magnetic resonance imaging of the normal and ischemic femoral head. AJR Am J Roentgenol 1984;143:1273–1280

44. Hayes CW, Balkissoon AA. Magnetic resonance imaging of the musculoskeletal system. II. The hip. Clin Orthop Relat Res 1996;322:297–309

45. Shimizu K, Moriya H, Akita T, Sakamoto M, Suguro T. Prediction of collapse with magnetic resonance imaging of avascular necrosis of the femoral head. J Bone Joint Surg Am 1994;76:215–223

46. Stoller DW, Sampson T, Bredella M. The hip. In: Stoller DW, ed. Magnetic Resonance Imaging in Orthopaedics and Sports Medicine. Philadelphia: Lippincott Williams & Wilkins; 2007:41–304.

47. Takatori Y, Kamogawa M, Kokubo T, et al. Magnetic resonance imaging and histopathology in femoral head necrosis. Acta Orthop Scand 1987;58:499–503

48. Khanna AJ, Yoon TR, Mont MA, Hungerford DS, Bluemke DA. Femoral head osteonecrosis: detection and grading by using a rapid MR imaging protocol. Radiology 2000;217:188–192

49. Lafforgue P, Dahan E, Chagnaud C, Schiano A, Kasbarian M, Acquaviva PC. Early-stage avascular necrosis of the femoral head: MR imaging for prognosis in 31 cases with at least 2 years of follow-up. Radiology 1993;187:199–204

50. Koo KH, Kim R. Quantifying the extent of osteonecrosis of the femoral head. A new method using MRI. J Bone Joint Surg Br 1995;77:875–880

51. Cherian SF, Laorr A, Saleh KJ, Kuskowski MA, Bailey RF, Cheng EY. Quantifying the extent of femoral head involvement in osteonecrosis. J Bone Joint Surg Am 2003;85:309–315

52. Beltran J, Herman LJ, Burk JM, et al. Femoral head avascular necrosis: MR imaging with clinical-pathologic and radionuclide correlation. Radiology 1988;166(1 Pt 1):215–220

53. Kalliakmanis AG, Pneumaticos S, Plessas S, Papachristou G. Transient hip osteoporosis. Orthopedics 2006;29:263–264

54. Beltran J, Opsha O. MR imaging of the hip: osseous lesions. Magn Reson Imaging Clin N Am 2005;13:665–676

55. Siebenrock KA, Wahab KHA, Werlen S, Kalhor M, Leunig M, Ganz R. Abnormal extension of the femoral head epiphysis as a cause of cam impingement. Clin Orthop Relat Res 2004;418:54–60

56. Siebenrock KA, Schoeniger R, Ganz R. Anterior femoro-acetabular impingement due to acetabular retroversion. Treatment with periacetabular osteotomy. J Bone Joint Surg Am 2003;85:278–286

57. Beck M, Leunig M, Parvizi J, Boutier V, Wyss D, Ganz R. Anterior femoroacetabular impingement: part II. Midterm results of surgical treatment. Clin Orthop Relat Res 2004;418:67–73

58. Ganz R, Parvizi J, Beck M, Leunig M, Nötzli H, Siebenrock KA. Femoroacetabular impingement: a cause for osteoarthritis of the hip. Clin Orthop Relat Res 2003;417:111–119

59. Lavigne M, Parvizi J, Beck M, Siebenrock KA, Ganz R, Leunig M. Anterior femoroacetabular impingement: part I. Techniques of joint preserving surgery. Clin Orthop Relat Res 2004;418:61–66

60. Ito K, Minka MA II, Leunig M, Werlen S, Ganz R. Femoroacetabular impingement and the cam-effect. A MRI-based quantitative anatomical study of the femoral head-neck offset. J Bone Joint Surg Br 2001;83:171–176

61. Tanzer M, Noiseux N. Osseous abnormalities and early osteoarthritis: the role of hip impingement. Clin Orthop Relat Res 2004;429:170–177

62. Beck M, Kalhor M, Leunig M, Ganz R. Hip morphology influences the pattern of damage to the acetabular cartilage: femoroacetabular impingement as a cause of early osteoarthritis of the hip. J Bone Joint Surg Br 2005;87:1012–1018

63. Nötzli HP, Wyss TF, Stoecklin CH, Schmid MR, Treiber K, Hodler J. The contour of the femoral head-neck junction as a predictor for the risk of anterior impingement. J Bone Joint Surg Br 2002;84:556–560

64. Reynolds D, Lucas J, Klaue K. Retroversion of the acetabulum. A cause of hip pain. J Bone Joint Surg Br 1999;81:281–288

65. Bredella MA, Stoller DW. MR imaging of femoroacetabular impingement. Magn Reson Imaging Clin N Am 2005;13:653–664

66. Shindle MK, Voos JE, Heyworth BE, et al. Hip arthroscopy in the athletic patient: current techniques and spectrum of disease. J Bone Joint Surg Am 2007;89(suppl 3):29–43

67. Sadro C. Current concepts in magnetic resonance imaging of the adult hip and pelvis. Semin Roentgenol 2000;35:231–248

68. Koulouris G, Morrison WB. MR imaging of hip infection and inflammation. Magn Reson Imaging Clin N Am 2005;13:743–755

69. Wilkinson M, Bywaters EGL. Clinical features and course of ankylosing spondylitis; as seen in a follow-up of 222 hospital referred cases. Ann Rheum Dis 1958;17:209–228

70. Szypryt P, Twining P, Preston BJ, Howell CJ. Synovial chondromatosis of the hip joint presenting as a pathological fracture. Br J Radiol 1986;59:399–401

71. Tyler WK, Vidal AF, Williams RJ, Healey JH. Pigmented villonodular synovitis. J Am Acad Orthop Surg 2006;14:376–385

8 The Knee

Brett M. Cascio, A. Jay Khanna, Sergio A. Glait, Andrew J. Cosgarea, Timothy S. Johnson, and John D. Reeder

■ Specialized Pulse Sequences and Protocols

For MRI of the knee, the patient is positioned with the leg in comfortable external rotation. Sagittal, coronal, and axial imaging is obtained with fat-suppressed acquisition in at least one plane. To optimize spatial resolution, thinner segments are preferred, but the choice of segment thickness must be balanced with signal-to-noise and scan time constraints. In general, MRI systems with higher field strengths can achieve thinner segments with a better signal-to-noise ratio in less time than can units with lower field strength. For most SE protocols designed for knee imaging, the effective segment thickness is 3 to 4 mm; that for gradient-echo imaging is 1 to 3 mm.

A typical low magnetic field strength protocol for knee imaging may include T1-weighted and T2-weighted sagittal acquisitions, a coronal STIR sequence, and an axial FSE T2-weighted sequence. A sagittal 3D gradient-echo sequence represents an additional option, particularly with low field strength systems; this high-resolution technique offers a relatively thin segment with a superior signal-to-noise ratio, useful for meniscal assessment. A high field strength approach to knee imaging may include the following sequences:

- Sagittal FSE proton-density fat-suppressed sequence to evaluate the following:
  - Menisci
  - Articular cartilage
  - Cruciate ligaments
  - Extensor mechanism
  - Articular fluid
- Coronal FSE fat-suppressed T2-weighted sequence to assess the following:
  - Osseous injury
  - Articular and meniscal cartilage
  - Collateral supporting structures
  - Fluid distribution
- Sagittal T1-weighted sequence to evaluate the following:
  - Evaluate marrow and subcutaneous fat
  - Detect heterotopic ossification
  - Provide further evaluation of meniscal integrity

- Axial FSE T2-weighted sequence primarily to assess the patellofemoral joint

■ Traumatic Pathology

Acute Hemarthrosis

Acute knee trauma commonly presents with pain and hemarthrosis. ACL tears are seen in more than 70% of acute hemarthroses.[1] Usually, ACL tears are associated with other injuries such as meniscal tears, osteochondral fractures, patellar dislocations, and ligament and tendon tears. MRI is commonly used to discern the etiology of an acute hemarthrosis, especially when the knee is too tender or the patient is too anxious for a thorough physical examination. MRI is especially helpful when conventional radiographs are negative. Typically, acute hemarthrosis appears as fluid within the joint with high signal intensity on T2-weighted images and intermediate signal intensity on T1-weighted images. Similar findings can be seen with inflammatory processes, resulting in a nontraumatic knee effusion, and the two processes may be differentiated by the clinician, based on the history and physical examination. The presence of blood in joint fluid causes a relatively brighter appearance on T1 imaging than that observed with nonhemorrhagic fluid because of the effect of methemoglobin. Hemosiderin deposition within joint fluid, associated with chronic hemorrhage or PVNS, appears dark on all pulse sequences.

Table 8.1 Grading of Meniscal Tears

Grade	Pathologic and MRI Findings
1	Degenerative process; focal, globular intrasubstance increased signal; no extension to articular surface
2	Degenerative process; horizontal, linear intrasubstance increased signal; no extension to articular surface
3	Meniscal tear; increased signal extends to or communicates with at least one articular surface
4	Complex tear/macerated meniscus

Source: From Khanna AJ, Cosgarea AJ, Mont MA, et al. Magnetic resonance imaging of the knee: current techniques and spectrum of disease. J Bone Joint Surg Am 2001;83:128–141. Reprinted by permission.

Meniscal Tears

Meniscal tears are a very common finding on MRI. Clinical suspicion of a meniscal tear is a common reason for ordering an MRI. Tears can be a source of pain and disability, or they can be incidental findings. The tears can range from in-trasubstance degeneration that can be seen only on MRI to complete tears that allow fragments of the meniscus to flip or displace.

Meniscal tears are graded according to how they appear on MRI (**Table 8.1**[2]; **Fig. 8.1**), and are best seen on T1-weighted, gradient-echo, and proton-density images. The menisci are

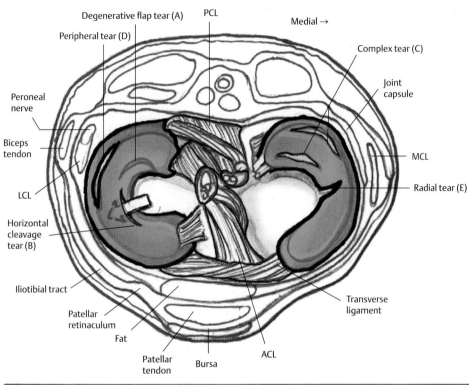

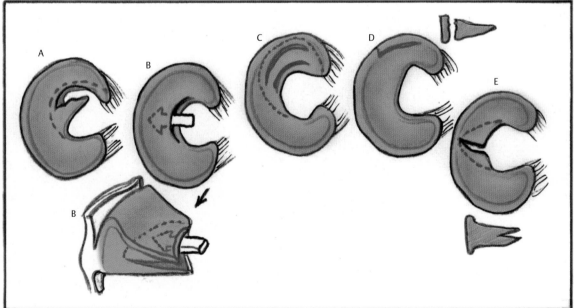

Fig. 8.1 Artist's sketch illustrating the morphology of meniscal tear patterns and relevant anatomy of the knee: **(A)** degenerative flap tear, **(B)** horizontal cleavage tear, **(C)** complex tear, **(D)** peripheral vertical longitudinal tear, and **(E)** vertical radial tear.

Table 8.2   Characteristics of Meniscal Tears on MRI

Meniscal Tear Morphology	Description	Appearance on MRI
Horizontal	Separates meniscus into superior (femoral) and inferior (tibial) fragments	Primarily horizontal signal on sagittal images
Vertical radial	Splits central margin of meniscus	Vertical signal oriented perpendicular to the curvature of the meniscus
Vertical longitudinal	Extends along length of meniscus; separates meniscus into inner and outer fragments	Vertical signal oriented parallel to the curvature of the meniscus.
Bucket handle	Subtype of the longitudinal tear in which the displaced central fragment resembles a bucket handle	"Double-PCL" sign; displaced fragment often seen parallel to the PCL in the intercondylar notch on sagittal images
Complex	Combination of multiple planes; commonly horizontal and radial	Characteristics of each tear type or fragmented/macerated
Meniscocapsular separation	Rupture of meniscus-capsule junction	Increased signal between the edge of the meniscus and the capsule

Source: Adapted from Khanna AJ, Cosgarea AJ, Mont MA, et al. Magnetic resonance imaging of the knee: current techniques and spectrum of disease. J Bone Joint Surg Am 2001;83:128–141, combined with information from Kelley EA, Berquist TH. Knee. In: Berquist TH, ed. MRI of the Musculoskeletal System. Philadelphia: Lippincott Williams & Wilkins; 2006:303–429. Adapted by permission.

low intensity on all sequences.[3-10] Most tears involve the medial meniscus, but most acute tears involve the lateral meniscus (**Table 8.2**[2,11]). Special attention should be given to the menisci in the presence of a chronic ACL tear because associated meniscus tears are common. The medial meniscus is commonly torn in the chronically ACL-deficient knee because the meniscus plays a secondary stabilizing role to anterior tibial translation.

The types of meniscal tear morphologies have been well described (**Table 8.2**[2,11]). In early publications on MRI evaluation of meniscal pathology, detection focused primarily on meniscal signal intensity patterns and their relationship to the meniscal surface.[12,13] Grade I and grade II[9] meniscal tears referred to increased intrameniscal signal that appeared punctate or linear, respectively, and were particularly evident on T1-weighted images. The grade III designation indicated

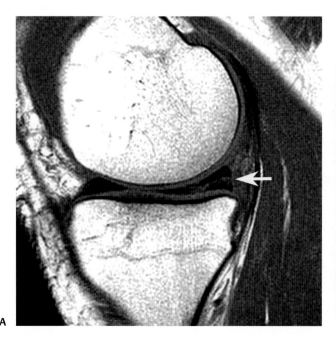

A

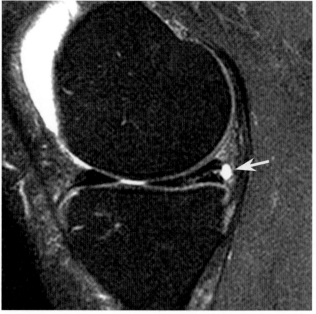

B

Fig. 8.2 Horizontal tear in the posterior horn of the medial meniscus. Sagittal T1-weighted **(A)** and fat-suppressed proton-density **(B)** images showing a horizontal tear (*arrow on each*) communicating with the undersurface of the meniscus. Note the small meniscal cyst posterior to the meniscus on the fat-suppressed proton-density image.

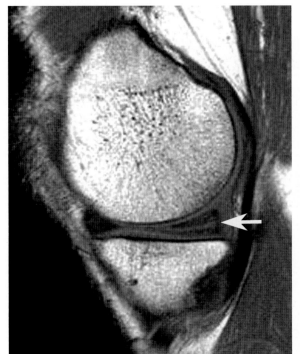

A

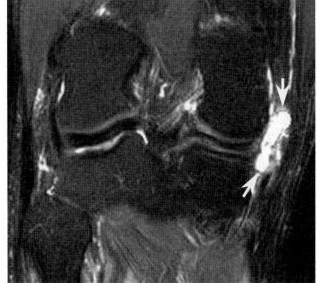

B

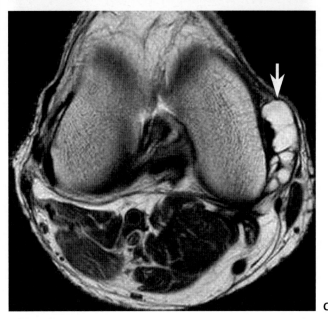

C

Fig. 8.3 Horizontal medial meniscal tear with large meniscal cyst in the right knee. **(A)** A sagittal T1-weighted image shows a horizontal tear (*arrow*) of the posterior horn of the medial meniscus. **(B)** A coronal fat-suppressed T2-weighted image shows a large meniscal cyst (*arrows*) extending medial to the medial compartment. **(C)** An axial T2-weighted image shows a multiloculated meniscal cyst (*arrow*).

that the signal intensity pattern communicated with the superior or inferior meniscal surface, and therefore most likely corresponded to an arthroscopically identifiable meniscal tear.[9] If grade II meniscal pathology was reported in an MRI interpretation as a grade II tear, however, it could create the erroneous impression that meniscal surface pathology existed. Although grade II intrameniscal signal can reflect the presence of a meniscal contusion or an intrameniscal tear, it may also denote myxoid internal meniscal degeneration, artifact (*magic angle effect* or truncation), or normal meniscal vascularity in a child or young adult.[14,15] This grading system also does not consider morphologic alterations in characterizing meniscal pathology. Because the morphology of a meniscal tear impacts its relative clinical significance and influences surgical planning, a more specific classification

system, currently afforded wide acceptance, uses MRI findings to categorize tears as follows[13]:

- Horizontal
- Vertical radial
- Vertical longitudinal with/without flap displacement
- Complex

Horizontal tears divide the meniscus into superior and inferior components, identified on sagittal and coronal imaging series (**Fig. 8.2**). The tear often communicates with the inferior meniscal surface; sometimes a concomitant meniscal cyst is identified, involving the perimeniscal soft tissue (**Fig. 8.3**).

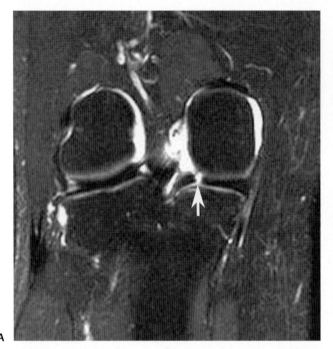

Fig. 8.4 Vertical radial meniscal tear in the posterior horn of the medial meniscus in the right knee. **(A)** A coronal fat-suppressed T2-weighted image shows a vertical defect (*arrow*) involving the posterior horn of the medial meniscus. **(B)** A sagittal fat-suppressed proton-density image, obtained in the plane of the tear, shows truncation (*arrow*) and abnormal signal intensity involving the posterior horn. Note the normal anterior horn.

Vertical radial tears exhibit a linear signal pattern. They violate the superior and inferior meniscal surfaces and are oriented perpendicular to the meniscal axis of curvature.[16] As such, if a vertical radial tear involves the anterior or posterior portion of the meniscus, the tear will show a linear vertical configuration on coronal images (**Fig. 8.4A**) and an abrupt truncation of the central meniscal contour on sagittal images (**Fig. 8.4B**). With this type of tear, the change in meniscal morphology, appreciated in the imaging plane oriented parallel to the tear, is equally as important as the surface communication of linear abnormal meniscal signal intensity, noted in the imaging plane perpendicular to the axis of the tear. If the vertical radial tear involves the midbody of the meniscus, a linear meniscal defect is noted on sagittal images (**Fig. 8.5A**), and blunting or truncation of the central meniscal contour is observed on coronal images (**Fig.**

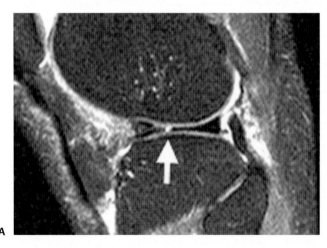

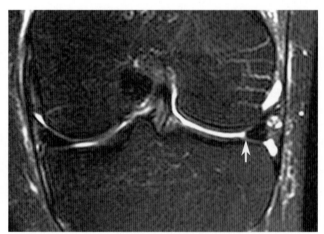

Fig. 8.5 Vertical radial meniscal tear in the mid-body lateral meniscus in the left knee. **(A)** A sagittal fat-suppressed proton-density image shows a vertical tear (*arrow*) of the central edge of the lateral meniscus, oriented perpendicular to the curvature of the meniscus. Note the superimposed horizontal tear of the anterior horn. **(B)** A coronal fat-suppressed T2-weighted image shows the same tear with truncation of the central meniscal margin (*arrow*).

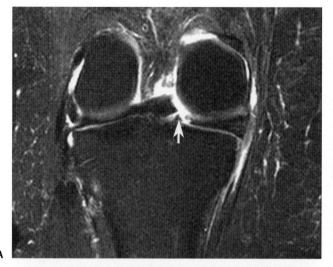

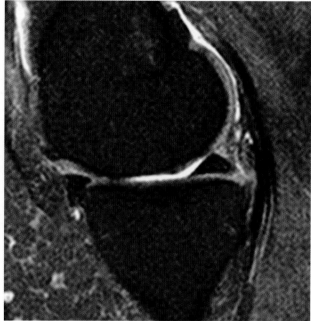

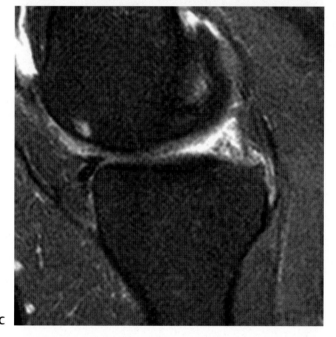

Fig. 8.6 Vertical radial tear of the meniscal root in the right knee. **(A)** A coronal fat-suppressed T2-weighted image shows a vertical radial defect (*arrow*) at the meniscal root. **(B)** A sagittal fat-suppressed proton-density image, obtained just medial to the tear, shows normal posterior horn morphology. **(C)** A sagittal fat-suppressed proton-density image, obtained in the plane of the tear, shows abrupt transition to markedly abnormal posterior meniscal morphology, corresponding to the meniscal root tear.

8.5B). A commonly overlooked vertical radial tear occurs at the root of the posterior horn of the medial meniscus (**Fig. 8.6**). This tear, particularly common in obese patients, destabilizes the meniscus, and medial extrusion of the meniscus is often identified on MRI. Chondromalacia and osseous stress injury are also frequently observed in association with these radial tears of the root of the posterior horn of the medial meniscus.[17]

Vertical longitudinal tears also exhibit a vertical signal orientation on MRI, but because the tear is oriented parallel to the axis of meniscal curvature, it is identified as a vertical linear signal intensity interfacing with the superior and inferior meniscal articular surfaces on sagittal and coronal imaging planes. Peripheral vertical longitudinal tears of the posterior horn of the medial meniscus and vertical longitudinal tears of the posterior horn of the lateral meniscus at the attachment of the meniscofemoral ligament are commonly associated with ACL tears (**Fig. 8.7**). Displacement of a meniscal flap associated with a vertical longitudinal tear may occur, and unstable meniscal tears are more likely to be symptomatic and impair biomechanics; in such circumstances, surgical intervention usually is necessary to restore

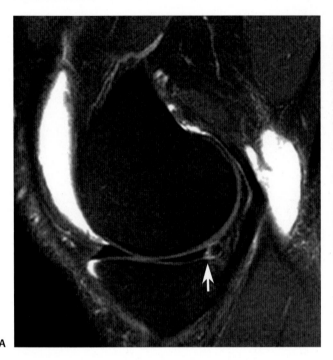

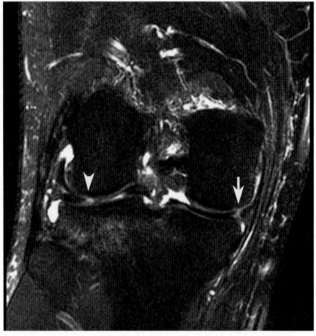

A   B

Fig. 8.7 Vertical longitudinal tear in the right knee. **(A)** A sagittal fat-suppressed proton-density image shows a peripheral vertical longitudinal tear (*arrow*) of the posterior horn of the medial meniscus. Note the effusion and Baker cyst. **(B)** A coronal fat-suppressed T2-weighted image shows the vertical longitudinal tear (*arrow*), propagating parallel to the meniscal curvature. Note the tear of the posterior horn of the lateral meniscus (*arrowhead*) with an adjacent lateral tibial plateau bone bruise in this patient with an acute ACL tear.

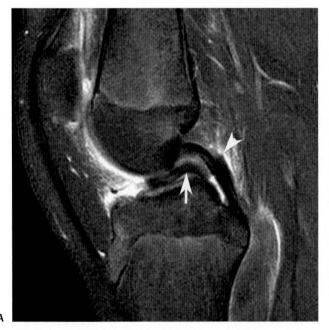

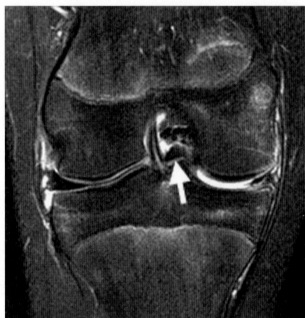

A   B

Fig. 8.8 Bucket-handle tear in the right knee. **(A)** A sagittal fat-suppressed proton-density image shows a meniscal flap (*arrow*), arising from the medial meniscus and displaced inferior to the PCL (*arrowhead*), exhibiting the double-PCL sign. **(B)** A coronal fat-suppressed T2-weighted image shows a centrally displaced meniscal flap (*arrow*) inferior to the PCL. Note the abnormal morphology of the nondisplaced medial meniscal remnant.

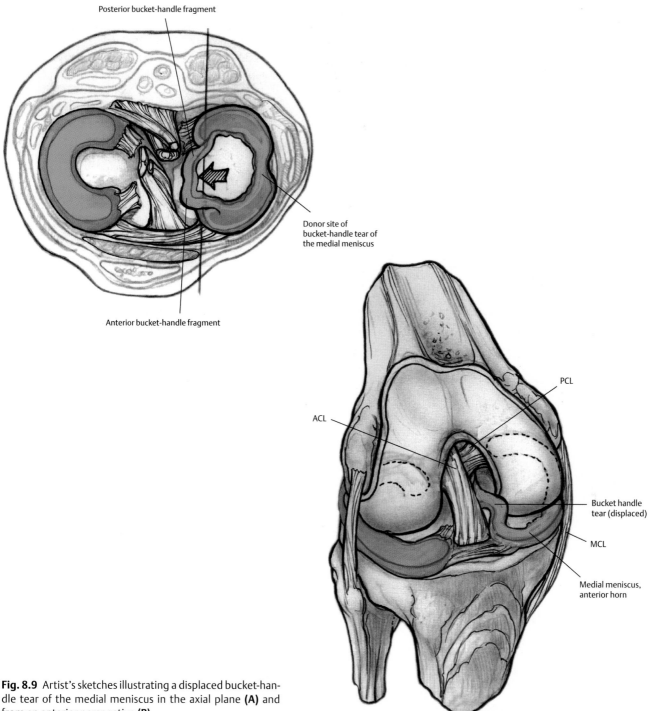

Fig. 8.9 Artist's sketches illustrating a displaced bucket-handle tear of the medial meniscus in the axial plane **(A)** and from an anterior perspective **(B)**.

function.[18] Failure to address surgically the presence of a displaced meniscal flap or fragment represents a cause of persistent joint pain and dysfunction after arthroscopy.[19] Unstable meniscal tears may exhibit central or peripheral flap displacement. A typical bucket-handle tear represents a vertical longitudinal tear with central displacement of meniscal tissue. If the medial meniscus is involved, the flap is displaced inferior to the PCL, creating the double-PCL

sign[20] (**Figs. 8.8** and **8.9**). Bucket-handle tears of the lateral meniscus often exhibit anterior central displacement of a flap arising from the posterior horn of the meniscus (**Fig. 8.10**). Displaced bucket-handle tears are a common cause of locked knee in an athlete. Posterior central flap displacement may also occur with a flap arising from the posterior horn of the medial meniscus and the displaced meniscal tissue positioned in the recess between the distal PCL and the medial meniscus (**Fig. 8.11**). Meniscal tissue may also displace peripherally into the recess between the capsule and the femoral condyle (**Fig. 8.12**) or between the capsule and the tibial plateau (**Fig. 8.13**). Although peripherally displaced tears are less likely than centrally displaced tears to result in locking, they tend to cause adjacent capsular inflammation and osseous stress reaction, contributing to pain related to the meniscal tear. Preoperative identification and

localization of the displaced meniscal flap with MRI contribute to a more expeditious operative procedure.[10]

The designation of a tear as complex, based on MRI findings, implies that the tear exhibits multiple vectors or that the meniscus appears macerated and fragmented. These tears are usually unstable and, if chronic, are associated with chondromalacia and osseous stress reaction, also identified on MRI.

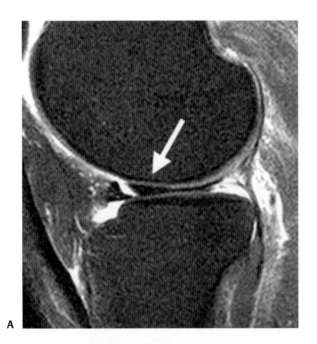

A

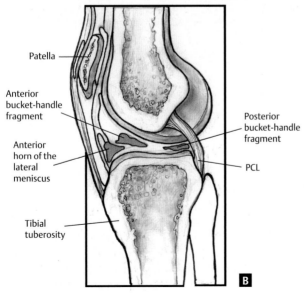

B

Fig. 8.10 A sagittal fat-saturated proton-density image **(A)** and artist's drawing **(B)** showing anterior displacement of the posterior horn of the lateral meniscus (*arrow*) with the displaced flap positioned just posterior to the anterior horn of the lateral meniscus.

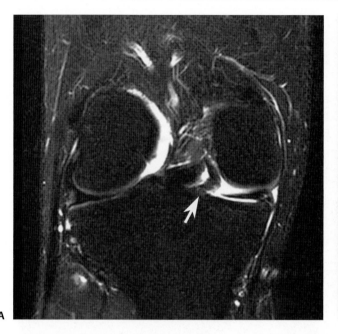
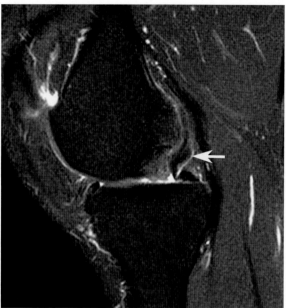

Fig. 8.11 Displaced meniscal tear in the right knee. Coronal fat-suppressed T2-weighted **(A)** and sagittal fat-suppressed proton-density **(B)** images show the posterior central displacement of a medial meniscal flap (*arrow on each*).

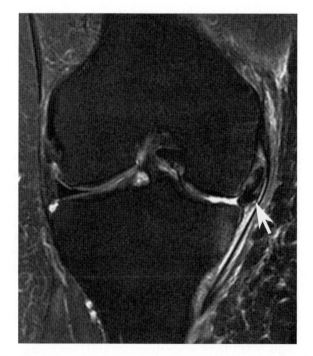

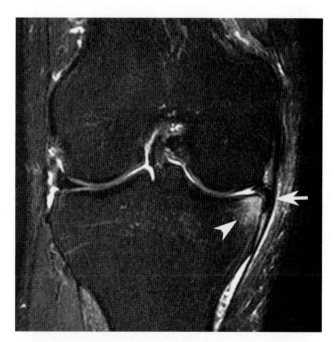

Fig. 8.12 This coronal fat-suppressed T2-weighted image of the right knee shows the peripheral superior displacement of a large meniscal flap (*arrow*), arising from the medial meniscus and extending into the recess medial to the medial femoral condyle.

Fig. 8.13 This coronal fat-suppressed T2-weighted image of the right knee shows the peripheral inferior displacement of a meniscal flap (*arrow*), arising from the medial meniscus and extending into the recess medial to the medial tibial plateau. Note the adjacent osseous stress reaction (*arrowhead*) and pericapsular edema.

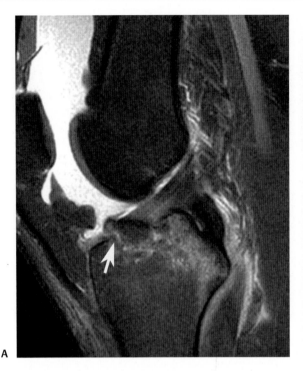
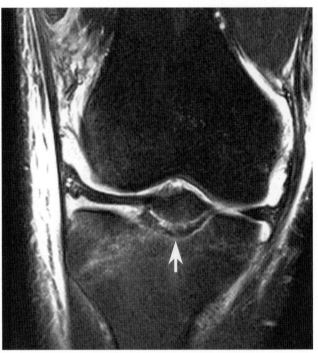

A   **B**

Fig. 8.14 ACL avulsion. Sagittal fat-suppressed proton-density **(A)** and coronal fat-suppressed T2-weighted **(B)** images of the right knee show an avulsion (*arrow on each*) of the tibial attachment of the ACL.

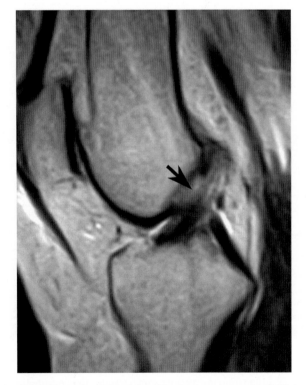

Fig. 8.15 This sagittal T2-weighted image shows a proximal ACL tear (*arrow*).

ACL Tears

ACL evaluation is one of the primary indications for MRI of the knee.[21] The patient usually describes a noncontact, twisting or valgus injury to the knee with a planted foot and often describes sensing a "pop" inside the knee. The patient may experience a subsequent lack of quadriceps function because of the resulting effusion. Physical examination findings include a positive Lachman test and pivot shift. The patient's anxiety may make the physical examination equivocal, increasing the importance of the MRI.

The adult ACL usually avulses from its femoral attachment or develops an intrasubstance tear. The tendon does not have to dissociate completely to become incompetent.[22] The presence of blood at the femoral avulsion can appear as a "pseudomass" because of volume averaging.[23] With skeletally immature patients, the ACL may remain intact and avulse a fragment of bone off of the tibial attachment (**Fig. 8.14**). Treatment is determined by the degree of displacement, but it usually requires surgical fixation via arthroscopic or open techniques.

The signs of an ACL injury on MRI include abnormal ligament signal and loss of the normal orientation and continuity of the ligament (**Fig. 8.15**). There are primary and secondary signs of ACL tears as visualized on MRI (summarized in **Table 8.3**[24–26]). MRI findings commonly associated with acute ACL injury include loss of ligament continuity and replacement of the ligament by a poorly marginated pseudomass

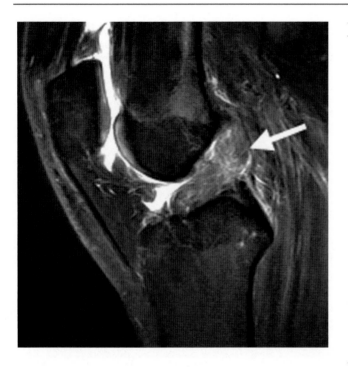

Fig. 8.16 This sagittal fat-suppressed proton-density image shows the pseudomass appearance (*arrow*) of an acute ACL tear.

Table 8.3 Signs of an ACL Tear on MRI

Primary signs

- Nonvisualization of ligament
- Complete disruption of a ligament segment
- Abnormal signal within ligament on T2-weighted images
- Alteration of normal linear configuration of ligament
- Alteration of normal angulation of ligament

Secondary signs

- Bone contusion (posterolateral and posteromedial tibia, lateral condyle of femur)
- Deepening of lateral femoral condyle notch or sulcus
- Anterior translation of tibia >5 mm from posterior margin of femoral condyle
- Buckling of the PCL (decreased angle of the PCL)
- Segond fracture
- Meniscal tear
- Posterior horn medial meniscus and tear of the lateral meniscus at the meniscofemoral ligament attachment
- Posterior displacement of posterior horn of lateral meniscus

that shows high signal on T2-weighted imaging and low signal on T1-weighted imaging (**Fig. 8.16**). With both acute and chronic ACL tears, the ligament may appear abnormal in angulation, typically because of inferior displacement of the proximal portion of the ligament. Acute tears of the ACL are often accompanied by bone bruises involving the posterior aspect of the lateral tibial plateau, the anterolateral aspect of the lateral femoral condyle with impaction of the articular surface notch, and the posterior aspect of the medial tibial plateau (**Fig. 8.17**). The osseous contusions are related to

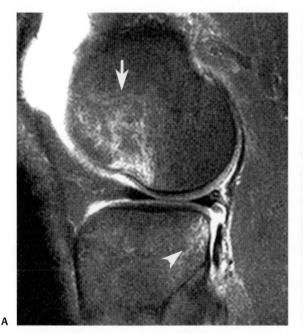

A

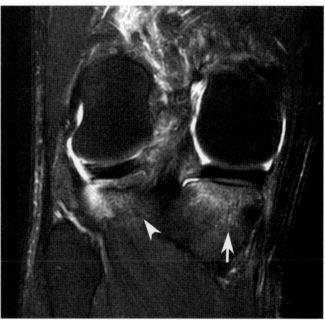

B

Fig. 8.17 Bone bruise pattern with ACL tear. **(A)** A sagittal fat-suppressed proton-density image shows a bone bruise (*arrow*) with osteochondral impaction involving the lateral femoral condyle and a bone bruise (*arrowhead*) involving the posterior aspect of the lateral tibial plateau. **(B)** A coronal fat-suppressed T2-weighted image of the right knee shows bone bruises involving the posterior aspect of the lateral tibial plateau (*arrowhead*) and medial tibial plateau (*arrow*).

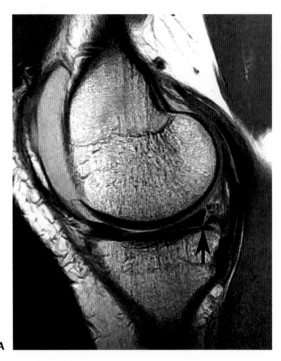
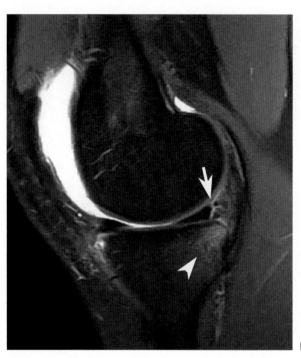

Fig. 8.18 Medial meniscal tear with ACL tear. Sagittal proton-density **(A)** and sagittal fat-suppressed T2-weighted **(B)** images show a peripheral tear (*arrow on each*) of the posterior horn of the medial meniscus. Note the bone bruise (*arrowhead on* **B**) of the posterior aspect of the medial tibial plateau.

the initial pivot shift rotational stress (lateral injuries) and the subsequent abrupt return to normal alignment (medial plateau injury). Additional findings include anterior translation of the tibia, resulting in increased PCL flexion, popliteus muscle strain, peripheral tears of the posterior horn of the medial meniscus (**Fig. 8.18**), and tears of the lateral meniscus associated with the attachment of the meniscofemoral ligament (**Fig. 8.19**).

Other knee structures are also commonly injured at the time of ACL injury, and it is imperative that the MRI be evaluated for these concomitant injuries. These injuries, such as meniscus tears, bone bruises, and cartilage injuries, not only may need to be addressed surgically, but also aid in the diagnosis when the ACL tear is not obvious.[27]

A variety of other radiographic findings seen in association with ACL tears are considered secondary signs (**Table 8.3**[24–26]). A relatively small avulsion fracture seen at the lateral tibial cortex (known as a Segond fracture) is caused by avulsion of the middle third of the lateral capsule[28] (**Fig. 8.20**).

When the ACL tears, the posterior tibial plateau translates anteriorly, impacting the anterior aspect of the lateral femoral condyle in the region of the terminal sulcus. The resulting contusion leaves a bone bruise pattern in these two locations, best seen on T2-weighted images (**Fig. 8.17**). This pathologic contact of the tibial and the femoral condyles may leave an

indentation or notch, also called a "deepened terminal sulcus," particularly when the patient experiences repeated instability episodes. Another sign of chronic ACL insufficiency is buckling of the PCL, which suggests that the tibia is positioned in an anteriorly displaced position. Patients with chronic ACL insufficiency also frequently develop secondary degenerative changes, including partial- and full-thickness chondral lesions, peripheral osteophytes, and peaking of the tibial spines.

When evaluating the MRI study of a patient with ACL injury, multiple factors should be taken into consideration and included in the description of the MRI findings, including the location and degree of disruption of the ACL. In addition, the collateral ligaments, PCL, and secondary restraints (including the menisci) should be carefully reviewed. It is also important to review the status of the osseous structures and articular cartilage because injuries to these structures can also be treated at the time of ACL reconstruction and repair. Lastly, the condition of any tissues that might be used when reconstructing the ACL should be evaluated, and injury to them should be ruled out.

Chronic degeneration of the ACL should be differentiated from an acute ACL injury or tear. Patients with chronic degeneration often present with chronic knee discomfort and a vague, nonspecific knee pain. The process is thought to be secondary to repetitive low-energy microtrauma as opposed

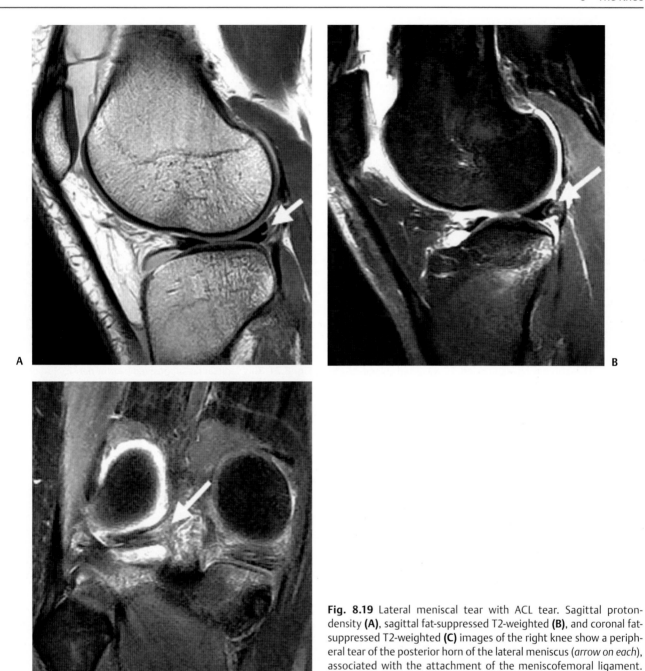

Fig. 8.19 Lateral meniscal tear with ACL tear. Sagittal proton-density **(A)**, sagittal fat-suppressed T2-weighted **(B)**, and coronal fat-suppressed T2-weighted **(C)** images of the right knee show a peripheral tear of the posterior horn of the lateral meniscus (*arrow on each*), associated with the attachment of the meniscofemoral ligament. Note the proximal tibial bone bruises, typical for an acute ACL injury.

to a single high-energy event that might produce an acute ACL tear. Minimal to no instability is seen on physical examination. The MRI may show evidence of advanced degeneration of the ACL with thickening of the ligament and less increase in T2-weighted signal than that which is typically seen with an acute tear (**Fig. 8.21**). Such patients also often have similar PCL involvement.

PCL Tears

The PCL is more robust and more consistently has lower signal on MRI than does the ACL. MRI is very sensitive for tears of the PCL because of its normal low signal (**Fig. 8.22**). Any increased signal within the PCL on T2-weighted images is suspicious for injury.[29–31] The PCL can be torn partially, indicated by increased signal on T2 images with the ligament in continuity (**Fig. 8.23**), or completely, visualized as a loss of

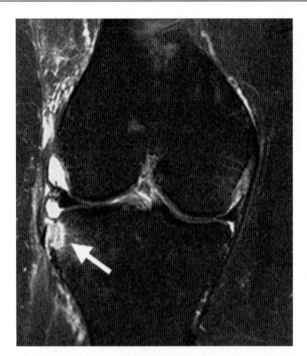

Fig. 8.20 This coronal fat-suppressed T2-weighted image of the right knee shows a Segond fracture (*arrow*) of the lateral aspect of the lateral tibial plateau at the capsular attachment in a patient with an acute ACL tear.

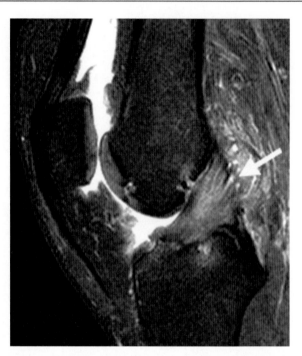

Fig. 8.21 This sagittal fat-suppressed proton-density image shows advanced degeneration (marked thickening) of the ACL (*arrow*).

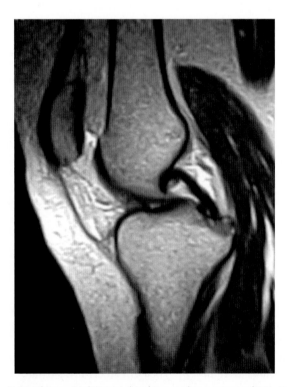

Fig. 8.22 This sagittal T2-weighted image shows a normal PCL. Note the absence of signal within the PCL.

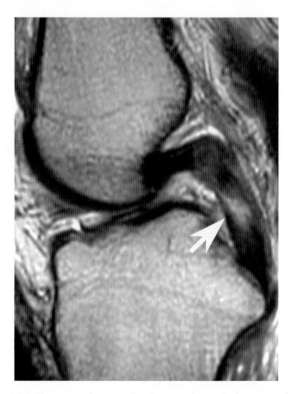

Fig. 8.23 This sagittal T2-weighted image shows thickening and abnormal signal intensity of the PCL (*arrow*), corresponding to a tear.

Table 8.4   Grading of PCL Laxity

Grade	Description of Posterior Drawer Examination
1.0	3- to 5-mm difference in tibial step-off; tibial plateau prominence remaining anterior to femoral condyles
1.5	6- to 8-mm difference in tibial step-off; tibial and femoral condyles not yet flush
2.0	9- to 10-mm difference in tibial step-off; anterior tibia and femoral condyles flush with each other
2.5	11- to 13-mm difference in tibial step-off; anterior tibia is posterior to femoral condyles
3.0	>13 mm difference in tibial step-off; anterior tibia is well posterior to femoral condyles; other ligamentous laxity most likely present

continuity of the ligament. Bone bruises may be present, depending on the mechanism of injury. A blow to the proximal tibia from a dashboard during a motor vehicle accident can produce soft-tissue edema and a bone contusion involving the tibial plateau, best seen on T2-weighted images. Bone bruises may be present on the anterior tibial plateaus and the femoral condyles if the PCL injury occurs from a hyperextension mechanism.

It is important to note evidence for avulsion injuries or multiple ligament injuries because both are indications for early operative repair (for avulsions) or reconstruction (for tears). A "reverse Segond" fracture on the medial side of the joint has been associated with PCL tears.[32] PCL tears can be graded according to the amount of laxity noted on the posterior drawer examination. Laxity grades of 2.5 or more usually are associated with other knee injuries, so a high index of suspicion is indicated when reviewing the MR images of such patients.[33]

The clinician can be alerted to the amount of PCL laxity by noting the resting position of the tibia in relation to the femur on midsagittal images (see **Table 8.4**[33] for a summary of one grading system for PCL laxity). The degree of posterior tibial subluxation relates to the severity of the PCL insufficiency. More severe PCL tears can benefit from reconstruction. As with ACL injuries, care should be taken to evaluate the MRI study for associated knee injuries.

Collateral Ligament Tears

Coronal images allow for optimal evaluation of collateral ligament injury. Collateral ligament injury can be classified as mild, moderate (**Fig. 8.24**), or severe (**Fig. 8.25; Table 8.5**[34,35]).[34] Injured ligaments should show varying amounts of increased signal intensity on T2-weighted images based on severity of tissue damage.

In general, complete MCL tears are treated nonoperatively, whereas complete LCL tears are addressed surgically with early repair and later reconstruction with allograft or autograft.

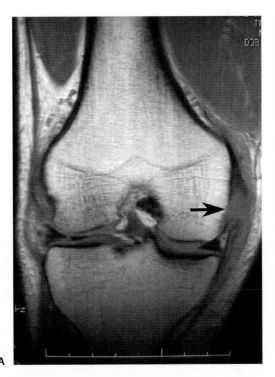
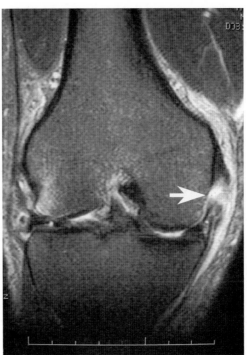

A   B

Fig. 8.24 Moderate MCL injury in the right knee. Coronal T1-weighted (**A**) and coronal fat-suppressed T2-weighted (**B**) images show a focal tear (*arrow on each*) of the proximal MCL. Note the corresponding impaction-related bone bruise of the lateral femoral condyle and the lateral meniscal tear.

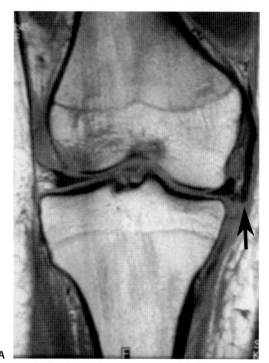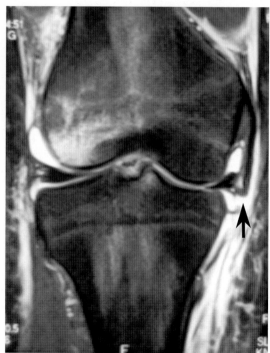

A   B

Fig. 8.25 Marked MCL injury in the right knee. Coronal T1-weighted **(A)** and fat-suppressed T2-weighted **(B)** images show a high-grade MCL injury (*arrow on each*). Note the marked lateral femoral condyle bone contusion.

MCL injuries comprise part of the "terrible triad"; the other two components are ACL tears and medial meniscus tears. However, it has been found that lateral meniscus tears, rather than medial meniscus tears, are more common with acute ACL tears.[36]

Posterolateral Corner

The posterolateral corner of the knee is complex from an anatomic and, therefore, imaging standpoint. The variability of the posterolateral structures makes the images of this area of the knee even more difficult to interpret. The posterolateral corner structures resist varus and external rotation forces. The structures that comprise the posterolateral corner are the following:

- LCL
- Arcuate ligament
- Popliteal tendon
- Lateral head of the gastrocnemius
- Posterolateral capsule
- Biceps tendon
- Meniscofibular ligament
- Popliteofibular ligament
- Fabellofibular ligament (when the fabella is present)

Although the biceps tendon and LCL usually are identifiable, identifying the popliteofibular ligament is more difficult.[37] This difficulty could contribute to the incidence of missed posterolateral corner injuries. Coronal oblique images offer the best imaging for evaluating and diagnosing the posterolateral structures (**Fig. 8.26**). Specific attention should be given to including imaging through the entire fibular head. A high-energy varus injury to the knee can place tension on, and even rupture, the peroneal nerve after the postero-

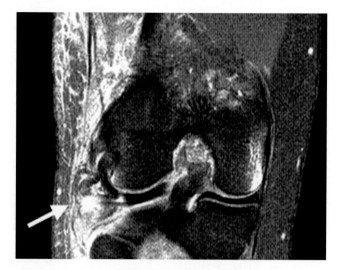

Fig. 8.26 This coronal fat-suppressed T2-weighted image of the right knee shows tears of the fibular collateral ligament (*arrow*) and biceps femoris tendon at the fibular head. Note the corresponding impaction injury of the medial femoral condyle.

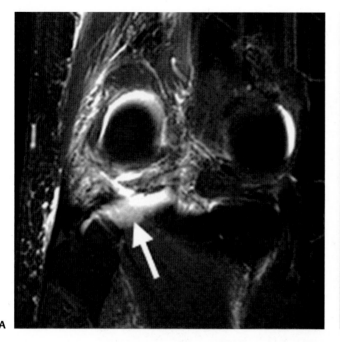
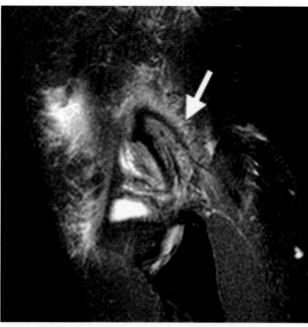

Fig. 8.27 Posterolateral corner injury in the right knee. Coronal fat-suppressed T2-weighted **(A)** and sagittal fat-suppressed proton-density **(B)** images of a patient with an acute ACL injury show marked soft-tissue edema (*arrow on each*) involving the posterolateral corner of the knee.

lateral knee structures are torn. Careful attention should also be given to noting discontinuity or edema of the peroneal nerve.

The arcuate complex is composed of the LCL, arcuate liga-

ment, and popliteus tendon. It provides posterolateral stability of the knee to varus and rotatory stress. The arcuate ligament is an inconsistent structure and is occasionally absent in individuals with large fabellae. Injury to this complex area of the knee is seen as increased signal intensity on T2-weighted images because of the underlying edema (**Fig. 8.27**).

Posteromedial Corner

The posteromedial corner is composed of the deep and superficial MCLs, the posterior oblique ligament, and the oblique popliteal ligament. Damage to the posteromedial corner can cause valgus instability of the knee and increased anteromedial subluxation. The posterior oblique ligament is attached to the posterior horn of the medial meniscus. Some authors have advocated surgical repair of damage to this complex.[38] Coronal images (**Fig. 8.28**) offer the best views of

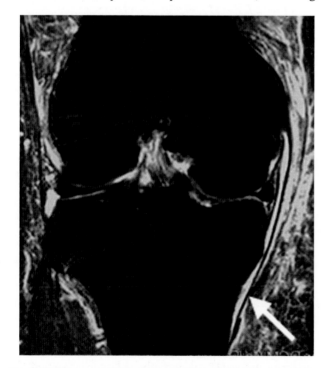

Fig. 8.28 This coronal fat-suppressed T2-weighted image of a patient with an MCL sprain in the right knee shows the deep and superficial (*arrow*) components of the MCL complex, separated by fluid and edema.

Table 8.5   Collateral Ligament Tears

Grade of Tear	Description	MRI Appearance
Mild	Ligament has some torn or stretched fibers	Periligamentous edema; ligament grossly intact, hematoma possible
Moderate	Incomplete tear with no laxity	Partial tear with edema, hematoma possible
Severe	Loss of ligament integrity, pathologic laxity	Complete tear, fibers not in continuity, considerable edema and hematoma

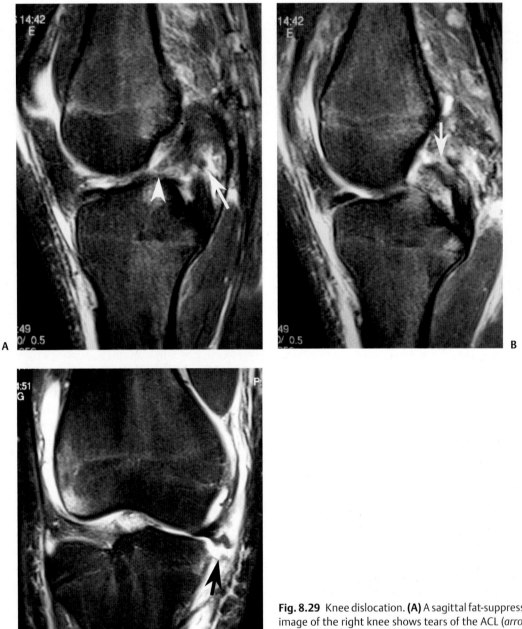

Fig. 8.29 Knee dislocation. **(A)** A sagittal fat-suppressed T2-weighted image of the right knee shows tears of the ACL (*arrowhead*) and PCL (*arrow*). **(B)** A sagittal fat-suppressed T2-weighted image shows a proximal PCL tear (*arrow*). **(C)** A coronal fat-suppressed T2-weighted image of the right knee shows severe MCL injury (*arrow*) and a lateral femoral condylar bone bruise.

these structures. The femoral and tibial attachments of the structures should be evaluated carefully for increased signal on T2-weighted images, which indicates edema and injury.

Knee Dislocation

Knee dislocation is a serious injury that may lead to compartment syndrome and rhabdomyolysis, with resultant loss of limb and even life. Vascular injury occurs in as many as 50% of knee dislocations, whereas peroneal or tibial nerve injuries occur in up to 30%.[39,40] Although angiography is the standard for diagnosing vascular injuries associated with knee dislocations, MR angiography is less invasive and can play a valuable role (see Chapter 16). Care must be taken to evaluate for peroneal nerve or tibial nerve edema or discontinuity. A careful neurovascular examination is essential. As

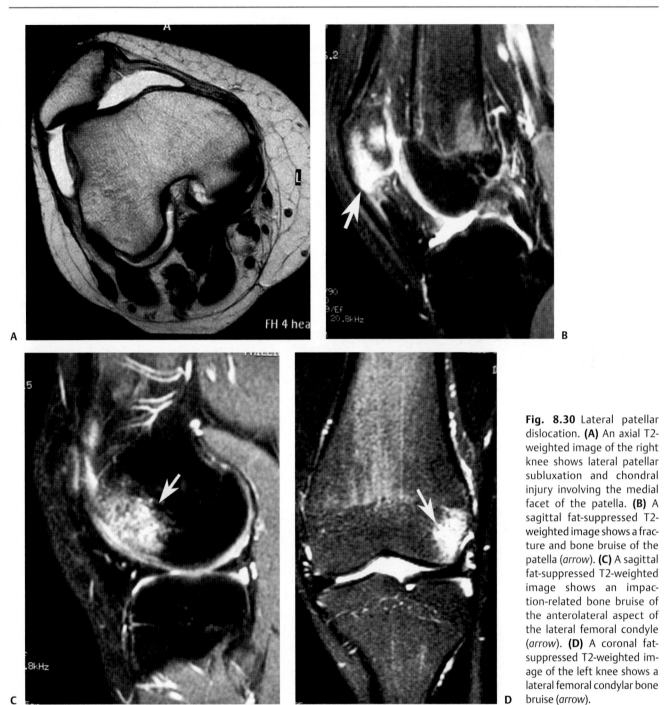

Fig. 8.30 Lateral patellar dislocation. **(A)** An axial T2-weighted image of the right knee shows lateral patellar subluxation and chondral injury involving the medial facet of the patella. **(B)** A sagittal fat-suppressed T2-weighted image shows a fracture and bone bruise of the patella (*arrow*). **(C)** A sagittal fat-suppressed T2-weighted image shows an impaction-related bone bruise of the anterolateral aspect of the lateral femoral condyle (*arrow*). **(D)** A coronal fat-suppressed T2-weighted image of the left knee shows a lateral femoral condylar bone bruise (*arrow*).

with many other diagnoses, the clinician has a substantial advantage over the radiologist, given that the clinician can correlate the clinical findings with the imaging findings to determine the most likely diagnosis with a high degree of certainty. Knee dislocations are associated with fractures, cartilage injury, and tears of the ACL, PCL, LCL, MCL, and posterolateral and posteromedial corners (**Fig. 8.29**); imaging studies should be scrutinized carefully for the presence or absence of these findings.

Extensor Mechanism

Traumatic injuries to the extensor mechanism include patellar dislocation, quadriceps tendon rupture, and patellar tendon rupture.[41]

Patellar Dislocation

Patellar dislocations occur through noncontact mechanisms such as rotation on a planted foot (e.g., as during batting in

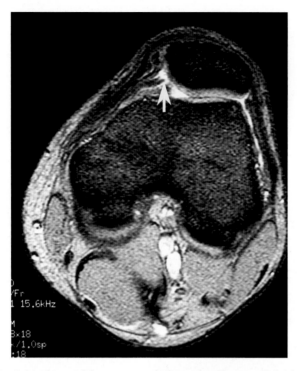

Fig. 8.31 This axial fat-suppressed T2-weighted image of the left knee shows a tear (*arrow*) of the medial patellar retinaculum at its patellar attachment.

baseball) and through contact mechanisms (e.g., laterally directed force to the medial side of the patella). Patients can be first-time dislocators, which implies acute trauma, or recurrent dislocators, implying chronicity and instability. The MRI findings in the recurrent dislocator without a history of trauma may not be as definitive. The patella has usually already reduced by the time the MRI study has been obtained, but it is frequently subluxated laterally. Images of acute patellar dislocations commonly show bone bruises of the lateral trochlea and the medial patella (**Fig. 8.30**). When the patella displaces over the lateral femoral condyle, varying sizes of osteochondral fragments may be fractured from the patella or trochlea, or both. On MRI, these loose bodies may be found in the joint, and fluid–fluid levels may be seen. MRI typically reveals a rupture of the medial patellar retinaculum, including the medial patellofemoral ligament (**Fig. 8.31**). Noting the location of the medial patellofemoral ligament is important because it can guide decisions about repair or reconstruction and may help identify the optimal location for the incision. Edema may also be seen in the region of the vastus medialis oblique. The only clue for chronic dislocators may be an attenuation or laxity of the medial retinaculum and medial patellofemoral ligament. Large effusions are commonly seen on MRI of these injuries. MRI also can help the clinician determine the degree of predisposition to patella dislocation. For instance, a hypoplastic lateral trochlea seen on axial images suggests instability secondary to insufficient osseous constraint. Identification of these predisposing factors assists with surgical planning and determination of prognosis.

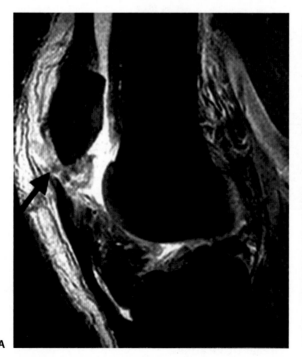

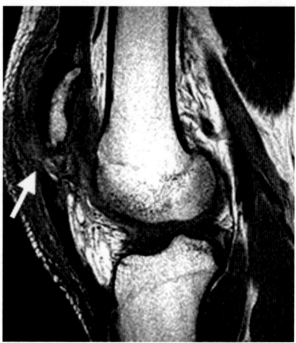

Fig. 8.32 Patellar tendon rupture. Sagittal fat-suppressed proton-density **(A)** and sagittal T1-weighted **(B)** images show a compete tear (*arrow on each*) of the proximal patellar tendon.

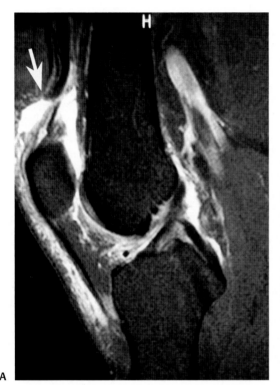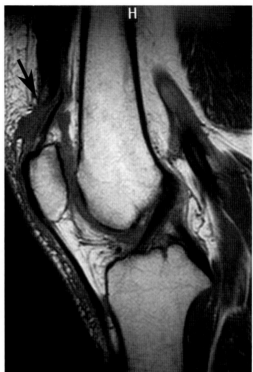

A   B

Fig. 8.33 Quadriceps tendon rupture. Sagittal fat-suppressed T2-weighted (**A**) and sagittal T1-weighted (**B**) images show a rupture of the quadriceps tendon (*arrow on each*).

Quadriceps and Patellar Tendon Ruptures

The quadriceps tendon has a laminated appearance on MRI because it is formed as a conjoined structure from four muscles. Understanding this concept allows the orthopaedic surgeon to avoid misreading the normal appearance of the quadriceps tendon as an intrasubstance injury or strain of the quadriceps tendon. Partial quadriceps tendon tears often are associated with increased T2-weighted signal, especially on fat-suppressed images, just anterior to the quadriceps tendon.

Patellar tendon ruptures (**Fig. 8.32**) usually occur in young patients (<50 years old), whereas quadriceps tendon ruptures (**Fig. 8.33**) occur in older patients, in patients with comorbidities such as diabetes mellitus and obesity, and in patients on steroids. Sagittal images are ideal for visualizing both types of ruptures. Tendon discontinuity with patella alta is seen on T1-weighted sagittal images with patellar tendon rupture. Discontinuity of the tendon and patella baja can be seen in patients with quadriceps tendon rupture.[42] Both types of rupture show edema on T2-weighted images. It is helpful to differentiate an avulsion from an intratendinous failure because bone-to-bone healing allows for a better prognosis. Although the diagnosis of quadriceps and patellar tendon rupture can frequently be made by history and physical examination (including palpation of a suprapatellar or infrapatellar defect), MRI may still provide valuable information regarding the presence or absence of other intraarticular injuries, such as cruciate ligament or meniscal tears, that may be treated at the time of ligament repair or reconstruction.

Muscle Strain

Muscle strains about the knee are common.[43] The biceps femoris (**Fig. 8.34**) is by far the most commonly strained muscle at the knee, followed by the semimembranosus and semitendinosus muscles.[44] A muscle strain is identified on MRI as a region of increased T2-weighted signal within the substance of the muscle without frank discontinuity of the muscle fibers. One third of all strains involve multiple muscles.[43] The length of abnormal signal in the strained muscle is predictive of the athlete's ability to return to play.[45] Care must be taken to differentiate an avulsion from a strain, given that avulsions often require surgical intervention.

Loose Bodies

Loose bodies are an indication for arthroscopic surgery. There are two typical sources for loose bodies:

- Osteophytes and degenerative cartilage debris in the osteoarthritic knee

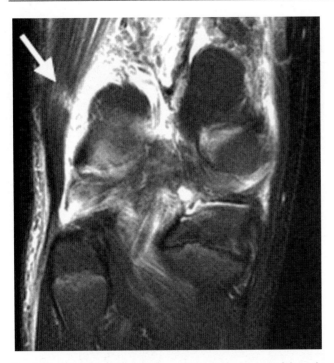

Fig. 8.34 This coronal fat-suppressed T2-weighted image of the right knee shows intramuscular edema (*arrow*), compatible with strain, involving the biceps femoris muscle.

• Osteochondral fragments from acute trauma, such as when the patella dislocates

The source of the loose body sometimes is recognizable; when it is, it offers valuable information. MRI is useful for locating chondral or osseous fragments in the knee, especially purely chondral and unmineralized lesions, which are not visible on conventional radiographs. Estimating the size of osteochondral fragments is important because the size dictates what treatment options are available. Loose bodies are found most frequently in the suprapatellar pouch, the medial and lateral gutters, and the posterior compartments[46] (**Fig. 8.35**). A good clue that allows for diagnosis of a loose body is identification of the osteochondral donor site. Multiple loose bodies seen on MRI without evidence of donor sites may suggest synovial osteochondromatosis, a benign proliferative disorder of the synovium.

MRI and MR arthrography can be used to evaluate loose bodies, which typically have low signal on T1-weighted and T2-weighted pulse sequences. Gradient-echo images are also frequently used, especially to help differentiate the diagnosis from PVNS. As with other diagnoses, it is important to correlate the MRI findings with those seen on conventional radiographs.

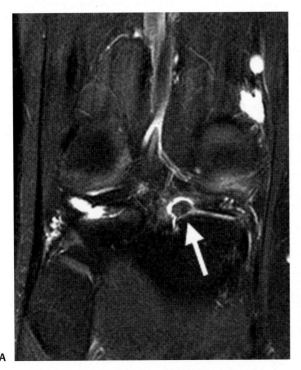
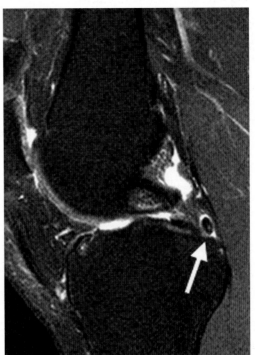

Fig. 8.35 Loose bodies. Coronal fat-suppressed T2-weighted **(A)** and sagittal fat-suppressed proton-density **(B)** images of the right knee show a loose body (*arrow on each*) located within the recess lateral to the posterior horn of the medial meniscus.

Meniscal ossicles, which may be mistaken for loose bodies, are typically located at the posterior horns of the menisci and, on MRI, appear as corticated structures with marrow signal characteristics on all sequences. Meniscal ossicles are rare and frequently asymptomatic. Their etiology and clinical significance are unclear.

Hoffa Disease

Hoffa disease (fat pad disease) has been described in young athletes, usually after traumatic events.[11] Acutely, edema is found in the patellar fat pad and can cause pain. The fat pad may hypertrophy, and repetitive trauma and fibrosis can ensue (see Anterior Interval Scarring, below).

■ Degenerative (Nonacute) Pathology

Stress Fracture

Stress fractures about the knee are often missed because this diagnosis may not be considered.[47] There may be no changes on conventional radiographs, especially early in the progression and before the sclerosis seen in the healing phase occurs. MRI findings of an acute stress fracture include a low signal intensity line on T1-weighted images and a high signal intensity linear region on T2-weighted images because of the presence of surrounding edema (**Fig. 8.36**). Although stress fractures of the femoral neck have more severe clinical consequences, stress fractures of the proximal tibia and distal femur must be identified early and treated appropriately.

Extensor Mechanism: Patellar Tendinitis

Also known as jumper's knee, patellar tendinitis is a common entity in patients participating in activities requiring explosive jumping motions, such as basketball, soccer, and volleyball. MR images may show variable amounts of focal thickening of the tendon and associated increased signal intensity on T2-weighted images (**Fig. 8.37**).[48,49] These partial tears usually are located at the proximal aspect of the tendon just distal to the inferior pole of the patella. The diagnosis of patellar tendinitis is important because the inflammatory process and associated tendon degeneration may proceed to complete rupture.

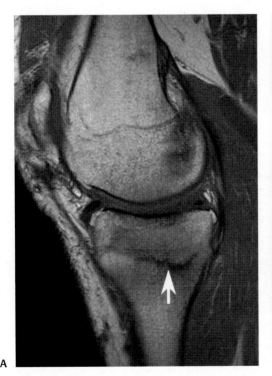
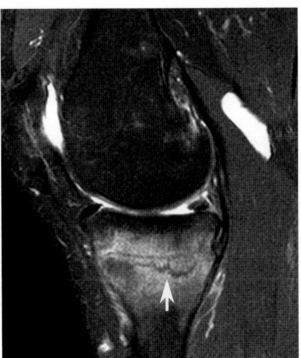

Fig. 8.36 Stress fracture. Sagittal T1-weighted **(A)** and fat-suppressed proton-density **(B)** images show a horizontal fracture (*arrow on each*) of the medial tibial metaphysis in a patient with a partial medial meniscectomy. Note the surrounding bone marrow edema pattern.

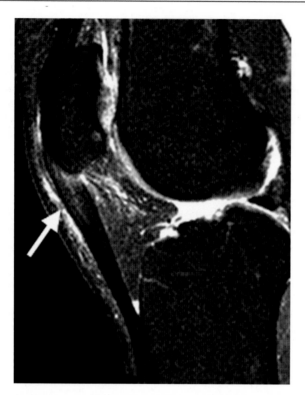

Fig. 8.37 This sagittal fat-suppressed proton-density image shows thickening and abnormal signal intensity (*arrow*) involving the proximal patellar tendon, indicative of a partial tear (jumper's knee).

Osteochondroses

Osgood-Schlatter Disease

Osgood-Schlatter disease is an osteochondrosis of the immature apophysis of the patellar insertion found commonly in adolescent males. The patella tendon insertion is tender to the touch. The adolescent can have severe pain with activity, especially with forceful extension of the flexed knee. MRI shows focal fragmentation of the patellar tendon insertion onto the tibia with associated edema (**Fig. 8.38**). Patients are treated with activity modification, rest, and occasionally casting. Very rarely, surgery is necessary to remove recalcitrant, painful fragments.

Sinding-Larsen-Johansson Disease

This entity, which is similar to but less common than Osgood-Schlatter disease, occurs at the inferior pole of the patella.

Discoid Meniscus

This entity occurs in approximately 5% of the population.[50-52] The lateral meniscus is much more commonly involved than is the medial meniscus.[53] Discoid menisci were first classified by Wantanabe et al[54] as follows:

- Grade I (complete)
- Grade II (incomplete)
- Grade III (Wrisberg or lateral meniscal variant, i.e., a meniscus that is not secured to the posterior tibia by coronary ligaments)

Monllau et al[55] described a fourth, ring-shaped type. Symptoms include a popping sensation in the knee and pain. Treatment includes arthroscopic contouring or stabilization of the discoid meniscus.

The discoid lateral meniscus is recognizable on sagittal and coronal MR images with central bridging of the anterior and posterior horns (**Fig. 8.39**). Particularly on sagittal images obtained through the central portion of the lateral compartment, the normally separate triangular anterior and posterior meniscal horns are connected by fibrocartilaginous tissue. The discoid meniscus may show increased signal intensity on T1-weighted images because of internal myxoid degeneration, even in children and young adults.

Plicae

Plicae are synovial folds that are embryologic remnants. Usually four plicae are described (**Fig. 8.40**):

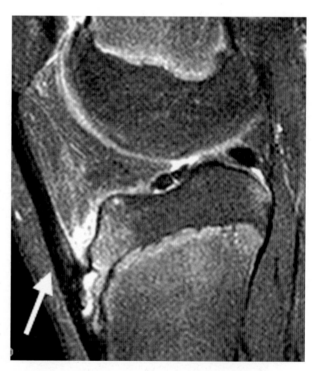

Fig. 8.38 This sagittal fat-suppressed proton-density image shows Osgood-Schlatter disease: thickening and abnormal signal intensity involving the distal patellar tendon (*arrow*); bone marrow edema and slight distraction of the tibial tubercle apophysis; and fluid accumulation and edema involving the deep infrapatellar bursa, posterior to the distal patellar tendon.

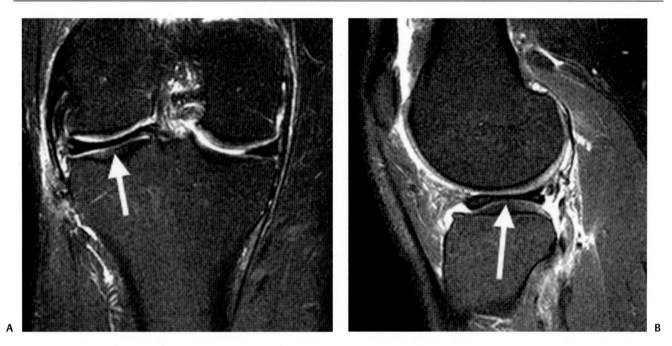

Fig. 8.39 Discoid lateral meniscus. Coronal fat-suppressed T2-weighted **(A)** and sagittal fat-suppressed proton-density **(B)** images of the right knee show central bridging (*arrow on each*) of the anterior and posterior horns of the lateral meniscus.

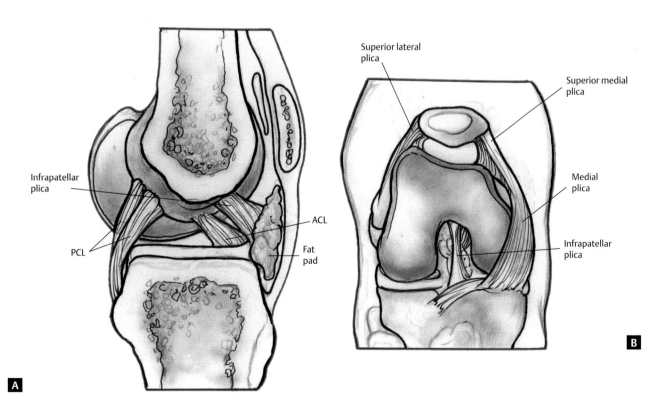

Fig. 8.40 Artist's sketch illustrating the location of superior, inferior, and medial plicae of the knee in the sagittal **(A)** and coronal **(B)** planes.

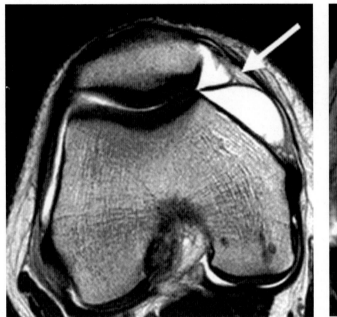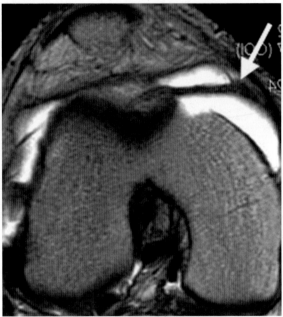

Fig. 8.41 Medial plica. **(A)** An axial T2-weighted image of the right knee showing a medial plica (*arrow*) with normal thickness. **(B)** An axial T2-weighted image of the right knee showing a medial plica (*arrow*) with thickening in a patient with plica syndrome.

- Suprapatellar
- Infrapatellar
- Lateral
- Medial

Plicae are a common source of atraumatic, activity-associated pain in young, active individuals. The medial plica is the most commonly symptomatic, and it may cause pain secondary to irritation and even abrasion of the medial femoral condyle at approximately 30 degrees of flexion as it rubs across the condyle (**Fig. 8.41**). The patient typically presents with a sharp, pinching pain, usually on the anteromedial aspect of the knee, associated with activity such as running. Well-developed and large plicae can present with a painful popping sensation in the knee. If nonoperative therapy fails to relieve symptoms, arthroscopic release of the offending plica is indicated. Chondroplasty of the abraded cartilage, if identified, is also indicated.

Bursitis

The pes anserine bursa lies over the tendinous attachment of the sartorius, gracilis, and semitendinosus tendons. The Voshell bursa is deep to the superficial MCL. T2-weighted MR images show fluid in inflamed bursae (**Fig. 8.42**). Aspiration of the fluid is an option if a collection of fluid is identified. The physical examination is indispensable for this diagnosis because pain on palpation of the pes bursa is the sine qua non of bursitis. Bursae can become infected, which

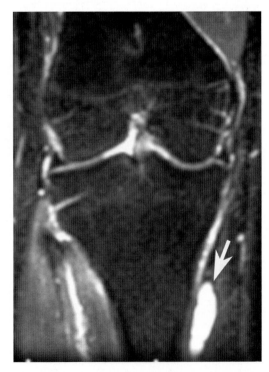

Fig. 8.42 This coronal fat-suppressed T2-weighted image of the right knee shows fluid accumulation within the bursa (*arrow*) associated with the insertion of the pes anserine tendons.

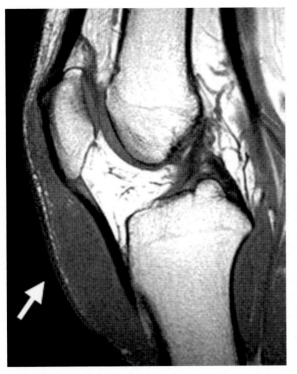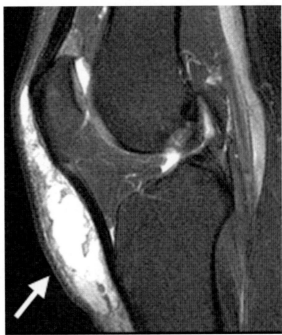

A   B

Fig. 8.43 Prepatellar bursitis. Sagittal T1-weighted (**A**) and fat-suppressed proton-density (**B**) images show distention of the prepatellar and superficial infrapatellar bursae (*arrow on each*).

makes treating them more difficult. Saphenous neuritis is in the differential diagnosis for pain in the proximal, antero-medial knee. If the bursa does not appear to be inflamed on MRI when bursitis is the suspected diagnosis, then a repeat physical examination is warranted and a diagnostic injection should be considered.

Prepatellar bursitis (**Fig. 8.43**) is a common clinical diagnosis that is seen in active individuals after an abrasion to the anterior aspect of the knee. MRI shows fluid in the prepatellar bursa. Aspiration and, rarely, surgical debridement are used to treat this condition. Similar to prepatellar bursitis, the infrapatellar bursa may also be affected.

ITB Syndrome

ITB syndrome is a common cause of lateral knee pain in runners. Other conditions in the differential diagnosis for lateral knee pain include the following:

- LCL injury
- Lateral meniscal tears and degeneration
- Popliteal tendon and hamstring strains

The presence or absence of each of these entities should be evaluated carefully, especially in patients presenting with lateral knee pain. The ITB is best seen on coronal and axial T2-weighted and fat-suppressed T2-weighted images. Edema is seen superficial to the lateral femoral epicondyle, involving the ITB. Small fluid collections, which are relatively poorly defined, and variable thickening of the ITB are often seen. The athlete has pain on palpation over the lateral femoral epicondyle. The classic Ober test is useful for diagnosing a tight ITB. If a tight ITB is found, then stretching is the first line of treatment. Activity modification, nonsteroidal anti-inflammatory medications, and modalities such as ultrasound are other options.

Osteonecrosis

Osteonecrosis (also known as avascular necrosis) in the knee is associated with many causative factors (**Table 8.6**[56-60]); most often, they are atraumatic in nature (**Fig. 8.44**). The most common atraumatic causes are alcohol abuse and steroid use, but others include the following:

- Gaucher disease
- Sickle cell disease
- Caisson disease

The exact pathophysiology has not been elucidated, but it may involve an increase in intramedullary pressure. Bone death in the femur can involve the epiphysis, metaphysis, and diaphysis. Occurring less commonly than true bone infarcts, osteonecrosis can develop secondary to an insufficiency fracture of the subchondral bone.[56] This process,

Table 8.6   Osteonecrosis

Parameter	SPONK	Atraumatic Osteonecrosis of the Knee*
Location	Medial femoral condyle	Multiple condyles, tibial involvement 20% to 30%
Distribution	Subcortical	Epiphyseal, metaphyseal, and diaphyseal common
Age	Usually >60 years	Usually <45 years
Bilateral knee involvement	<1%	>80%
Hip involvement	None	90%
Associated risk factors	Rare	>80% (e.g., steroids, alcohol)
Pathogenesis	May represent microtrauma, osteoarthritis, or osteopenia	Multiple theories regarding etiology

*Synonym: secondary or steroid-associated osteonecrosis.

termed *SPONK*, usually occurs in female patients >60 years old and involves the medial femoral condyle.[57] Lesions >2.3 cm^2 have been found to lead to osteoarthritis.[58]

MRI is the most sensitive and specific imaging modality for the early detection of osteonecrosis (**Table 8.6**[56–60]). Early diagnosis is an important consideration because patients usually do not feel pain until the joint surface collapses, and early detection may make it possible to prevent this collapse. MRI also can help distinguish osteonecrosis and SPONK. On MRI, SPONK appears as a wedge-shaped lesion in the epiphysis that can extend into the metaphysis and diaphysis. In contrast, atraumatic osteonecrosis shows a serpiginous zone demarcating the extent of the necrosis and bone marrow edema. There can be marrow conversion from red to fatty marrow. The fatty marrow shows high signal intensity on T1-weighted images.[61] The lesion in SPONK is subchondral and usually involves collapse and flattening of the medial femoral condyle. It is important to distinguish between these two forms of osteonecrosis because the treatments differ.

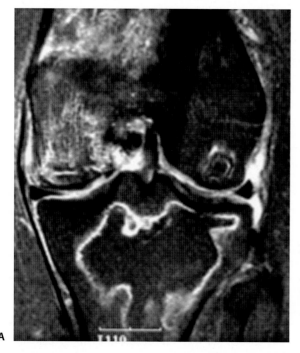
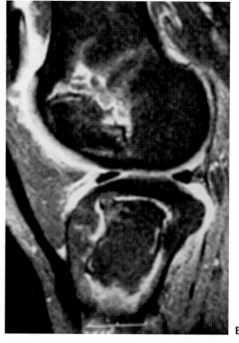

Fig. 8.44 Osteonecrosis. Coronal **(A)** and sagittal **(B)** fat-suppressed T2-weighted images of the left knee show findings typical for osteonecrosis of the distal femur and proximal tibia. Note the extensive reactive and stress-related bone marrow edema involving the medial femoral condyle. (From Khanna AJ, Cosgarea AJ, Mont MA, et al. Magnetic resonance imaging of the knee: current techniques and spectrum of disease. J Bone Joint Surg Am 2001;83:128–141. Reprinted by permission.)

Degenerative Joint Disease

Traditionally, much of the evaluation of degenerative knee disease is accomplished with conventional radiographs. In the past, when the findings and symptoms of degenerative knee disease were severe enough, patients were offered total joint arthroplasty. Currently, for active, physiologically young patients with unicompartmental disease, there are other options, including the following:

- High tibial osteotomy
- Unicompartmental arthroplasty
- Arthroscopy (for selected patients)

In the active patient with degenerative knee disease, there are findings on MRI that potentially can be addressed, at least temporarily, with less extensive procedures than total knee arthroplasty; these findings include the following:

- Scarring of the suprapatellar pouch
- Complex meniscus tears with flap formation
- Localized cartilage lesions
- Scarring and adhesions of the infrapatellar fat pad

Osteophyte formation is a common finding in degenerative disease and contributes to the painful loss of motion of the knee. Typically, flexion contractures occur, which substantially hinder a patient's gait. When flexion contractures occur because of a mechanical block to extension, identification of these offending osteophytes allows for planning for their surgical removal.

Degenerative Meniscus

Degenerative meniscus refers to a meniscus with complex tears and attenuation. Eventually, the meniscus can be extruded out of the compartment and into the medial or lateral gutter. Initially, primarily one compartment is affected, depending on the alignment of the knee. Because varus alignment is more common, the medial compartment, which receives most of the forces, usually is affected primarily. Typically, associated cartilage changes also occur.

It is useful to note whether the meniscus appears to have degenerated severely and is not functional, or is still essentially intact. This determination helps with patient counseling and surgical planning.

Adhesion Formation

Part of the degenerative process is the formation of adhesions, especially in the suprapatellar pouch. Adhesions appear as dark gray or black bands on MRI. These bands can be seen in the suprapatellar pouch, usually on sagittal T2-weighted images, running from the quadriceps tendon posteriorly to the synovium on the anterior aspect of the femur. The adhesions are thought to affect the biomechanics of the knee adversely and are a source of ongoing investigation. Pli-

cae and adhesions combine to decrease the volume of the knee joint and create pseudocompartments. If the steroid and anesthetic are injected into a pseudocompartment, then the painful areas of the knee are not exposed to the medications, which provides an explanation for why an injection into the knee may not relieve symptoms. Arthroscopic release of adhesions increases the volume of the knee joint and may restore more normal knee mechanics.[62]

Anterior Interval Scarring

The anterior interval of the knee is the space between the patellar tendon and the intermeniscal ligament. It usually is filled with a mobile, compliant fat pad. Surgery and senescent degeneration of the knee are associated with scarring and decreased compliance of this space. Physical examination of such patients reveals an immobile, noncompliant patellar tendon. If the patient complains of pain in the anterior aspect of the knee in the presence of fat pad scaring, then an excision or release of this scar tissue may be beneficial. Similar to suprapatellar adhesions, anterior interval scarring appears as linear bands. These bands begin on the patellar tendon and traverse the fat pad to insert on the anterior aspect of the proximal tibia, anterior to the ACL.

Baker (Popliteal) Cyst

A Baker cyst (**Fig. 8.45**), a classic finding in degenerative knee disease, is a collection of fluid that has escaped from the joint posteromedially and rests between the medial head of gastrocnemius and semimembranosus. Although the term *Baker cyst* is commonly used to describe all popliteal or synovial cysts in the region of the knee, it should be noted that the term is intended for those cases in which the gastrocnemiosemimembranous bursa is involved.[63] The typical MRI findings include a mass in the posterior fossa with uniform low signal on T1-weighted images and high signal on T2-weighted images. The walls of the cyst are well circumscribed.

These collections can decompress spontaneously into the lower leg. Operative treatment is not usually recommended, but when the cyst is present for an extended period of time, the contents may become gelatinous, and then open or arthroscopic intervention may be beneficial.

■ Infectious Conditions: Osteomyelitis and Septic Effusion

Osteomyelitis and septic effusion are common forms of infection involving the knee. MRI is the most sensitive and specific test for the presence of osteomyelitis.[64-66] Osteomyelitis causes an intense reaction of the surrounding tissue

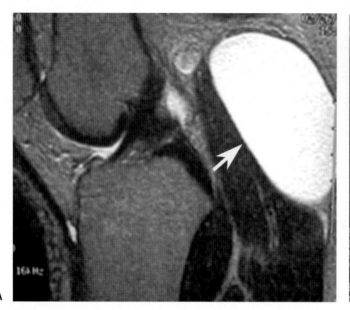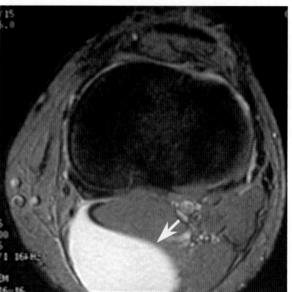

Fig. 8.45 Baker cyst. Sagittal **(A)** and axial **(B)** T2-weighted images show distension of the gastrocnemiosemimembranosus bursa (*arrow on each*).

characterized by edema that is seen on T2-weighted images. A septic effusion can be seen on T2-weighted images as a fluid collection within the joint. Septic arthritis also causes associated bone marrow edema. The diagnosis can be confirmed with aspiration or biopsy, and surgical intervention and antibiotics usually are necessary for treatment. Periarticular osteomyelitis involving the knee joint exhibits a bone marrow edema pattern, hyperintense relative to normal marrow on T2-weighted and STIR images and hypointense on T1-weighted images. Loss of the normally sharply defined low signal intensity cortical margin may occur with osteolysis secondary to infection. An intraosseous fluid collection, surrounded by edema, suggests the presence of focal bone abscess. Septic arthritis may simply exhibit features of a knee joint effusion, but frequently synovial thickening is observed, particularly conspicuous on contrast-enhanced fat-suppressed T1-weighted imaging. Also, a periarticular bone marrow edema pattern may be identified secondary to generalized hyperemia, independent of actual osseous infection.

■ Postoperative Findings

Postoperative Meniscus: Partial Meniscectomy, Repair, and Allograft Replacement

Surgical approaches to the treatment of meniscal tears include meniscal debridement or partial meniscec-

tomy, meniscal repair, and meniscal allograft placement. These techniques are designed to stabilize the meniscus while maintaining its shock-absorbing and loading-force-distributing properties. The procedures share the clinical goals of pain relief, restoration of mechanical function, and prevention or mitigation of the development of chondromalacia and osteoarthritis.

With partial meniscectomy, as little meniscal tissue as possible is resected to stabilize the articular margin of the meniscus without excessively exposing the articular cartilage to unprotected impaction forces. Thus, on MRI, it is common to identify the presence of a small tear involving the meniscal remnant (**Fig. 8.46**). The tear may be stable and asymptomatic. Also, because the process of meniscal debridement creates a new articular surface, intrameniscal MRI findings related to myxoid degeneration may abut the surgically recontoured articular margin, converting internal meniscal signal (noted on T1-weighted or proton-density images) into surface-communicating signal and potentially creating the false impression of a meniscal tear.[4] Although T2-weighted imaging and MR arthrography may be used to differentiate converted intrameniscal signal intensity from a true surface defect into which fluid can dissect, evidence of a surface tear does not necessarily translate to a clinically relevant cause of a patient's symptoms. However, if, after a conservative partial meniscectomy, a large tear involving the meniscal remnant is noted on MRI, its clinical significance probably is similar to that of a tear in a nondebrided meniscus. After partial meniscectomy, severe tears identified with MRI typically exhibit a complex signal pattern, flap, or

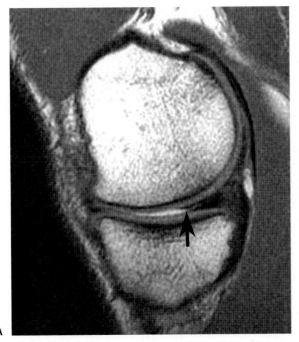
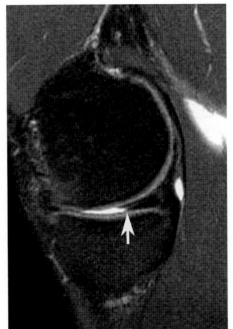

Fig. 8.46 Partial meniscectomy. Sagittal proton-density **(A)** and sagittal fat-suppressed T2-weighted **(B)** images show blunting of the anterior margin of the posterior horn of the medial meniscus, con-sistent with meniscal debridement. The small horizontal tear (*arrow*) is unlikely to be clinically symptomatic.

fragment displacement or show progressive enlargement on serial postoperative MRI studies[67] (**Fig. 8.47**).

Meniscal repairs, typically performed in the context of a vertical longitudinal tear, often continue to manifest abnormal signal, communicating with the meniscal articular surfaces despite successful stabilization of the meniscus (**Fig. 8.48**).[4,67–69]

On serial follow-up MRI examinations, the apparent surface defect may remain, but if progressive development of adjacent chondromalacia or osseous stress reaction is not identified on subsequent postoperative studies and the morphology of the tear remains unchanged, surgical stabilization of the meniscus probably has been achieved (**Fig. 8.49**). In the case of a displaced meniscal tear that has been repaired, the MRI study should reveal normal meniscal morphology and positioning but, again, the linear tear may remain evident. MR arthrography does not statistically improve accuracy in detecting postoperative meniscal tears and, like nonarthrographic techniques, cannot distinguish between residual and recurrent tears.[70] Additionally, the penetration or imbibition

of gadolinium contrast material in a repaired meniscal defect does not necessarily indicate that the tear is unstable or responsible for a patient's symptoms.

With meniscal allograft procedures, MRI is used to evaluate the positioning of the graft. A graft may be displaced by loading, shearing, or rotational forces that exceed its surgical attachments; by traction related to capsular adhesions or contracture; or by adjacent arthrofibrosis (**Fig. 8.50**). On MRI, tears involving the meniscal allograft exhibit the same features as do tears in a native meniscus.[71]

In summary, care must be taken when assessing the clinical significance of MRI findings after meniscal surgery. Most importantly, a meniscal tear involving a debrided or repaired meniscus, even when observed with MR arthrography, does not necessarily correlate with the presence of clinical symptoms or functional impairment. In a patient with knee pain and a history of meniscal surgery, the role of MRI includes evaluation of the knee for other potential symptom-producing pathology, especially chondromalacia, osseous stress injury, and osteonecrosis.[72,73]

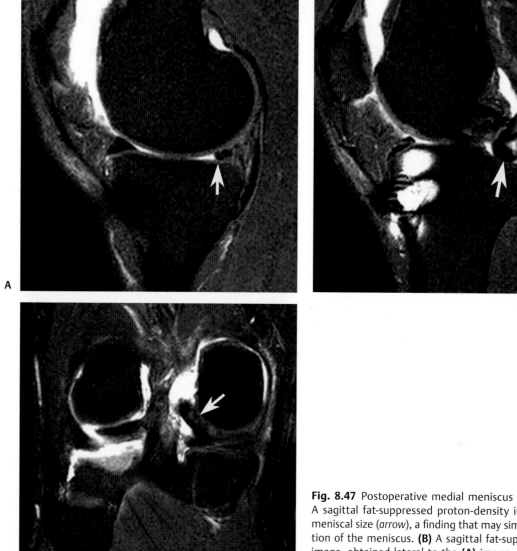

Fig. 8.47 Postoperative medial meniscus with displaced flap. **(A)** A sagittal fat-suppressed proton-density image shows decreased meniscal size (*arrow*), a finding that may simply reflect partial resection of the meniscus. **(B)** A sagittal fat-suppressed proton-density image, obtained lateral to the **(A)** image, shows posterior central displacement of a large meniscal flap, arising from the posterior horn remnant (*arrow*). **(C)** A fat-suppressed coronal T2-weighted image of the right knee shows central displacement of a large posterior medial meniscal flap (*arrow*).

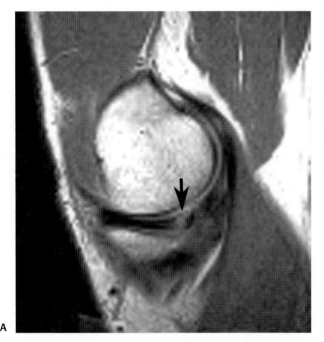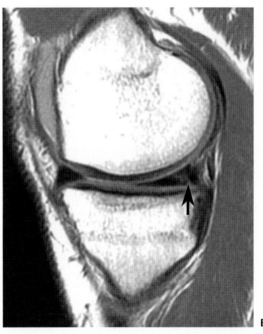

A

B

Fig. 8.48 Meniscal repair. **(A)** A preoperative sagittal T1-weighted image shows a peripheral vertical longitudinal tear (*arrow*) of the posterior horn of the medial meniscus. **(B)** A postoperative sagittal T1-weighted image in the same patient shows persistent signal communication with the articular surface of the meniscus (*arrow*).

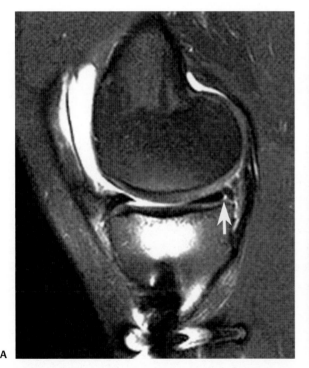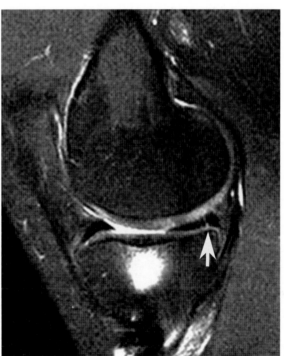

A

B

Fig. 8.49 Meniscal repair. **(A)** A sagittal fat-suppressed proton-density image, obtained after repair of a peripheral vertical longitudinal tear, shows persistent signal communication with the articular surface of the posterior horn of the medial meniscus (*arrow*). **(B)** A sagittal fat-suppressed proton-density image, obtained 1 year later in the same patient, shows stability of the meniscal signal pattern (*arrow*).

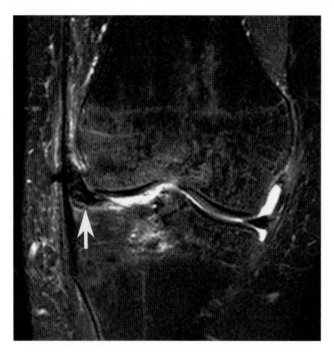

Fig. 8.50 This coronal fat-suppressed T2-weighted image of the right knee shows fibrous adherence of the meniscal allograft (*arrow*) to the ITB with lateral displacement of the allograft.

ACL Reconstruction

The ACL graft is a low signal intensity structure that should run in continuity along approximately the same trajectory as the native ACL (**Fig. 8.51**). Metallic screws can be identified on MRI by their very dark appearance. Ferromagnetic artifact is a major problem because it can conceal local pathology. Bioabsorbable interference screws and transfixion pins do not cause such artifact. Absorption of bioabsorbable implants varies but takes at least 1 year.[74] Cyst formation is a normal finding around these screws as they are absorbed.[75] Bone graft incorporation, which can take 3 years or more,[75] also can be seen on MRI.

MRI is useful in the evaluation of the patient who has had an ACL reconstruction or repair. The study should be evaluated for the following (**Fig. 8.52**):

- Presence or absence of graft failure
- Impingement
- Arthrofibrosis
- Placement and orientation of the graft, hardware, and tunnels

Most ACL grafts are 8 to 10 mm wide, and the associated tunnel should not be more than 10 mm wide on MRI. Widening of the graft tunnel can be seen with chronic remodeling secondary to the presence of a ganglion cyst or other process, such as infection, within the graft.

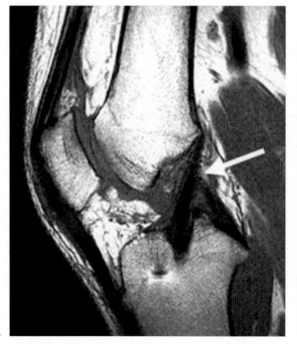

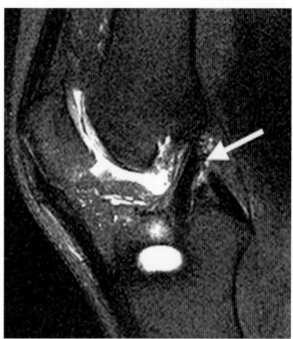

Fig. 8.51 ACL reconstruction. Sagittal T1-weighted **(A)** and fat-suppressed proton-density **(B)** images show normal ACL graft trajectory (*arrow on each*).

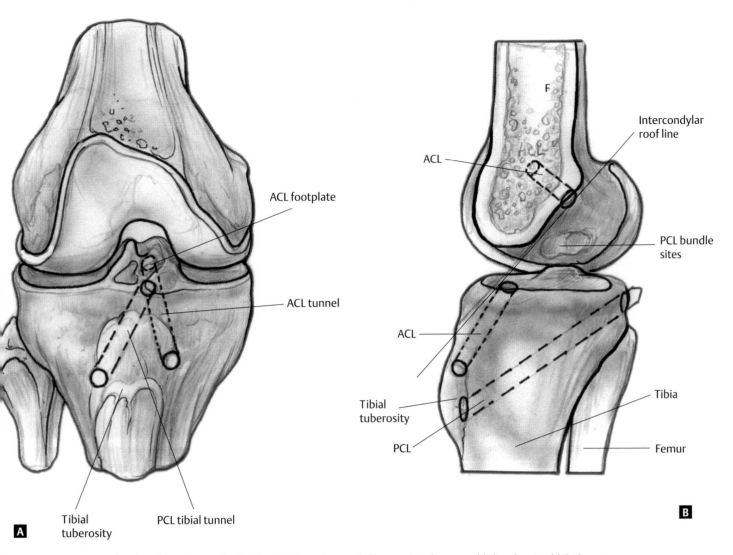

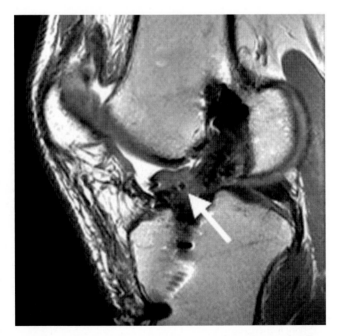

Fig. 8.52 Artist's sketches illustrating optimal ACL and PCL graft tunnel placement in the coronal **(A)** and sagittal **(B)** planes.

Fig. 8.53 This sagittal proton-density image shows focal arthrofibrosis, consistent with a cyclops lesion (*arrow*), anterior to an ACL graft.

All of the potential sites of osseous impingement should be evaluated carefully, including the following:

- Intercondylar roof
- Intraarticular entrance zones of the bone tunnels
- Side walls of the intercondylar fossa

The MRI findings in roof impingement include posterior bowing of the graft caused by contact of the graft against the roof, increased signal in the distal two thirds of the graft, and placement of the tibial tunnel anterior to the slope of the intercondylar roof when the knee is in an extended position.[76]

Cyclops Lesion

The cyclops lesion results from granulation tissue overgrowth of remnant ACL. This entity, which can cause a painful block to full extension, is found anterior to the ACL graft and is easily seen on MRI (**Fig. 8.53**). Patients with a cyclops lesion often also have associated anterior compartment degenerative changes, which should be evaluated carefully on the MRI study.

References

1. Hardaker WT Jr, Garrett WE Jr, Bassett FH III. Evaluation of acute traumatic hemarthrosis of the knee joint. South Med J 1990;83:640–644

2. Khanna AJ, Cosgarea AJ, Mont MA, et al. Magnetic resonance imaging of the knee: current techniques and spectrum of disease. J Bone Joint Surg Am 2001;83:128–141

3. Cheung LP, Li KC, Hollett MD, Bergman AG, Herfkens RJ. Meniscal tears of the knee: accuracy of detection with fast spin-echo MR imaging and arthroscopic correlation in 293 patients. Radiology 1997;203:508–512

4. Deutsch AL, Mink JH, Fox JM, et al. Peripheral meniscal tears: MR findings after conservative treatment or arthroscopic repair. Radiology 1990;176:485–488

5. Justice WW, Quinn SF. Error patterns in the MR imaging evaluation of menisci of the knee. Radiology 1995;196:617–621

6. Kaplan PA, Nelson NL, Garvin KL, Brown DE. MR of the knee: the significance of high signal in the meniscus that does not clearly extend to the surface. AJR Am J Roentgenol 1991;156:333–336

7. Kornick J, Trefelner E, McCarthy S, Lange R, Lynch K, Jokl P. Meniscal abnormalities in the asymptomatic population at MR imaging. Radiology 1990;177:463–465

8. Rubin DA, Paletta GA Jr. Current concepts and controversies in meniscal imaging. Magn Reson Imaging Clin N Am 2000;8:243–270

9. Stoller DW, Martin C, Crues JV III, Kaplan L, Mink JH. Meniscal tears: pathologic correlation with MR imaging. Radiology 1987;163:731–735

10. Wright DH, De Smet AA, Norris M. Bucket-handle tears of the medial and lateral menisci of the knee: value of MR imaging in detecting displaced fragments. AJR Am J Roentgenol 1995;165:621–625

11. Kelley EA, Berquist TH. Knee. In: Berquist TH, ed. MRI of the Musculoskeletal System. Philadelphia: Lippincott Williams & Wilkins; 2006:303–429

12. De Smet AA, Norris MA, Yandow DR, Quintana FA, Graf BK, Keene JS. MR diagnosis of meniscal tears of the knee: importance of high signal in the meniscus that extends to the surface. AJR Am J Roentgenol 1993;161:101–107

13. Rubin DA. MR imaging of the knee menisci. Radiol Clin North Am 1997;35:21–44

14. Peterfy CG, Janzen DL, Tirman PFJ, van Dijke CF, Pollack M, Genant HK. "Magic-angle" phenomenon: a cause of increased signal in the normal lateral meniscus on short-TE MR images of the knee. AJR Am J Roentgenol 1994;163:149–154

15. Turner DA, Rapoport MI, Erwin WD, McGould M, Silvers RI. Truncation artifact: a potential pitfall in MR imaging of the menisci of the knee. Radiology 1991;179:629–633

16. Tuckman GA, Miller WJ, Remo JW, Fritts HM, Rozansky MI. Radial tears of the menisci: MR findings. AJR Am J Roentgenol 1994;163:395–400

17. Costa CR, Morrison WB, Carrino JA. Medial meniscus extrusion on knee MRI: is extent associated with severity of degeneration or type of tear? AJR Am J Roentgenol 2004;183:17–23

18. Vande Berg BC, Malghem J, Poilvache P, Maldague B, Lecouvet FE. Meniscal tears with fragments displaced in notch and recesses of knee: MR imaging with arthroscopic comparison. Radiology 2005;234:842–850

19. Lecas LK, Helms CA, Kosarek FJ, Garret WE. Inferiorly displaced flap tears of the medial meniscus: MR appearance and clinical significance. AJR Am J Roentgenol 2000;174:161–164

20. Vande Berg BC, Poilvache P, Duchateau F, et al. Lesions of the menisci of the knee: value of MR imaging criteria for recognition of unstable lesions. AJR Am J Roentgenol 2001;176:771–776

21. Gentili A, Seeger LL, Yao L, Do HM. Anterior cruciate ligament tear: indirect signs at MR imaging. Radiology 1994;193:835–840

22. Umans H, Wimpfheimer O, Haramati N, Applbaum YH, Adler M, Bosco J. Diagnosis of partial tears of the anterior cruciate ligament of the knee: value of MR imaging. AJR Am J Roentgenol 1995;165:893–897

23. Cone RO III. Knee. Section B. Imaging sports-related injuries of the knee. In: DeLee JC, Drez D Jr, Miller MD, eds. DeLee and Drez's Orthopaedic Sports Medicine: Principles and Practice. Philadelphia: WB Saunders; 2003:1595–1652

24. Graf BK, Cook DA, De Smet AA, Keene JS. "Bone bruises" on magnetic resonance imaging evaluation of anterior cruciate ligament injuries. Am J Sports Med 1993;21:220–223

25. Robertson PL, Schweitzer ME, Bartolozzi AR, Ugoni A. Anterior cruciate ligament tears: evaluation of multiple signs with MR imaging. Radiology 1994;193:829–834

26. Tung GA, Davis LM, Wiggins ME, Fadale PD. Tears of the anterior cruciate ligament: primary and secondary signs at MR imaging. Radiology 1993;188:661–667

27. McCauley TR, Moses M, Kier R, Lynch JK, Barton JW, Jokl P. MR diagnosis of tears of anterior cruciate ligament of the knee: importance of ancillary findings. AJR Am J Roentgenol 1994;162:115–119

28. Goldman AB, Pavlov H, Rubenstein D. The Segond fracture of the proximal tibia: a small avulsion that reflects major ligamentous damage. AJR Am J Roentgenol 1988;151:1163–1167

29. Gross ML, Grover JS, Bassett LW, Seeger LL, Finerman GA. Magnetic resonance imaging of the posterior cruciate ligament. Clinical use to improve diagnostic accuracy. Am J Sports Med 1992;20:732–737

30. Sonin AH, Fitzgerald SW, Friedman H, Hoff FL, Hendrix RW, Rogers LF. Posterior cruciate ligament injury: MR imaging diagnosis and patterns of injury. Radiology 1994;190:455–458

31. Sonin AH, Fitzgerald SW, Hoff FL, Friedman H, Bresler ME. MR imaging of the posterior cruciate ligament: normal, abnormal, and associated injury patterns. Radiographics 1995;15:551–561

32. Escobedo EM, Mills WJ, Hunter JC. The "reverse Segond" fracture: association with a tear of the posterior cruciate ligament and medial meniscus. AJR Am J Roentgenol 2002;178:979–983

33. Shelbourne KD, Rubinstein RA Jr. Methodist Sports Medicine Center's experience with acute and chronic isolated posterior cruciate ligament injuries. Clin Sports Med 1994;13:531–543

34. O'Donoghue DH. Treatment of acute ligamentous injuries of the knee. Orthop Clin North Am 1973;4:617–645

35. Yao L, Dungan D, Seeger LL. MR imaging of tibial collateral ligament injury: comparison with clinical examination. Skeletal Radiol 1994;23:521–524

36. D'Amato MJ, Bach BR Jr. Knee. Section J: Anterior cruciate ligament injuries. Part 1: Anterior cruciate ligament reconstruction in the adult. In: DeLee JC, Drez D Jr, Miller MD, eds. DeLee and Drez's Orthopaedic Sports Medicine: Principles and Practice. Philadelphia: WB Saunders; 2003:2012–2067

37. LaPrade RF, Gilbert TJ, Bollom TS, Wentorf F, Chaljub G. The magnetic resonance imaging appearance of individual structures of the posterolateral knee. A prospective study of normal knees and knees with surgically verified grade III injuries. Am J Sports Med 2000;28:191–199

38. Hughston JC, Eilers AF. The role of the posterior oblique ligament in repairs of acute medial (collateral) ligament tears of the knee. J Bone Joint Surg Am 1973;55:923–940

39. Green NE, Allen BL. Vascular injuries associated with dislocation of the knee. J Bone Joint Surg Am 1977;59:236–239

40. Good L, Johnson RJ. The dislocated knee. J Am Acad Orthop Surg 1995;3:284–292

41. Sonin AH, Fitzgerald SW, Bresler ME, Kirsch MD, Hoff FL, Friedman H. MR imaging appearance of the extensor mechanism of the knee: functional anatomy and injury patterns. Radiographics 1995;15:367–382

42. Zeiss J, Saddemi SR, Ebraheim NA. MR imaging of the quadriceps tendon: normal layered configuration and its importance in cases of tendon rupture. AJR Am J Roentgenol 1992;159:1031–1034

43. De Smet AA, Best TM. MR imaging of the distribution and location of acute hamstring injuries in athletes. AJR Am J Roentgenol 2000;174:393–399

44. Koulouris G, Connell D. Evaluation of the hamstring muscle complex following acute injury. Skeletal Radiol 2003;32:582–589

45. Connell DA, Schneider-Kolsky ME, Hoving JL, et al. Longitudinal study comparing sonographic and MRI assessments of acute and healing hamstring injuries. AJR Am J Roentgenol 2004;183:975–984

46. Brossman J, Preidler KW, Daenen B, et al. Imaging of osseous and cartilaginous intraarticular bodies in the knee: comparison of MR imaging and MR arthrography with CT and CT arthrography in cadavers. Radiology 1996;200:509–517

47. Capps GW, Hayes CW. Easily missed injuries around the knee. Radiographics 1994;14:1191–1210

48. Yu JS, Petersilge C, Sartoris DJ, Pathria MN, Resnick D. MR imaging of injuries of the extensor mechanism of the knee. Radiographics 1994;14:541–551

49. Yu JS, Popp JE, Kaeding CC, Lucas J. Correlation of MR imaging and pathologic findings in athletes undergoing surgery for chronic patellar tendinitis. AJR Am J Roentgenol 1995;165:115–118

50. Kato Y, Oshida M, Aizawa S, Saito A, Ryu J. Discoid lateral menisci in Japanese cadaver knees. Mod Rheumatol 2004;14:154–159

51. Rao PS, Rao SK, Paul R. Clinical, radiologic, and arthroscopic assessment of discoid lateral meniscus. Arthroscopy 2001;17:275–277

52. Rohren EM, Kosarek FJ, Helms CA. Discoid lateral meniscus and the frequency of meniscal tears. Skeletal Radiol 2001;30:316–320

53. Berquist TH. Musculoskeletal Imaging Companion. Philadelphia: Lippincott Williams & Wilkins; 2002

54. Wantanabe M, Takeda S, Ikeuchi H. Atlas of Arthroscopy. Berlin: Springer-Verlag; 1979

55. Monllau JC, León A, Cugat R, Ballester J. Ring-shaped lateral meniscus. Arthroscopy 1998;14:502–504

56. Yamamoto T, Bullough PG. Spontaneous osteonecrosis of the knee: the result of subchondral insufficiency fracture. J Bone Joint Surg Am 2000;82:858–866

57. Ecker ML, Lotke PA. Spontaneous osteonecrosis of the knee. J Am Acad Orthop Surg 1994;2:173–178

58. Rozing PM, Insall J, Bohne WH. Spontaneous osteonecrosis of the knee. J Bone Joint Surg Am 1980;62:2–7

59. Ramnath RR, Kattapuram SV. MR appearance of SONK-like subchondral abnormalities in the adult knee: SONK redefined. Skeletal Radiol 2004;33:575–581

60. Yates PJ, Calder JD, Stranks GJ, Conn KS, Peppercorn D, Thomas NP. Early MRI diagnosis and non-surgical management of spontaneous osteonecrosis of the knee. Knee 2007;14:112–116

61. Vande Berg BC, Gilon R, Malghem J, Lecouvet F, Depresseux G, Houssiau FA. Correlation between baseline femoral neck marrow status and the development of femoral head osteonecrosis in corticosteroid-treated patients: a longitudinal study by MR imaging. Eur J Radiol 2006;58:444–449

62. Millett PJ, Steadman JR. The role of capsular distention in the arthroscopic management of arthrofibrosis of the knee: A technical consideration. Arthroscopy 2001;17:E31

63. Lindgren PG, Willén R. Gastrocnemio-semimembranosus bursa and its relation to the knee joint. I. Anatomy and histology. Acta Radiol Diagn (Stockh) 1977;18:497–512

64. Bancroft LW. MR imaging of infectious processes of the knee. Magn Reson Imaging Clin N Am 2007;15:1–11

65. Kapoor A, Page S, Lavalley M, Gale DR, Felson DT. Magnetic resonance imaging for diagnosing foot osteomyelitis: a meta-analysis. Arch Intern Med 2007;167:125–132

66. Pineda C, Vargas A, Rodríguez AV. Imaging of osteomyelitis: current concepts. Infect Dis Clin North Am 2006;20:789–825

67. Farley TE, Howell SM, Love KF, Wolfe RD, Neumann CH. Meniscal tears: MR and arthrographic findings after arthroscopic repair. Radiology 1991;180:517–522

68. Davis KW, Tuite MJ. MR imaging of the postoperative meniscus of the knee. Semin Musculoskelet Radiol 2002;6:35–45

69. Lim PS, Schweitzer ME, Bhatia M, et al. Repeat tear of postoperative meniscus: potential MR imaging signs. Radiology 1999;210:183–188

70. White LM, Schweitzer ME, Weishaupt D, Kramer J, Davis A, Marks PH. Diagnosis of recurrent meniscal tears: prospective evaluation of conventional MR imaging, indirect MR arthrography, and direct MR arthrography. Radiology 2002;222:421–429

71. Potter HG, Rodeo SA, Wickiewicz TL, Warren RF. MR imaging of meniscal allografts: correlation with clinical and arthroscopic outcomes. Radiology 1996;198:509–514

72. Brahme SK, Fox JM, Ferkel RD, Friedman MJ, Flannigan BD, Resnick DL. Osteonecrosis of the knee after arthroscopic surgery: diagnosis with MR imaging. Radiology 1991;178:851–853

73. Dandy DJ, Jackson RW. Meniscectomy and chondromalacia of the femoral condyle. J Bone Joint Surg Am 1975;57:1116–1119

74. Cossey AJ, Kalairajah Y, Morcom R, Spriggins AJ. Magnetic resonance imaging evaluation of biodegradable transfemoral fixation used in anterior cruciate ligament reconstruction. Arthroscopy 2006;22:199–204

75. Macarini L, Murrone M, Marini S, Mocci A, Ettorre GC. [MRI in ACL reconstructive surgery with PDLLA bioabsorbable interference screws: evaluation of degradation and osteointegration processes of bioabsorbable screws]. Radiol Med (Torino) 2004;107:47–57

76. Watanabe BM, Howell SM. Arthroscopic findings associated with roof impingement of an anterior cruciate ligament graft. Am J Sports Med 1995;23:616–625

9 The Foot and Ankle

Daniel J. Durand, John A. Carrino, Meena W. Shatby, Ali Moshirfar, and John T. Campbell

■ Specialized Pulse Sequences and Imaging Protocols

Indiscriminate use of MRI can confuse the clinical situation by identifying findings that are not necessarily pathologic or that are poorly correlated with clinical symptoms; these findings in turn can lead to unnecessary and costly interventions and can delay proper diagnosis and treatment.[1] MRI of the foot and ankle has improved with the development of high-field systems and enhanced surface coil technology. Most centers use a standard screening examination, consisting of an array of specified imaging planes and pulse sequences. For the ankle, the patient is imaged in a supine, feet-first position with the malleoli several centimeters inferior to the center of the coil; images are obtained in the axial, coronal, and sagittal planes relative to the tabletop. Imaging of the foot is performed in so-called oblique planes, which are parallel and perpendicular to the long axis of the metatarsals, and with minimal plantarflexion to accentuate the fat plane between the peroneal tendons, improve visualization of the calcaneofibular ligament, and decrease the *magic angle effect.*[2]

In addition to standard T1-weighted and T2-weighted sequences, fat-suppressed T2-weighted and STIR sequences are extremely sensitive for detecting marrow and soft-tissue pathology by accentuating the increased signal of fluid and edema relative to the surrounding structures. A proton-density pulse sequence is occasionally used, often with fat suppression; it combines characteristics of T1-weighted and T2-weighted images. These sequences are acquired with an FSE technique that produces the desired contrast in a fraction of the time needed for conventional T2-weighted sequences, minimizing patient motion, improving throughput, and providing great benefit for claustrophobic patients. Novel developments such as parallel imaging techniques,[3] combined with increased signal-to-noise ratio at higher field strengths, may continue to reduce scan times.

Imaging parameters can also be refined for optimal cartilage visualization (see Chapter 14). Gradient-echo sequences are often used to evaluate ligaments and articular cartilage (see Chapter 14), particularly in the coronal plane, allowing for optimal visualization of the articular cartilage within the mortise joint. However, early reports comparing cartilage imaging within the ankle at 3.0 T and 1.5 T have suggested that coronal intermediate-weighted FSE sequences result in better images than do fat-suppressed gradient-echo–based sequences at 3.0 T, primarily because of increased artifact at higher field strength on gradient-echo sequences.[4] In addition, gradient-echo sequences should be avoided in the presence of indwelling metal hardware because of the technique's inherent increased artifact (see Chapter 1).

MR arthrography can be performed as a direct or indirect method. Direct MR arthrography is performed by injecting approximately 10 mL of diluted gadolinium contrast agent into the ankle joint from an anterior approach, entering just medial to the tibialis anterior tendon with slight cranial angulation; care should be taken to avoid the course of the dorsalis pedis artery.[5] Postinjection imaging sequences typically include fat-suppressed T1-weighted and T2-weighted images. Indirect MR arthrography is performed by injecting gadolinium intravenously and imaging the joint after contrast has been taken up by the synovium and then diffused into the joint.

Direct MR arthrography of the ankle can improve visualization of acute and chronic ligamentous injuries, particularly those involving the LCL complex, although arthrography can also be useful for visualizing syndesmotic and deltoid ligament tears. MR arthrography has also been shown to be an accurate technique for visualizing intraarticular pathology in the various ankle impingement syndromes, in differentiating stage II from stage III osteochondral talar lesions, and in identifying loose bodies and synovial disorders.[5] Indirect MR arthrography is limited by the lack of joint distention and by inferior contrast relative to direct arthrography, although it can be a useful adjunct to MRI for the assessment of the following[5]:

- Subtle cartilage defects
- Osteochondral talar lesions
- Ligamentous injuries
- Synovitis
- Sinus tarsi syndrome

However, with the advent of high-field, high-resolution imaging and novel noncontrast MR techniques, direct and indirect MR arthrography techniques may be rendered obsolete in the future.

■ Traumatic Conditions

Bone Contusion

Bone contusion represents an injury to the internal bone structure with microtrabecular disruption, but no gross cortical fracture. On MRI, bone contusion appears as a focal area of low signal on T1-weighted images with ill-defined margins; high signal on T2-weighted images signifies edema within the bone marrow but an intact cortical structure[6] (**Fig. 9.1**). Bone bruises may be seen after direct trauma or after acute ankle sprains.[6,7] Certain bone-bruise patterns are characteristic for specific injury mechanisms. For example, inversion injuries are associated with contusion of the medial malleolus and medial talus (with signal changes seen in those structures), whereas a plantarflexion mechanism can result in a posterior tibial bone bruise. Jamming injuries of the hallux may result in a bone contusion of the first metatarsal head dorsally, but direct impact on the ball of the foot may result in contusion of a sesamoid. Acute bone bruises typically resolve within 2 to 3 months unless there is ongoing repetitive injury.

Ligament Sprains

Ankle sprains are an extremely common injury, both during sports and during daily activities. The vast majority can be diagnosed with a detailed history, careful physical examination, and ankle radiographs to exclude acute fracture. MRI

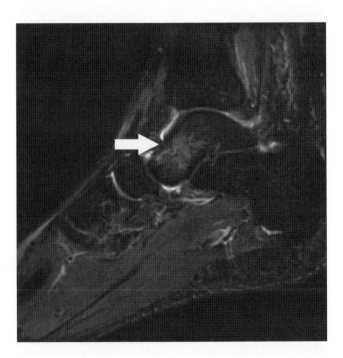

Fig. 9.1 A sagittal T2-weighted image with fat suppression showing a talar contusion. Note the focus of high signal within the talus (*arrow*), which signifies edema within the bone marrow. The cortex is intact.

is not necessary for most acute ankle sprains, but it can be of use in certain cases of atypical presentation or to rule out other injuries such as an OCD or tendon injury. Within the first week after an ankle sprain, MRI usually reveals prominent subcutaneous edema and juxtaarticular hematoma; these findings present as high signal fluid in the ankle joint and adjacent tendon sheaths on T2-weighted images, indicating the presence of blood within these compartments.[6,8] The edema typically diminishes rapidly thereafter, although fascial edema around the injured ligament may persist.[6,8] After the first several weeks, the ligament becomes thickened and may appear in continuity despite a tear, which may confound accurate interpretation. Two months after injury, fascial edema is resolved and the torn ligaments may appear intact, thinned, attenuated, or even completely absent, depending on the degree of initial injury.[6,8]

Lateral Ankle Sprains

Ankle sprains are the most common athletic injury, and specifically, lateral ankle ligament sprains are the most common type.[9] Ankle sprains account for 45% of basketball injuries,[10] and are commonly seen in football, soccer, rugby, and volleyball players. These injuries vary in severity from mild to severe[6,10]; lateral ligament injuries are more common than medial ones.[9,10] The most commonly injured ligament is the anterior talofibular ligament, followed by a combination injury of the calcaneofibular and anterior talofibular ligaments. An isolated posterior talofibular ligament tear is rare. The most common mechanism of injury is inversion and internal rotation. It must be noted that this mechanism can also produce other common injuries, in isolation or in combination with ankle sprain, such as the following:

- Fibular or talar fractures
- Osteochondral lesions
- Peroneal tendon tears
- Fifth metatarsal fractures

The diagnosis of ankle sprain is usually accomplished with a thorough history and physical examination. Conventional radiographs may reveal any associated avulsion fractures or osteochondral injuries, and stress views can be obtained to evaluate structural instability. Occasionally, MRI is used to confirm the diagnosis or for the evaluation of associated injuries. Ligament injuries are best evaluated on T2-weighted and fat-suppressed T2-weighted MR images. These images usually show increased signal intensity that represents the edema and fluid collection secondary to trauma.[6,8] Discontinuity of the ligament on T1-weighted and T2-weighted images signifies disruption.[6,8] The anterior talofibular ligament is the weakest and the most vulnerable of all ankle ligaments. Tears in this ligament are best diagnosed on axial images (**Fig. 9.2**).

The second most common pattern of ankle injury is a combined injury to the anterior talofibular ligament and

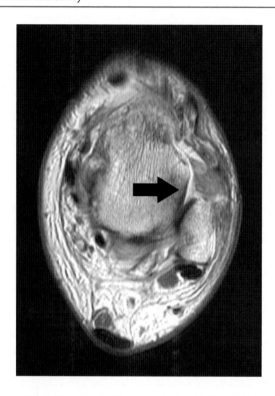

Fig. 9.2 An axial T1-weighted image of the left ankle at the level of the superior talus. No ligament is seen at the expected location of the attachment of the anterior talofibular ligament (*arrow*). Instead, there are ill-defined fibers extending anteriorly from the fibula, representing a grade III tear.

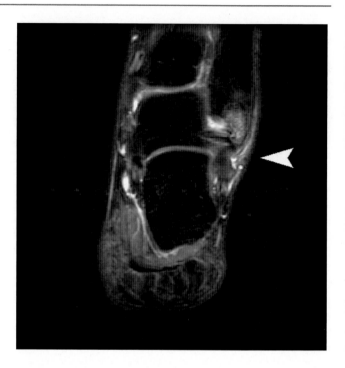

Fig. 9.3 A coronal STIR image of the left ankle showing edema and fluid (*arrowhead*) tracking longitudinally along the fibers of the calcaneofibular ligament, representing a grade II tear. There is also edema of the distal fibula.

the calcaneofibular ligament.[10] Isolated tears of the calcaneofibular ligament are extremely uncommon.[10] Unlike the anterior talofibular ligament, tears of the calcaneofibular ligament are best seen on the coronal T2-weighted, fat-suppressed T2-weighted, and fat-suppressed STIR images (**Fig. 9.3**). MRI grading of the ligamentous injury can be categorized as follows[6]:

- Grade I, intact ligament structure but surrounding edema as seen on T2-weighted images
- Grade II, thickening or partially torn fibers of the ligament and surrounding edema
- Grade III, complete disruption of the ligament and loss of its attachment as seen on T1-weighted and T2-weighted images

Medial Ankle Sprains

Isolated injuries of the deltoid ligament are uncommon.[10] They often occur in conjunction with a fibular fracture or a purely ligamentous syndesmotic injury. Deltoid ligament injuries are best viewed on coronal T2-weighted and fat-suppressed T2-weighted images (**Fig. 9.4**). Occasionally, medial edema and deltoid thickening are seen on T2-weighted images secondary to an inversion injury.[6] This medial

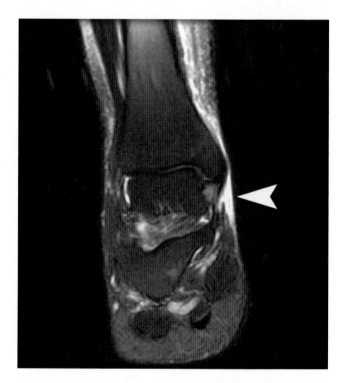

Fig. 9.4 A coronal fat-suppressed T2-weighted image of the right ankle showing a grade II or grade III tear (*arrowhead*) of the deltoid ligament.

impaction is usually associated with lateral soft-tissue edema or evidence of a lateral ligament tear. MR images must be correlated carefully with clinical examination to avoid treatment of false-positive findings.

Syndesmotic Injuries[11,12]

Also sometimes called high ankle sprains, syndesmotic sprains are reported to occur in as many as 18% of all ankle sprains in athletes.[13] Syndesmotic injury usually is associated with a fibular fracture, but it can occur as a purely ligamentous diastasis.[12,14] The major contributors to the distal tibiofibular syndesmotic structure are the following:

- Anteroinferior tibiofibular ligament
- Posteroinferior tibiofibular ligament
- Interosseous membrane

The anteroinferior tibiofibular ligament is most commonly involved in syndesmotic injuries. External rotation is the typical mechanism of injury, and many of these injuries are not recognized initially unless the clinician has a high level of suspicion for them.[13] Patients typically present with severe edema, ecchymosis, and tenderness more laterally than would be expected with a standard lateral ligament sprain.

Clinical examination is supplemented with radiographic studies to exclude fibular fracture or diastasis of the syndesmosis. One study has indicated that the measurements on static ankle radiographs are poorly predictive of syndesmotic injury.[11] Dynamic stress radiographs may identify instability of the syndesmosis, but they may be limited in the acute setting because of patient discomfort.

MRI has been found to very useful in identifying these injuries. In one study, MRI had a sensitivity of 100%, a specificity of 93%, and an accuracy of 97% in diagnosing syndesmotic injuries.[12] The anteroinferior tibiofibular ligament and posteroinferior tibiofibular ligament are best viewed in axial images at the level of the tibial plafond. When injured, the ligaments can be seen as edematous, wavy, absent, or discontinuous on T1-weighted and T2-weighted sequences (**Fig. 9.5A**). Extension of fluid into the syndesmosis on axial T2-weighted images can also assist in the diagnosis of syndesmotic disruption (**Fig. 9.5B**).

OCD of the Talus

OCD, also known as an osteochondral fragment of the talus, is a disruption of that structure's cartilage surface. Analogous lesions are common in the knee and elbow. Many occur

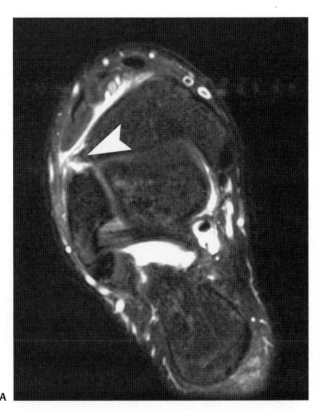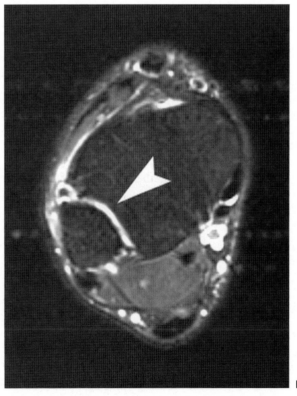

A   B

Fig. 9.5 MRI can reveal direct or indirect evidence of syndesmotic injury. **(A)** An axial fat-suppressed T2-weighted image of the right ankle shows ill-defined, wavy fibers of a torn anteroinferior tibiofibular ligament (*arrowhead*), direct evidence of a syndesmotic sprain.

(B) More superiorly on the same patient, there is extension of fluid into the syndesmosis (*arrowhead*), providing indirect evidence of syndesmotic disruption.

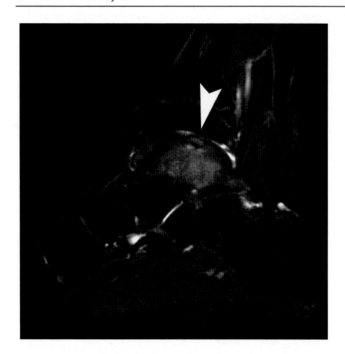

Fig. 9.6 A sagittal fat-suppressed T2-weighted image showing the typical MRI appearance of an OCD, with osseous edema and irregularity of the subchondral bone plate and overlying cartilage (*arrowhead*).

can be useful in assessing OCD lesions. The AP location can be determined on axial and sagittal images, whereas the mediolateral location can be assessed on coronal and axial views. The depth of the lesion can be viewed on sagittal and coronal images. The MRI appearance of an OCD lesion typically shows osseous edema along with irregularity of the subchondral bone plate and overlying cartilage (**Fig. 9.6**). Specialized cartilage-specific sequences can improve imaging of the chondral surface to identify subtle disruption[20] (see the detailed discussion in Chapter 14). In some cases, the surrounding bone edema may cause overestimation of the true size of the lesion. MRI appearance also may assist in predicting the stability of the lesion; fluid or granulation tissue beneath the lesion at the interface with the osseous crater appears bright on T2-weighted imaging and implies instability[21–23] (**Fig. 9.7**). MRI has also been shown to be of use in evaluating healing of the OCD lesion after surgery, with some normalization of signal changes noted.[24,25]

Stress Fractures

Osseous stress fractures occur from repetitive stress that is below the threshold for acute fracture but substantial enough to cause microtrabecular failure. They often occur

after a traumatic injury, although some patients do not recall a specific injury. An OCD lesion often is misdiagnosed clinically as an ankle sprain.[15,16] Patients typically present with pain located deep within the joint that is worsened with activity or sports; patients may also complain of ankle swelling, giving way, or locking.

OCD lesions can occur anywhere on the surface of the talar dome; the classic literature notes anterolateral and posteromedial lesions as the most common.[15,17] A recent MRI study identified the centromedial and centrolateral locations as the most common.[18]

A spectrum of OCD lesions exists, including the following[16,19]:

- Softening of the cartilage
- Partial detachment of an osteochondral fragment
- Complete detachment of an osteochondral fragment
- Free-floating fragment within the joint
- Subchondral cystic lesion

Stable lesions may respond to nonsurgical treatment, whereas unstable lesions and cystic OCD lesions typically are treated surgically.

MRI is a very useful modality for diagnosing OCD lesions, particularly if the lesion is not visualized on standard radiographs. MRI can also assess other pathologic entities, such as tendon or ligamentous injuries, in the patient with persistent pain after ankle sprain. All three imaging planes

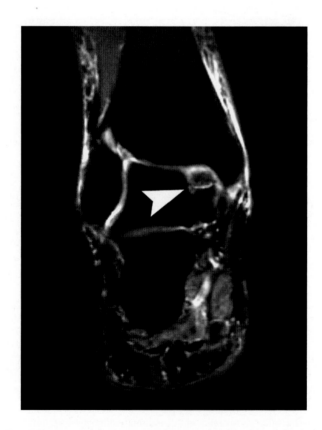

Fig. 9.7 A coronal fat-suppressed T2-weighted image of the right ankle showing an unstable OCD with fluid beneath the lesion at the interface with the osseous crater of the medial talus (*arrowhead*).

secondary to overuse situations, such as in an athlete with a sudden, dramatic increase in running or other training. The bone is unable to heal adequately because of ongoing insult, and a stress fracture results. These fractures are typically diagnosed based on a history of repetitive overuse and are differentiated from acute fractures by the lack of an acute traumatic event. The location of lower extremity stress fractures in a group of military recruits has been reported to vary by gender: the most common sites in males were the metatarsals (66%), calcaneus (20%), and lower leg (13%), whereas the most common sites in females were the calcaneus (39%), metatarsals (31%), and lower leg (27%).[26] Furthermore, conventional radiographs usually are negative early in the process until callus appears or the stress fracture progresses to a frank fracture. One study found a rate of positive radiographic findings of only 10% in patients with stress fractures.[27] MRI is a very helpful tool in evaluating these injuries, with high sensitivity and specificity. Typically, the osseous structures have a linear region of low signal intensity on T1-weighted and T2-weighted images; T2-weighted images also show surrounding high signal intensity consistent with bone marrow edema.[6]

Calcaneal Stress Fractures

A patient with a calcaneal stress fracture presents with posterior heel pain and, occasionally, swelling. On physical examination, pain is elicited with medial-lateral compression of the heel. Sometimes conventional radiographs can show a radiolucent line at the posterior aspect of the calcaneus perpendicular to the trabecular cancellous lines. MRI is useful if radiographs are negative, with T1-weighted images showing a linear fracture line and T2-weighted images revealing associated marrow edema (**Fig. 9.8**).

Navicular Stress Fractures

Navicular stress fractures commonly present in an athlete who complains of vague arch pain that is worsened with running or sports activities. The stress fracture usually occurs in the middle third of the navicular secondary to increased stresses in that region along with poor local vascular supply to the bone. MRI typically shows edema within the navicular on T2-weighted and fat-suppressed T2-weighted images (**Fig. 9.9A**). T1-weighted images show a low intensity linear lesion representing a fracture line (**Fig. 9.9B**). If MRI suggests a navicular stress fracture, a CT scan may be indicated to define more clearly the osseous structure and extent of the fracture.

Metatarsal Stress Fractures

Metatarsal stress fractures are also called *march fractures* because they often present in military recruits who participate in extended marching drills. Metatarsal stress fractures also commonly present in female dancers who are often in the

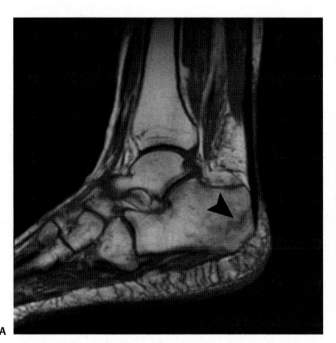
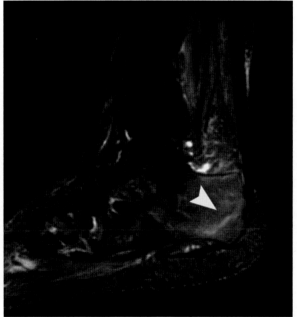

A   B

Fig. 9.8 Calcaneal stress fracture. **(A)** A sagittal T1-weighted image showing an oblique fracture line in the posterior calcaneus (*arrow-head*). **(B)** A sagittal fat-suppressed T2-weighted image shows marrow edema and edema tracking along the fracture line (*arrowhead*).

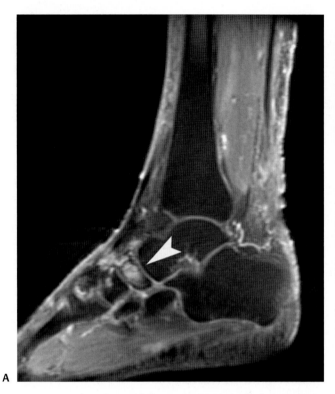

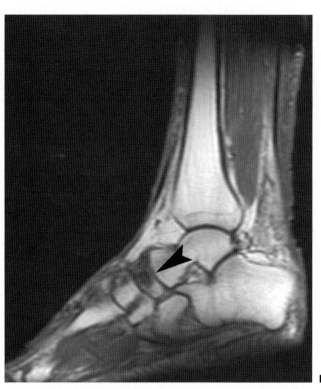

Fig. 9.9 Navicular stress fracture. **(A)** A sagittal fat-suppressed T2-weighted image showing marrow edema (*arrowhead*) within the navicular. **(B)** A sagittal T1-weighted image showing a hypointense region within the dorsal aspect of the navicular with a faint horizontally oriented fracture line (*arrowhead*).

en-pointe position and in female athletes, both of whom subject the central metatarsals to increased mechanical load. The second metatarsal is the most frequent location for fracture (more than half of all metatarsal stress fractures), followed by the third and fourth metatarsals.[28] Stress fractures of the central metatarsals typically occur in the diaphysis, whereas a stress fracture of the first metatarsal occurs in the proximal metaphysis and a stress fracture of the fifth metatarsal occurs at the diaphyseal-metaphyseal junction.[28] Patients typically complain of aching pain related to weight-bearing activities, running, or sports. Conventional radiographs often are diagnostic, although they may be negative early in the process. MRI can be useful in such cases and to rule out other causes of pain such as synovitis. The metatarsal shows the characteristic linear density on T1-weighted images with high signal on corresponding T2-weighted and fat-suppressed T2-weighted images (**Fig. 9.10**).

■ Degenerative Conditions

Tendon Disorders

Tendon disorders can represent traumatic injuries, inflammatory conditions, or degenerative tendinosis. Regardless of the etiology, MRI is the ideal method of evaluating tendon

disorders and is best achieved by obtaining images perpendicular to the tendon's course.[29–33] At the ankle and hindfoot levels, axial views are ideal for tendon imaging, whereas coronal images are best for visualizing more distal structures in

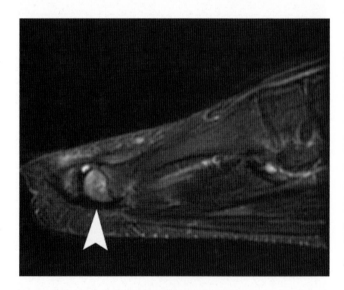

Fig. 9.10 A sagittal fat-suppressed T2-weighted image showing edema of the head of the second metatarsal (*arrowhead*) in a patient with a stress fracture.

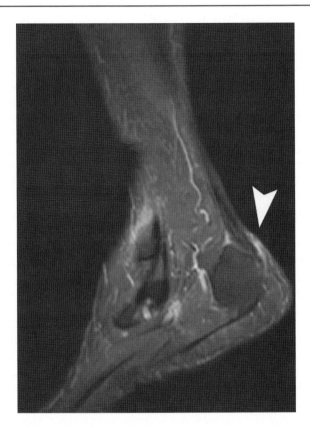

Fig. 9.11 Adventitial bursitis as seen on a sagittal fat-suppressed T2-weighted image showing soft-tissue inflammation posterior to the calcaneus (*arrowhead*).

the midfoot. The magic angle effect is a phenomenon seen in tissues with well-ordered collagen fibers, such as a tendon.[34] This phenomenon occurs when the images are obtained with the magnetic field at an oblique angle (55 degrees) relative to the fibers of the tendon, and it shows abnormal signal intensity on T1-weighted images. T2-weighted images are unaffected by this phenomenon, so corresponding T2-weighted images are scrutinized in the affected areas to determine if the signal abnormality seen on T1-weighted images represents true pathology or simply artifact. The magic angle effect is seen most notably in the posterior tibialis and peroneal tendons as they course around the malleoli. Knowledge that this magic angle effect exists, combined with assessment of the T2-weighted images, assists the radiologist or surgeon in accurately identifying pathology of the tendons about the ankle.

Achilles Tendon Disorders

Achilles tendon disorders represent a spectrum of disease, including the following:

- Retrocalcaneal bursitis
- Paratenonitis
- Insertional tendinosis
- Noninsertional tendinosis
- Rupture

Isolated retrocalcaneal bursitis can be seen secondary to systemic inflammatory disease or localized soft-tissue irritation from impingement by the posterosuperior process of the calcaneus (Haglund process). Sagittal MR images show decreased signal intensity on T1-weighted images and increased intensity on T2-weighted and fat-suppressed T2-weighted images, consistent with soft-tissue inflammation[6] (**Fig. 9.11**). Paratenonitis represents a diffuse inflammation of the investing paratenon layer that surrounds the Achilles tendon. Sagittal T2-weighted and fat-suppressed T2-weighted images show loss of the normal sharp interface between the Achilles and surrounding soft tissues but normal intrasubstance appearance and morphology of the tendon itself (**Fig. 9.12**).

The term *Achilles tendinitis* now is believed to be a misnomer because the tendon typically does not show an inflammatory component. Instead, *tendinosis* is the preferred term, which more accurately reflects the disorganized collagen fibers, myxoid degeneration, and microscopic intrasubstance tearing seen histologically.[35] Achilles tendinosis

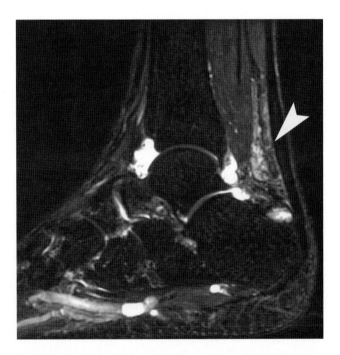

Fig. 9.12 The MRI appearance of Achilles paratenonitis is defined by diffuse inflammation of the investing paratenon layer that surrounds the Achilles tendon. This sagittal fat-suppressed T2-weighted image shows inflammation of the soft tissues surrounding the Achilles (including Kager's fat pad) (*arrowhead*) but normal intrasubstance appearance and morphology of the tendon itself. An ankle joint effusion is also seen.

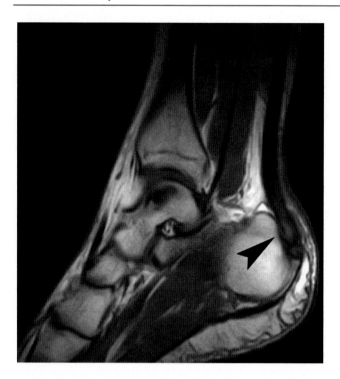

Fig. 9.13 This sagittal T1-weighted image shows tendon hypertrophy and heterogeneity of the substance (*arrowhead*), the characteristic MRI appearance of Achilles tendinosis.

is believed to be secondary to age-related degeneration and can also occur from repetitive strain or overuse, as is seen in running athletes.[36] Achilles tendinosis can occur at the insertion on the posterior calcaneus or more proximally in the noninsertional tendon, approximately 3 to 6 cm above the insertion point.[6,35] In Achilles tendinosis, there is a loss of the sharp tendon interface with the surrounding tissues, and the tendon may appear thickened and dysmorphic with loss of the normal concave appearance on axial images.[6] Axial and sagittal T1-weighted images show tendon hypertrophy and heterogeneity of the substance (**Fig. 9.13**), whereas T2-weighted and fat-suppressed T2-weighted images show intratendinous edema and splitting.[6] Insertional tendinosis may have an associated intratendinous spur on the calcaneus.

MRI is usually not necessary to diagnose acute rupture of the Achilles, which is often apparent clinically. The tear is typically located several centimeters above the insertion, but it may show complex patterns, including avulsion off the calcaneus or longitudinal splitting. MRI may be helpful for differentiating partial and complete tears, or chronic ruptures that present in a delayed fashion.[6] Sagittal and axial images show a gap between the torn ends with intervening fluid seen on T2-weighted images[6] (**Fig. 9.14**). In chronic cases, fibrous tissue is present between the distal stump and the proximally retracted tendon.

Posterior Tibial Tendon Dysfunction

Posterior tibial tendon dysfunction is the most common cause of adult-onset flatfoot deformity.[30,37] It results from degenerative tendinosis, inflammatory disease, or, more rarely, trauma. The pathophysiology involves microscopic tears, collagen disorganization, and myxoid degenerative changes within the tendon. Clinically, patients present with flatfoot deformity, medial ankle pain, swelling, and weakness of the tendon.[37]

Conventional radiographs are useful in determining the severity of the deformity and the presence of secondary arthritis of the hindfoot and ankle. Although not necessary in all cases, MRI is a useful adjunct in assessing the posterior tibialis tendon and is superior to other modalities in detecting inflammation and tears within the tendon.[37] Typically, the posterior tibial tendon is two to three times larger than the flexor digitorum longus tendon. It may have a small amount of synovial fluid around it, but usually no more than 1 to 2 mm.[31] The tendon should have a homogeneous signal on both T1-weighted and T2-weighted images.[31] Posterior tibial tendon tears are typically seen around the medial malleolus, or distally within 2 to 3 cm of its insertion on the navicular.[29–31] Posterior tibial tendon tears are best diagnosed on T2-weighted and fat-suppressed axial images, which show morphologic changes and intratendinous signal changes (**Fig. 9.15**). Sagittal images may be useful for assessing the distal insertion site on the navicular. Additionally, some

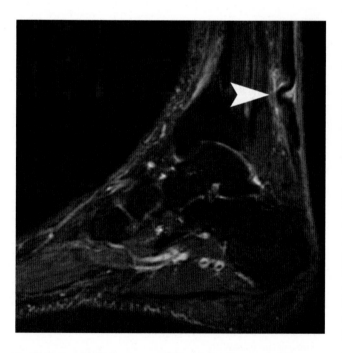

Fig. 9.14 A sagittal fat-suppressed T2-weighted image showing a tear of the Achilles tendon with overlapping ends and fluid and edema at the site of the tear (*arrowhead*).

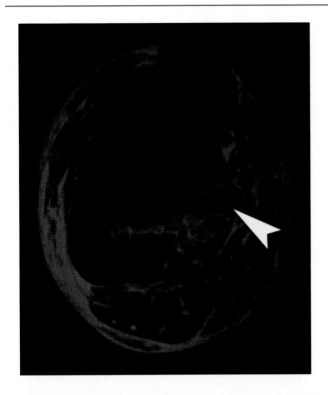

Fig. 9.15 An axial fat-suppressed T2-weighted image of the right ankle showing a posterior tibial tendon tear with hypertrophy and prominent intratendinous signal changes (*arrowhead*).

at the level of the cuboid or fifth metatarsal base. The pathophysiology at each level differs, but all three areas can be evaluated effectively with MRI.

Peroneal tenosynovitis or tear can occur at the retrofibular groove behind the lateral malleolus secondary to acute injury or chronic involvement. Axial MR images are ideal for revealing evidence of tendon sheath effusion and tenosynovitis.[32] A small amount of fluid can normally be observed in the peroneal sheaths.[6] However, if the amount of fluid is larger than the tendon or if there is complexity to the tendon sheath fluid, the abnormality can be considered tenosynovitis (**Fig. 9.18**). In progressive cases, tendon thickening can be seen, as can increased signal on T1-weighted or T2-weighted images, consistent with chronic tendinopathy.

Acute peroneal tendon ruptures, although uncommon, can occur as a result of trauma, chronic oral corticosteroid use, or inflammatory arthritis. Axial MR images are most helpful, with irregular tendon appearance noted on T1-weighted images, and fluid within the sheath and surrounding tissues noted on T2-weighted and fat-suppressed T2-weighted im-

patients have posterior tibialis tendon dysfunction secondary to an accessory navicular. T2-weighted and fat-suppressed images may show bone marrow edema within the accessory bone or the fibrous connection (synchondrosis) to the main navicular body[6] (**Fig. 9.16**).

Posterior tibialis tendon tears can be classified into three types on the basis of their MRI characteristics[30]:

- Type I tears have longitudinal splits in the tendon resulting in hypertrophy, scar formation, and thickening of the tendon. The posterior tibial tendon can be enlarged up to four to five times the size of the adjacent flexor digitorum longus (**Fig. 9.17A**).
- Type II tears are more severe, with longitudinal splits that cause the tendon to attenuate to one half to one third of its original thickness (**Fig. 9.17B**).
- Type III tears represent a complete rupture of the tendon with retraction of the stump and a visible gap (**Fig. 9.17C**).

Peroneal Tendon Disorders

Peroneal tendon disorders include tenosynovitis, tears, and subluxation. Pathology of the peroneal tendons can develop posterior to the lateral malleolus, on the lateral side of calcaneus inferior to the tip of the lateral malleolus, and distally

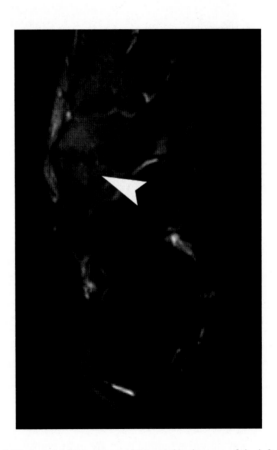

Fig. 9.16 An axial fat-suppressed T2-weighted image of the left foot shows marrow edema within an accessory navicular bone, superficial soft tissues, and the fibrous connection (synchondrosis) to the main navicular body (*arrowhead*). An accessory navicular bone is an occasional cause for posterior tibialis tendon dysfunction.

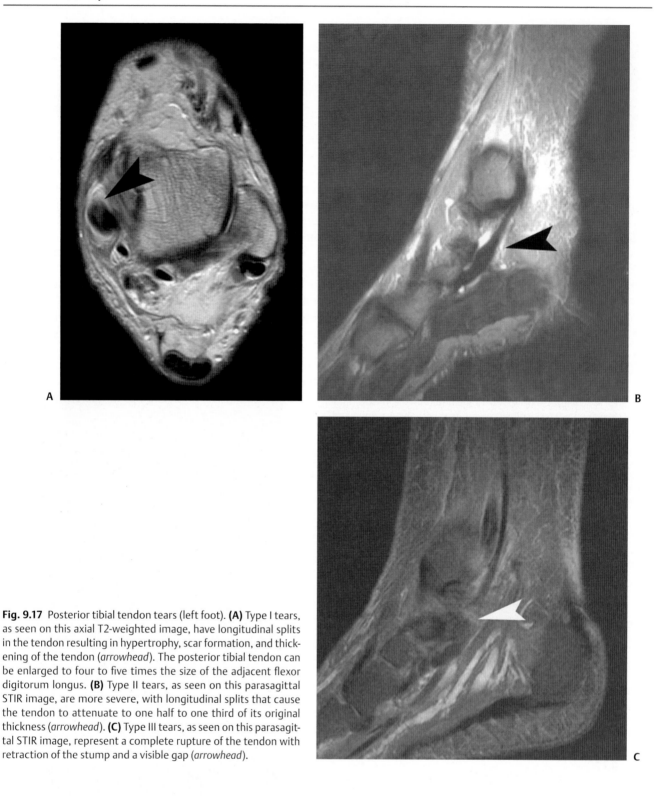

Fig. 9.17 Posterior tibial tendon tears (left foot). **(A)** Type I tears, as seen on this axial T2-weighted image, have longitudinal splits in the tendon resulting in hypertrophy, scar formation, and thickening of the tendon (*arrowhead*). The posterior tibial tendon can be enlarged to four to five times the size of the adjacent flexor digitorum longus. **(B)** Type II tears, as seen on this parasagittal STIR image, are more severe, with longitudinal splits that cause the tendon to attenuate to one half to one third of its original thickness (*arrowhead*). **(C)** Type III tears, as seen on this parasagittal STIR image, represent a complete rupture of the tendon with retraction of the stump and a visible gap (*arrowhead*).

ages. Chronic peroneal tendon tears are more common than acute rupture. Chronic longitudinal split tears of the peroneus brevis can occur from chronic abrasion of the tendon against the posterolateral ridge of the fibula secondary to instability of the tendons.[38] Another proposed mechanism for a peroneus brevis longitudinal tear is compression of the peroneus brevis by the peroneus longus against the posterior surface of the fibula, with central tendon attenuation and damage. Axial MR images reveal an irregular shape of the peroneus brevis tendon, such as a chevron or bilobed

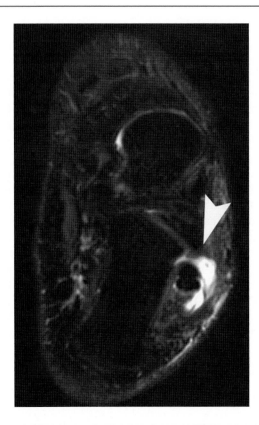

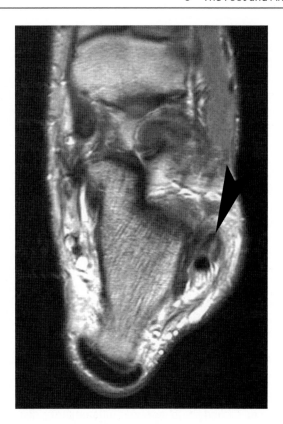

Fig. 9.18 In tenosynovitis of the peroneal longus tendon, the cross-sectional area of the peritendinous fluid collection must be larger than the tendon itself (as seen on this axial STIR image of the left foot) (*arrowhead*) or complex.

Fig. 9.19 An axial T1-weighted image of the left foot showing a "split" peroneus brevis tendon with an irregular, bilobed shape (*arrowhead*).

appearance (**Fig. 9.19**); other suggestive findings include fluid within the sheath, a flat retrofibular groove, and spurring of the lateral edge of the fibula.[32,39–41]

Chronic peroneal tendon subluxation or instability has been reported with attenuation of the superior peroneal retinaculum and a shallow retrofibular groove. Both of these features can be well visualized on axial T1-weighted images[39–41] (**Fig. 9.20**). The tendons may even be noted to be grossly dislocated on the lateral side of the lateral malleolus.[39–41] Crowding of the retrofibular groove secondary to mass effect, leading to peroneal instability, is another proposed mechanism. Such crowding can occur secondary to a low-lying peroneus brevis muscle belly, a ganglion cyst arising from the posterolateral ankle, or an accessory peroneus quartus muscle. A peroneus quartus muscle is present in 10% to 20% of individuals and occurs more commonly in men than in women.[39,42] It is found posterior to the peroneus brevis and longus and inserts onto the calcaneus, cuboid, or peroneal tendons themselves.[42] It is visualized on axial T1-weighted images as a tendon separate from the brevis and longus tendons (**Fig. 9.21**).

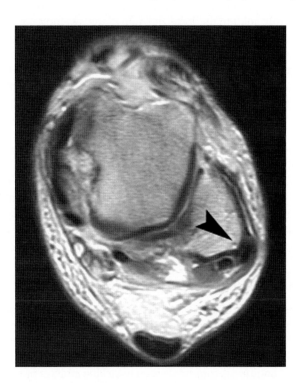

Fig. 9.20 An axial T1-weighted image of the left ankle showing the peroneal tendon laterally subluxed over the lateral aspect of the retrofibular groove (*arrowhead*).

Distal peroneal pathology is less common; tenosynovitis or tear can occur inferior to the tip of the lateral malleolus or at the insertion sites of either tendon. Impingement of the peroneals can occur between the tip of the fibula and the peroneal tubercle on the lateral side of the calcaneus secondary to valgus hindfoot alignment or malunion of a previous calcaneal fracture. Distally, tenosynovitis can occur at the base of the fifth metatarsal at the insertion of the brevis tendon. Distal peroneus longus pathology can present as painful os peroneum syndrome (POPS).[43] Patients with this entity present with pain and tenderness in the region of the cuboid inferolaterally secondary to tenosynovitis or tearing of the longus tendon. With complete rupture of the peroneus longus tendon, the associated os peroneum may retract proximal to the calcaneocuboid joint. Radiographically, a retracted or fragmented os peroneum may be seen. On MRI, there is fluid and edema in the sheath of the peroneus longus at the level of the cuboid, with edema and fragmentation of the os peroneum (**Fig. 9.22**).

Anterior Tibial Tendon Disorders

Disorders of the anterior tibialis tendon are relatively less common than those of the tendons listed above. Tendinitis can occur secondary to systemic inflammatory disease or overuse syndromes. Acute anterior tibialis tendon rupture can occur from trauma or laceration, and chronic attritional tear can present in elderly patients. Patients present with anterior ankle pain, localized soft-tissue swelling, and diminished dorsiflexion strength.[33] Tendinitis appears as soft-tissue edema on axial and sagittal T2-weighted images[33,44] (**Fig. 9.23**). As with tendinosis in other tendons, anterior tibial tendinosis appears on T1-weighted and T2-weighted images as hypertrophy, heterogeneous signal changes within the tendon substance, and even partial longitudinal splitting.[33,44] In complete rupture, sagittal T1-weighted images show discontinuity of the tendon, with proximal retraction and intervening fluid on T2-weighted images.[33,44]

Signal abnormality sometimes is seen on T1-weighted images distally at the insertion site because of the magic angle effect. This phenomenon can occur when the foot is imaged in a neutral position.[44] In addition, a longitudinal split of the tendon is occasionally seen at its insertion.

FHL and Posterior Impingement (Os Trigonum)

Tenosynovitis of the FHL tendon typically occurs at the posterior ankle at the level of the FHL tendon sheath posterior to the talus. Usually, patients present with deep ankle posteromedial pain, particularly with the ankle in plantarflexion. This condition is commonly seen in kicking athletes or ballet dancers performing in the en-pointe position.[45] Clinically, tenosynovitis can overlap with posterior ankle impingement syndrome because of a prominent posterior process or

os trigonum. The os trigonum becomes impacted between the posterior tibia and calcaneus with ankle plantarflexion, which can cause osseous edema and localized inflammation; this impaction and inflammation can also lead to secondary FHL tenosynovitis and, potentially, a partial longitudinal tear. Passive plantarflexion on physical examination elicits posterior pain; passive dorsiflexion of the hallux stretches the FHL and may cause posterior ankle pain, also suggestive of FHL tendon pathology.

Conventional radiographs may show a large posterior talar process or an os trigonum. MRI shows fluid and soft-tissue signal intensity posteriorly around the region of the os trigonum, extending into the posterior portions of the ankle and the subtalar joints.[6] The fibrous synchondrosis between the os trigonum and talus may show increased signal intensity on T2-weighted axial and sagittal images because of fluid traversing the articulation and forming a pseudarthrosis[6] (**Fig. 9.24**). Edema also can be seen in the ossicle, posterior tibia, and dorsal calcaneus secondary to impaction. The FHL sheath appears enlarged and fluid-filled, and it may

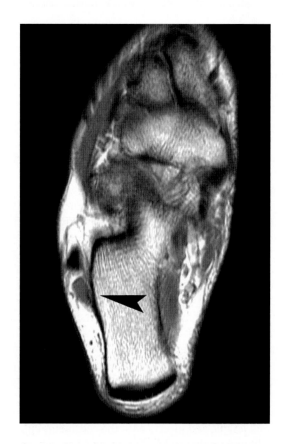

Fig. 9.21 An axial T1-weighted image of the right foot showing an accessory peroneus quartus muscle posterior to the peroneus longus and brevis muscles (*arrowhead*).

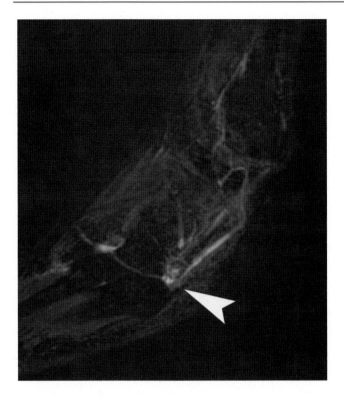

Fig. 9.22 A sagittal T2-weighted image showing an edematous os peroneum with fluid and edema of the sheath of the distal peroneus longus tendon (*arrowhead*).

show loculation or a ganglion cyst; on rare occasions, the tendon may show intratendinous signal change consistent with a partial tear[6] (**Fig. 9.25**).

Anterolateral Impingement

Impingement of the anterolateral aspect of the ankle joint is seen after a lateral ankle sprain in which hypertrophic scar tissue proliferates in the lateral gutter. This proliferation is sometimes called a *meniscoid lesion* because of its appearance as a meniscus-shaped focus of fibrous and synovial tissue that can lead to pain with dorsiflexion or eversion of the ankle.[6,46] On physical examination, the patient exhibits tenderness at the anterolateral corner of the ankle that can be exacerbated by passive dorsiflexion. MRI findings in anterolateral impingement include the presence of inflamed soft tissue or increased fluid against the inner margin of the anteroinferior tibiofibular ligament and the anterior talofibular ligament instead of a small fat pad that sits anterior to the fibula on axial imaging[6,46] (**Fig. 9.26**). MR arthrography with gadolinium contrast may help to outline this synovial tissue more accurately and confirm the diagnosis.[46]

Osteonecrosis of the Talus

Osteonecrosis (also termed *avascular necrosis*) of the talus typically occurs after talus fracture secondary to disruption

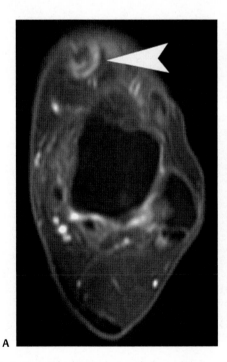
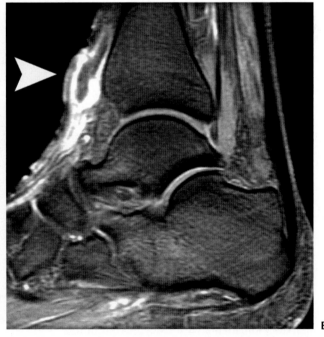

Fig. 9.23 Anterior tibialis tendon pathology. **(A)** An axial fat-suppressed T2-weighted image of the left ankle showing anterior tibial tendinitis with soft-tissue edema (*arrowhead*). **(B)** A sagittal fat-suppressed T2-weighted image showing a complete rupture of the anterior tibialis tendon with discontinuity of the tendon, proximal retraction, and intervening fluid (*arrowhead*).

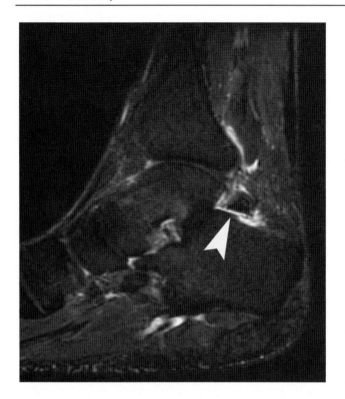

Fig. 9.24 A sagittal fat-suppressed T2-weighted image shows fluid signal within the fibrous synchondrosis between the os trigonum and talus (*arrowhead*), representing formation of a pseudarthrosis.

of the osseous blood supply.[47] Atraumatic osteonecrosis can also occur in various medical conditions (such as vasculitis, sickle cell disease, or excessive alcohol use) or secondary to oral corticosteroid use.[47] Patients complain of severe pain and difficulty with ambulation. Conventional radiographs may show sclerosis, cystic changes, or bone collapse, although they are believed to have low sensitivity. MRI is a very sensitive test for making the diagnosis of osteonecrosis of the talus and has the added advantage of better anatomic resolution than bone scintigraphy.[48] On T1-weighted images, low signal is seen with osteonecrosis secondary to marrow fat replacement, whereas T2-weighted images typically show edema in the avascular lesion (**Fig. 9.27**). Because there is a risk of osteonecrosis after talar neck fractures, titanium screws are recommended for surgical fixation to minimize the metallic artifact on postoperative MRI studies.[47]

■ Infectious Processes

Infections in the foot and ankle are typically seen in the pediatric population, in patients with diabetes, and in immunocompromised individuals. Patients with infections present with pain, erythema, and swelling and can have fevers and other systemic responses. Physical examination reveals swelling, erythema, induration, tenderness, and warmth. Many infections in the foot and ankle result from a direct spread from contiguous ulceration, which occurs often in diabetic patients; penetrating trauma is another common cause.

Cellulitis and Abscess

An MRI study is often obtained in the setting of cellulitis to rule out deep-space abscess or associated osteomyelitis. Cellulitis typically shows low signal intensity in the subcutaneous fat on T1-weighted images and increased signal intensity on T2-weighted images. Fat-suppressed T2-weighted images are particularly sensitive in detecting subcutaneous edema; the underlying osseous structures appear normal. An abscess appears as a well-defined fluid collection that is low signal on T1-weighted and higher signal on T2-weighted and fat-suppressed images[49] (**Fig. 9.28**). Administration of gadolinium contrast results in enhancement of the abscess rim.[49] Cellulitis or abscess in the foot is best imaged on coronal and sagittal images; cellulitis at the ankle level is better visualized with sagittal and axial images. In cases of cellulitis or abscess secondary to penetrating trauma, a retained foreign

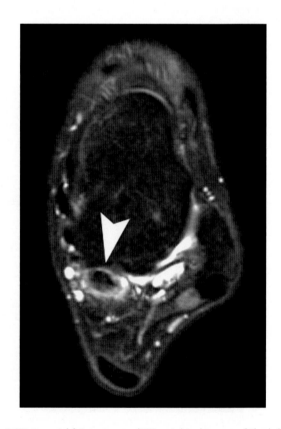

Fig. 9.25 An axial fat-suppressed T2-weighted image of the left ankle showing an enlarged and fluid-filled FHL with intratendinous signal change consistent with a partial tear (*arrowhead*).

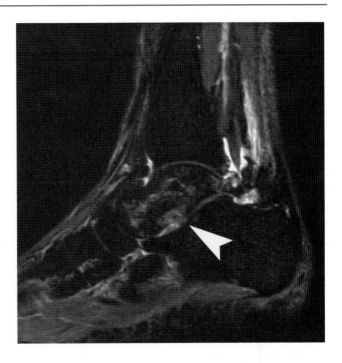

Fig. 9.27 A sagittal fat-suppressed T2-weighted image showing osteonecrosis of the talus with patchy areas of bone marrow edema (*arrowhead*), some of which contain devitalized bone.

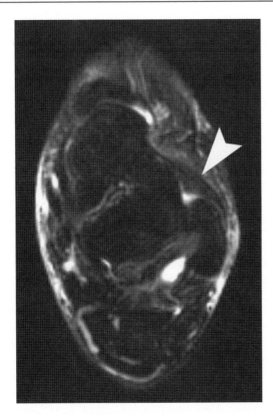

Fig. 9.26 An axial fat-suppressed T2-weighted image of the left ankle showing a nidus of inflammatory soft tissue adjacent to the inner margin of the anteroinferior tibiofibular ligament (*arrowhead*), suggestive of anterolateral impingement.

body may be difficult to identify but can present as a signal void in the midst of the edema pattern or fluid collection.

Septic Arthritis

Septic arthritis can occur secondary to direct penetration of a foreign body into the joint or secondary to hematogenous spread from a noncontiguous source. Occasionally, when the diagnosis is unclear, MRI may be helpful in identifying a joint effusion and may exclude a deep abscess or associated bone changes indicative of osteomyelitis. On MRI, septic arthritis shows a joint effusion with distention of the synovial recesses and intense contrast enhancement.[50] Aspiration of the involved joint confirms the diagnosis and provides fluid for microscopic examination, culture, and sensitivity examination to help guide antibiotic management. The treatment involves drainage of the involved joint with repeated aspiration or open surgical drainage.

Osteomyelitis

Osteomyelitis, or bone infection, can be acute or chronic. In the foot and ankle, osteomyelitis is usually seen in the presence of a contiguous ulcer as in the diabetic or neuropathic patient. Radiographs in the early stages of osteomyelitis often are normal, and changes (including osteolysis, periosteal reaction, and osseous destruction) may not be seen until

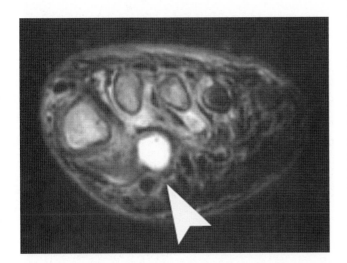

Fig. 9.28 A coronal fat-suppressed T2-weighted image of the left foot showing a well-defined fluid collection within the plantar forefoot (*arrowhead*), representing an abscess. Note that there is inflammation and edema of the surrounding tissues and probable osteomyelitis involving the first, second, and third metatarsals.

several weeks later. MRI has become an extremely useful tool in the diagnosis of osteomyelitis, with a reported sensitivity and specificity of more than 90%.[49] Low-intensity bone marrow signal is seen on T1-weighted images and high signal is seen on T2-weighted images, particularly if fat suppression is used[49] (**Fig. 9.29**). In addition, periosteal reaction will be seen as circumferential high signal on T2-weighted images with disproportionate enhancement on postgadolinium T1-weighted images. Cortical disruption also is seen in more advanced cases and may be associated with surrounding soft-tissue abscess or fluid collection.[49] These changes are usually seen adjacent to the associated ulcer, which can be labeled with a skin marker at the time of scanning to assist with interpretation.

The MRI changes seen in osteomyelitis are somewhat nonspecific, however, and can be confused with neuroarthropathic fractures, which also can occur in patients with neuropathy, diabetes, and ulceration.

■ Other Pathologic Conditions

Charcot Neuroarthropathy

Charcot neuroarthropathy is most commonly seen in patients with diabetes or those with other forms of peripheral neuropathy; the reported rate of Charcot arthropathy in individuals with diabetes is 0.1% to 0.4%.[51,52] Charcot neuroarthropathy is hypothesized to occur secondary to repeti-

tive trauma on insensate joints (leading to degeneration and fractures), combined with autonomic dysfunction (leading to altered local osseous circulation and osteopenia). Osseous fragmentation and destruction lead to progressive foot deformity and ulceration with increased risk of infection. The midfoot is most commonly involved, but Charcot arthropathy can also affect the hindfoot or ankle. Careful history and physical examination are supplemented by conventional radiographs to confirm the diagnosis, determine the extent of involvement and deformity, and monitor the progression of the disease.

The clinical scenario becomes more complicated in the setting of concomitant Charcot arthropathy and contiguous ulceration from deformity and osseous pressure. Distinguishing osteomyelitis from underlying Charcot arthropathy can be difficult because both show osseous edema, soft-tissue inflammation, and bone destruction. Distinguishing osteomyelitis from neuroarthropathy via imaging has been difficult. Osteomyelitis typically occurs secondary to contiguous spread from an adjacent ulcer. Osseous changes seen on MRI that are not adjacent to an ulcer have a lower likelihood of signifying infection and instead suggest neuropathic arthropathy. In settings with neuroarthropathic changes, contiguous ulceration, and clinical findings of infection, a potentially useful MRI finding is the "ghost" sign.[49] Bones that appear to be "dissolved" on T1-weighted images but appear more morphologically normal on T2-weighted or contrast-enhanced imaging with diffusely abnormal marrow signal often contain infection, and these findings are more specific for osteomyelitis.[49]

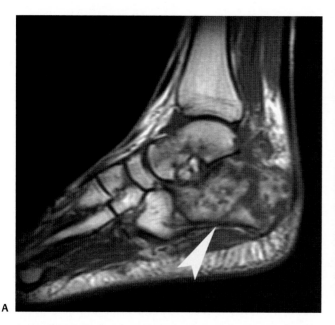
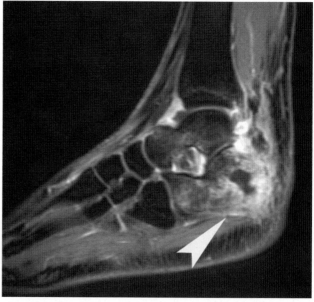

Fig. 9.29 Osteomyelitis. **(A)** A sagittal T1-weighted image showing diffuse foci of low signal throughout the calcaneus and talus (*arrowhead*). **(B)** A sagittal fat-suppressed T2-weighted image of the same patient showing diffuse foci of high signal in the same distribution (*arrowhead*). There is devitalization of a portion of the calcaneus.

Tumors

MRI is a crucial component in the diagnosis and characterization of tumors of the foot and ankle (see Chapter 15, for a more detailed review of MRI for this disease process). MRI is extremely helpful in determining the size and morphology of benign and malignant lesions of bone and soft tissues. As in other areas of the body, certain lesions have characteristic appearances on MRI that can aid in the diagnosis and can suggest appropriate treatment. The following discussion focuses on the most common lesions seen in the foot and ankle.

A ganglion cyst is a benign lesion that occurs next to a joint capsule or tendon sheath. Weakening or degeneration of the capsule or tendon sheath secondary to underlying arthritis or inflammation results in an outpouching of retained fluid and mucoid degeneration. Such ganglion cysts, which can be simple or multilocular, are frequently seen about the ankle, in the sinus tarsi area, and on the dorsal midfoot. The cyst shows high signal intensity consistent with fluid on T2-weighted images[53] (**Fig. 9.30A**). On T1-weighted images, the cyst exhibits intermediate signal intensity (**Fig. 9.30B**). Cysts may also show rim enhancement after intravenous gadolinium contrast.

Plantar fibromatosis is a benign nodular proliferation of fibroblasts arising from the plantar fascia.[54] The nodule typically arises from the superficial (plantar) side of the fascia and may infiltrate the subcutaneous tissues and skin of the plantar foot in a manner similar to that of a Dupuytren contracture of the hand. It does not undergo malignant transfor-

mation, but it can be locally infiltrative and may have a high recurrence rate after surgical excision. Plantar fibromatosis is best seen on coronal and sagittal MR images of the foot; the lesion typically has low to intermediate signal intensity on T1-weighted and T2-weighted images and is directly contiguous to the plantar fascia, with minimal soft-tissue edema or signal alternation in the deep musculature (**Fig. 9.31**).

Hemangiomas have a tendency to involve the muscular components of the lower extremities, often with a multicompartmental distribution. In the region of the foot and ankle, hemangiomas tend to involve the plantar aspect. They produce pain, focal swelling, and paresthesia. On MRI, they show increased signal intensity on T2-weighted and fat-suppressed T2-weighted images, with intermediate signal on T1-weighted images. With gadolinium enhancement, hemangiomas show a marked increase in signal intensity.[53]

PVNS and giant cell tumor of the tendon sheath are characterized by inflammatory proliferation of the synovium associated with deposits of hemosiderin. PVNS often occurs in individuals 20 to 50 years old and can manifest as a focal mass or as a generalized lesion involving the entire joint space. It can develop in any joint of the foot but is most frequently found in the ankle.[53] The characteristic appearance on MRI is inhomogeneous signal intensity within the synovial proliferation. The lesion has low signal intensity on T1-weighted and T2-weighted images and may show diffusely inhomogeneous enhancement with gadolinium contrast[53] (**Fig. 9.32**). Although histologically similar to PVNS, giant cell tumor of the tendon sheath originates in a tendon sheath rather than a joint. In the foot, giant cell tumor of the

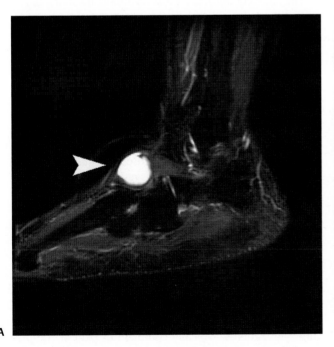
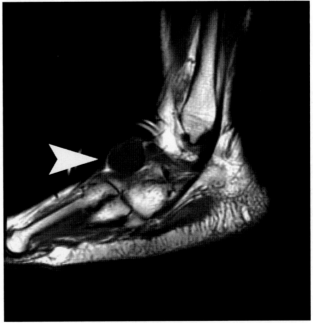

A   B

Fig. 9.30 Ganglion cysts. These lesions have high signal intensity (*arrowhead*) on T2-weighted images **(A)** and intermediate signal intensity (*arrowhead*) on T1-weighted images **(B)**, consistent with fluid.

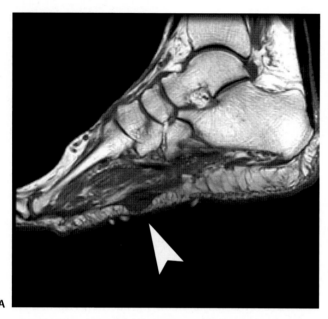
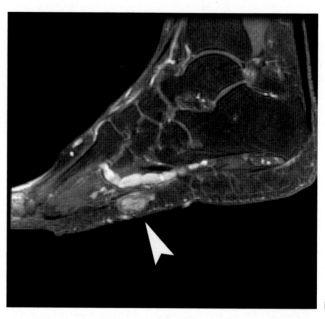

Fig. 9.31 Plantar fibromatosis is best seen on coronal and sagittal MR images of the foot. **(A)** The lesion typically has low to intermediate signal intensity (*arrowhead*) on T1-weighted images and is directly contiguous to the plantar fascia. **(B)** On T2-weighted images, there is low to intermediate signal and soft-tissue edema and/or signal alternation in the deep musculature. On this fat-suppressed T2-weighted image, the signal within the mass (*arrowhead*) seems relatively high because of fat suppression.

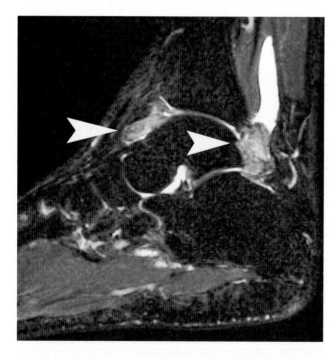

Fig. 9.32 A sagittal fat-suppressed T2-weighted image of the ankle in a patient with PVNS shows heterogeneous signal intensity within a region of synovial proliferation in the anterior (*left arrowhead*) and posterior (*right arrowhead*) tibiotalar joint. There is also a large posterosuperior extension of the synovial space.

tendon sheath predominantly affects the peroneal and flexor tendon sheaths. The MRI appearance is similar to that of intraarticular PVNS, but the lesion is typically less diffuse and more defined.[53]

The more common benign bone tumors involving the foot and ankle are the following:

- Simple bone cyst
- Aneurysmal bone cyst
- Intraosseous lipoma
- Giant cell tumor
- Enchondroma
- Osteoid osteoma

Malignant bone tumors of the foot and ankle are rare, but metastasis, Ewing sarcoma, chondrosarcoma, and osteosarcoma are occasionally seen in this region.

Plantar Fasciitis

Plantar fasciitis is a degenerative condition that occurs at the origin of the medial calcaneal tuberosity.[54] Less commonly, it can also occur secondary to an enthesopathy from systemic disease (such as RA, diabetes, or lupus) or after trauma, but typically it does not involve an inflammatory infiltrate, so "fasciitis" is a misnomer. The diagnosis is usually made clinically. Patients typically complain of pain at the plantar medial aspect of the heel that is severe first thing in the morning, after prolonged sitting, and toward the end of the

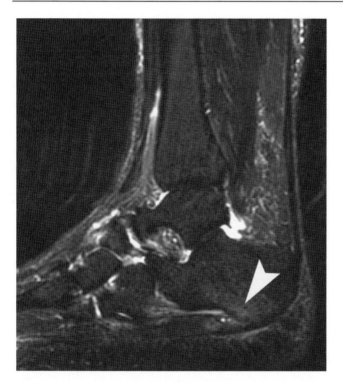

Fig. 9.33 A sagittal fat-suppressed T2-weighted image of a patient with plantar fasciitis, showing thickening of the fascia at its origin, intrasubstance changes, and edema of the calcaneus (*arrowhead*).

day after activity. The patient has point tenderness at the medial edge of the calcaneal tuberosity. Although not necessary at early presentation, MRI may be useful in differentiating plantar fasciitis from other conditions such as calcaneal stress fractures. Sagittal images are most helpful in assessing the plantar fascia. MRI shows thickening of the fascia at its origin, intrasubstance changes, and sometimes edema of the calcaneus (**Fig. 9.33**).

Morton Neuroma

Morton neuroma refers to entrapment or impingement of an interdigital nerve between two adjacent metatarsals near the MTP joint.[55] The nerve emerges from beneath the intermetatarsal ligament to bifurcate and course distally to the two adjacent toes at that web space. It most commonly affects the third interspace; the second interspace is the second most often affected area.[56] The patient typically complains of stabbing, burning, or radiating pain and often numbness in the corresponding toes.[57] Histologically, the nerve shows thickening, perineural fibrosis, and axonal demyelination.[57] MRI can be a useful diagnostic adjunct to clinical examination because conventional radiographs do not image the soft tissues effectively. Axial images are best for evaluating the interspaces (**Fig. 9.34**). On cross-sectional imaging, the nerve appears enlarged and spindle-shaped plantar to the inter-

metatarsal ligament.[58] The neuroma is isointense compared with muscle on T1-weighted images and hypointense to fat on non–fat-suppressed T2-weighted images.[58]

■ Postoperative Findings

Although radiography remains the predominant postoperative imaging modality for the ankle and foot, the excellent soft-tissue contrast of MRI is particularly useful for assessment after ligament and tendon surgery.

Tendon Repair

The treatment of tendon injuries consists primarily of immobilization and surgical reconnection of the apposed tendon ends. During the first month after tendon repair, granulation tissue bridges the anastomosis (week 1), followed by increased vascularization of the paratenon zone (week 2),

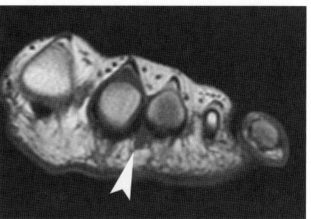

A

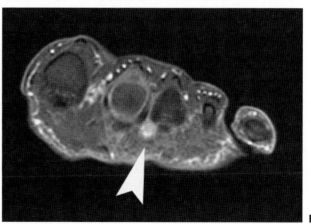

B

Fig. 9.34 Morton neuroma. **(A)** A coronal T1-weighted image of the left foot shows a small nodular mass (*arrowhead*) plantar to the intermetatarsal ligament connecting the second and third metatarsals. **(B)** A coronal fat-suppressed T2-weighted image of the same patient shows relative hyperintensity of the lesion (*arrowhead*).

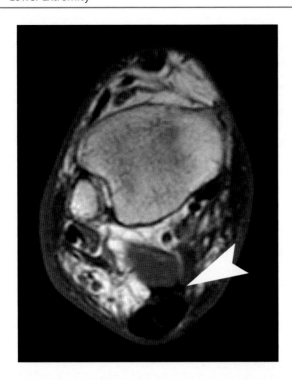

Fig. 9.35 An axial T1-weighted image of the right ankle showing an intact anastomosis (*arrowhead*) between the FHL and the Achilles tendon after tendon transfer surgery for Achilles repair.

collagen fibril formation (week 3), and, ultimately, the resolution of edema (week 4).[59] In cases where tendon rupture is left untreated for extended periods of time, the muscle becomes retracted and grafting may be required.[60] In such cases, available grafting strategies include free tendon grafts, tendon lengthening, and tendon transfers.

In the early postoperative period, the repaired tendon appears to be thickened.[59] In the late postoperative period, the principal findings can include generalized thickening and moderate heterogeneity of signal.[61] In the presence of a tendon transfer, the postoperative MR appearance includes nonanatomic connections between the relevant tendons (**Fig. 9.35**). Recurrent and new tears can be diagnosed as new areas of focal high signal on proton-density and T2-weighted images. T1-weighted images can also be reviewed for anatomic detail (**Fig. 9.36**). Comparison with previous studies is often useful for distinguishing postoperative intrasubstance changes and degeneration from re-tears. Postoperative infections such as abscess formation and osteomyelitis are best imaged using sequences before and after contrast enhancement.

Lateral Ankle Ligament Reconstruction

Surgical reconstruction of the lateral ligament complex is indicated for patients with chronic lateral instability as a sequela of ankle sprain.[62] In such cases, knowledge of the relevant surgical procedure is essential because the post-

operative appearance is characterized by nonanatomic anastomoses and osseous tunnels.[63] In the modified Evans procedure, the peroneus brevis tendon is transected, passed through a fibular tunnel, and anastomosed at the transaction site.[63] In the Lee procedure, the peroneus brevis is transected proximally, and the distal portion is looped through a fibular tunnel and anastomosed to its distal portion. The proximal peroneus brevis is then anastomosed to the peroneus longus.[63] In the Watson-Jones procedure, the peroneus brevis tendon is transected proximally, looped through two fibular tunnels and a tarsal tunnel, and sutured to itself distally.[63] As in the Lee procedure, the proximal portion is anastomosed to the peroneus longus. In the Christman-Sook procedure, the peroneus brevis is split, and the free half is passed beneath the talar periosteum, fibula tunnel, and calcaneal periosteum where it is anastomosed to the tethered portion of the peroneus brevis and adjacent peroneus longus in the region of the distal fibula (**Fig. 9.37**).[63]

Other Foot and Ankle Surgical Procedures

Other common surgical procedures of the foot and ankle include plantar fasciotomy, tarsal tunnel surgery, arthrod-

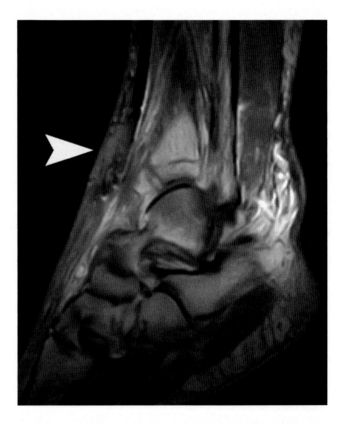

Fig. 9.36 A sagittal T1-weighted image showing several foci of susceptibility artifact within the anterior tibialis tendon, suggestive of previous repair. In addition, there is discontinuity within the anterior tibialis tendon (*arrowhead*), representing recurrent tear with some retraction.

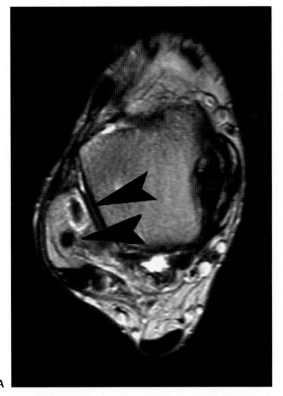

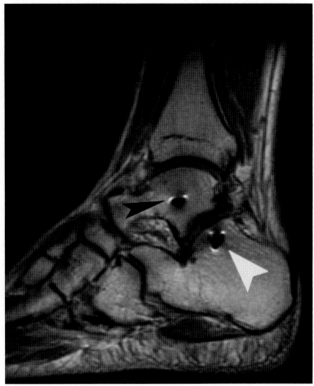

Fig. 9.37 Postoperative imaging in lateral ankle ligament reconstruction in a patient after a Chrisman-Snook procedure. **(A)** An axial T1-weighted image of the right ankle showing the split peroneus brevis tendon traversing two osseous tunnels through the fibula (*ar-rowheads*). **(B)** A sagittal T1-weighted image showing the split peroneus brevis tendon traversing through additional tunnels traversing the talus (*black arrowhead*) and calcaneus (*white arrowhead*).

esis, and hallux valgus repair.[59] After fasciotomy, the plantar fascia is thickened with indistinct margins, with a lack of the fascial edema that characterizes plantar fasciitis.[64] After tarsal tunnel surgery, MR shows scarring of the subcutaneous fat and fascia medial to the tarsal tunnel visible as abnormal areas of low T1 signal.[54] Postoperative imaging after arthrodesis typically involves using radiography or CT to assess the extent of osseous fusion, although MRI can be useful for assessing soft-tissue complications such as infection, secondary degenerative changes, and tendinous and ligamentous stability. Lastly, MR is a useful adjunct in postoperative assessment of hallux valgus repair to evaluate for complications such as infection, osteonecrosis, and nonunion.[59]

References

1. Tocci SL, Madom IA, Bradley MP, Langer PR, DiGiovanni CW. The diagnostic value of MRI in foot and ankle surgery. Foot Ankle Int 2007;28:166–168

2. Rosenberg ZS, Beltran J, Bencardino JT. From the RSNA Refresher Courses. MR imaging of the ankle and foot. Radiographics 2000;20(Suppl 1):S153–S179

3. Bauer JS, Banerjee S, Henning TD, Krug R, Majumdar S, Link TM. Fast high-spatial-resolution MRI of the ankle with parallel imaging using GRAPPA at 3 T. AJR Am J Roentgenol 2007;189:240–245

4. Barr C, Bauer JS, Malfair D, et al. MR imaging of the ankle at 3 Tesla and 1.5 Tesla: protocol optimization and application to cartilage, ligament and tendon pathology in cadaver specimens. Eur Radiol 2007;17:1518–1528

5. Cerezal L, Abascal F, García-Valtuille R, Canga A. Ankle MR arthrography: how, why, when. Radiol Clin North Am 2005;43:693–707

6. Morrison WB. Magnetic resonance imaging of sports injuries of the ankle. Top Magn Reson Imaging 2003;14:179–197

7. Pinar H, Akseki D, Kovanlikaya I, Araç S, Bozkurt M. Bone bruises detected by magnetic resonance imaging following lateral ankle sprains. Knee Surg Sports Traumatol Arthrosc 1997;5:113–117

8. Schneck CD, Mesgarzadeh M, Bonakdarpour A. MR imaging of the most commonly injured ankle ligaments. Part II. Ligament injuries. Radiology 1992;184:507–512

9. Fong DTP, Hong Y, Chan LK, Yung PSH, Chan KM. A systematic review on ankle injury and ankle sprain in sports. Sports Med 2007;37:73–94

10. Clanton TO, Schon LC. Athletic injuries to the soft tissues of the foot and ankle. In: Mann RA, Coughlin MJ, eds. Surgery of the Foot and Ankle. St. Louis: Mosby-Year Book; 1993:1095–1224

11. Nielson JH, Gardner MJ, Peterson MGE, et al. Radiographic measurements do not predict syndesmotic injury in ankle fractures: an MRI study. Clin Orthop Relat Res 2005;436:216–221

12. Oae K, Takao M, Naito K, et al. Injury of the tibiofibular syndesmosis: value of MR imaging for diagnosis. Radiology 2003;227:155–161

13. Boytim MJ, Fischer DA, Neumann L. Syndesmotic ankle sprains. Am J Sports Med 1991;19:294–298

14. Edwards GS Jr, DeLee JC. Ankle diastasis without fracture. Foot Ankle 1984;4:305–312

15. Flick AB, Gould N. Osteochondritis dissecans of the talus (transchondral fractures of the talus): review of the literature and new surgical approach for medial dome lesions. Foot Ankle 1985;5:165–185

16. Berndt AL, Harty M. Transchondral fractures (osteochondritis dissecans) of the talus. J Bone Joint Surg Am 1959;41:988–1020

17. Canale ST, Belding RH. Osteochondral lesions of the talus. J Bone Joint Surg Am 1980;62:97–102

18. Raikin SM, Elias I, Zoga AC, Morrison WB, Besser MP, Schweitzer ME. Osteochondral lesions of the talus: localization and morphologic data from 424 patients using a novel anatomical grid scheme. Foot Ankle Int 2007;28:154–161

19. Scranton PE Jr, McDermott JE. Treatment of type V osteochondral lesions of the talus with ipsilateral knee osteochondral autografts. Foot Ankle Int 2001;22:380–384

20. Mintz DN, Tashjian GS, Connell DA, Deland JT, O'Malley M, Potter HG. Osteochondral lesions of the talus: a new magnetic resonance grading system with arthroscopic correlation. Arthroscopy 2003;19:353–359

21. Stroud CC, Marks RM. Imaging of osteochondral lesions of the talus. Foot Ankle Clin 2000;5:119–133

22. De Smet AA, Fisher DR, Burnstein MI, Graf BK, Lange RH. Value of MR imaging in staging osteochondral lesions of the talus (osteochondritis dissecans): results in 14 patients. AJR Am J Roentgenol 1990;154:555–558

23. Dipaola JD, Nelson DW, Colville MR. Characterizing osteochondral lesions by magnetic resonance imaging. Arthroscopy 1991;7:101–104

24. Lahm A, Erggelet C, Steinwachs M, Reichelt A. Arthroscopic management of osteochondral lesions of the talus: results of drilling and usefulness of magnetic resonance imaging before and after treatment. Arthroscopy 2000;16:299–304

25. Higashiyama I, Kumai T, Takakura Y, Tamail S. Follow-up study of MRI for osteochondral lesion of the talus. Foot Ankle Int 2000;21:127–133

26. Pester S, Smith PC. Stress fractures in the lower extremities of soldiers in basic training. Orthop Rev 1992;21:297–303

27. Matheson GO, Clement DB, McKenzie DC, Taunton JE, Lloyd-Smith DR, Macintyre JG. Scintigraphic uptake of 99mTc at non-painful sites in athletes with stress fractures. The concept of bone strain. Sports Med 1987;4:65–75

28. Weinfeld SB, Haddad SL, Myerson MS. Metatarsal stress fractures. Clin Sports Med 1997;16:319–338

29. Khoury NJ, El-Khoury GY, Saltzman CL, Brandser EA. MR imaging of posterior tibial tendon dysfunction. AJR Am J Roentgenol 1996;167:675–682

30. Rosenberg ZS, Cheung Y, Jahss MH, Noto AM, Norman A, Leeds NE. Rupture of posterior tibial tendon: CT and MR imaging with surgical correlation. Radiology 1988;169:229–235

31. Schweitzer ME, Karasick D. MR imaging of disorders of the posterior tibialis tendon. AJR Am J Roentgenol 2000;175:627–635

32. Khoury NJ, El-Khoury GY, Saltzman CL, Kathol MH. Peroneus longus and brevis tendon tears: MR imaging evaluation. Radiology 1996;200:833–841

33. Khoury NJ, El-Khoury GY, Saltzman CL, Brandser EA. Rupture of the anterior tibial tendon: diagnosis by MR imaging. AJR Am J Roentgenol 1996;167:351–354

34. Erickson SJ, Cox IH, Hyde JS, Carrera GF, Strandt JA, Estkowski LD. Effect of tendon orientation on MR imaging signal intensity: a manifestation of the "magic angle" phenomenon. Radiology 1991;181:389–392

35. Puddu G, Ippolito E, Postacchini F. A classification of Achilles tendon disease. Am J Sports Med 1976;4:145–150

36. Kvist M. Achilles tendon injuries in athletes. Sports Med 1994;18:173–201

37. Rosenberg ZS. Chronic rupture of the posterior tibial tendon. Magn Reson Imaging Clin N Am 1994;2:79–87

38. Sobel M, Geppert MJ, Olson EJ, Bohne WH, Arnoczky SP. The dynamics of peroneus brevis tendon splits: a proposed mechanism, technique of diagnosis, and classification of injury. Foot Ankle 1992;13:413–422

39. Major NM, Helms CA, Fritz RC, Speer KP. The MR imaging appearance of longitudinal split tears of the peroneus brevis tendon. Foot Ankle Int 2000;21:514–519

40. Rosenberg ZS, Beltran J, Cheung YY, Colon E, Herraiz F. MR features of longitudinal tears of the peroneus brevis tendon. AJR Am J Roentgenol 1997;168:141–147

41. Schweitzer ME, Eid ME, Deely D, Wapner K, Hecht P. Using MR imaging to differentiate peroneal splits from other peroneal disorders. AJR Am J Roentgenol 1997;168:129–133

42. Cheung YY, Rosenberg ZS, Ramsinghani R, Beltran J, Jahss MH. Peroneus quartus muscle: MR imaging features. Radiology 1997;202:745–750

43. Sobel M, Pavlov H, Geppert MJ, Thompson FM, DiCarlo EF, Davis WH. Painful os peroneum syndrome: a spectrum of conditions responsible for plantar lateral foot pain. Foot Ankle Int 1994;15:112–124

44. Mengiardi B, Pfirrmann CWA, Vienne P, et al. Anterior tibial tendon abnormalities: MR imaging findings. Radiology 2005;235:977–984

45. Sammarco GJ, Cooper PS. Flexor hallucis longus tendon injury in dancers and nondancers. Foot Ankle Int 1998;19:356–362

46. Rubin DA, Tishkoff NW, Britton CA, Conti SF, Towers JD. Anterolateral soft-tissue impingement in the ankle: diagnosis using MR imaging. AJR Am J Roentgenol 1997;169:829–835

47. Adelaar RS, Madrian JR. Avascular necrosis of the talus. Orthop Clin North Am 2004;35:383–395

48. Brody AS, Strong M, Babikian G, Sweet DE, Seidel FG, Kuhn JP. John Caffey Award paper. Avascular necrosis: early MR imaging and histologic findings in a canine model. AJR Am J Roentgenol 1991;157:341–345

49. Schweitzer ME, Morrison WB. MR imaging of the diabetic foot. Radiol Clin North Am 2004;42:61–71

50. Ledermann HP, Morrison WB, Schweitzer ME. MR image analysis of pedal osteomyelitis: distribution, patterns of spread, and frequency of associated ulceration and septic arthritis. Radiology 2002;223:747–755

51. Fabrin J, Larsen K, Holstein PE. Long-term follow-up in diabetic Charcot feet with spontaneous onset. Diabetes Care 2000;23:796–800

52. Klenerman L. The Charcot joint in diabetes. Diabet Med 1996;13(suppl 1):S52–S54

53. Woertler K. Soft tissue masses in the foot and ankle: characteristics on MR Imaging. Semin Musculoskelet Radiol 2005;9:227–242

54. Recht MP, Donley BG. Magnetic resonance imaging of the foot and ankle. J Am Acad Orthop Surg 2001;9:187–199

55. Morton TG. The Classic. A peculiar and painful affection of the fourth metatarso-phalangeal articulation. Clin Orthop Relat Res 1979;142: 4–9

56. Levitsky KA, Alman BA, Jevsevar DS, Morehead J. Digital nerves of the foot: anatomic variations and implications regarding the pathogenesis of interdigital neuroma. Foot Ankle 1993;14:208–214

57. Kay D, Bennett GL. Morton's neuroma. Foot Ankle Clin 2003;8: 49–59

58. Zanetti M, Weishaupt D. MR imaging of the forefoot: Morton neuroma and differential diagnoses. Semin Musculoskelet Radiol 2005;9:175–186

59. Bergin D, Morrison WB. Postoperative imaging of the ankle and foot. Radiol Clin North Am 2006;44:391–406

60. Platt MA. Tendon repair and healing. Clin Podiatr Med Surg 2005;22:553–560

61. Reinig JW, Dorwart RH, Roden WC. MR imaging of a ruptured Achilles tendon. J Comput Assist Tomogr 1985;9:1131–1134

62. Alparslan L, Chiodo CP. Lateral ankle instability: MR imaging of associated injuries and surgical treatment procedures. Semin Musculoskelet Radiol 2008;12:346–358

63. Chien AJ, Jacobson JA, Jamadar DA, Brigido MK, Femino JE, Hayes CW. Imaging appearances of lateral ankle ligament reconstruction. Radiographics 2004;24:999–1008

64. Woelffer KE, Figura MA, Sandberg NS, Snyder NS. Five-year follow-up results of instep plantar fasciotomy for chronic heel pain. J Foot Ankle Surg 2000;39:218–223

IV Spine

10 The Cervical Spine

Lukas P. Zebala, Jacob M. Buchowski, Aditya R. Daftary, Joseph R. O'Brien, John A. Carrino, and A. Jay Khanna

■ Specialized Pulse Sequences and Protocols

Although imaging protocols of the cervical spine for specific indications can vary among institutions, standard MRI of the cervical spine for degenerative pathologies usually includes the following pulse sequences:

- Sagittal T1-weighted SE
- Sagittal T2-weighted FSE
- Axial gradient-echo
- Axial T2-weighted FSE

A detailed discussion of all the imaging sequences used in the cervical spine is beyond the scope of this chapter; however, salient features of commonly used sequences are discussed below.

T1-weighted images are useful in identifying fracture lines. Because they are sensitive to the presence of gadolinium contrast, they are also used for contrast-enhanced imaging, which is helpful in assessing neoplasms, infections, and the postoperative spine. Typically, fat-suppressed postgadolinium T1-weighted images are used to make lesions more conspicuous. T2-weighted images are sensitive to water (and thus edema) and are useful in identifying areas of potential pathology. However, care must be taken with regard to interpreting bone marrow edema because it may be seen with a variety of conditions, including infection, inflammation, trauma, and degeneration. Although edema may focus attention toward an abnormality, many of these conditions can coexist, so additional analysis is required before finalizing a conclusion. FSE is now routinely used to acquire T2-weighted images at speeds up to 64 times faster than conventional SE T2-weighted images. Sometimes the differentiation of fat, water, and lesions can be difficult, especially on T2-weighted FSE images, and therefore fat suppression is used to make these areas more conspicuous. This sequence can be obtained by applying a fat-suppression pulse to produce fat-suppressed T2-weighted images or by obtaining a STIR sequence. Visualizing edema is helpful in identifying ligamentous injuries, and such visualization is best achieved with STIR or fat-suppressed T2-weighted images. T2-weighted images are also most sensitive for evaluating the cord parenchyma for lesions and edema, which are seen as abnormally bright signal, although the sagittal orientation is subject to linear bright artifact within the cord (Gibbs phenomenon). For this reason, axial T2-weighted images serve as a useful tool for detecting cord abnormalities and confirming lesions suspected on sagittal T2-weighted images.

Gradient-echo images are very susceptible to magnetic artifacts; this important characteristic makes them useful for detecting small areas of hemorrhage, such as with cervical spine trauma and vascular malformations. However, these images can also overestimate the degree of canal and foraminal stenosis secondary to artifact from the adjacent bone. Because of the rapidity with which gradient-echo images are acquired, studies can be obtained with higher resolution than that required for other pulse sequences and even as a 3D volume set, which allows for isotropic voxels and reformations in multiple planes. This volume set can then allow one to characterize the cervical foramina in the appropriate oblique plane.

For evaluation of vascular structures in the neck, MR angiography can be obtained without contrast, using 2D or 3D time-of-flight or phase-contrast imaging. These sequences create contrast between flowing and stationary structures. Phase-contrast imaging may also provide flow-velocity information. As a result of the technique, time-of-flight imaging shows fat or subacute thrombus as bright signal and may be useful in detecting small, subtle thrombi. The 3D techniques require more time and are slightly less sensitive to slow flow states. Gadolinium-enhanced MR angiography may also be obtained and is extremely accurate.

■ Traumatic Conditions

Although the cervical spine is injured in only 2% to 3% of blunt trauma accidents,[1] the potential for instability and critical neurologic injury makes prompt identification and management of cervical spine injuries important. Patients with suspected cervical spine injury should be evaluated initially with conventional radiographs (AP, lateral, and open-mouth odontoid views). CT imaging offers greater osseous detail than does conventional radiography and may reveal fractures or details that are not detected with radiography. CT is especially helpful in assessing fractures of the occipital condyles and cervicothoracic junction, where osseous overlap on conventional radiographs makes fracture detection difficult. MRI provides soft-tissue visualization superior to that of conventional radiography or CT and is useful for the assessment of spinal cord injury, ligamentous injury, degree of spinal stenosis, and additional fracture evaluation. Occult fractures not visible on conventional radiographs or CT images may be detected by the presence of vertebral body edema on MR images. Although MRI is extremely sensitive in identifying cervical spine fractures, their characteristics and the exact appearance of the osseous components can be challenging; CT may be a better choice for assessing such details. In addition, MRI is useful for the evaluation of obtunded patients or those with cervical spine injury, neurologic deficits, or an unreliable physical examination.[2-7]

MRI is indicated specifically when neurologic deficit, vascular injury, or soft-tissue injury is suspected in the setting of trauma. It is also useful in assessing posttraumatic sequelae.[8] Imaging spinal gunshot injuries is controversial. Theoretically, a ferrous gunshot fragment may become mobile, but most bullets are nonferrous, and therefore such patients can usually be imaged without consequences. Unfortunately, the exact composition of a gunshot fragment is seldom known, and therefore MRI remains controversial and dependent on the clinical need.[9,10]

It should be noted that there are obstacles to obtaining MRI studies in the trauma setting, especially with regard to cervical spine trauma, because patients may have clinically significant neurologic deficits. These obstacles include the following:

- Lack of availability of MRI capabilities on an urgent basis
- MR-incompatibility of some ventilators, traction devices, and other equipment
- Lack of clinical access to patients during the imaging study

MRI protocols vary by institution, but commonly used sequences in trauma evaluation include the following[11]:

- Sagittal T1-weighted images to assess the alignment of the cervical spine, vertebral body integrity, fractures, and spinal cord caliber
- Sagittal T2-weighted images to assess for the presence of cord edema, compression, and spondylotic changes
- Sagittal STIR images to assess for the presence of paraspinal ligamentous injury and bone marrow edema
- Axial T1-weighted and T2-weighted images to assess for the presence of posterior element fractures, to evaluate for spinal stenosis, to better define disc pathology, and to confirm the precise location of abnormalities detected on sagittal images
- Sagittal T2-weighted gradient-echo images (in some institutions) to assess for the presence of acute spinal cord hemorrhage and disc herniation (high signal in the disc even with severe osseous degeneration, which

Table 10.1 Evaluation of Cervical Spine Trauma

Anatomy	Evaluation
Spinal column/ vertebral bodies	Alignment Vertebral body fracture Posterior element fracture Edema Degenerative change
Ligaments	Anterior longitudinal ligament Posterior longitudinal ligament Interspinous and supraspinous ligaments Ligamentum flavum Evaluation for edema/rupture
Spinal cord	Edema Hemorrhage Compression Syrinx
Epidural space	Hematoma Disc herniation Osseous fragment
Vascular	Vertebral artery

Source: Takhtani D, Melhelm ER. MR imaging in cervical spine trauma. Magn Reson Imaging Clin N Am 2000;8:615–634. Modified with permission.

enables the distinction between bone fragments and a disc herniation)

Regardless of the specific institutional MRI protocol, a systematic approach (see Chapter 3) for the evaluation of cervical spine MRI should be used to avoid missing pathologic conditions (see **Table 10.1** for important cervical spine structures to evaluate). In addition, it is essential that the interpretation of the MRI findings be performed in conjunction with that of the other available imaging modalities, including conventional radiographs (with flexion and extension views if clinically indicated) and CT (see Chapter 17).

Classification of Cervical Spine Trauma

Cervical spine injuries can be classified based on the mechanism of injury. Although six categories have been described (vertical compression, compressive flexion, distractive flexion, lateral flexion, compressive extension, and distractive extension[12]) (**Fig. 10.1**), the classification scheme is simplified here into three broad categories:

- Hyperflexion
- Hyperextension
- Axial loading

In many instances, the mechanism of injury can be difficult to determine from an analysis of the clinical situation (in the absence of imaging findings), and therefore clinicians may choose to broadly classify cervical spine injuries as follows:

- Secondary to blunt trauma
- Secondary to penetrating trauma

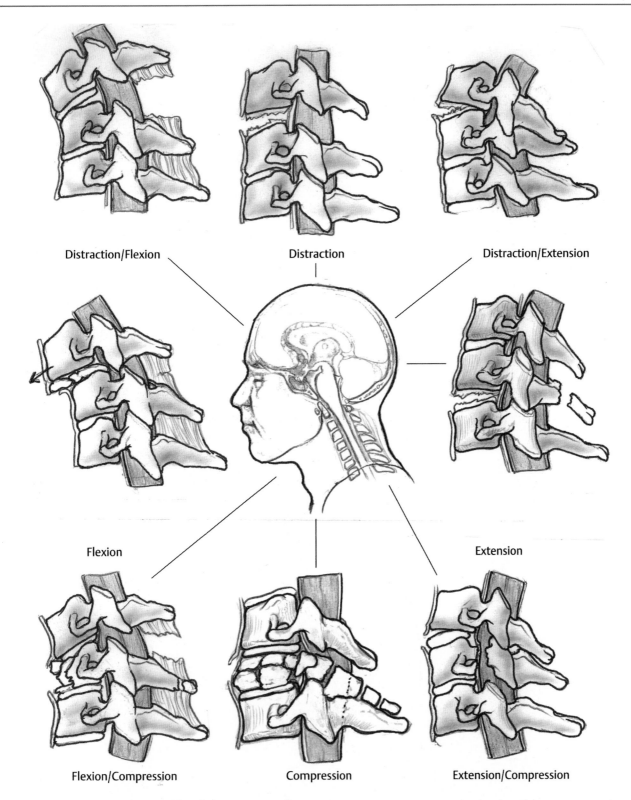

Distraction/Flexion

Distraction

Distraction/Extension

Flexion

Extension

Flexion/Compression

Compression

Extension/Compression

Fig. 10.1 An artist's representation of the Allen-Ferguson mechanistic classification system for subaxial cervical spine fractures. (From Chapman JR, Anderson PA. Cervical spine trauma. In: Frymoyer J, Ducker TB, Hadler NM et al, eds. The Adult Spine: Principles and Practice. 2nd ed. Philadelphia: 1997:1245–1295. Reprinted with permission.)

In addition, cervical spine injuries can be subdivided based on the region of injury within the occipitocervical spine:

- Occipitocervical junction
- Suboccipital cervical spine (C1-C2)
- Subaxial cervical spine (C3-C7)

More recently, the subaxial cervical spine injury classification system has been described as an approach that recognizes the importance of fracture morphology, neurologic injury, and integrity of the discoligamentous complex.[13] A systematic evaluation of these three components can be used to guide the treatment of patients with cervical spine fractures.

Hyperflexion Injuries

Flexion-compression injuries range from the minor anterior compression of the anterosuperior end plate (**Fig. 10.2**) to a severe teardrop or quadrangular fracture. These injuries are associated with retrolisthesis, kyphosis, and circumferential soft-tissue disruption. The radiographic evaluation

of flexion-compression injuries includes inspection for the following:

- Anterior and middle column compromise
- Vertebral body-height loss
- Translation
- Angulation
- Posterior element competence

Although conventional radiographs and CT scans can evaluate fracture pattern, alignment, angulation, and translation, MRI provides additional diagnostic value and can assist with the determination of treatment options for such patients because it facilitates the assessment of spinal cord compression and posterior element compromise.

Flexion-distraction forces can lead to facet subluxations, dislocations, or fracture-dislocations. These injuries represent a spectrum of osteoligamentous pathology, ranging from the purely ligamentous dislocation to fracture of the facet and lateral mass. MRI helps assess the compromise of posterior musculature, interspinous ligaments, ligamentum flavum, and facet capsules that is often seen with flexion-distraction injuries.[14] The role of MRI in the treatment algo-

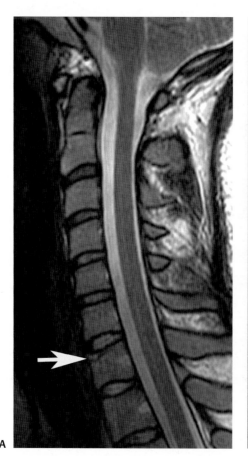
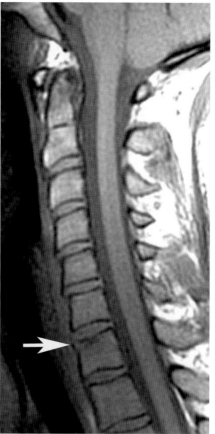

Fig. 10.2 C7 vertebral compression fracture. Sagittal T2-weighted (A) and T1-weighted (B) images showing the fracture (*arrow on each*) with minimal loss of height.

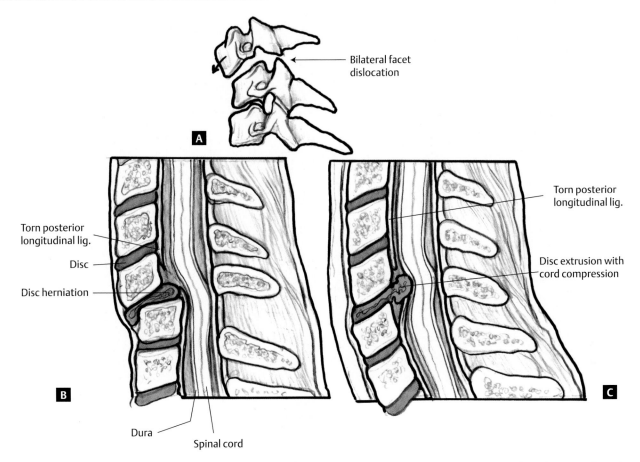

Fig. 10.3 Artist's sketches illustrating the pathology in bilateral facet dislocation. **(A)** A lateral view of osseous structures shows that the facets are perched and that additional translation will lead to complete dislocation. **(B)** A lateral view before reduction shows approximately 50% translation of the superior vertebral body relative to the inferior one and displacement of the intervertebral disc. **(C)** A lateral view after reduction shows that the intervertebral disc has displaced into the spinal canal and compressed the spinal cord during the reduction maneuver.

rithm of patients who present with bilateral cervical facet dislocations (**Fig. 10.3**) without neurologic compromise is the subject of substantial debate in the literature and among spine surgeons.[14–16] The treatment options include MRI before attempting closed reduction or surgical intervention; closed reduction with traction while monitoring the patient's neurologic examination; and surgical intervention via anterior, posterior, or combined approaches.[14–16] One of the purposes of obtaining an MRI study before the reduction of bilateral facet dislocations is to rule out the possibility of an extruded disc fragment that may displace into the spinal canal during a closed reduction (**Fig. 10.4**).

Most flexion injuries are well visualized on MRI, and MRI is particularly effective for the assessment of the following[11]:

- Alignment
- Fractures
- Ligamentous injury
- Cord abnormalities
- Acute disc herniations
- The cause of anterior subluxation, either chronic degenerative changes or hyperflexion sprain

Facet joint injuries may be seen on parasagittal or axial images, which show increased signal on T2-weighted images secondary to edema from facet capsule tears.[11,17–19] Injury to posterior ligaments may be seen as areas of hyperintensity on T2-weighted images, especially fat-suppressed T2-weighted or STIR images (**Fig. 10.5**).

Hyperextension Injuries

Cervical spine extension injury results in the posterior translation or rotation of a vertebral body in the sagittal plane.[6,11,20] Hyperextension injuries often are produced by rear-impact motor-vehicle collisions or direct facial trauma.

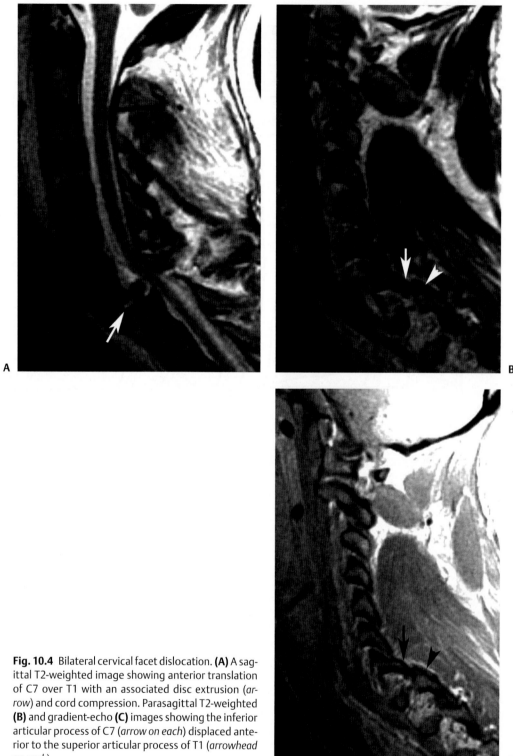

Fig. 10.4 Bilateral cervical facet dislocation. **(A)** A sagittal T2-weighted image showing anterior translation of C7 over T1 with an associated disc extrusion (*arrow*) and cord compression. Parasagittal T2-weighted **(B)** and gradient-echo **(C)** images showing the inferior articular process of C7 (*arrow on each*) displaced anterior to the superior articular process of T1 (*arrowhead on each*).

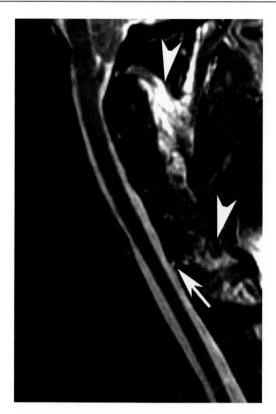

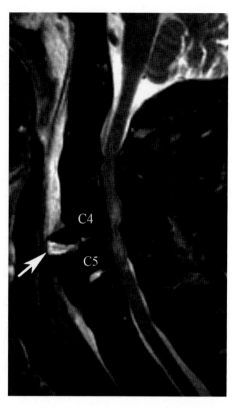

Fig. 10.5 A sagittal STIR image shows edema in the supraspinous ligament region (*arrowhead*) and interspinous region at C6-C7 and C7-T1, with a small, focal region of increased T2-weighted signal in the ligamentum flavum at the C7-T1 level (*arrow*) compatible with a partial tear.

Fig. 10.6 A sagittal STIR image showing an intervertebral disc rupture at C4-C5 (*arrow*) in a patient who sustained a hyperextension injury to the cervical spine. Note the associated prevertebral hematoma and the severe multilevel degenerative stenosis with associated cord signal change.

In cervical spine hyperextension injuries, potential findings include the following[6,11,17,19,20]:

- Tear(s) of the anterior longitudinal ligament
- Avulsion of the intervertebral disc from an adjacent vertebral body
- Horizontal intervertebral disc rupture (**Fig. 10.6**)

More severe and potentially unstable hyperextension injuries may be associated with the following[6]:

- Prevertebral hematoma
- Widening of the disc space
- Posterior ligament complex edema
- Herniated disc

Elderly patients with spondylosis and kyphosis of the cervical spine may suffer spinal cord injury without fracture or ligamentous injury because of posterior infolding of the ligamentum flavum upon a spinal canal already narrowed by posterior vertebral osteophytes.[6]

Whiplash injuries often have no associated osseous injury on standard radiographs or CT images, and flexion-extension radiographs may be nondiagnostic because of poor excursion secondary to pain. However, MRI is of limited value for the assessment of whiplash; several studies have failed to show positive MRI findings in the absence of neurologic symptoms.[18,21] In contrast, patients with a fused cervical spine secondary to ankylosing spondylitis or diffuse idiopathic skeletal hyperostosis may benefit from an MRI examination to assess for acute fracture, instability, or neurologic compromise. In such patients, the fused cervical spine acts like a long-bone fracture, and even minimally displaced fractures may be unstable (**Fig. 10.7**).[22]

Finally, MRI can assess intervertebral disc injury and subtle fractures caused by any of the above-mentioned mechanisms.[11,17–19,23] Intervertebral disc injury may range from tear(s) of the outer annulus fibrosis (seen as increased T2-weighted signal in the outer annular fibers) to frank intervertebral disc herniation. The identification of an annular tear on MRI does not indicate acute traumatic injury and can be seen in asymptomatic individuals.[24,25] Intervertebral disc separation from the adjacent vertebral body may be seen as a horizontal hyperintense T2-weighted signal.[11,17,19] Subtle fractures, such as vertebral end-plate fractures, may be best visualized with MRI because it can detect osseous edema and hemorrhage not seen on conventional radiographs or CT images.[11,17,19]

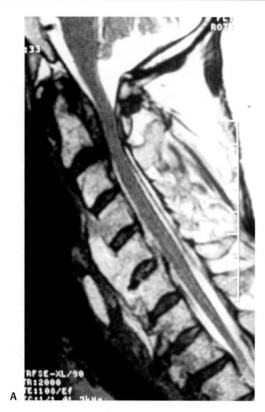

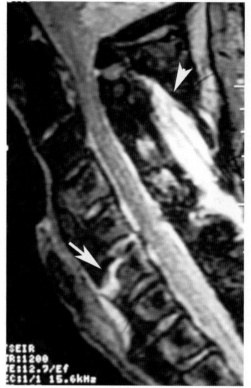

Fig. 10.7 Ankylosing spondylitis. **(A)** A T2-weighted image shows multilevel ankylosis of the cervical spine and ossification of the posterior longitudinal ligament posterior to the body of C2 but no specific evidence of fracture. (Conventional radiographs and CT images also showed no evidence of fracture.) **(B)** A sagittal STIR image shows a nondisplaced "fracture" or injury through the anterior column at C6 (*arrow*) and posterior column injury; both injuries manifested as regions of increased signal intensity with the use of this fluid-sensitive pulse sequence.

Axial Load Injuries

Axial load injuries are caused by the axial transmission of force through the skull, through the occipital condyles, and into the spine. This force transmission can cause a Jefferson burst fracture or burst fractures of the subaxial cervical spine. MRI is useful for the assessment of C1 compression fractures and associated pathologies such as lateral mass displacement on coronal images, atlantodental interval increase on sagittal images, and transverse ligament disruption on axial images.[11] For burst fractures, MRI is useful for diagnosing associated spinal cord injury caused by an acute herniated disc or retropulsion of osseous fragments (**Fig. 10.8**). Because a purely axial force subjects the posterior capsuloligamentous structures to compression only, these posterior structures should remain intact.[11,20] However, there often is some degree of spine flexion during the traumatic event that may cause injury to the posterior spinal elements, which can be detected by MRI.[20] It is important to carefully scrutinize the fat-suppressed T2-weighted and other images for evidence of injury to the posterior ligamentous and osseous structures because such injury will lead to consideration of posterior fusion in addition to the anterior decompression and fusion that is often performed for patients with cervical burst fractures.

Occipitocervical Junction Injuries

Although injury to the occipitocervical junction occurs in a small percentage of blunt trauma victims (0.8% in one study[26]), recognition of such injuries is crucial because of their devastating effects.[27-30] A detailed discussion of occipitocervical craniotomy and the various measurement techniques for evaluation of occipitocervical pathology is beyond the scope of this chapter, but presented here is an overview of the major types of occipitocervical traumatic findings as seen on MRI. It is important to keep in mind that MRI studies of the occipitocervical junction should be reviewed in conjunction with conventional radiographic and CT imaging.

Atlantooccipital Dissociation

Atlantooccipital dissociation is any separation of the atlantooccipital articulation. The skull may displace anteriorly, posteriorly, or superiorly, and may be complete (disloca-

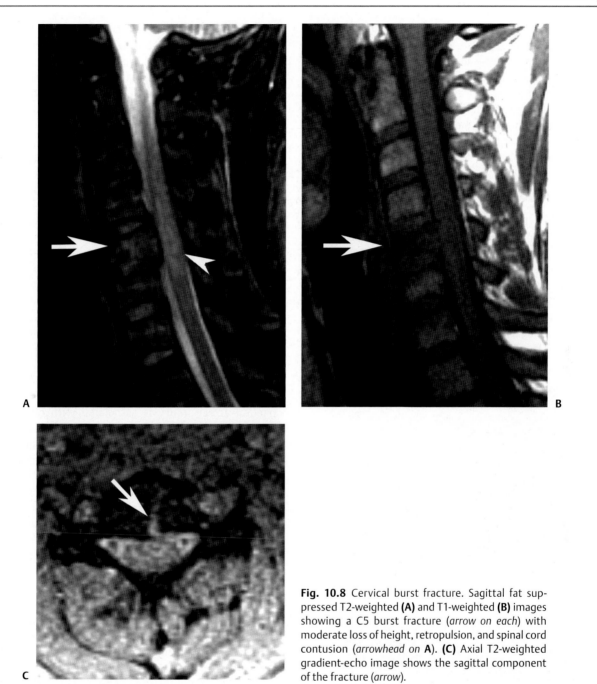

Fig. 10.8 Cervical burst fracture. Sagittal fat suppressed T2-weighted **(A)** and T1-weighted **(B)** images showing a C5 burst fracture (*arrow on each*) with moderate loss of height, retropulsion, and spinal cord contusion (*arrowhead on* **A**). **(C)** Axial T2-weighted gradient-echo image shows the sagittal component of the fracture (*arrow*).

tion) or partial (subluxation). Atlantooccipital dissociation can be a devastating injury.[27–30] The primary injury is to the ligaments that provide structural support to the cervicocranial junction. In addition, even without frank dislocation, the occiput–C1 junction may be injured, as indicated by postmortem studies.[27,28] Although this injury may be fatal, improvement in resuscitative and medical treatment has increased survival rates. CT imaging may be used to assess associated fractures or relationships among the basion, dens, occipital condyles, and atlas in conjunction with atlanto-

occipital dissociation, whereas MRI is better at detecting injury to the cervicocranial ligaments (e.g., transverse, apical, cruciate, atlantooccipital membrane and capsular ligaments, tectorial membrane), brainstem, or spinal cord.[11,19,31]

Trauma to the Atlas

Axial load to the occipitocervical junction at the atlas may result in a burst fracture of the atlas. The injury is visualized on open-mouth odontoid radiographs or coronal CT images.[32,33]

As indicated by the cadaver study of Spence et al.,[34] combined overhang of the lateral masses of C1 over C2 of ≥6.9 mm is associated with transverse ligament rupture and indicates a relatively unstable Jefferson burst fracture. The axial T2-weighted images can be critically evaluated to rule in or rule out injury to the transverse ligament. These images should be carefully scrutinized for increased T2-weighted signal in or along the course of the transverse ligament. The ligament should also be evaluated for regions of discontinuity.

Trauma to the Axis

C2 is the most commonly fractured cervical spine level.[26] In the elderly, odontoid fractures tend to be posteriorly displaced. Fracture location, displacement, and angulation are important factors that assist with clinical decision-making. Lateral cervical radiographs and CT scans can be used to characterize such fractures and better evaluate the osseous detail. MRI can assist in the evaluation of these fractures by providing assessment of the degree of edema at the fracture site (**Fig. 10.9**). This information provides insight into the age of the fracture (acute versus subacute versus chronic), which can be used to guide treatment. The sagittal and axial T2-weighted images should also be carefully evaluated to determine the degree of neural compression, from either a displaced fracture or underlying degenerative changes.

Atlantoaxial Dissociation

Atlantoaxial dissociation may be caused by distraction with superior migration of the atlas away from the axis or by odontoid fractures with anterior or posterior displacement of C1 relative to C2. MRI clearly depicts the associated pathology seen with atlantoaxial dissociation.[11] As noted above, MRI is very useful for detecting ligamentous and spinal cord injury. The relationship of the atlas to axis is clearly visible with MRI. Specifically, the integrity of the transverse ligament should be evaluated along with the approximate size of the anterior atlantodens interval. This measurement is more frequently evaluated on flexion and extension lateral cervical spine radiographs (**Fig. 10.10**).

Vertebral Artery Injury

Vertebral artery injury is associated with blunt cervical trauma, with an incidence as high as 11%.[35] This potentially devastating injury may occur with cervical spine fractures extending into the transverse foramen, but it is associated most often with unilateral or bilateral facet dislocations.[19,36] MR angiography may be used to assess vertebral artery patency, especially with such fractures.[19] MR angiography may show areas of vascular stenosis or occlusion. Flowing blood creates a signal void on axial SE images and is seen as a bright signal on gradient-echo images; merging the data from these two modalities can help determine the status of blood flow in the vertebral arteries[19,37] (**Fig. 10.11**).

The types of vertebral artery injuries are thrombosis, dissection, and transection (rare). MR angiography shows vertebral artery thrombosis as the absence of flow-related enhancement on images in the expected course of the vertebral artery and as an acute thrombus in the foramen transversarium, dissections as a tapering of the vessel, and transections as a focal discontinuity of the vessel. Major clues to vascular injury include changes in vessel caliber, loss of the normal rounded shape, increase in caliber from proximal to distal (except at the carotid bulb), or the presence of an extraluminal thrombus or a slit or dark band through the lumen.

Penetrating Trauma

Penetrating injury to the cervical spine can be caused by projectiles (e.g., bullets) or puncture mechanisms. Missiles can cause spinal cord injury by direct penetration, displacement of bone fragments into the spinal canal compressing

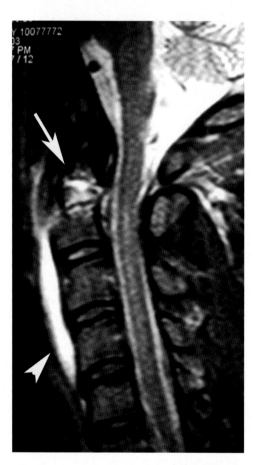

Fig. 10.9 A sagittal T2-weighted image of a type II odontoid fracture showing edema at the fracture site (*arrow*), indicating an acute or subacute fracture. Note the prevertebral edema or hematoma (*arrowhead*).

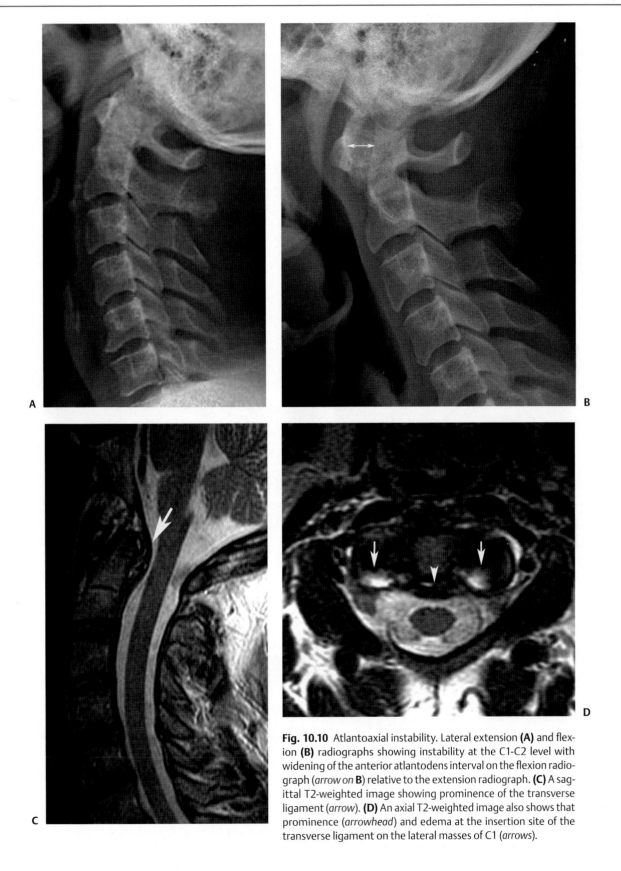

Fig. 10.10 Atlantoaxial instability. Lateral extension **(A)** and flexion **(B)** radiographs showing instability at the C1-C2 level with widening of the anterior atlantodens interval on the flexion radiograph (*arrow on* **B**) relative to the extension radiograph. **(C)** A sagittal T2-weighted image showing prominence of the transverse ligament (*arrow*). **(D)** An axial T2-weighted image also shows that prominence (*arrowhead*) and edema at the insertion site of the transverse ligament on the lateral masses of C1 (*arrows*).

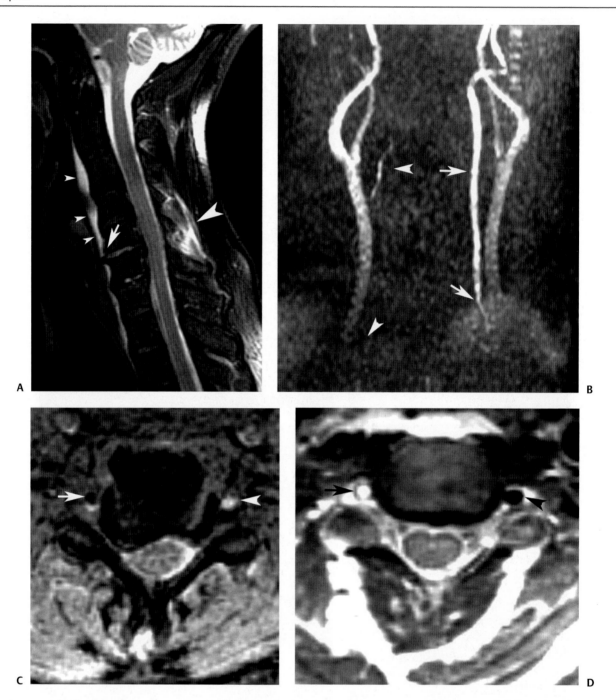

Fig. 10.11 Vertebral artery injury after unilateral facet dislocation at C5-C6 without spinal cord injury. **(A)** A sagittal T2-weighted image shows an injured disc at C5-C6 with increased signal intensity in the disc and probable avulsion of the anterior longitudinal ligament (*arrow*). Prevertebral edema (*small arrowheads*) and edema in the posterior paraspinal musculature (*large arrowhead*) are present. **(B)** An MR angiogram (anterior view) from a 2D time-of-flight acquisition shows absence of signal intensity in the expected course of the right vertebral artery (*arrowheads*). Note the normal course of the left vertebral artery (*arrows*). **(C)** An axial image from a 3D gradient-echo acquisition shows an oval area of low signal intensity in the right foramen transversarium (*arrow*) corresponding to a thrombus in the right vertebral artery. Note the normal flow-related enhancement in the left foramen transversarium (*arrowhead*). **(D)** An axial FSE image obtained at a similar level to that in **C** shows a high-signal-intensity thrombus (*arrow*) in the right foramen transversarium, indicative of a thrombosed vertebral artery. Note the normal flow void of the left vertebral artery in the left foramen transversarium (*arrowhead*). (From Torina PJ, Flanders AE, Carrino JA, et al. Incidence of vertebral artery thrombosis in cervical spine trauma: correlation with severity of spinal cord injury. AJNR Am J Neuroradiol 2005;26:2645–2651. Reprinted with permission.)

the spinal cord, or a blast effect. The osseous architecture of the spine often protects the spinal cord from direct injury from a stabbing mechanism because the lamina and spinous processes can deflect the penetrating object into the paraspinal soft tissues. MRI is useful for assessing the specific location, extent, and type of cord injury from penetrating trauma.

Characterization of Spinal Cord Injury

The severity of spinal cord injury depends on the characteristics of the traumatic event (including the amount, duration, and location of the applied force) and the underlying health of the spinal cord. Spinal cord insult may range from a concussive injury (purely functional and reversible) to complete transection (irreversible). Spinal cord concussive injury often has no MRI evidence of edema (increased T2-weighted signal), or the edema is transient and resolves with time.[11] Spinal cord contusion is a more severe injury and may be caused by transient compression or stretching of the spinal cord. Spinal cord compression may show injury characteristics similar to those of spinal contusion, but it can be associated with a specific compressive lesion such as disc herniation (**Fig. 10.12**) or osseous fragment.

An injured spinal cord segment may have an increase in cord diameter because of swelling, edema, or hemorrhage. MRI characteristics of an injured spinal cord segment are based on the degree of swelling, edema, or hemorrhage, each of which may have a different pattern of signal changes on various pulse sequences.[7] On T2-weighted images, edema and acute hemorrhage are seen as bright signal, whereas chronic hemorrhage is seen as darker signal. Gradient-echo images show dark areas that are larger than the abnormality on the T2-weighted images. This enlargement, or "blooming," is the result of the magnetic susceptibility artifact from methemoglobin.[7] The anatomic location, morphology, and length of the spinal cord lesion are important factors in determining the degree of neurologic loss. Initial neurologic deficit and potential for recovery are related directly to the extent of spinal cord damage by hemorrhage or edema.[7] Evidence of parenchymal hemorrhage on MRI may predict worse functional outcomes or neurologic recovery than is associated with a spinal cord injury with predominantly edematous changes.[7]

Highly T2-weighted images offer a myelographic effect for the assessment of spinal cord compression. These images should be carefully evaluated in the sagittal and axial planes for regions of effacement of the ventral or dorsal CSF spaces, which indicate spinal stenosis and cord compression. Trauma patients who have underlying degenerative or congenital stenosis are at increased risk for spinal cord injury because of the decrease in the cross-sectional area available for the spinal cord.

Clinical and experimental evidence has shown that surgical decompression of stenotic areas has a beneficial effect

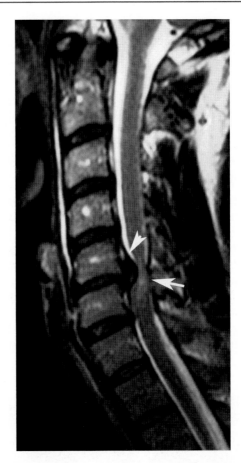

Fig. 10.12 A sagittal T2-weighted image showing a large central disc extrusion at the C5-C6 level with associated increased cord signal intensity (*arrow*) compatible with myelomalacia. Note the elevation of the posterior longitudinal ligament (*arrowhead*).

on neurologic recovery, which makes prompt identification of stenotic areas and distinguishing these areas from simple contusions important.[11] In addition, MRI assessment of cervical spine fractures in obtunded or uncooperative patients may identify disc herniations that may cause spinal cord compression and iatrogenic or progressive neurologic injury during fracture reduction.[20,38,39]

Characterization of Cervical Spine Instability

White et al.[40] defined cervical spine instability as the inability to maintain a normal association between vertebral segments while under a physiologic load. Cervical spine instability may be caused by damage to the osseous and/or ligamentous structures. Conventional radiographs and CT scans often provide the best assessment of osseous injuries. Ligamentous injury contributing to cervical spine instability may be assessed with flexion and extension lateral cervical spine radiographs and by physical examination. MRI can also be used to evaluate for ligamentous injury; the sensitivity for detection of such injuries is greatest within 24 to 72 hours postinjury.[5,17,19,41] Important ligaments to assess include the following[20]:

- Anterior longitudinal ligament
- Posterior longitudinal ligament
- Posterior column ligament complex (supraspinous ligament, interspinous ligament, and ligamentum flavum), which has been recognized as an important restraint to spinal instability (especially kyphosis)
- Transverse ligament

MRI characteristics of ligamentous injury include increased T2-weighted signal (from edema) within the ligamentous and other posterior structures (**Fig. 10.13**) or loss of ligament continuity (normally a low intensity continuous signal). Ligamentous injury is best assessed on STIR or fat-suppressed T2-weighted images.[20] A ligament strain, without complete disruption, may be seen as an elongated or redundant ligament on sagittal MR images. Despite the capability of MRI to detect ligamentous injury, not all MRI-detected ligamentous injuries result in spinal instability or warrant treatment.[20,21]

For example, minor motor-vehicle accidents that result in acute whiplash injury of the cervical spine without fracture do not need emergent MRI evaluation for ligamentous injury and may be treated symptomatically only.[21]

With the increasing availability of flexion–extension (kinematic) cervical spine MRI, a dynamic assessment of cervical spinal instability and associated stenosis can be obtained.[42] Although such information provides insight into the degree of spinal instability, it tends to be most useful for the evaluation of patients with degenerative disorders of the cervical and lumbar spine (**Fig. 10.14**).[43] Patients who have sustained severe trauma to the cervical spine are likely to be immobilized. After a period of immobilization and after frank instability of the cervical spine has been ruled out with patient-controlled flexion–extension cervical spine radiographs, a kinematic cervical spine MRI study can be considered. The information obtained from such kinematic studies can be used to guide surgical treatment and may allow the surgeon to decide among anterior, posterior, or combined surgical approaches.

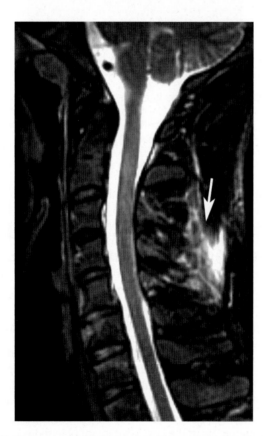

Fig. 10.13 A sagittal STIR image of a patient who sustained a hyperflexion injury to the cervical spine shows increased signal intensity within the region of the supraspinous and interspinous ligaments between C3 and C6 (*arrow*). These findings are compatible with injury to the posterior ligamentous structures.

■ Degenerative Conditions

Degenerative changes of the cervical spine are common after the fourth decade of life.[44] Cervical spine degeneration may be asymptomatic or have acute or insidious onset of symptoms; it may result in pain, stiffness, radiculopathy, myelopathy, and even permanent disability. Degenerative pathology may affect multiple areas in the cervical spine, including the following:

- Intervertebral discs
- Facet joints
- Uncovertebral joints of Luschka
- Ligaments
- Paravertebral musculature

Because these elements are biomechanically linked, a single cervical spine level may have multiple degenerative pathologies and cause adjacent-level degenerative changes. Conventional radiographs often are the initial screening studies for evaluating cervical spine degeneration and may guide the selection of more advanced imaging techniques.[45] MRI usually is considered the preferred initial advanced imaging modality for the evaluation of symptomatic cervical spine degeneration; it has a reported sensitivity and specificity of 91% for the detection of cervical degenerative changes.[45,46] Despite this high sensitivity and specificity, it is important to understand that radiographic and MRI abnormalities do not always correlate with a symptomatic degenerative lesion.[47] Boden et al.[44] reported that almost 60% of their asymptomatic patients more than 40 years old had cervical spine degenerative disc disease on MRI.

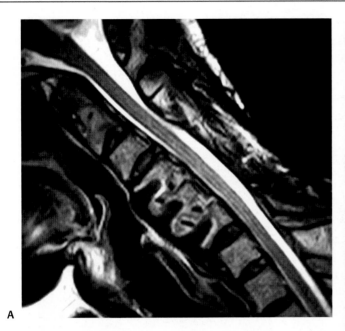

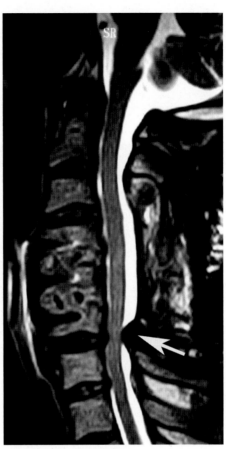

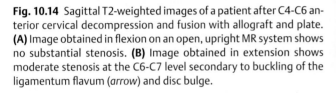

Fig. 10.14 Sagittal T2-weighted images of a patient after C4-C6 anterior cervical decompression and fusion with allograft and plate. **(A)** Image obtained in flexion on an open, upright MR system shows no substantial stenosis. **(B)** Image obtained in extension shows moderate stenosis at the C6-C7 level secondary to buckling of the ligamentum flavum (*arrow*) and disc bulge.

Although one should always correlate the patient's history and physical examination with the imaging findings (see Chapter 3), this practice is especially important when evaluating the MRI studies of a patient with a suspected cervical or lumbar spine degenerative disorder. Specifically, one should know whether a patient is presenting with neck pain, radiculopathy, myelopathy, or a more focal neurologic deficit. The laterality and level of the symptoms should also be assessed, and this information should be taken into consideration, along with the imaging findings, when making a choice among the various nonoperative and surgical treatment options.

Degenerative Disc Disease

An intervertebral disc is composed of an outer annulus fibrosus, an inner nucleus pulposus, and superior and inferior cartilaginous end plates. The structural composition of the intervertebral disc changes with age: the water content of the nucleus pulposus and annulus fibrosis decreases from approximately 90% in the first year of life to 70% to 75% in the eighth decade.[17,48,49] The remainder of the nucleus pulposus consists of proteoglycans and collagen that attract water and allow the nucleus pulposus to resist axial loading. The collagen fibers in the annulus are abundant anteriorly but deficient posterolaterally, creating a potential weak area at risk for degenerative tears and disc herniation.[49] The posterior longitudinal ligament reinforces this deficient area.[49]

With advancing age, the proteoglycan composition of the intervertebral disc changes and water is lost, diminishing the disc's ability to support load. The nucleus pulposus is replaced with more fibrous structures and blends with the adjacent annulus fibrosus into amorphous fibrocartilaginous tissue.[46] Disc desiccation leads to bulging of the annulus fibrosus and loss of disc height, causing increased stress transfer to adjacent facet and uncovertebral joints.[46] This increased stress on facet and uncovertebral joints propagates osteocartilaginous hypertrophy and osteophyte formation. In addition, the loss of intervertebral disc elasticity exposes these small vertebral joints to increased motion and instability, furthering their degeneration. Nerve root compression may occur secondary to the decreased width and height of the adjacent neural foramina caused by disc height loss, annulus bulging, and uncinate process and facet hypertrophy. On MRI, a normal intervertebral disc has intermediate signal intensity on T1-weighted images and high signal intensity on T2-weighted sequences, whereas disc desiccation shows as low signal intensity on T1-weighted and T2-weighted images (**Fig. 10.15**).[45,46]

As the disc degenerates and desiccates, degenerative changes also affect the annulus fibrosus and result in delamination of and change in the architecture of the concentric annular fibers.[17] These changes may lead to annular

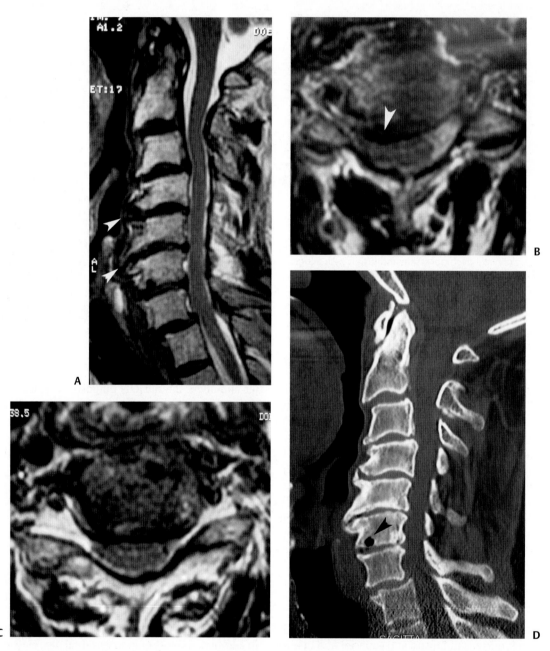

Fig. 10.15 Multilevel degenerative disc disease. **(A)** A sagittal T2-weighted image shows multilevel degenerative disc disease as evidenced by the loss of the normal high signal intensity within the discs. Note the degenerative spondylolisthesis at C2-C3, C3-C4 (subtle), and C7-T1, and the multilevel anterior osteophyte formation (*arrowheads*). There is also a loss of the normal cervical lordosis. **(B)** An axial T2-weighted image at the C3-C4 level shows a right paracentral disc bulge (*arrowhead*), resulting in moderate stenosis with asymmetric cord compression. **(C)** An axial T2-weighted image at the C5-C6 level shows moderate central stenosis. **(D)** A sagittal reconstructed CT image also shows multilevel degenerative disc disease and provides improved osseous detail that complements the information seen on the MR images. Note the gas-containing subchondral cyst at the inferior end plate of C6 (*arrowhead*) and the multilevel anterior osteophyte formation.

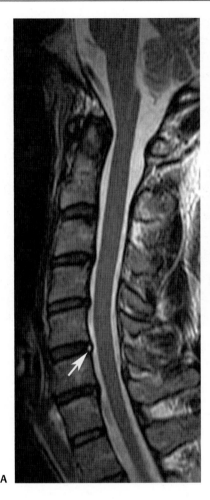

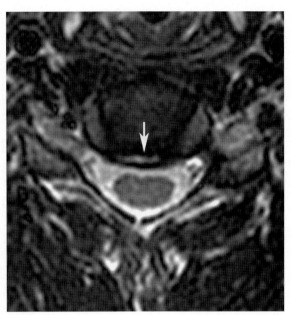

Fig. 10.16 Annular tear. Sagittal **(A)** and axial **(B)** T2-weighted images showing a high-intensity zone in the posterior annulus at C5-C6 (*arrows*). This finding is compatible with an annular tear that may be responsible for the patient's discogenic neck pain.

tears. Discogenic pain may be associated with transverse, radial, or complete tears.[46] On T2-weighted images, tears are seen as areas of high signal intensity within the annulus (**Fig. 10.16**).[45,46] A weakened annulus fibrosus may

Table 10.2   Intervertebral Disc Pathology

Disc Pathology	MRI Findings
Bulge	Symmetric extension of annulus beyond confines of adjacent end plates
Protrusion	Focal area of disc material that extends beyond vertebral margin but remains contained within the outer annular fibers
Extrusion	Herniation of nucleus pulposus beyond confines of annulus with disc attached to remainder of nucleus pulposus by a narrow pedicle
Sequestration	Portion of disc fragment entirely separated from parent disc

Source: Khanna AJ, Carbone JJ, Kebaish KM, et al. Magnetic resonance imaging of the cervical spine. J Bone Joint Surg Am 2002;84:70–80. Modified with permission.

lead to a spectrum of intervertebral disc pathology based on the extent of annulus bulging and disc herniation (**Table 10.2**). The findings of degenerative disc disease seen on MRI should also be correlated with the degenerative changes seen on cervical spine radiographs. Specifically, the degree of vertebral body end-plate sclerosis can be best evaluated on radiographs, and oblique radiographs will best show foraminal stenosis secondary to osteophyte formation.

Disc Displacement

Along with the degenerative disc disease and the normal aging process described above, elevated pressures within the nucleus pulposus and compromise of the structural integrity of the annulus fibrosis can lead to migration of disc material toward the neural elements and produce the clinical findings of radiculopathy or myelopathy. Patients with large central disc herniations tend to present with symptoms of myelopathy, whereas those with posterolateral disc herniations tend to present with radiculopathy.

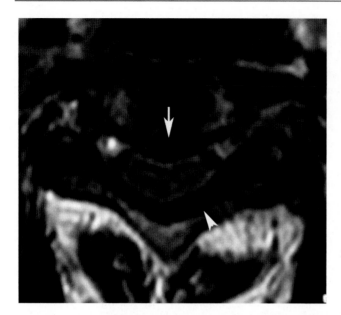

Fig. 10.17 An axial T2-weighted image at the C5-C6 level showing a central disc bulge (*arrow*) with moderate stenosis. The disc bulge and ligamentum flavum hypertrophy (*arrowhead*) act to produce effacement of the ventral and dorsal CSF spaces and deformity of the spinal cord.

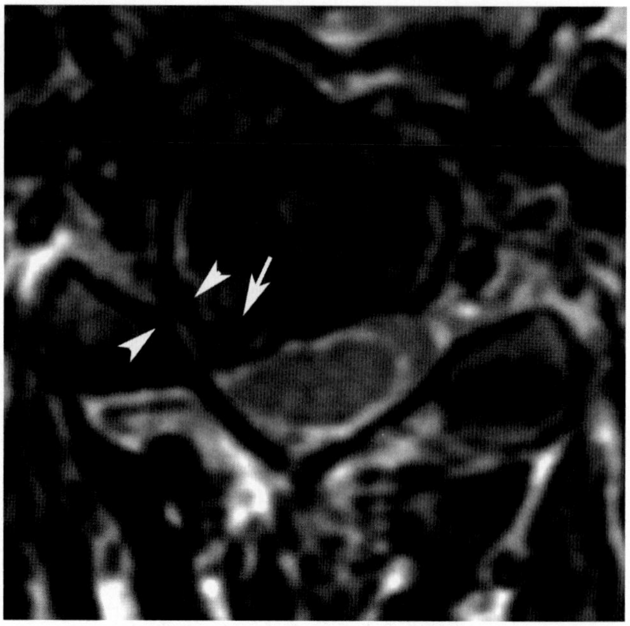

Fig. 10.18 An axial T2-weighted image at the C5-C6 level showing a right posterolateral disc protrusion with associated uncovertebral joint hypertrophy (*arrow*), which produces mild deformity of the right side of the spinal cord and severe foraminal stenosis (*between arrowheads*). Note the normal size of the neural foramen on the left side.

Disc herniations most commonly occur at the levels with greatest motion (C5-C6 and C6-C7) and may be generally classified as the following:

- Central (compression of the medial portion of the spinal cord) (**Fig. 10.17**)
- Posterolateral (compression of the lateral portion of spinal cord and nerve root) (**Fig. 10.18**)
- Lateral (compression of the nerve root only) (**Fig. 10.19**)

The nomenclature used to describe cervical disc displacements varies widely among radiologists and clinicians. Although a task force has provided formal guidelines for the description of lumbar disc pathology[50] (see Chapter 11), similar guidelines have not been widely adopted for the cervical spine. The terms *bulge, protrusion, extrusion,* and *sequestration* are commonly used to describe cervical disc pathology (**Table 10.2**). It should be noted that the anatomy of the cervical facet joints (which are located more laterally than those in the lumbar spine) essentially makes them the posterior wall of the intervertebral nerve root canals, and there is no subarticular recess in the cervical spine. Thus, disc herniation positions in the cervical spine are described as central, paracentral (left or right), foraminal, and far lateral.

With regard to the size of the disc abnormality, it may be more important to note the degree of mass effect on neural structures than the size of the abnormality itself. For example, a small protrusion in a person with developmental spinal stenosis will be more likely to produce symptoms

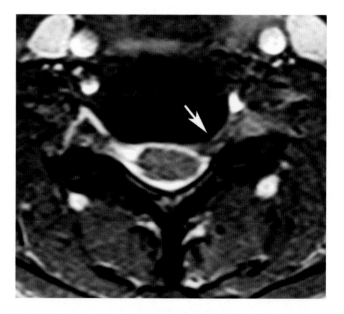

Fig. 10.19 An axial T2-weighted image at the C5-C6 level showing a lateral or foraminal disc protrusion (*arrow*) on the left side that produces severe foraminal stenosis and compresses the nerve root. Note that the signal is different than that of the bone.

than a similar protrusion in a patient with a capacious spinal canal.

In addition to an evaluation of the level, direction, and configuration of disc displacement, the MRI study should also be scrutinized for the presence or absence of areas of calcium deposition, anterior or posterior osteophyte formation, and vertebral end-plate changes.[45,46,51,52] These findings should be correlated with the findings seen on lateral and oblique cervical spine radiographs.

Additional scrutiny of the imaging findings also allows the surgeon to determine whether a cervical disc protrusion can be classified as a "soft" or "hard" disc (**Fig. 10.20**). This information may help in determining whether an anterior or posterior approach is chosen for the treatment of a patient with unilateral cervical radiculopathy. Such a determination can be made by reviewing the images for increased T2-weighted signal within the displaced disc, which would be expected in a patient with a relatively well-hydrated soft disc herniation. Conversely, a hard disc herniation shows low signal on T2-weighted images and may also show associated osteophytes on gradient-echo and other pulse sequences. This

combination of hard disc disease and associated osteophyte is often referred to as a *disc–ridge complex* and may preclude the performance of a posterior keyhole foraminotomy and discectomy for the treatment of a patient with unilateral radiculopathy.

The findings on MR images should be used to differentiate cervical disc disease and protrusions from ossification of the posterior longitudinal ligament. On most MR images showing cervical stenosis secondary to disc displacement (for example, **Figs. 10.12** and **10.15**), the pathology and stenosis is based at the level of the disc, and stenosis is seen only behind the vertebral body in cases of disc extrusion and migration (**Fig. 10.21**). Conversely, MRI in patients with ossification of the posterior longitudinal ligament shows stenosis at the level of the disc and also along the course of the posterior longitudinal ligament, which runs along the posterior aspect of the vertebral bodies (**Fig. 10.22**). In patients with suspected ossification of the posterior longitudinal ligament, CT imaging can be obtained to rule in or rule out this diagnosis, given that it provides optimal visualization of calcification and osseous detail. The importance of this

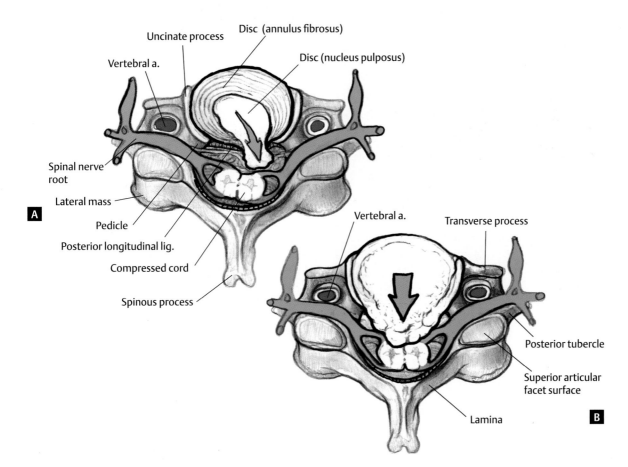

Fig. 10.20 Axial illustrations showing the difference between soft and hard disc pathology in the subaxial cervical spine. **(A)** A left posterolateral disc protrusion (*arrow*) resulting in mild deformity of the cord and compression of the exiting nerve root. **(B)** Moderate central stenosis secondary to a large central disc protrusion with an associated osteophyte complex (*arrow*); the osteophyte creates most of the stenosis.

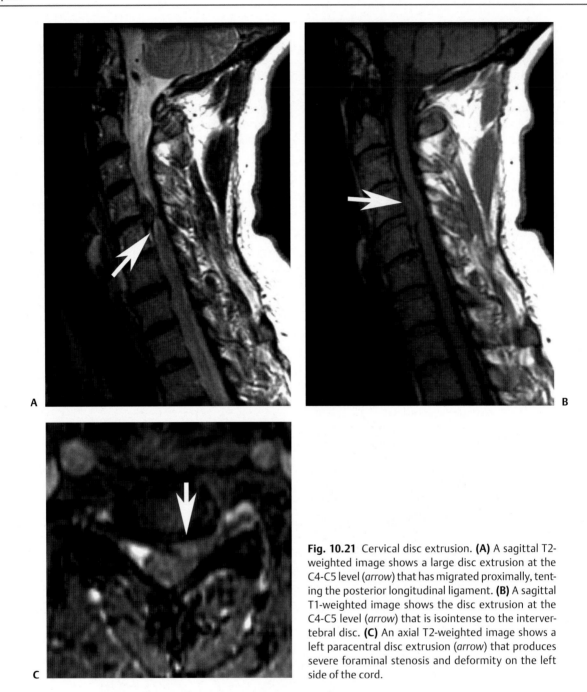

Fig. 10.21 Cervical disc extrusion. **(A)** A sagittal T2-weighted image shows a large disc extrusion at the C4-C5 level (*arrow*) that has migrated proximally, tenting the posterior longitudinal ligament. **(B)** A sagittal T1-weighted image shows the disc extrusion at the C4-C5 level (*arrow*) that is isointense to the intervertebral disc. **(C)** An axial T2-weighted image shows a left paracentral disc extrusion (*arrow*) that produces severe foraminal stenosis and deformity on the left side of the cord.

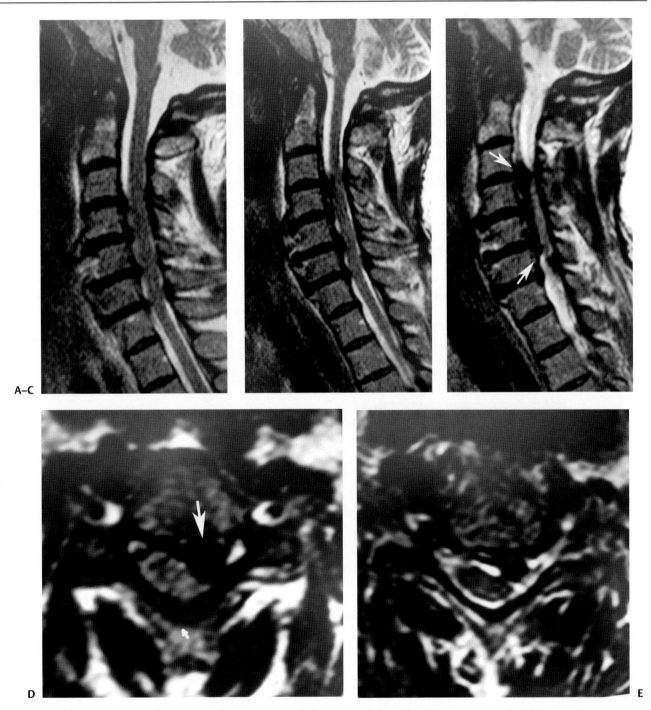

A–C

D
E

Fig. 10.22 Ossification of the posterior longitudinal ligament. **(A)** A midline sagittal T2-weighted image showing multilevel degenerative disc disease and moderate stenosis from C3-C4 to C6-C7. The stenosis appears to be centered at the level of the disc spaces on this midline image. **(B)** A parasagittal T2-weighted image obtained a few millimeters lateral to the midline suggests that the posterior longitudinal ligament is thickened and that the stenosis is present at the level of the vertebral bodies and discs from C3 to C7. **(C)** A parasagittal T2-weighted image obtained farther from the midline shows that the posterior longitudinal ligament is markedly hypertrophied and nearly fills the spinal canal (*between arrows*). **(D)** An axial T2-weighted image shows severe left paracentral stenosis secondary to what appears to be a disc protrusion (*large arrow*) but is actually a focal region of ossification of the posterior longitudinal ligament at the level of the C4 vertebral body. (The *small arrow* is a pointer from the computer workstation and should be ignored.) **(E)** An axial T2-weighted image at the level of the C4-C5 disc shows similar findings. (Continued on page 250)

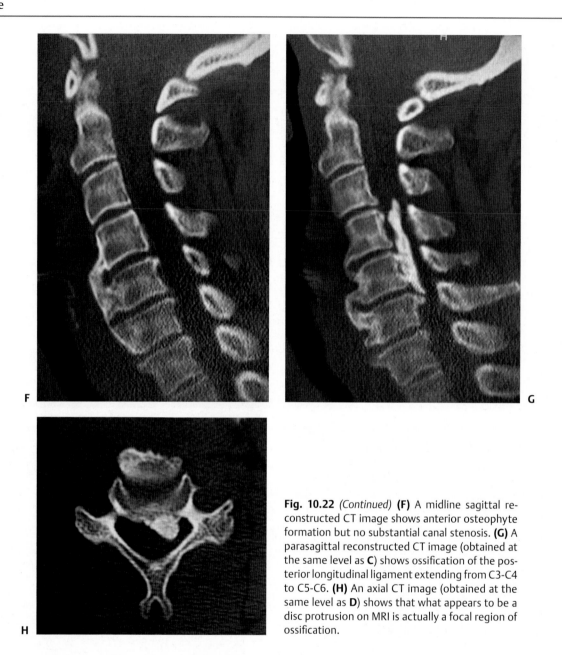

Fig. 10.22 *(Continued)* **(F)** A midline sagittal reconstructed CT image shows anterior osteophyte formation but no substantial canal stenosis. **(G)** A parasagittal reconstructed CT image (obtained at the same level as **C**) shows ossification of the posterior longitudinal ligament extending from C3-C4 to C5-C6. **(H)** An axial CT image (obtained at the same level as **D**) shows that what appears to be a disc protrusion on MRI is actually a focal region of ossification.

differentiation lies in the fact that anterior decompression for patients with ossification of the posterior longitudinal ligament tends to be difficult and is associated with higher rates of durotomy and bleeding, and therefore surgeons may prefer to proceed with posterior decompression even though the primary compression is located ventral to the spinal cord.

Spinal Stenosis

The term *spinal stenosis* describes the compression of the neural elements in the spinal canal, lateral recesses, or neu-

ral foramina (**Fig. 10.23**). Spinal stenosis can develop from congenital or acquired causes (**Table 10.3**); patients can also develop degenerative stenosis superimposed on preexisting congenital stenosis (**Fig. 10.24**).

Foraminal stenosis may be caused by a disc herniation or uncovertebral or facet joint hypertrophy. Central canal stenosis is most often caused by a combination of two or more of the following (**Fig. 10.25**):

- Disc bulge or herniation
- Uncovertebral joint osteophyte formation

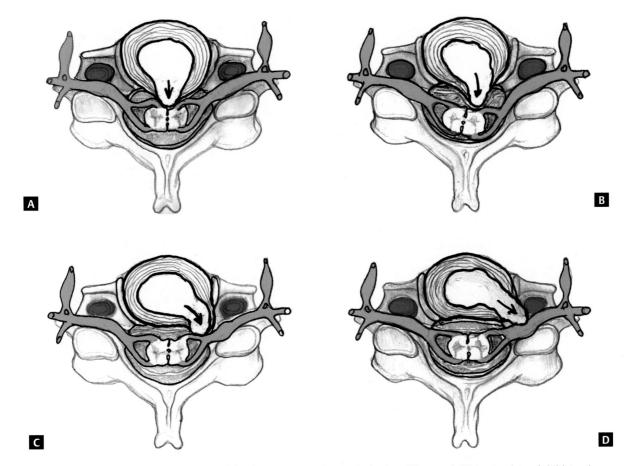

Fig. 10.23 Artist's sketches showing four types of disc herniations in the cervical spine: **(A)** central, **(B)** posterolateral, **(C)** lateral recess, and **(D)** foraminal.

Table 10.3 Acquired and Congenital Factors Associated with Spinal Stenosis

Type	Factor
Acquired	Intervertebral disc pathology
	Uncovertebral joint hypertrophy
	Facet joint hypertrophy
	Ligamentous (ligamentum flavum hypertrophy/ ossification, ossification of the posterior longitudinal ligament, diffuse idiopathic skeletal hyperostosis)
	Spondylosis
	Metabolic
	Postinflammatory
	Spondylolisthesis
	Postoperative
	Neoplastic
Congenital	Idiopathic with short pedicles
	Skeletal growth disorders
	Down syndrome
	Achondroplasia
	Mucopolysaccharidosis
	Scoliosis

- Ligamentum flavum hypertrophy
- Facet arthrosis
- Thickening, calcification, or ossification of the posterior longitudinal ligament or other structures

On MRI, central canal stenosis is characterized by compression of the thecal sac, best seen on the sagittal and axial T2-weighted images. Such images provide a "myelographic effect," in which the CSF is seen as bright signal anterior and posterior to the spinal cord on sagittal images and circumferentially around the spinal cord on axial images. Effacement, discontinuity, or displacement of this CSF space is seen in patients with focal and concentric spinal stenosis.

The degree of central canal stenosis can range from mild encroachment on the ventral subarachnoid space to severe compression and flattening of the spinal cord with myelomalacia. MRI findings may correspond to the severity and duration of the compression.[45] Early changes of spinal cord compression can be seen as cord edema (high signal areas on T2-weighted images); progressive compression may cause spinal cord necrosis and atrophy (**Fig. 10.26**), cystic degeneration, and syrinx formation (low signal on T1-weighted and high signal on T2-weighted images).[45]

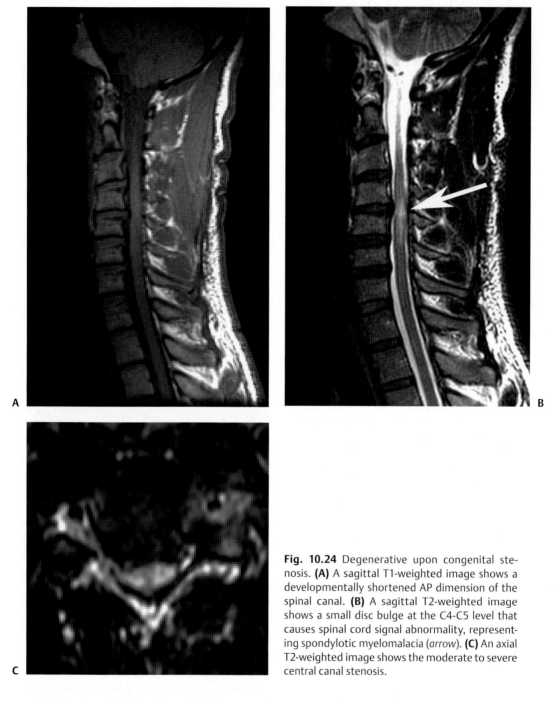

Fig. 10.24 Degenerative upon congenital stenosis. **(A)** A sagittal T1-weighted image shows a developmentally shortened AP dimension of the spinal canal. **(B)** A sagittal T2-weighted image shows a small disc bulge at the C4-C5 level that causes spinal cord signal abnormality, representing spondylotic myelomalacia (*arrow*). **(C)** An axial T2-weighted image shows the moderate to severe central canal stenosis.

Given that the great majority of cervical spine MRI studies are obtained to evaluate for the presence, location, and degree of degenerative cervical spinal stenosis, one should have a systematic approach to the evaluation of these studies. The authors' suggested approach for the evaluation of a cervical spine MRI study (see Chapter 3) includes a critical evaluation of the degree of spinal cord and nerve root compression on the sagittal, parasagittal, and axial T2-weighted images. The midline sagittal T2-weighted images provide a global view of the levels and degree of effacement

of the CSF column and spinal cord compression, whereas the parasagittal images allow for visualization of lateral recess and foraminal stenosis (**Fig. 10.27**). The information from these images should be correlated with that from the axial images, which show the same pathology in an orthogonal plane.

There are several objective measures of cervical spinal stenosis. Relative stenosis is defined as an AP canal diameter of <13 mm, and absolute stenosis is defined as an AP canal diameter of <10 mm. The Torg or Pavlov ratio is calculated

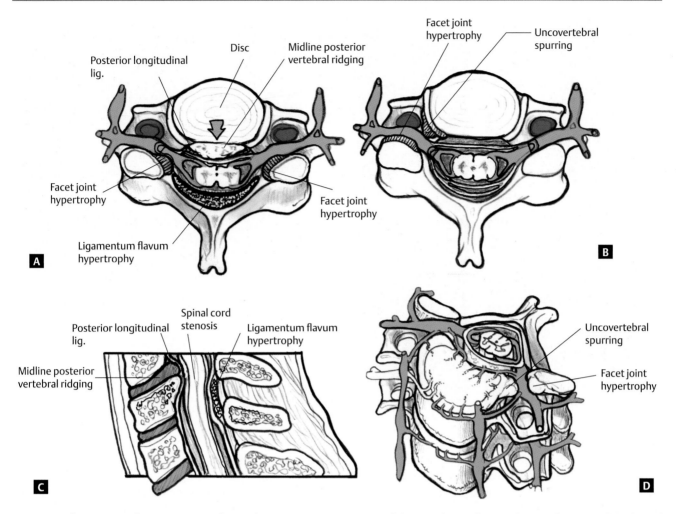

Fig. 10.25 Illustrations of various potential contributors to cervical spinal stenosis: central disc bulge, facet joint hypertrophy, and ligamentum flavum hypertrophy. **(A)** An axial view showing central stenosis. **(B)** An axial view showing foraminal stenosis. **(C)** A lateral view showing central stenosis with cord compression. **(D)** A 3D view showing foraminal stenosis.

by dividing the AP canal diameter by the AP vertebral body diameter, with a ratio <0.8 defined as stenotic.[53] This ratio is often used to evaluate for congenital stenosis in athletes. Although such definitions are well known, most clinicians and radiologists tend to grade the degree of spinal stenosis using the terms *mild*, *moderate*, and *severe*, as well as gradations such as *moderate–severe*. The authors tend to use the following terms and definitions (**Figs. 10.28** and **10.29**):

- Mild—stenosis occupying less than one third of normal canal dimension in which the ventral and dorsal CSF spaces are partially effaced by disc bulging, ligamentum flavum hypertrophy, and facet arthropathy; no mass effect on the cord
- Moderate—stenosis occupying between one and two thirds of normal canal dimension; findings similar to those of mild stenosis but with compression and minimal flattening and deformity of the spinal cord

- Severe—stenosis occupying more than two thirds of normal canal dimension, with advanced stenosis with very pronounced flattening and deformity of the spinal cord that is obvious on both sagittal and axial T2-weighted images

Occipitocervical Stenosis

Occipitocervical stenosis is not typically degenerative; it can occur secondary to congenital and developmental processes, such as Arnold Chiari malformation and cranial settling, in patients with RA. Other nontraumatic causes of occipitocervical stenosis and instability include occipital, C1, and C2 dysplasia and anomalies; Down syndrome; and tumors. Because of the complexity of the occipitocervical junction, normal relationships are defined using landmarks originally described on conventional radiography.[54,55] Many of these

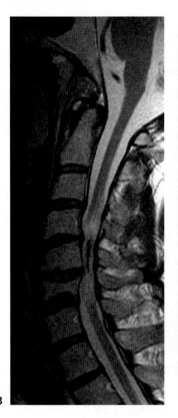
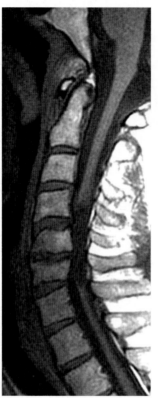
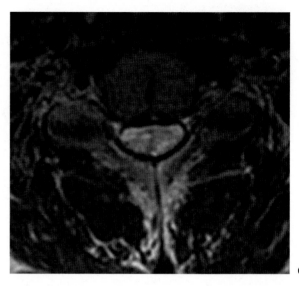

A, B

C

Fig. 10.26 Spinal cord atrophy. **(A)** A sagittal T2-weighted image showing moderate-severe stenosis at C4-C6, with resultant atrophy of the spinal cord at the level of C5 and regions of cord edema proximal and distal to the region of atrophy. **(B)** A sagittal T1-weighted image showing a segment of low signal intensity within the spinal cord from C4-C5 to C6-C7. **(C)** An axial T2-weighted image at the C4-C5 level showing atrophy of the spinal cord and indistinct margins between the spinal cord and the surrounding CSF.

relationships and lines have now been extrapolated for use with MR and CT imaging and can be used to diagnose and quantify the degree of basilar invagination and cranial settling (**Table 10.4**; **Fig. 10.30**).

Chiari Malformations

Chiari malformations result in a caudal migration of the cerebellar tonsils to and through the foramen magnum with resultant occipitocervical stenosis. Although many such malformations are minor, incidentally noted findings, advanced lesions can produce symptoms, and thus may benefit from a neurosurgical evaluation and eventual suboccipital decompression. Three types of Chiari malformations have been described[56,57]:

- Type I (**Fig. 10.31**)
  - Defined as a defect in the cerebellum with a downward displacement of the tonsils >5 mm below the plane of the foramen magnum[58,59]
  - Associated with basilar invagination in 50%, atlantooccipital assimilation in 10%, and Klippel-Feil syndrome in 5%[58,59]
- Type II
  - Results from dysgenesis of the hindbrain[60]
  - Involves herniation of the inferior cerebellar vermis, fourth ventricle, and medulla

- Associated with spina bifida aperta and myelomeningocele
- Not usually associated with atlantooccipital assimilation or basilar invagination[60]
- Type III
  - Defined as herniation of the hindbrain into a high cervical encephalocele
  - Occurs rarely[60,61]

RA

RA is a systemic disease that causes inflammation of synovial joints. The synovial joints develop pannus secondary to erosion of supporting ligamentous structures and the associated instability.[60,62,63] In the cervical spine, this condition may affect the craniocervical junction as well as the subaxial cervical spine, as described below.[60,62-65] Most commonly, atlantoaxial instability develops secondary to erosion of the ligaments at the occipitocervical junction.[62,63] As the disease progresses, erosion of the lateral masses of C1, the occipital condyles, and facets of C2 occurs, resulting in cranial settling.[60,62,63] As the odontoid process begins to occupy a relatively more rostral position, it compresses the brainstem and vertebrobasilar system. This pathologic process is postulated by some as the etiology of sudden death in those with advanced RA.[60,62,63,66] It is important to note that in contrast to other disorders, the C1 arch migrates with the skull base

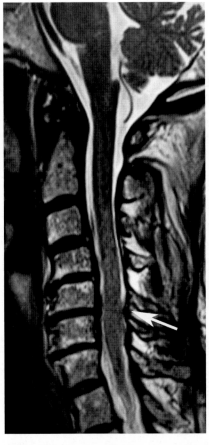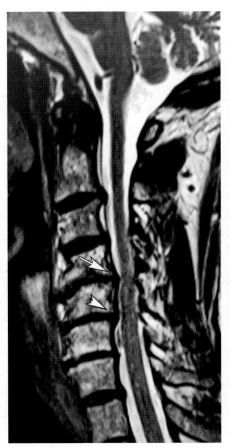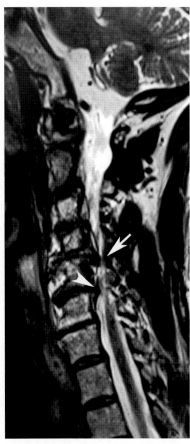

A–C

Fig. 10.27 Cervical stenosis. **(A)** A midline sagittal T2-weighted image shows multilevel degenerative disc disease with mild spondylolisthesis at C3-C4 and thickening of the posterior longitudinal ligament at multiple levels. There is focal thickening of the ligamentum flavum at the C5-C6 level (*arrow*). **(B)** A parasagittal T2-weighted image obtained several millimeters lateral to the midline shows effacement of the ventral CSF space and moderate stenosis at the C4-C5 level (*arrow*) from osteophyte formation and thickening of the posterior longitudinal ligament. Similar, but less severe, changes are seen at the C5-C6 level (*arrowhead*). **(C)** A parasagittal T2-weighted image obtained farther laterally in the plane of the neuroforamina shows severe foraminal stenosis at the C4-C5 level (*arrow*) and moderate foraminal stenosis at the C5-C6 level (*arrowhead*).

to lie in a more caudal position.[60] In some cases, it has been reported to be as inferior as the C2-C3 disc space.[60,62,63,67] Two studies reported on the use of MRI to measure the space available for the cord as a technique for predicting recovery after cervical stabilization for patients with RA and atlantoaxial instability.[62,63] A cord space, or space available for the cord, of >14 mm on MRI was associated with better clinical outcomes than was a space of <10 mm, which was associated with a poor prognosis.[62,63] Flexion–extension MRI is particularly useful for evaluating patients with RA and specifically those with instability at the occipitocervical junction and suboccipital cervical spine (**Fig. 10.32**), especially because supine extension MRI does not account for the commonly occurring subluxations in such patients that are exaggerated with movement. Similar information can be obtained by combining the information obtained from a static (conventional) MRI study and flexion–extension cervical spine radiographs (**Fig. 10.10**).

MRI can detect pannus formation in the cervical spine well before conventional radiographic signs become evident. In addition, involvement of the facet joints (inflammation, edema, and fusion) may be detected on MRI. Patients with RA may also present with a rheumatoid discitis that manifests as increased T2-weighted and decreased T1-weighted signal in the disc. The substantial differences between imaging and clinical features of RA in the spine have been documented and are well known.[68,69]

■ Infectious Conditions

The treatment of spinal infections continues to be a challenge despite advances in imaging, diagnostic testing, and antimicrobial therapy. A delay in diagnosis is common because spinal infections often have an early indolent course and early symptoms may be nonspecific (neck pain, muscle

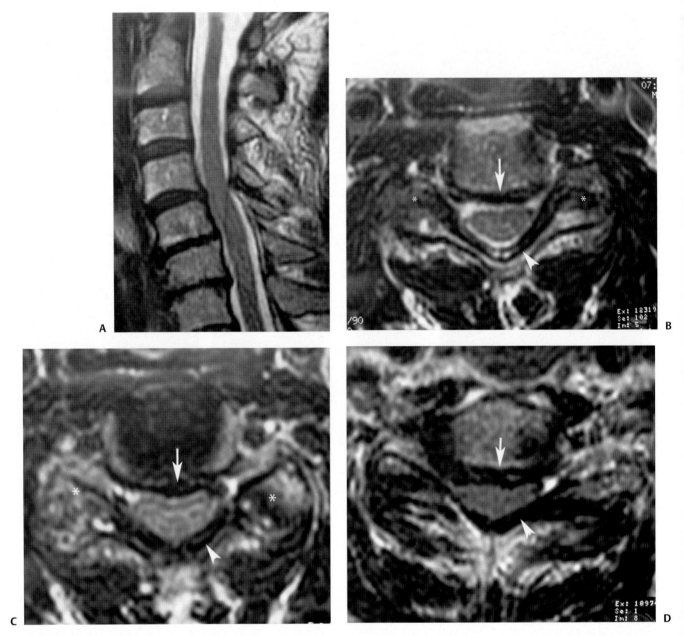

Fig. 10.28 Grading of cervical stenosis: mild to moderate-severe. **(A)** A sagittal T2-weighted image showing minimal spondylolisthesis at C4-C5 with **moderate** stenosis at this level. **(B)** An axial T2-weighted image at the C5-C6 level showing **mild** stenosis secondary to a central disc bulge (*arrow*), ligamentum flavum hypertrophy (*arrowhead*), and facet arthropathy (*asterisk*). **(C)** Axial T2-weighted image at the C4-C5 level shows **moderate** stenosis secondary to more substantial central disc bulge (*arrow*), ligamentum flavum hypertrophy (*arrowhead*), and facet arthropathy (*asterisk*). **(D)** Axial T2-weighted image (different patient) showing **moderate-severe** stenosis at the C5-C6 level as a result of even greater central disc bulge (*arrow*) and ligamentum flavum hypertrophy (*arrowhead*).

spasm), leading to a misdiagnosis of more common spinal ailments (e.g., muscle strain, degenerative disease). Spine infections may involve the vertebral body, posterior elements, intervertebral discs, epidural space, subdural space, subarachnoid space, or the spinal cord.

Cervical Vertebral Osteomyelitis and Discitis

Infections of the cervical spine account for approximately 10% of spine infections and are less common than thoracic (approximately 40%) or lumbar (approximately 50%) spine

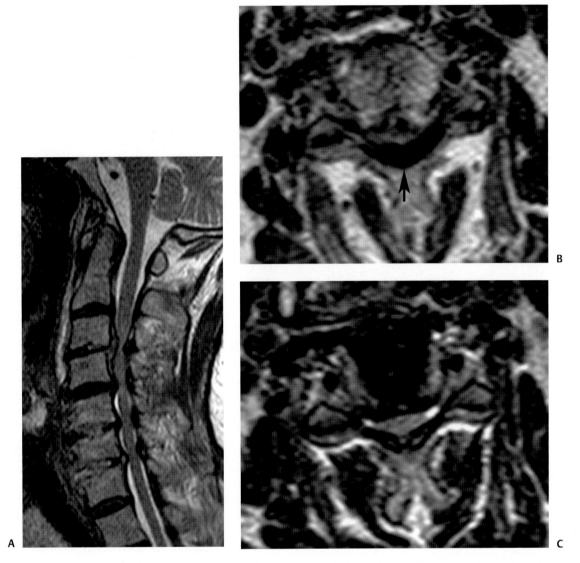

Fig. 10.29 Grading of cervical stenosis: severe. **(A)** A sagittal T2-weighted image showing **severe** stenosis at the C3-C4 level and **moderate** to **moderate-severe** stenosis at the C4-C5, C5-C6, and C6-C7 levels. **(B)** An axial image at the C3-C4 level shows **very severe** stenosis with complete obliteration of the CSF space and compression of the spinal cord to an AP diameter of 2 mm secondary to a cen-tral disc bulge and severe ligamentum flavum hypertrophy (*arrow*). **(C)** An axial T2-weighted image at the C4-C5 level showing **severe** (but less severe than in **B**) stenosis with compression and deformity of the spinal cord with minimal CSF seen in the lateral recesses bilat-erally. (Images courtesy of Mesfin A. Lemma, MD.)

infections.[70] Anatomic differences between the cervical and thoracolumbar spine (smaller canal diameter, intervertebral discs, and epidural space, and a vast venous plexus) may al-low cervical spine infections to have a more aggressive and rapid progression that requires expedited treatment.[71] In general, the clinical presentation of vertebral osteomyelitis and discitis has variable signs and symptoms, including fe-ver (approximately 50% of the time), weight loss, and neck or back pain, that do not vary with activity level. Neuro-logic symptoms may vary based on the level of spinal in-volvement, spinal cord compression, spinal instability, or deformity.[17,18,70–73] Neurologic deficits secondary to spinal

infection are more common in patients more than 50 years old and in those with comorbidities such as diabetes, RA, and immunodeficiency.[17,70]

Bacterial inoculation of the spine may occur through he-matogenous seeding, direct inoculation, or contiguous spread from local infection. *Staphylococcus aureus* is the most com-monly cultured organism causing cervical osteomyelitis and discitis.[70,74] It is found in 50% to 65% of culture-positive cases and accounts for >80% of pediatric spinal infections.[74] Gram-negative infections (*Escherichia coli, Pseudomonas, Proteus*) may occur after genitourinary infections. Immunocompro-mised patients are susceptible to infections with atypical

Table 10.4   Occipitocervical Junction: Anatomic Relationships, and Lines for Use with MRI, CT, and Conventional Radiographs

Eponym	Parameters	Pathology
Wackenheim's clivus baseline	Tangent drawn along the superior surface of the clivus	Dens should be below the line.
Clivus canal angle	Angle formed between Wackenheim's line and the posterior vertebral body line	Normal ranges are 180 degrees in extension to 150 degrees in flexion; an angle of <150 degrees is considered abnormal.
Chamberlain's line	Between the hard palate and the opisthion	Protrusion of the dens >3 mm above this line is considered abnormal.
McRae's line	Basion to the opisthion	Protrusion of the dens above this line is abnormal.
McGregor's line	From the hard palate to the most caudal point on the midline occipital curve	Odontoid process rising >4.5 mm above this line is considered abnormal.
Ranawat criterion	Distance between the center of the pedicle of C2 and the transverse axis of C1	Measurement of <15 mm in males and <13 mm in females is abnormal.
Welcher's basal angle	Tangent to the clivus as it intersects a tangent to the sphenoid bone	The normal range is 125 to 143 degrees; platybasia exists when the basal angle is >143 degrees.

bacteria, such as *Aspergillus, Candida, Nocardia asteroides,* and *Mycobacterium. Pseudomonas* infections may occur in intravenous drug abusers. Children with sickle cell disease may develop spine infections secondary to *Salmonella.*

Isolated discitis is common in the pediatric population because vascularity extends through the cartilaginous growth plate into the nucleus pulposus, allowing direct deposition of bacteria into the disc center. In adults, blood vessels reach only the annulus fibrosus, limiting bacterial deposition to the vertebral body metaphysis and end plate. In adult infections, intervertebral disc destruction may occur through bacterial proteolytic enzyme infiltration.

MRI is the imaging modality of choice for the diagnosis and evaluation of spinal infections and for monitoring the response to treatment.[71] High sensitivity (96%), specificity (93%), and accuracy (94%) have been reported for the MRI diagnosis of vertebral osteomyelitis.[51] MRI is more sensitive than conventional radiographs or CT and more specific than nuclear scintigraphy in identifying vertebral osteomyelitis.[71] Infectious spondylitis may present with findings such as low T1-weighted signal with or without high T2-weighted signal (high signal is often more evident on fat-suppressed T2-weighted or STIR images); increased T2-weighted signal within the intervertebral disc; contrast enhancement in the disc, subchondral marrow, and epidural space; erosion of end plates; epidural fluid collections; paraspinous soft-tissue abnormalities; and posterior element involvement[17,71,73,75] (**Fig. 10.33**). Unfortunately, these imaging characteristics are the same as those of many spine pathologies, including neoplastic disease. One can differentiate infection from other processes affecting the vertebral body bone marrow by noting that the epicenter of the former pathology tends to be at the intervertebral disc. Conversely, neoplastic processes tend to have their epicenters within the vertebral body, and the edema tends not to cross the intervertebral disc. In addition, the vertebral end plate may have an irregular appearance because of infectious destruction, and disc height loss or collapse may occur with progressive infection. On gadolinium-enhanced images, disc enhancement is an essential factor for the diagnosis of discitis, and enhancement of the vertebral subchondral bone may indicate a well-established and chronic infection.[17,71,73]

In comparison with other bacterial infections, *Mycobacterium tuberculosis* infection of the spine has some distinct differences:

- Intervertebral discs are damaged less or completely spared and may not show signal enhancement on T2-weighted images.[71]
- Tuberculous spondylodiscitis is a slow-growing process that often results in marked collapse of the vertebral bodies.
- Subligamentous spread of infection is often observed.
- Telescoping of one vertebral body disc into an adjacent level may be seen.

Gadolinium-enhanced MRI also is essential for monitoring the efficacy of treatment of vertebral infection.[76] With appropriate treatment of the infection, a regression of the T2-weighted signal hyperintensity is observed.[73] Scar formation within the intervertebral disc is seen as a region of low signal intensity. A region of mottled signal intensity may also develop within the area of previous infection with associated contrast enhancement. Over time, osteophytic bridging may occur, followed by segmental fusion.[73] It should be noted, however, that a lack of improvement on MRI and even deterioration of MRI features in the setting of clinical improvement do not necessarily indicate failure of treatment.[77,78]

In the postoperative patient, evaluation for cervical spine infection may be complicated by the normal enhancement of the uninfected disc. MRI findings of infection in a postoperative patient include contrast enhancement of the subchon-

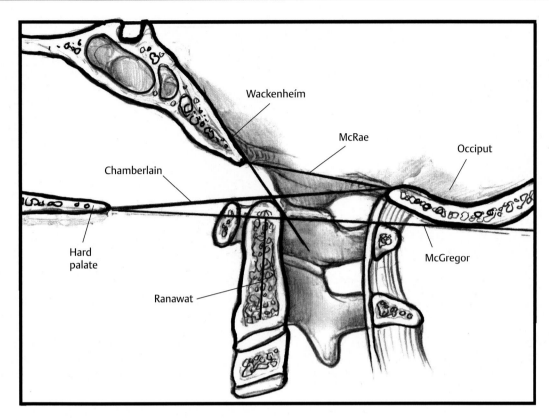

Fig. 10.30 Lines and measurements for evaluation of basilar invagination.

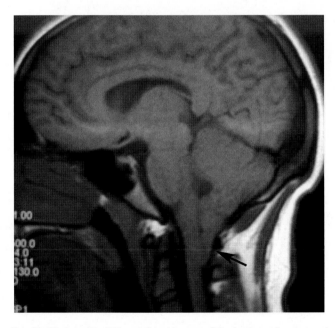

Fig. 10.31 A sagittal T1-weighted image of the brain and upper cervical spine shows inferior migration of the cerebellar tonsils (*arrow*) below the level of the foramen magnum compatible with a type 1 Arnold Chiari malformation.

dral bone and marrow adjacent to the infected disc.[71] Graft material and native vertebra should not enhance within the first few days after spinal surgery. After several months, graft enhancement occurs, but it is often less intense and less uniform than that caused by infection. Bone graft usually has high signal intensity on T2-weighted images during the first postoperative year, and the signal gradually decreases with time as the bone graft is vascularized and fused.[71] An enhancing mass adjacent to the graft or a graft dislodgment is a sign of potential infection.[71]

Epidural Abscess

A spinal epidural abscess is a collection of purulent material outside the dura mater. An epidural abscess is usually associated with vertebral osteomyelitis, and direct extension from an adjacent infected vertebral body is the most common source for an epidural abscess.[71] Epidural abscesses are less common in the cervical spine than in the thoracic or lumbar spine and may be located anterior or posterior to the spinal cord.[71] Multiple spinal segments are usually involved (most commonly, C4 to C7).[71]

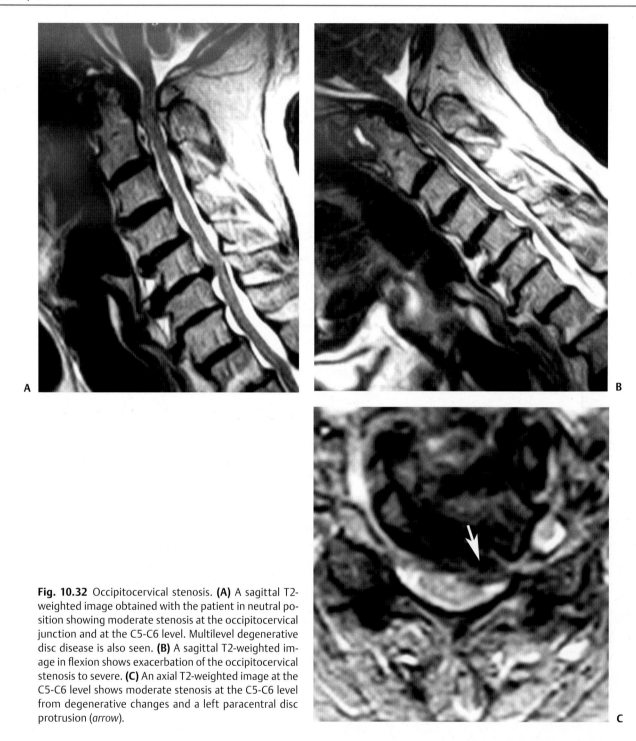

Fig. 10.32 Occipitocervical stenosis. **(A)** A sagittal T2-weighted image obtained with the patient in neutral position showing moderate stenosis at the occipitocervical junction and at the C5-C6 level. Multilevel degenerative disc disease is also seen. **(B)** A sagittal T2-weighted image in flexion shows exacerbation of the occipitocervical stenosis to severe. **(C)** An axial T2-weighted image at the C5-C6 level shows moderate stenosis at the C5-C6 level from degenerative changes and a left paracentral disc protrusion (*arrow*).

Along with the increase in the number of patients with risk factors for spinal infections, the number of patients with cervical epidural abscess is also increasing. The risk factors associated with vertebral osteomyelitis include the following:

- Age >50 years
- Alcoholism
- Diabetes
- Immunodeficiency (e.g., from medications, HIV)
- Intravenous drug abuse
- Male gender
- Malignancy
- Malnutrition
- Obesity
- Previous spinal procedure

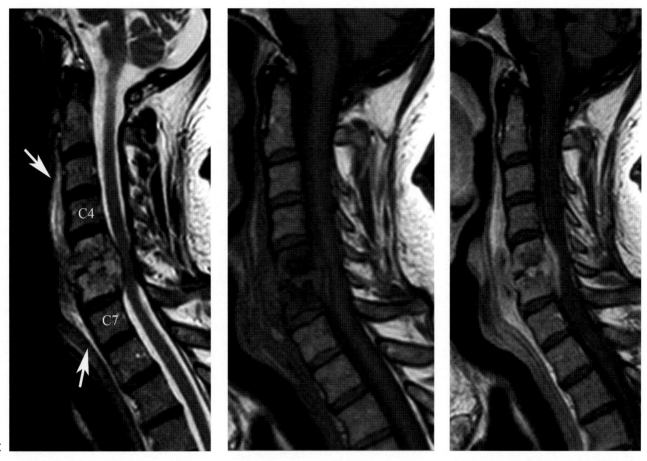

Fig. 10.33 Cervical spine discitis and osteomyelitis. **(A)** A sagittal T2-weighted image showing obliteration of the C5-C6 disc space with associated edema in the C5-C6 vertebral bodies and an associated epidural component, which produces moderate spinal stenosis in a patient with infectious symptoms and findings. Note the preverte- bral edema and soft-tissue fullness (*between arrows*). Pregadolinium **(B)** and postgadolinium **(C)** T1-weighted images show enhancement at the disc space, in the vertebral body's epidural component, and in the prevertebral space.

- Recent systemic illness
- Tobacco use
- Trauma

These factors also increase the risk for development of an epi- dural abscess. The clinical presentation for an epidural abscess may be similar to that of vertebral osteomyelitis. Mass effect from the abscess compressing the spinal cord or nerve roots may present as radiculopathy, myelopathy, or paralysis.

As it is for vertebral osteomyelitis, MRI is the diag- nostic study of choice for the evaluation of an epidural abscess.[17,71,73] Gadolinium-enhanced, fat-suppressed, T1- weighted images provide anatomic detail of the location and extension of the abscess and any associated vertebral infections.[71] T2-weighted and fat-suppressed T2-weighted images also show the boundaries of the epidural abscess and allow for the assessment of the degree of spinal cord com-

pression. Gadolinium enhancement patterns may vary from a thin, peripheral pattern (which may represent a collection of liquefied pus with a surrounding rim) to a homogeneous pattern seen with a phlegmon. The spinal cord may be evalu- ated for the level and amount of compression, as described above.

Intradural Infections

Intradural infections may be categorized as subdural ab- scess, leptomeningitis, or myelitis. A subdural abscess, which is clinically indistinguishable from an epidural ab- scess, is caused by direct extension from an epidural ab- scess, hematogenous spread, or iatrogenic contamination. Gadolinium-enhanced MRI shows the enhancing intradural– extramedullary abscess next to a compressed spinal cord. T2- weighted images show an associated signal intensity change within the spinal cord secondary to compression, ischemia, or myelitis.

Spinal leptomeningeal infections can be caused by many organisms, including *Neisseria meningitidis*, *Coccidioides immitis*, *Cryptococcus* sp., *Treponema pallidum*, and viral organisms. Gadolinium-enhanced MRI shows abnormal meningeal enhancement along the surface of the cord or nerve roots.[79] Meningeal enhancement can be seen incidentally over the brain, but meningeal enhancement of the spinal cord is abnormal.

Spinal cord infections and abscesses are uncommon but are associated with a high mortality rate.[71,73] Hematogenous seeding of bacteria is the most common etiology. Early cord infection shows increased T2-weighted signal and poorly defined enhancement with gadolinium.[71,73] Progressive infection may cause spinal cord cavitation, depicted as areas of low signal intensity on T1-weighted images and high signal intensity on T2-weighted images. In addition, the spinal cord may become edematous and enlarged from the infection, with MRI characteristics as described above.

■ Other Pathologic Conditions

Tumors

Spine tumors are categorized by their anatomic location (see Chapter 12) as follows[72]:

- Extradural
- Intradural–extramedullary
- Intramedullary

A reasonable differential diagnosis may be established by incorporating a clinical history, physical examination, a basic understanding of possible tumor location, and the MRI examination findings.[72] A definitive diagnosis often requires a biopsy of the lesion.

MRI is an effective technique for imaging spine tumors because it:

- Provides unparalleled soft-tissue detail
- Evaluates the neural elements
- Reveals important tissue characteristics of the tumor (vascularity, density, vascular perfusion, extent of marrow involvement)
- Assesses the extent of spinal cord compression

The entire spine needs to be evaluated because of possible skip lesions from intrathecal seeding, multiple primary sites, or a syrinx. The spinal cord can be screened with sagittal T1-weighted SE images and sagittal T2-weighted FSE images to obtain a myelogram-like examination of the spinal cord. Axial images may be helpful for specific areas of interest. Contrast enhancement is beneficial for increasing the detec-

tion of most intramedullary and intradural-extramedullary tumors.[72] However, gadolinium enhancement may obscure the contrast between metastatic lesions and normal bone marrow if fat suppression is not applied.[80] Gradient-echo images usually are not beneficial for imaging spinal cord tumors because of the limited ability to distinguish between soft tissue or tumor and CSF. For osseous tumors, gradient-echo imaging may reveal areas of calcification or hemorrhage within the tumor (see Chapter 12 for a more detailed discussion).[80]

Intrinsic Inflammatory Myelopathies

The most common cause of myelopathy is extrinsic compression, as noted above. Although orthopaedic surgeons typically do not treat intrinsic inflammatory myelopathies, they should realize that they exist and can be differentiated from myelopathy secondary to extrinsic compression. A basic understanding of these processes is important, specifically so that surgery is not considered for the treatment of a patient who presents with an intrinsic inflammatory myelopathy in the presence of incidentally noted or minimal stenosis. Briefly described below are the most common inflammatory myelopathies affecting the cervical spinal cord and their MRI findings.[72]

Multiple Sclerosis

Approximately 60% to 75% of multiple sclerosis plaques outside of the brain occur in the cervical spinal cord, and 90% of patients with cord plaques also have brain plaques.[81,82] Most plaques span two or fewer vertebral levels, occupy less than half the spinal cord diameter, and are located peripherally in the spinal cord.[82] MRI findings may include increased signal on T2-weighted sequences, decreased signal on T1-weighted images, patchy cord enhancement with gadolinium administration, and cord swelling or atrophy with larger plaques (**Fig. 10.34**).[83]

Acute Transverse Myelopathy

Acute transverse myelitis is a monophasic, acute inflammatory condition of the entire spinal cord that produces motor, sensory, and sphincter impairment. There are multiple causes, including inflammatory processes, viral infections, vascular disorders, collagen vascular disease, postinfectious states, and idiopathic processes.[81] MRI findings vary, with T2-weighted pulse sequences showing areas of hyperintensity of various length and width, often involving more than three or four spinal segments.[84] Enlargement of the spinal cord and gadolinium enhancement also vary.[85]

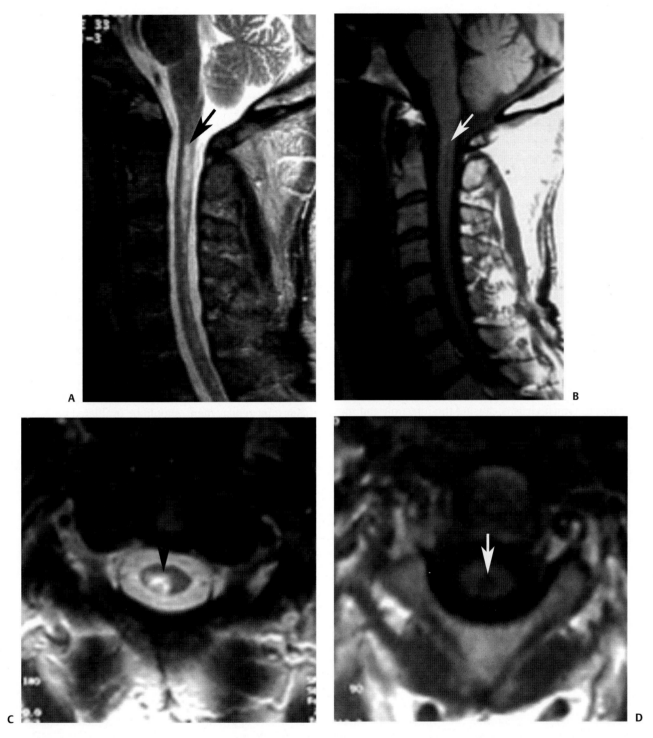

Fig. 10.34 Multiple sclerosis. Sagittal T2-weighted **(A)**, sagittal T1-weighted **(B)**, axial T2-weighted **(C)**, and axial T1-weighted **(D)** images showing a focal region of increased **(A, C)** and decreased **(B, D)** signal within the spinal cord (*arrow on each*). In the appropriate clinical setting, these findings are compatible with multiple sclerosis; the diagnosis can be confirmed with lumbar puncture and CSF analysis.

Subacute Necrotizing Myelopathy

Subacute necrotizing myelopathy is a rare, progressive myelopathy that occurs most often in elderly persons and often is attributed to spinal dural arteriovenous fistula, causing venous congestion, ischemia, and infarction of the spinal cord. Symptoms range from spastic to flaccid paraparesis, sensory abnormalities, and bowel and bladder dysfunction. MRI typically reveals a long segment of fusiform cord swelling and edema with peripheral contrast enhancement.[81]

AIDS

Spinal cord disease in patients with AIDS is common and includes HIV myelitis and vacuolar myelopathy. HIV myelitis may be caused by direct HIV infection, lymphoma, opportunistic infections, or metabolic and vascular disorders. Vacuolar myelopathy, a spongy degeneration primarily involving the posterior and lateral spinal columns causing progressive ataxia and paraparesis,[81] is the most common spinal cord disease associated with AIDS.[86] T2-weighted MRI images reveal cord atrophy and symmetric hyperintense focal lesions in the dorsal and lateral columns.[87] There is no cord swelling or gadolinium enhancement.

Viral Diseases

Viral infections of the spinal cord may be caused by multiple viruses affecting immunocompetent and immunocompromised patients. MRI characteristics of viral infection vary according to which virus is causing the infection and may include hyperintense areas on T2-weighted images, nerve root thickening, clumping and enhancement, and diffuse atrophy.[81] Gadolinium enhancement varies by spinal cord area and characteristic, depending on which virus is the underlying cause of the infection.

Bacterial, Parasitic, and Granulomatous Diseases

Clinical symptoms of myelitis, meningitis, and radiculitis can result from spinal cord invasion by bacterial, parasitic, or granulomatous infection. MRI findings vary and may include cord swelling, cord edema, rim-enhancing lesions, and nerve enhancement.[81]

Metabolic or Toxic Diseases

Subacute combined degeneration is a complication of vitamin B_{12} deficiency or nitrous oxide poisoning. The dorsal and lateral spinal columns show demyelination, axonal loss, and gliosis. MRI may show increased signal in the dorsal and lateral columns on T2-weighted images.[81] Radiation myelopathy is a progressive myelopathy most often seen in patients treated with radiation therapy for head and neck cancer. MRI may reveal cord swelling, edema, and contrast enhancement corresponding to cord necrosis, demyelination, and gliosis.[88]

Arthritides

Common arthritic conditions that affect the cervical spine and characteristic MRI findings are described below. Imaging evaluation of these conditions often begins with conventional radiographs to assess the pattern and extent of osseous involvement. MRI is the preferred modality for the assessment of the spinal cord and neural elements.

RA

RA is the most common inflammatory arthropathy, and the cervical spine is the most common area of spinal involvement.[89] The destructive process is through an inflammatory synovitis, leading to bone, cartilage, ligament, and periarticular destruction. Clinical symptoms include pain, deformity, loss of mobility, paresthesias, myelopathy, radiculopathy, paralysis, and sudden death. MRI is useful for the evaluation of the craniocervical junction and for the assessment of atlantoaxial and subaxial subluxation, basilar invagination, and spinal cord compression (**Fig. 10.35**).[89] In addition, MRI depicts the extent of periodontoid pannus formation, associated dens fractures, nodular fibrosis, and perivertebral erosions.[89] Patients with RA who are undergoing elective surgery for another musculoskeletal condition, such as major joint replacement, should be evaluated with cervical spine radiographs with flexion and extension views. If evidence of instability is noted on conventional radiographs, MRI should be considered to evaluate further, especially for atlantoaxial instability.

Juvenile RA

Juvenile RA is the most common connective tissue disorder in children and may present as one of three types: oligoarthritis (60%), polyarthritis (30%), or systemic disease (10%).[89] As it is for the adult form, MRI is excellent for identifying synovial hypertrophy, cartilage and bone destruction, and joint effusion in the juvenile form.[89]

Ankylosing Spondylitis

Ankylosing spondylitis, a seronegative spondyloarthropathy, is a chronic inflammatory arthropathy of unknown origin that affects approximately 1% of the general population[89] and predominantly involves the axial skeleton. Males are affected more often than are females, and symptoms appear in late adolescence and early adulthood. The disease begins in the thoracolumbar and lumbosacral junctions and ascends to involve the thoracic and cervical spine.[89] MRI is useful for the evaluation of early development of ankylosing spondylitis, acute fractures, pseudarthrosis, advanced degenerative changes, vertebral body subluxations, epidural hematoma, cord compression, and deformity.[89] MRI

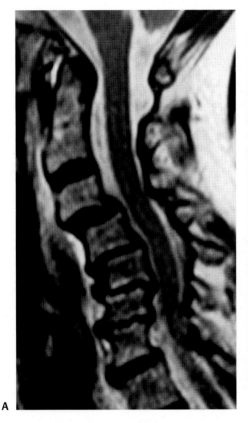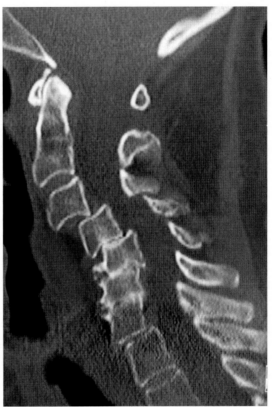

A

B

Fig. 10.35 Subaxial subluxation in RA. Sagittal T2-weighted MR image **(A)** and sagittal reconstructed CT image **(B)** show multilevel subaxial subluxation and degenerative disc disease. Specifically, there is spondylolisthesis at C3-C4 and C4-C5 and retrolisthesis at C5-C6. Note the improved osseous detail provided by the CT image compared with the MR image.

findings often provide guidance for medical and surgical treatment.

A common clinical scenario is one in which a patient with known or previously unknown ankylosing spondylitis presents with a complaint of neck pain after minor trauma. Conventional radiographs may show ankylosis of the cervical (or lumbar) spine but no evidence of fracture or displacement. It is important to note that such patients may have an unrecognized nondisplaced fracture. MRI can be obtained to rule out the presence of a nondisplaced fracture through the ankylosed spine. Such fractures are best seen on fat-suppressed T2-weighted images (**Fig. 10.7**).

Psoriatic Arthritis

Psoriatic arthritis may present before skin lesions. Axial skeleton radiographic findings are similar to those seen with RA.[89] MRI may reveal disc space narrowing and erosions of the apophyseal joints, vertebral end plates, and spinous process. On MRI, the atlantoaxial damage in patients with psoriatic arthritis is indistinguishable from that of patients with RA.[89]

Amyloidosis

Amyloidosis is characterized by extracellular deposition of insoluble fibrillar proteins throughout the body.[89] In addition, amyloidosis displays primary, secondary, familial, and dialysis-associated patterns. The dialysis-associated form, β_2-microglobulin, has a particular affinity for the musculoskeletal system and mimics inflammatory arthritis in its destructive nature.[89] Although the classic triad of β_2-microglobulin deposition includes shoulder pain, carpal tunnel syndrome, and scapulohumeral arthritis, it is also associated with destructive spondyloarthropathy of the cervical spine.[90] Amyloid deposits are found in the intervertebral discs, ligaments, and synovial tissue; the deposits have affinity for the atlantoaxial region.[89,90] Amyloid arthritis findings may mimic those of degenerative change, infectious destruction, inflammatory arthritides, or tumor. MRI is useful for distinguishing amyloid deposition destruction from others in the differential diagnosis. Amyloid deposits exhibit low signal intensity on MRI sequences and have variable enhancement patterns on contrast-supplemented sequences.[89]

Gout

Gout, which is caused by an imbalance in uric acid metabolism, is characterized by polyarticular inflammation, soft-tissue tophi, gouty nephritis, and renal stones. The classic presentation is monoarticular inflammation involving the first MTP joint. Gouty involvement of the spine, especially cervical and lumbar regions, is rare and is seen in patients with long-standing peripheral articular manifestations.[89] MRI characteristics of gouty tophi include intermediate signal intensity on T1-weighted images, variable signal intensity on T2-weighted sequences, and variable contrast enhancement patterns.[91]

Calcium Pyrophosphate Dihydrate Deposition Disease

This common crystal-induced arthritis affects peripheral joints and occasionally the spine. Spinal involvement may include calcium deposition in the intervertebral discs or ligaments. Areas affected with calcium pyrophosphate dihydrate deposition appear as isointense or hypointense signal on T1-weighted images relative to brain tissue, mixed signal intensity on T2-weighted images, and marked peripheral enhancement with gadolinium.[89] Sometimes, calcification may surround the dens, producing a characteristic "crowned dens" sign.

References

1. Lowery DW, Wald MM, Browne BJ, Tigges S, Hoffman JR, Mower WR; NEXUS Group. Epidemiology of cervical spine injury victims. Ann Emerg Med 2001;38:12–16

2. Rizzolo SJ, Vaccaro AR, Cotler JM. Cervical spine trauma. Spine (Phila Pa 1976) 1994;19:2288–2298

3. Carrino JA, Manton GL, Morrison WB, Vaccaro AR, Schweitzer ME, Flanders AE. Posterior longitudinal ligament status in cervical spine bilateral facet dislocations. Skeletal Radiol 2006;35:510–514

4. Ackland HM, Cooper DJ, Malham GM, Stuckey SL. Magnetic resonance imaging for clearing the cervical spine in unconscious intensive care trauma patients. J Trauma 2006;60:668–673

5. Stassen NA, Williams VA, Gestring ML, Cheng JD, Bankey PE. Magnetic resonance imaging in combination with helical computed tomography provides a safe and efficient method of cervical spine clearance in the obtunded trauma patient. J Trauma 2006;60: 171–177

6. Davis SJ, Teresi LM, Bradley WG Jr, Ziemba MA, Bloze AE. Cervical spine hyperextension injuries: MR findings. Radiology 1991;180:245–251

7. Flanders AE, Spettell CM, Tartaglino LM, Friedman DP, Herbison GJ. Forecasting motor recovery after cervical spinal cord injury: value of MR imaging. Radiology 1996;201:649–655

8. Silberstein M, Tress BM, Hennessy O. Delayed neurologic deterioration in the patient with spinal trauma: role of MR imaging. AJNR Am J Neuroradiol 1992;13:1373–1381

9. Smith AS, Hurst GC, Duerk JL, Diaz PJ. MR of ballistic materials: imaging artifacts and potential hazards. AJNR Am J Neuroradiol 1991;12:567–572

10. Teitelbaum GP, Yee CA, Van Horn DD, Kim HS, Colletti PM. Metallic ballistic fragments: MR imaging safety and artifacts. Radiology 1990;175:855–859

11. Takhtani D, Melhem ER. MR imaging in cervical spine trauma. Magn Reson Imaging Clin N Am 2000;8:615–634

12. Allen BL Jr, Ferguson RL, Lehmann TR, O'Brien RP. A mechanistic classification of closed, indirect fractures and dislocations of the lower cervical spine. Spine (Phila Pa 1976) 1982;7:1–27

13. Vaccaro AR, Hulbert RJ, Patel AA, et al; Spine Trauma Study Group. The subaxial cervical spine injury classification system: a novel approach to recognize the importance of morphology, neurology, and integrity of the disco-ligamentous complex. Spine (Phila Pa 1976) 2007;32:2365–2374

14. Vaccaro AR, Madigan L, Schweitzer ME, Flanders AE, Hilibrand AS, Albert TJ. Magnetic resonance imaging analysis of soft tissue disruption after flexion-distraction injuries of the subaxial cervical spine. Spine (Phila Pa 1976) 2001;26:1866–1872

15. Hart RA. Cervical facet dislocation: when is magnetic resonance imaging indicated? Spine (Phila Pa 1976) 2002;27:116–117

16. Lee JY, Nassr A, Eck JC, Vaccaro AR. Controversies in the treatment of cervical spine dislocations. Spine J 2009;9:418–423

17. Boden SD, Lee RR, Herzog RJ. Magnetic resonance imaging of the spine. In: Frymoyer JW, ed. The Adult Spine: Principles and Practice. 2nd ed. Philadelphia: Lippincott-Raven; 1997:563–629

18. Kaiser JA, Holland BA. Imaging of the cervical spine. Spine (Phila Pa 1976) 1998;23:2701–2712

19. Mirvis SE. Use of MRI in acute spinal trauma. In: Uhlenbrock D, ed. MR Imaging of the Spine and Spinal Cord. New York: Thieme; 2004:437–465

20. Kwon BK, Vaccaro AR, Grauer JN, Fisher CG, Dvorak MF. Subaxial cervical spine trauma. J Am Acad Orthop Surg 2006;14:78–89

21. Ronnen HR, de Korte PJ, Brink PRG, van der Bijl HJ, Tonino AJ, Franke CL. Acute whiplash injury: is there a role for MR imaging?—a prospective study of 100 patients. Radiology 1996;201:93–96

22. Kwon BK, Hilibrand AS. Management of cervical fractures in patients with diffuse idiopathic skeletal hyperostosis. Curr Opin Orthop 2003;14:187–192

23. White ML. Cervical spine: MR imaging techniques and anatomy. Magn Reson Imaging Clin N Am 2000;8:453–469

24. Quencer RM. The abnormal annulus fibrosus: can we infer the acuteness of an annular injury? AJNR Am J Neuroradiol 2002;23:1069

25. Stadnik TW, Lee RR, Coen HL, Neirynck EC, Buisseret TS, Osteaux MJC. Annular tears and disc herniation: prevalence and contrast enhancement on MR images in the absence of low back pain or sciatica. Radiology 1998;206:49–55

26. Goldberg W, Mueller C, Panacek E, Tigges S, Hoffman JR, Mower WR; NEXUS Group. Distribution and patterns of blunt traumatic cervical spine injury. Ann Emerg Med 2001;38:17–21

27. Adams VI. Neck injuries: I. Occipitoatlantal dislocation—a pathologic study of twelve traffic fatalities. J Forensic Sci 1992;37: 556–564

28. Adams VI. Neck injuries: III. Ligamentous injuries of the craniocervical articulation without occipito-atlantal or atlanto-axial facet

dislocation. A pathologic study of 21 traffic fatalities. J Forensic Sci 1993;38:1097–1104

29. Ahuja A, Glasauer FE, Alker GJ Jr, Klein DM. Radiology in survivors of traumatic atlanto-occipital dislocation. Surg Neurol 1994;41: 112–118

30. Alker GJ Jr, Oh YS, Leslie EV. High cervical spine and craniocervical junction injuries in fatal traffic accidents: a radiological study. Orthop Clin North Am 1978;9:1003–1010

31. Goldberg AL, Baron B, Daffner RH. Atlantooccipital dislocation: MR demonstration of cord damage. J Comput Assist Tomogr 1991;15:174–175

32. Bono CM, Vaccaro AR, Fehlings M, et al; Spine Trauma Study Group. Measurement techniques for upper cervical spine injuries: consensus statement of the Spine Trauma Study Group. Spine (Phila Pa 1976) 2007;32:593–600

33. Lee C, Woodring JH. Unstable Jefferson variant atlas fractures: an unrecognized cervical injury. AJNR Am J Neuroradiol 1991;12: 1105–1110

34. Spence KF Jr, Decker S, Sell KW. Bursting atlantal fracture associated with rupture of the transverse ligament. J Bone Joint Surg Am 1970;52:543–549

35. Hadley MN. Management of vertebral artery injuries after non-penetrating cervical trauma. Neurosurgery 2002;50(3, Suppl): S173–S178

36. Kathol MH. Cervical spine trauma. What is new? Radiol Clin North Am 1997;35:507–532

37. Bowen BC, Pattany PM. Contrast-enhanced MR angiography of spinal vessels. Magn Reson Imaging Clin N Am 2000;8:597–614

38. Robertson PA, Ryan MD. Neurological deterioration after reduction of cervical subluxation. Mechanical compression by disc tissue. J Bone Joint Surg Br 1992;74:224–227

39. Eismont FJ, Arena MJ, Green BA. Extrusion of an intervertebral disc associated with traumatic subluxation or dislocation of cervical facets. Case report. J Bone Joint Surg Am 1991;73:1555–1560

40. White AA, Southwick WO, Panjabi MM. Clinical instability in the lower cervical spine. A review of past and current concepts. Spine (Phila Pa 1976) 1976;1:15–27

41. D'Alise MD, Benzel EC, Hart BL. Magnetic resonance imaging evaluation of the cervical spine in the comatose or obtunded trauma patient. J Neurosurg Spine 1999;91:54–59

42. Miyazaki M, Hymanson HJ, Morishita Y, et al. Kinematic analysis of the relationship between sagittal alignment and disc degeneration in the cervical spine. Spine (Phila Pa 1976) 2008;33: E870–E876

43. Miura J, Doita M, Miyata K, et al. Dynamic evaluation of the spinal cord in patients with cervical spondylotic myelopathy using a kinematic magnetic resonance imaging technique. J Spinal Disord Tech 2009;22:8–13

44. Boden SD, McCowin PR, Davis DO, Dina TS, Mark AS, Wiesel S. Abnormal magnetic-resonance scans of the cervical spine in asymptomatic subjects. A prospective investigation. J Bone Joint Surg Am 1990;72:1178–1184

45. Boutin RD, Steinbach LS, Finnesey K. MR imaging of degenerative diseases in the cervical spine. Magn Reson Imaging Clin N Am 2000;8:471–489

46. Uhlenbrock D. Degenerative disorders of the spine. In: Uhlenbrock D, ed. MR Imaging of the Spine and Spinal Cord. New York: Thieme; 2004:159–268

47. Matsumoto M, Fujimura Y, Suzuki N, et al. MRI of cervical intervertebral discs in asymptomatic subjects. J Bone Joint Surg Br 1998;80: 19–24

48. Boos N, Weissbach S, Rohrbach H, Weiler C, Spratt KF, Nerlich AG. Classification of age-related changes in lumbar intervertebral discs: 2002 Volvo Award in basic science. Spine (Phila Pa 1976) 2002;27:2631–2644

49. Mercer S, Bogduk N. The ligaments and annulus fibrosus of human adult cervical intervertebral discs. Spine (Phila Pa 1976) 1999;24:619–626, discussion 627–628

50. Fardon DF, Milette PC; Combined Task Forces of the North American Spine Society, American Society of Spine Radiology, and American Society of Neuroradiology. Nomenclature and classification of lumbar disc pathology. Recommendations of the Combined task Forces of the North American Spine Society, American Society of Spine Radiology, and American Society of Neuroradiology. Spine (Phila Pa 1976) 2001;26:E93–E113

51. Modic MT, Feiglin DH, Piraino DW, et al. Vertebral osteomyelitis: assessment using MR. Radiology 1985;157:157–166

52. Modic MT, Steinberg PM, Ross JS, Masaryk TJ, Carter JR. Degenerative disc disease: assessment of changes in vertebral body marrow with MR imaging. Radiology 1988;166:193–199

53. Pavlov H, Torg JS, Robie B, Jahre C. Cervical spinal stenosis: determination with vertebral body ratio method. Radiology 1987;164: 771–775

54. Redlund-Johnell I, Pettersson H. Radiographic measurements of the cranio-vertebral region. Designed for evaluation of abnormalities in rheumatoid arthritis. Acta Radiol Diagn (Stockh) 1984;25:23–28

55. McGregor M. The significance of certain measurements of the skull in the diagnosis of basilar impression. Br J Radiol 1948;21: 171–181

56. Batzdorf U. Pathogenesis and development theories. In: Anson JA, Benzel EC, Awad IA, eds. Syringomyelia and the Chiari Malformations. Park Ridge, IL: American Association of Neurological Surgeons; 1997:35–40

57. Schenk M, Ruggieri PM. Imaging of syringomyelia and the Chiari malformations. In: Anson JA, Benzel EC, Awad IA, eds. Syringomyelia and the Chiari Malformations. Park Ridge, IL: American Association of Neurological Surgeons; 1997:41–56

58. Aboulezz AO, Sartor K, Geyer CA, Gado MH. Position of cerebellar tonsils in the normal population and in patients with Chiari malformation: a quantitative approach with MR imaging. J Comput Assist Tomogr 1985;9:1033–1036

59. Barkovich AJ, Wippold FJ, Sherman JL, Citrin CM. Significance of cerebellar tonsillar position on MR. AJNR Am J Neuroradiol 1986;7: 795–799

60. Smoker WRK. MR imaging of the craniovertebral junction. Magn Reson Imaging Clin N Am 2000;8:635–650

61. Castillo M, Quencer RM, Dominguez R. Chiari III malformation: imaging features. AJNR Am J Neuroradiol 1992;13:107–113

62. Boden SD, Dodge LD, Bohlman HH, Rechtine GR. Rheumatoid arthritis of the cervical spine. A long-term analysis with predictors of paralysis and recovery. J Bone Joint Surg Am 1993;75:1282–1297

63. Boden SD. Rheumatoid arthritis of the cervical spine. Surgical decision making based on predictors of paralysis and recovery. Spine (Phila Pa 1976) 1994;19:2275–2280

64. Dreyer SJ, Boden SD. Natural history of rheumatoid arthritis of the cervical spine. Clin Orthop Relat Res 1999;366:98–106

65. Reiter MF, Boden SD. Inflammatory disorders of the cervical spine. Spine (Phila Pa 1976) 1998;23:2755–2766

66. Oda T, Fujiwara K, Yonenobu K, Azuma B, Ochi T. Natural course of cervical spine lesions in rheumatoid arthritis. Spine (Phila Pa 1976) 1995;20:1128–1135

67. Ross JS. Cervicomedullary and craniovertebral junctions. In: Modic MT, Masaryk TJ, Ross JS, eds. Magnetic Resonance Imaging of the Spine. St. Louis: Mosby-Year Book; 1994:191–215

68. Bundschuh C, Modic MT, Kearney F, Morris R, Deal C. Rheumatoid arthritis of the cervical spine: surface-coil MR imaging. AJR Am J Roentgenol 1988;151:181–187

69. Oostveen JCM, Roozeboom AR, van de Laar MAFJ, Heeres J, den Boer JA, Lindeboom SF. Functional turbo spin echo magnetic resonance imaging versus tomography for evaluating cervical spine involvement in rheumatoid arthritis. Spine (Phila Pa 1976) 1998;23: 1237–1244

70. Tay BKB, Deckey J, Hu SS. Spinal infections. J Am Acad Orthop Surg 2002;10:188–197

71. Ruiz A, Post MJ, Sklar EM, Holz A. MR imaging of infections of the cervical spine. Magn Reson Imaging Clin N Am 2000;8:561–580

72. Khanna AJ, Carbone JJ, Kebaish KM, et al. Magnetic resonance imaging of the cervical spine. Current techniques and spectrum of disease. J Bone Joint Surg Am 2002;84(Suppl 2):70–80

73. Uhlenbrock D, Henkes H, Weber W, Felber S, Kuehne D. Inflammatory disorders of the spine and spinal canal. In: Uhlenbrock D, ed. MR Imaging of the Spine and Spinal Cord. New York: Thieme; 2004: 357–435

74. Harris LF, Haws FP. Disc space infection. Ala Med 1994;63:12–14

75. Renfrew DL. Infectious spondylitis. In: Renfrew DL, ed. Atlas of Spine Imaging. Philadelphia: Saunders; 2003:259–280

76. DiGiorgio ML, Sklar EML, Donovan Post MJ. Role of MR in determining the efficacy of medical therapy in spine infections. Radiology 1997;189:193

77. Carragee EJ. The clinical use of magnetic resonance imaging in pyogenic vertebral osteomyelitis. Spine (Phila Pa 1976) 1997;22: 780–785

78. Gillams AR, Chaddha B, Carter AP. MR appearances of the temporal evolution and resolution of infectious spondylitis. AJR Am J Roentgenol 1996;166:903–907

79. Murphy KJ, Brunberg JA, Quint DJ, Kazanjian PH. Spinal cord infection: myelitis and abscess formation. AJNR Am J Neuroradiol 1998;19:341–348

80. Keogh C, Bergin D, Brennan D, Eustace S. MR imaging of bone tumors of the cervical spine. Magn Reson Imaging Clin N Am 2000;8: 513–527

81. Finelli DA, Ross JS. MR imaging of intrinsic inflammatory myelopathies. Magn Reson Imaging Clin N Am 2000;8:541–560

82. Tartaglino LM, Friedman DP, Flanders AE, Lublin FD, Knobler RL, Liem M. Multiple sclerosis in the spinal cord: MR appearance and correlation with clinical parameters. Radiology 1995;195: 725–732

83. Wiebe S, Lee DH, Karlik SJ, et al. Serial cranial and spinal cord magnetic resonance imaging in multiple sclerosis. Ann Neurol 1992;32: 643–650

84. Choi KH, Lee KS, Chung SO, et al. Idiopathic transverse myelitis: MR characteristics. AJNR Am J Neuroradiol 1996;17:1151–1160

85. Pardatscher K, Fiore DL, Lavano A. MR imaging of transverse myelitis using Gd-DTPA. J Neuroradiol 1992;19:63–67

86. Budka H. Neuropathology of myelitis, myelopathy, and spinal infections in AIDS. Neuroimaging Clin N Am 1997;7:639–650

87. Chong J, Di Rocco A, Tagliati M, Danisi F, Simpson DM, Atlas SW. MR findings in AIDS-associated myelopathy. AJNR Am J Neuroradiol 1999;20:1412–1416

88. Wang PY, Shen WC, Jan JS. Serial MRI changes in radiation myelopathy. Neuroradiology 1995;37:374–377

89. Janssen H, Weissman BN, Aliabadi P, Zamani AA. MR imaging of arthritides of the cervical spine. Magn Reson Imaging Clin N Am 2000;8:491–512

90. Brzeski M, Fox JG, Boulton-Jones JM, Capell HA. Vertebral body collapse due to primary amyloidosis. J Rheumatol 1990;17:1701–1703

91. Yu JS, Chung C, Recht M, Dailiana T, Jurdi R. MR imaging of tophaceous gout. AJR Am J Roentgenol 1997;168:523–527

11 The Lumbar and Thoracic Spine

Gbolahan O. Okubadejo, Aditya R. Daftary, Jacob M. Buchowski, John A. Carrino, and A. Jay Khanna

■ Specialized Pulse Sequences and Imaging Protocols

Although imaging protocols of the lumbar spine for specific indications can vary among institutions, standard MRI studies of the lumbar spine for degenerative pathologies usually include the following sequences:

- Sagittal T1-weighted SE
- Sagittal T2-weighted FSE
- Sagittal T2-weighted with fat suppression or sagittal STIR
- Axial T2-weighted FSE
- Axial T1-weighted SE or axial gradient echo

T1-weighted images are good for identifying anatomy and assessing the quantity of fat in neural foramina and the epidural spaces. They also help identify the presence of fracture lines. However, edema has low signal on T1-weighted images and may be difficult to identify. Signal on T1-weighted images increases in the presence of gadolinium contrast, so these images are used to assess for contrast enhancement. Contrast enhancement is particularly useful in differentiating recurrent disc pathology from scar tissue and in assessing infection, neoplasms, and vascular malformations. Contrast enhancement may be made more conspicuous by obtaining postcontrast fat-suppressed images.

T2-weighted images are sensitive to edema, which is usually one of the early signs of pathology. Distinction between fat and fluid (edema) may be difficult on T2-weighted images. For this reason, fat suppression via a fat-suppressed T2-weighted or STIR image may be obtained to make edema more conspicuous. STIR images are preferred over fat-suppressed T2-weighted images for patients with spinal instrumentation because STIR images are less prone to magnetic susceptibility artifacts. T2-weighted and fat-suppressed T2-weighted or STIR images are extremely helpful in identifying ligamentous injury, subtle fractures, neoplasms, infection, and fluid collections, including joint effusions.

Highly T2-weighted images produce an "MR myelogram" that provides a nice perspective, which is similar to that of images obtained with conventional myelography and CT myelography. As with other myelographic images, these MR images can be used to evaluate for spinal stenosis. However, such images should always be interpreted in conjunction with other MR pulse sequences because they may be prone to artifacts that exaggerate or underestimate abnormalities, including the degree of stenosis.

By decreasing the degree to which protons are "flipped" during image acquisition (compared with T1-weighted and T2-weighted images in which they are flipped by 90 to 180 degrees), gradient-echo images can be acquired much more quickly. Adjustments in the "flip angle," TR, and TE can create T1 and T2 weighting in these images. Gradient-echo images are very susceptible to magnetic susceptibility artifacts, which make them quite useful for the detection of small areas of hemorrhage, such as those that occur with trauma and vascular malformations. On the other hand, this susceptibility also causes gradient-echo images to overestimate canal and foraminal stenosis because of artifact from the adjacent bone. Advances in MRI techniques are decreasing the latter problem.[1] Because of the rapidity with which images are acquired, they can be obtained with higher resolution and even as a 3D volume, which allows for isotropic voxels and reformations in multiple planes.

■ Traumatic Conditions

Patients with suspected lumbar spine injuries should be evaluated initially with conventional radiographs. CT imaging offers greater osseous detail than do conventional radiographs and may reveal fractures or details that are not detected with radiography. MRI provides superior visualization of soft tissues compared with conventional radiographs or CT images and is useful for the assessment of ligamentous injury, degree of spinal stenosis, additional fracture evaluation, and associated findings such as epidural hematomas. Occult fractures not visible on conventional radiographs or CT images may be detected by the presence of vertebral body edema on MR images. Although MRI is extremely sensitive in identifying thoracolumbar spine fractures, their characteristics and the exact appearance of the osseous components can be challenging; CT may be a better choice for assessing these aspects of the fractures. MRI is indicated when neurologic deficit, vascular injury, or soft-tissue injury is suspected in the setting of trauma. It is also useful for the assessment of posttraumatic sequelae.

Table 11.1 Evaluation of Lumbar and Thoracic Spine Trauma

Anatomy	Evaluation
Spinal column/ vertebral bodies	Alignment, vertebral body fracture, posterior element fracture, edema, degenerative change
Ligaments	Anterior longitudinal ligament, posterior longitudinal ligament, interspinous ligament, edema/rupture
Spinal cord	Edema, hemorrhage, compression, syrinx
Epidural space	Hematoma, disc herniation, osseous fragment

Source: Takhtani D, Melhelm ER. MR imaging in cervical spine trauma. Magn Reson Imaging Clin N Am 2000;8:615–634. Modified with permission.

A systematic approach (see Chapter 3) for the evaluation of lumbar spine MRI should be used to avoid missing pathologic conditions (see **Table 11.1** for important lumbar spine structures to evaluate). In addition, it is essential that the interpretation of the MRI findings be performed in conjunction with that of other available imaging modalities, including conventional radiographs (with flexion and extension views if clinically indicated) and CT (see Chapter 17).

Classification of Thoracolumbar Spine Trauma

Thoracolumbar spine trauma is a common and complex condition. There are many classification systems, all of which are based on a variety factors such as mechanism of injury, morphology of fracture, involvement of columns, and pres-

ence, absence, or degree of neural compromise.[2–4] As with many classification systems, those for the evaluation of thoracolumbar spine trauma have not been universally accepted. This lack of acceptance may be the result of their complexity, lack of reproducibility, or poor validity, or any combination thereof.

Recently, the Thoracolumbar Injury Classification and Severity Score has recognized the importance of the following three factors[5]:

- Fracture morphology (**Fig. 11.1**)
- Integrity of the posterior ligamentous complex (stability or potential for neurologic compromise)
- Neurologic status of the patient[5]

Although a detailed review of this classification system is outside the scope of this chapter, these three components are used here to review and highlight the role of MRI in the evaluation of patients with thoracolumbar spine trauma. In addition, a systematic evaluation of these three components and calculation of an injury severity score[5] can be used to guide the treatment of patients with thoracolumbar spine fractures.

Role of MRI in Thoracolumbar Spine Trauma

Evaluation of Fracture Morphology

The first element in the MRI evaluation of a thoracolumbar injury is the assessment of fracture morphology. The morphology description includes the type of fracture (compression, burst, etc.) and the position of various osseous fragments relative to their anatomic origin and to the spinal canal. As discussed above, for the assessment of the osse-

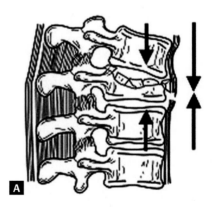
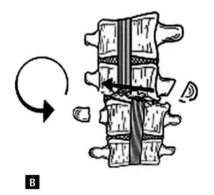
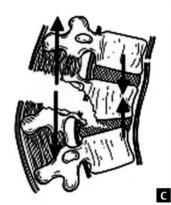

A **B** **C**

Fig. 11.1 Artist's sketches of the three major morphologic descriptors in the Thoracolumbar Injury Classification and Severity Score (compression, translation/rotation, and distraction). These descriptors are determined from a combination of conventional radiographs, CT images, and MRI sequences. **(A)** In compression, the vertebral body buckles under load to produce a compression or burst fracture. **(B)** In translation/rotation, the vertebral column is subjected to shear or torsional forces that cause the rostral part of the spinal column to translate or rotate with respect to the caudal part. **(C)** In distraction, the rostral spinal column becomes separated from the caudal segment because of distractive forces. Combinations of these morphologic patterns may occur. (From Vaccaro AR, Lehman RA Jr, Hurlbert RJ, et al. A new classification of thoracolumbar injuries. The importance of injury morphology, the integrity of the posterior ligamentous complex, and neurologic status. Spine 2005;30:2325–2333. Reprinted with permission.)

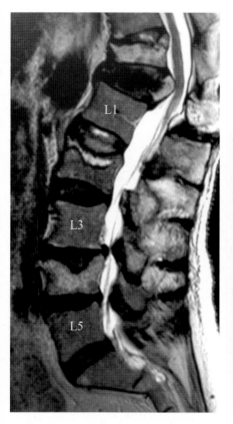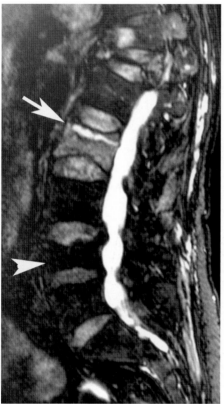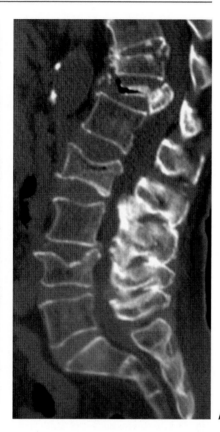

A–C

Fig. 11.2 Osteoporotic vertebral fractures. **(A)** A sagittal T2-weighted image showing multiple vertebral fractures, including vertebral compression fractures at L4, L2, and T11, and a burst fracture at T12. Note the bright T2-weighted signal fracture line at L2, characteristic of a benign osteoporotic fracture. **(B)** A sagittal STIR image shows a linear region of increased signal intensity compatible with edema in the L2 vertebral body (*arrow*), which is compatible with an acute fracture. Note the diffuse edema in the vertebral body that could be mistaken for diffuse bone marrow involvement by a neoplastic process. There is no increase in signal intensity in the L4 vertebral body (*arrowhead*), which is compatible with a chronic fracture. **(C)** A sagittal reconstructed CT image shows the osseous details of the fractures. The osseous margins are clearly defined, and the retropulsed posterior fragment characteristic of a benign osteoporotic fracture is evident at T12.

ous components of a fracture, CT is superior to conventional radiography and MRI because of the excellent spatial resolution and osseous detail it provides (**Fig. 11.2**). MRI may help provide additional information regarding the morphology of a fracture in a limited number of situations.

For example, subtle fractures may be difficult to identify on CT or conventional radiographs, especially in patients with degenerative disc disease where end-plate anatomy and vertebral morphology are affected by the degenerative changes. Furthermore, osteoporotic and osteopenic patients may show less osseous reactive change, which typically allows for the detection of subtle or subacute fractures on conventional radiographs. Fluid-sensitive pulse sequences such as fat-suppressed T2-weighted or STIR images are excellent for identifying areas of subtle bone marrow edema and focusing attention on an area of potential osseous injury. This bone marrow edema often appears almost immediately after injury and can persist for several months or even a year thereafter.[6,7] It should be noted, however, that the differential

considerations for bone marrow edema in a vertebral body are varied and include other entities such as tumors, end-plate degeneration, and infection. For this reason, correlation with other imaging findings, imaging techniques, and clinical information is important for making a definitive diagnosis.

For patients in whom vertebral compression fractures are associated with pain, vertebral augmentation procedures such as vertebroplasty or kyphoplasty may be considered as a treatment option. In a study of patients with chronic (1 year) vertebral compression fractures treated with vertebroplasty, Brown et al.[7] found that clinical improvement was definitively correlated with the presence of preprocedural bone marrow edema. Thus, it is essential that the MR images be reviewed for the absence, presence, and degree of bone marrow edema for each fracture (**Fig. 11.2**).

Differentiating posttraumatic and osteoporotic fractures from neoplastic or pathologic fractures can be challenging (**Figs. 11.2** and **11.3**), especially in elderly patients. Neoplastic processes tend to fracture when most of the vertebral

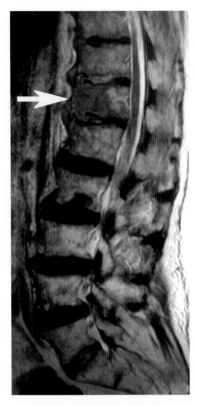
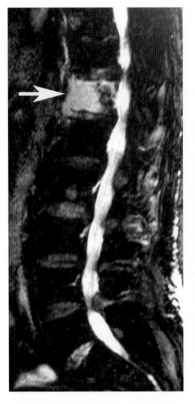
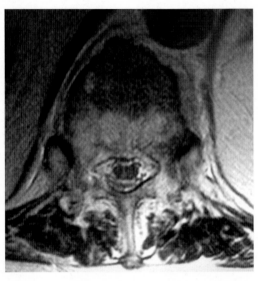

A–C

Fig. 11.3 Vertebral body metastasis in a patient with lung cancer. **(A)** A sagittal T2-weighted image showing heterogeneous bone marrow signal intensity in multiple vertebral bodies (which can be seen with osteoporosis) but most prominently within the anterior half of the T12 vertebral body (*arrow*). Note that the anterior aspect of the vertebral body appears expanded as it is infiltrated with tumor. **(B)** A sagittal STIR image shows intensely increased signal intensity in the same region (*arrow*). **(C)** An axial T2-weighted image shows heterogeneous signal intensity within the vertebral body. A percutaneous biopsy confirmed evidence of metastatic lung cancer.

body is infiltrated with tumor (**Fig. 11.3**). Key MRI features that suggest the presence of a malignant fracture include the following[8]:

- Convex posterior margin of the vertebral body (from tumor infiltration) (**Fig. 11.4**)
- Abnormal signal in the posterior elements
- Epidural mass and neural encasement by the same focal paraspinal mass
- Presence of other osseous lesions

In the search for other lesions, care should be taken not to mistake additional osteoporotic vertebral fractures for metastatic lesions. A horizontal linear bright fracture line on T2-weighted images is considered the most reliable sign of a nonmalignant fracture (**Fig. 11.2**). Other signs that decrease the likelihood of underlying tumor include a retropulsed fragment off of the posterior aspect of the vertebral body, multiple fractures, and normal bone marrow signal.[8,9] Because contrast enhancement is often seen with acute benign fractures, it is no longer considered diagnostic for an underlying lesion or malignancy.[8,10]

Assessment of Stability

The term *spinal stability* refers to the ability of the spine to limit neurologic compromise under physiologic loads. Panjabi et al.[11] have defined spinal stability as the degree of motion that prevents pain, neurologic deficit, and abnormal angulation. The definition can also be extended to include the ability of the spine to avoid the development of spinal deformity. Two key concepts in the MRI determination of spinal stability are the three-column concept and the assessment of the posterior ligamentous complex.

Three-Column Concept

More than 25 years ago, Denis[4] introduced the concept of the three-column spine and its clinical significance in the evaluation of spinal stability in patients with acute thoracolumbar injuries. Although the reliability and validity of the Denis system have been questioned,[12] it is still used frequently to help evaluate the degree of spinal instability. Spinal instability may be assessed based on the number of columns involved in an injury. The three columns are defined as follows:

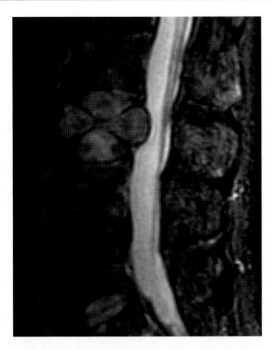

Fig. 11.4 A sagittal STIR image showing a pathologic burst fracture of the L3 vertebral body in a patient with metastatic lung cancer. Note the diffusely increased signal within the vertebral body and the convex posterior margin of the vertebral body.

- *Anterior*: anterior longitudinal ligament and the anterior portion of the vertebral body and annulus
- *Middle*: posterior vertebral body and annulus, and the posterior longitudinal ligament
- *Posterior*: facet joints, posterior elements, and posterior ligaments (supraspinous and interspinous ligaments and ligamentum flavum)

If one column is involved, the spine is generally considered stable; with two-column involvement, the spine is variably stable, depending on the degree of involvement; and the involvement of all three columns leads to a highly unstable spine.

Posterior Ligamentous Complex

The posterior column and posterior ligamentous complex is an area of increasing concern in spinal stability (**Fig. 11.1C**).[5,13,14] The components of the posterior ligamentous complex include the supraspinous ligament, interspinous ligament, ligamentum flavum, and the facet joint capsules.[5] The three ligaments that comprise the posterior ligamentous complex normally appear as dark and continuous bands on T1-weighted and T2-weighted images. When traumatized, they may show increased signal on fluid-sensitive pulse sequences (T2-weighted fat-suppressed and STIR) (**Fig. 11.5**) or associated hematomas. Discontinuity of the dark signal of the fibers is also seen on MRI. It has been sug-

gested that the MR images be reviewed with the intent of describing these ligaments to be intact, indeterminate, or disrupted.[5]

Subtle fractures and dislocations of the facet joints and posterior elements are detected well on CT, but in some instances the edema identified on MRI may be helpful in combination with close scrutiny of the CT images to identify subtle fractures. However, the true role of MRI in these instances is in identifying ligamentous injuries and hematomas; 28% to 47% of patients with thoracolumbar burst fractures are estimated to have disruption of the posterior ligamentous complex.[15]

Assessment of Neural Compromise

MRI plays its most vital role in the assessment of neural compromise and is excellent in its ability to determine the cause

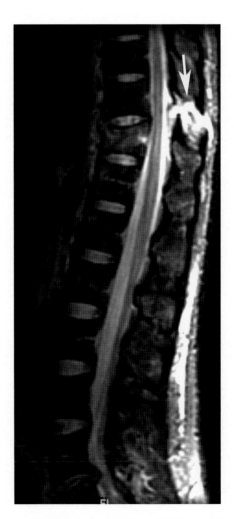

Fig. 11.5 A sagittal STIR image showing a T11 flexion-distraction injury with compression fracture of T11 and an associated injury of the interspinous and supraspinous ligaments, as evidenced by increased signal intensity in the interspinous and supraspinous region between T10 and T11 (*arrow*).

of compression. Neural compromise can be graded on MRI as mild, moderate, or severe (see Lumbar Spinal Stenosis, below). In addition to an evaluation of the degree of stenosis, the type of stenosis should also be described (central, lateral recess, or foraminal). In addition, one should note whether there is compression of specific neurologic structures, such as the spinal cord or a specific nerve root. Common causes of neural compromise in patients after thoracolumbar spine trauma include the following:

- Burst fractures
- Disc pathology
- Epidural hematoma
- Vertebral translation or dislocation
- Penetrating trauma (**Fig. 11.6**)

Burst Fracture

Although CT is excellent in assessing the osseous component of a burst fracture, the associated neural compression and hematoma may be difficult to assess on CT, and MRI is far more accurate. It is important to differentiate a burst fracture (**Fig. 11.7**) from a compression fracture (**Fig. 11.2**). The former involves injury to the anterior and middle columns, whereas the latter involves injury to the anterior column only. The MR images should be carefully evaluated for the absence or presence and degree of stenosis, which can be secondary to the fracture alone or to preexisting degenerative changes, or to any combination thereof. Specifically, the sagittal T2-weighted images should be evaluated in the midline for the degree of posterior vertebral body wall en-

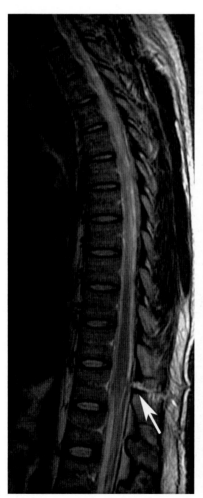
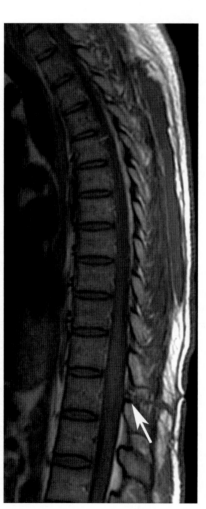
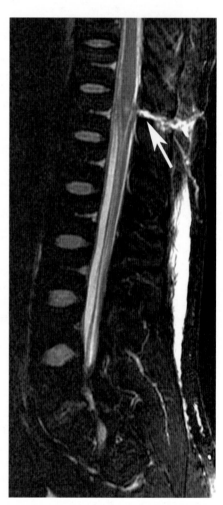

A–C

Fig. 11.6 Cord injury from a stab injury to the conus medullaris. **(A)** A sagittal T2-weighted image of the thoracic spine showing a linear track (*arrow*) from the skin to the conus medullaris with an associated region of increased signal within the conus medullaris, compatible with edema. **(B)** A sagittal T1-weighted image of the thoracic spine also showing the track (*arrow*) but not showing the edema within the conus medullaris. **(C)** A sagittal STIR image of the lumbar spine accentuates the edema along the track (*arrow*) and also that within the conus medullaris.

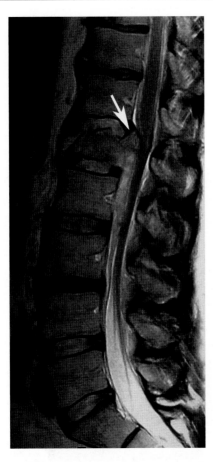

Fig. 11.7 A sagittal T2-weighted image showing an L1 burst fracture. Note that the posterior-superior margin of the vertebral body has displaced and rotated into the spinal canal. This displaced and rotated fragment (*arrow*) has been termed the *sentinel* or *culprit* fragment.

croachment on the spinal canal, CSF column, spinal cord, or cauda equina. Next, the parasagittal images should be evaluated for the same. Finally, the axial T2-weighted images can be reviewed to determine the location and degree of neural compromise in an orthogonal plane.

Disc Pathology

Traumatic compressive forces on the disc may lead to annular tears (also known as annular fissures), disc protrusions, extrusions, and sequestrations. Rupture of a few annular fibers leads to a small amount of fluid tracking from the nucleus pulposus to between the annular fibers, leading to a focus of high intensity on T2-weighted images. This finding of focal high intensity in the annulus is referred to as a *high-intensity zone* (**Fig. 11.8**) and is suggestive of an annular tear. Although this finding may be seen in association with trauma, its level of importance is controversial because it is also seen as a natural process of disc degeneration and may or may not be associated with acute pain.[16–18] MRI is the modality of choice for assessing such abnormalities and associated areas

for potential neurologic compromise (see Degenerative Disc Disease, below). The sagittal and axial T2-weighted images should be carefully evaluated for the presence of disc pathology such as protrusion, extrusions, and sequestrations. If present, the degree of neural compromise should be noted (see below).

Epidural Hematomas

Hematomas may occasionally be seen in association with thoracolumbar spine trauma, and they can be difficult to differentiate from disc protrusions and extrusions. Hematomas often resolve spontaneously and may provide an explanation for patients who show a rapid and spontaneous resolution of apparent disc herniations.[19–21] Key differentiating features between a disc extrusion and hematoma or fluid collection are a hematoma's larger size, different signal, obtuse margin along the posterior aspect of the vertebral body with maximum dimension at midvertebral body level, and possible containment by the central septum (which attaches the posterior longitudinal ligament to the vertebral body).[22,23]

The signal pattern associated with epidural hemorrhage is related directly to the state of the oxygenation of the blood that pools in the regions of interest adjacent to the cord. In the acute phase, T1-weighted images show signal that is isointense compared with that of the adjacent spinal

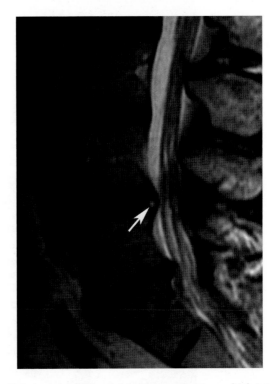

Fig. 11.8 A sagittal T2-weighted image showing a high-intensity zone at the posterior annulus of L4-L5 (*arrow*). Also noted is degenerative disc disease at L5-S1 with moderate loss of disc height. The L3-L4 disc is normal.

cord, and T2-weighted images show heterogeneous areas of increased and decreased signal intensity. During the acute phase, deoxyhemoglobin is the main component of the he-matoma. Deoxyhemoglobin appears isointense or slightly low in signal intensity compared with that of the normal spinal cord on T1-weighted images and as a hypointense sig-

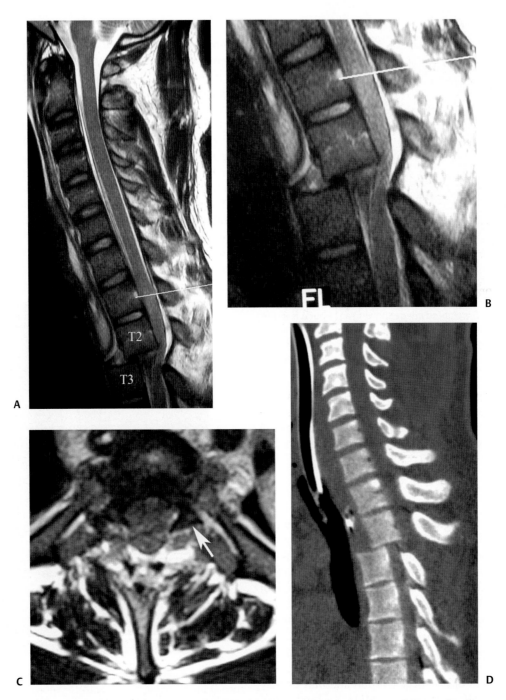

Fig. 11.9 T2-T3 dislocation. This sagittal T2-weighted image **(A)** and zoom-in **(B)** show anterior dislocation of T3 relative to T2 without fracture with resultant severe cord compression, deformity, and acute signal change within the cord; the *line* on each points to the L1 vertebral body. **(C)** An axial T2-weighted image shows that the facets are "naked" or dissociated, a finding better seen on the left side (*arrow*). **(D)** A sagittal reconstructed CT image also shows the dislocation and confirms the absence of a fracture.

nal on T2-weighted images. Within 2 to 4 days after injury, T1-weighted and T2-weighted images may show increased signal intensity.[15] By 8 to 10 days, the primary component of the hemorrhage is methemoglobin, which is hyperintense on T1-weighted images.[24]

Vertebral Translation or Dislocation

The posttraumatic translation of vertebral bodies may produce canal or foraminal narrowing with associated neural compression. Dislocation of the spine indicates an alteration of spinal alignment in all three planes and the displacement of one vertebral body relative to an adjacent one. Typical MRI signs of dislocations include the following:

- Altered facet joint anatomy with increased T2-weighted signal (or fluid) in the facet joints: the osseous anatomy is often better seen on CT, but as mentioned above, edema and fluid on MRI help focus the search for a subtle injury.
- Disc herniation or pseudoherniation: with translation of one vertebral body in relation to the adjacent one, there may be uncovering of the disc, which gives the appearance of a herniation (pseudoherniation).
- Vertebral body translation: sagittal and coronal images are excellent in determining translation of vertebral bodies (**Fig. 11.9**). Care should be taken in determining if translations are the result of facet degeneration, osseous injury, facet joint displacement, or pars defects.

■ Nomenclature and Classification of Lumbar Disc Pathology

The nomenclature used for describing lumbar disc pathology should be consistent and uniformly applied. Fardon and Milette[25] provide a comprehensive review of the nomenclature and classification of lumbar disc pathology. This nomenclature and classification scheme represents the recommendations of the combined task forces of the North American Spine Society, American Society of Spine Radiology, and American Society of Neuroradiology. Several other societies, including the American Academy of Orthopaedic Surgery, now support and recommend the use of the nomenclature described below. Surgeons and radiologists involved in the care of patients with known or suspected lumbar disc pathology and the evaluation of their MR images should consider reviewing this publication[25] for additional detail.

With this system, disc lesions are classified as follows:

- *Normal*: a young disc that is morphologically normal (no lesion)
- *Congenital/developmental variant*: discs that are congenitally abnormal or that have undergone changes in morphology secondary to abnormal growth of the spine
- *Degenerative/traumatic lesion*: annular tear, degeneration, herniation
- *Inflammation/infection*: inflammatory spondylitis of subchondral end plate and bone marrow manifested as Modic type 1 MRI changes[26–29]
- *Neoplasia*: all pathologic entities that may be primary or metastatic
- *Morphologic variant of unknown importance*

In the degenerative category, annular tears (also called annular fissures) are separations between annular fibers, avulsion of fibers from their vertebral body insertions, or other injuries of the fibers that involve one or multiple layers of the annular lamellae (**Fig. 11.10**).

The degenerative process includes desiccation, fibrosis, narrowing of the disc space, diffuse bulging of the annulus beyond the disc space, extensive fissuring, mucinous degeneration of the annulus, defects and sclerosis of the end plates, and osteophytes at the vertebral apophyses. Degenerative changes can also be subcategorized as spondylosis deformans (changes in the disc associated with a normal aging process) and intervertebral osteochondrosis (consequences of a more clearly pathologic process) (**Fig. 11.11**).

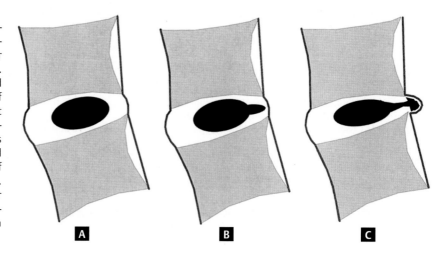

Fig. 11.10 Schematic sagittal drawings showing differentiating MRI features of disc pathology. **(A)** A normal disc. **(B)** An annular tear (radial tear, in this case). **(C)** A disc herniation. The term *tear* is used to refer to a localized radial, concentric, or horizontal disruption of the annulus without associated displacement of disc material beyond the limits of the intervertebral disc space. Nuclear material is shown in black, and the annulus (internal and external) corresponds to the white portion of the intervertebral space. (From Milette PC. The proper terminology for reporting lumbar intervertebral disc disorders. AJNR Am J Neuroradiol 1997;18:1859–1866. Reprinted with permission.)

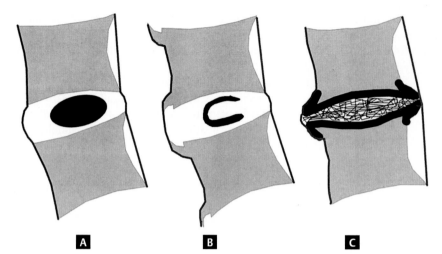

Fig. 11.11 Schematic sagittal drawings showing differentiating disc MRI characteristics. **(A)** Normal disc. **(B)** Spondylosis deformans. **(C)** Intervertebral osteochondrosis. The distinction between these three entities is usually possible on all imaging modalities, including conventional radiographs. (From Milette PC. The proper terminology for reporting lumbar intervertebral disc disorders. AJNR Am J Neuroradiol 1997;18:1859–1866. Reprinted with permission.)

Herniation is defined as a localized displacement of disc contents beyond the borders of the intervertebral disc space (**Fig. 11.12A**). The disc material may include nucleus, cartilage, fragmented apophyseal bone, or annular tissue, or a combination of those materials. Most clinicians tend to describe disc pathology using the terms *bulge, herniation, ex-trusion*, and *sequestration*. Although the last two terms are often used correctly, there seems to be a high degree of interobserver variability in the use of the first two terms.

The currently accepted nomenclature is as follows: A herniation is considered "localized" if it involves ≤50% of the disc circumference and "generalized" if it involves >50%. A

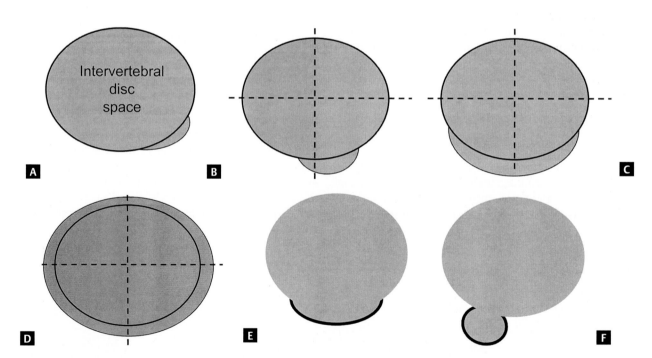

Fig. 11.12 In disc herniation, the interspace is defined, peripherally, by the edges of the vertebral ring apophyses, exclusive of osteophytic formations. **(A)** Localized extension of disc material beyond the intervertebral disc space, in a left posterior direction, which qualifies as a disc herniation. **(B)** By convention, a focal herniation involves <25% (90 degrees) of the disc circumference. **(C)** By convention, a broad-based herniation involves between 25% and 50% (90 to 180 degrees) of the disc circumference. **(D)** Symmetrical presence (or apparent presence) of disc tissue "circumferentially" (50% to 100%) beyond the edges of the ring apophyses may be described as a "bulging disc" or "bulging appearance" and is not considered a form of herniation. *Bulging* is a descriptive term for the shape of the disc contour and not a diagnostic category. **(E)** Protrusion (see definition in text). **(F)** Extrusion (see definition in text). (From Fardon DF, Milette PC. Nomenclature and classification of lumbar disc pathology. Recommendations of the Combined Task Forces of the North American Spine Society, American Society of Spine Radiology, and American Society of Neuroradiology. Spine 2001;26:E93–E113. Reprinted with permission.)

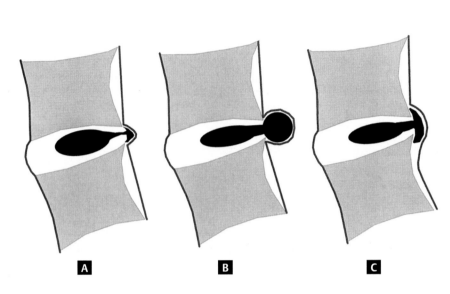

A **B** **C**

Fig. 11.13 Protrusion and extrusion. When a relatively large amount of disc material is displaced, distinction between protrusion **(A)** and extrusion **(B,C)** is usually possible only on sagittal MR sections or sagittal CT reconstructions. **(C)** Although the shape of the displaced material is similar to that of a protrusion, the greatest craniocaudal diameter of the fragment is greater than the craniocaudal diameter of its base at the level of the parent disc, and the lesion therefore qualifies as an extrusion. In any situation, the distance between the edges of the base, which serves as reference for the definition of protrusion and extrusion, may differ from the distance between the edges of the aperture of the annulus, which cannot be assessed on CT images and is seldom appreciated on MR images. In the craniocaudal direction, the length of the base cannot exceed, by definition, the height of the intervertebral space. (From Milette PC. Classification, diagnostic imaging, and imaging characterization of a lumbar herniated disc. Radiol Clin North Am 2000;38:1267–1292. Reprinted with permission.)

localized displacement is considered "focal" if <25% of the disc circumference is involved (**Fig. 11.12B**) and "broad-based" if the herniating disc content is between 25% and 50% (**Fig. 11.12C**). Disc tissue noted circumferentially, between 50% and 100%, and beyond the edges of the ring apophyses is termed *bulging*, which is not considered by some to be a form of herniation (**Fig. 11.12D**). The terms *protrusion* (**Fig. 11.12E**) and *extrusion* (**Fig. 11.12F**) are also commonly used in the context of disc herniation. A protrusion is present if the greatest distance between the edges of the disc material beyond the disc space is less than the distance between the edges of the base in the same plane. The base is the cross-sectional area of disc material at the outer margin of the disc space of origin, where disc material displaced beyond the disc space is continuous with disc material within the disc space. An extrusion is present when any one distance between the edges of the disc material beyond the disc space is greater than the distance between the edges of the base (**Fig. 11.13**) or when there is no continuity between the disc space and the disc fragment. Extrusion may be further classified as sequestered and migrated. Sequestration is noted if the displaced disc material is completely discontinuous with the parent disc. Migration refers to displacement of disc material away from the site of extrusion, regardless of whether or not there is sequestration (**Fig. 11.14**).

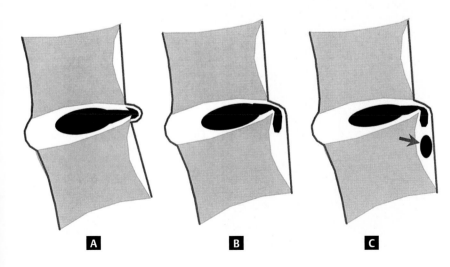

A **B** **C**

Fig. 11.14 Schematic representations of various types of posterior central herniations. **(A)** A small subligamentous herniation (or protrusion) without substantial disc material migration. **(B)** A subligamentous herniation with downward migration of disc material under the posterior longitudinal ligament. **(C)** A subligamentous herniation with downward migration of disc material and sequestered fragment (*arrow*). (From Milette PC. Classification, diagnostic imaging, and imaging characterization of a lumbar herniated disc. Radiol Clin North Am 2000;38:1267–1292. Reprinted with permission.)

Intravertebral herniation refers to a herniated disc in the craniocaudal direction through a defect in the vertebral body end plate. Herniations can also be described as contained or uncontained. Contained herniations are displaced disc material that is retained by the outer annulus. Uncontained herniations are not retained by the outer annulus. Each abnormal presentation of disc pathology has specific features that can be detected with MRI (see below).

■ Degenerative Conditions

Along with cervical degenerative disorders, lumbar degenerative disc disease and the associated stenosis are the most common indications for MRI of the spine. Most patients present with low back pain, lower extremity pain, or symptoms of neurogenic claudication. They usually have had at least 6 weeks of unsuccessful nonoperative management and often have already been evaluated with conventional radiography. The purpose of MRI in this situation is most frequently to evaluate for the presence or absence of spinal stenosis, disc herniation, and degenerative disc disease.

Lumbar spine degeneration typically includes a constellation of changes, such as degenerative disc disease, arthritic and hypertrophic changes involving the facet joints, and hypertrophy of the ligamentum flavum (see Chapter 10 for a discussion of inflammatory arthropathies, including ankylosing spondylitis). It is important to note that patients exhibiting MRI changes may not necessarily be symptomatic.[30] A study of 33 asymptomatic, elite tennis players showed that 15.2% had a normal MRI evaluation and 84.8% had abnormalities: 27.3% had pars lesions and 39.4% showed evidence of disc desiccation and bulging.[30] The high incidence of abnormal lumbar spine MRI studies was described by Boden et al.[31] in 67 asymptomatic patients. A follow-up study of those 67 patients concluded that the MRI findings were not predictive of the development or duration of low back pain.[32]

Disc and End Plates

Degenerative Disc Disease

As noted above, Fardon and Milette[25] have suggested the use of the terms *normal*, *spondylosis deformans*, and *intervertebral osteochondrosis* to describe the degenerative lumbar disc (**Fig. 11.11**). The specific changes seen on MRI correlate with the pathogenesis of degenerative disc disease, which results from the spectrum of changes that occur in the various parts of the vertebrodiscal complex. The nucleus pulposus becomes increasingly hypointense on T2-weighted images because of desiccation. An alternative finding is the inter-

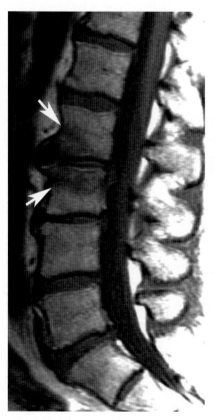 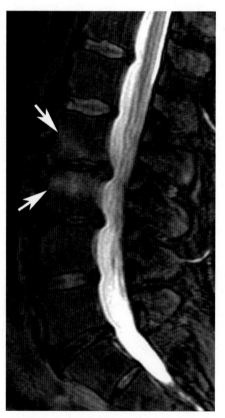

A, B

Fig. 11.15 Modic type 1 (fibrovascular) changes. Sagittal T1-weighted **(A)** and fat-suppressed T2-weighted **(B)** images showing the typical pattern (*arrow on each*) of decreased signal intensity on the T1-weighted image and increased signal on the T2-weighted image at the L2-L3 level that is seen with Modic type 1 end-plate changes.

vertebral disc vacuum phenomenon secondary to a collection of intradiscal nitrogen, which manifests as a linear area of signal void on T1-weighted and T2-weighted sequences. Gradient-echo sequences may show this particular finding even better than do T1-weighted and T2-weighted images.[33] Early signs of disc degeneration on MRI include infolding of the anterior annulus and a hypointense central region often seen before any loss of disc signal intensity, which may be associated with reproduction of pain at discography.[33] Advanced degeneration may present with a linear hyperintensity parallel to the end plate, which is thought to represent separation of the nucleus pulposus from the hyaline cartilage end plate.[33]

Pfirrmann et al[34] introduced a grading system for lumbar degenerative disc disease based on MRI findings on sagittal T2-weighted images. This classification system, which describes five grades of progressively increasing degenerative disc disease, is complex, which may be the reason it is not commonly used by most clinicians. To summarize, the grading system describes the lumbar disc degenerative process as a continuum that progresses from a normal disc, to loss of the normal disc signal on T2-weighted images, to increasing loss of disc height, to degenerative end-plate changes and sclerosis.

Modic et al.[26,29] described signal changes within the vertebral body bone marrow and end plate adjacent to degenerating discs. The first finding in the sequence of changes is fibrovascular ingrowth that results in diminished signal intensity on T1-weighted images and a corresponding increase in signal intensity on T2-weighted images (type 1) (**Fig. 11.15**). The more chronic, type 2 changes involve a change from hematopoietic (red) to fatty (yellow) marrow, leading to relatively increased signal on T1-weighted images and slightly diminished signal intensity on T2-weighted images (**Fig. 11.16**). Type 3 changes consist of decreased signal intensity on T1-weighted and T2-weighted sequences and are associated with subchondral sclerosis on radiographs[27,33] (**Fig. 11.17**). Among the three types of degenerative end-plate changes, type 1 changes have been found to have the greatest correlation with the presence of discogenic back pain.[28,35,36]

In addition to an assessment of the type of lumbar degenerative disc disease using the methods described above, one should also describe the degree of lumbar disc degeneration by noting the amount of disc space height loss (**Fig. 11.18**).

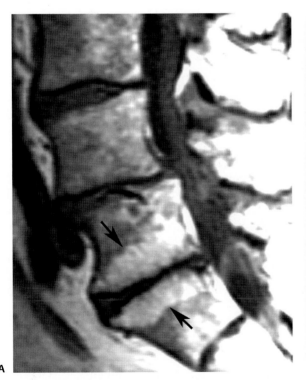

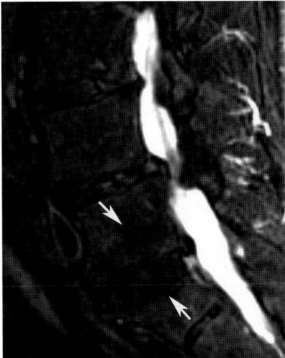

Fig. 11.16 Modic type 2 (fatty) changes. Sagittal T1-weighted **(A)** and fat-suppressed T2-weighted **(B)** images showing the typical pattern (*arrows on each*) of increased signal intensity on the T1-weighted image and decreased signal on the T2-weighted image at the L5-S1 level that is seen with Modic type 2 end-plate changes. Note that degenerative changes and stenosis are also seen at other levels.

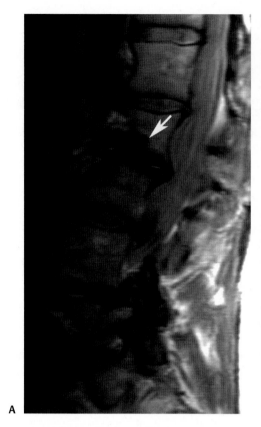 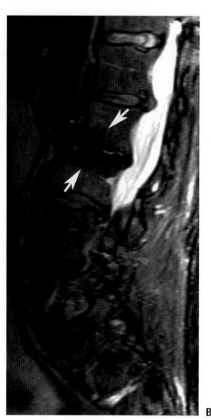

Fig. 11.17 Modic type 3 (sclerotic) changes. Sagittal T1-weighted **(A)** and fat-suppressed T2-weighted **(B)** images showing the typical pattern (*arrow[s] on each*) of decreased signal intensity at the L2-L3 level that is seen with Modic type 3 end-plate changes. Note that degenerative changes are seen at other levels and that there is also evidence of lumbar scoliosis.

Annular Tears

Annular tears on MRI have a variable appearance, ranging from intermediate to high signal intensity on T2-weighted images. Studies have shown a correlation between high signal intensity annular tears in the lumbar spine and painful concordant annular tears seen at provocative discography.[37,38] Some investigators have suggested that the inflammation associated with these annular tears results in irritation of the adjacent nerve root, potentially leading to radiculopathy without overt mechanical nerve root compression.[38] T2-weighted sequences have been used to show the following three types of annular tears:

- Concentric
- Radial
- Transverse

Concentric tears involve the entire extent of the annulus. Transverse tears occur at the periphery of the disc as a result of disruption of Sharpey's fibers. Radial tears extend from the nucleus through the annulus and may extend into the outer annulus, manifested on MRI as a high-intensity zone

(**Fig. 11.8**). The high-intensity zone is defined as a focal area of high signal intensity within the posterior annulus of the degenerating disc, separate from the nucleus. These high-intensity zones may also enhance after intravenous gadolinium administration.[33]

Discography can be used to further evaluate patients with annular tears. In addition to the morphologic information provided on fluoroscopic images and on post-discography CT, the patient's pain response can be used to help predict whether an annular tear or other degenerative pathology is the patient's pain generator.[39,40] It is important to keep in mind, however, that the use of discography in the diagnosis of discogenic low back pain continues to be debated and is not uniformly accepted at all centers.

Lumbar Herniated Nucleus Pulposus

The terms used to describe the progressive states of herniated nucleus pulposus have been addressed above (see Nomenclature and Classification of Lumbar Disc Pathology). Shown here are the MRI appearances of each:

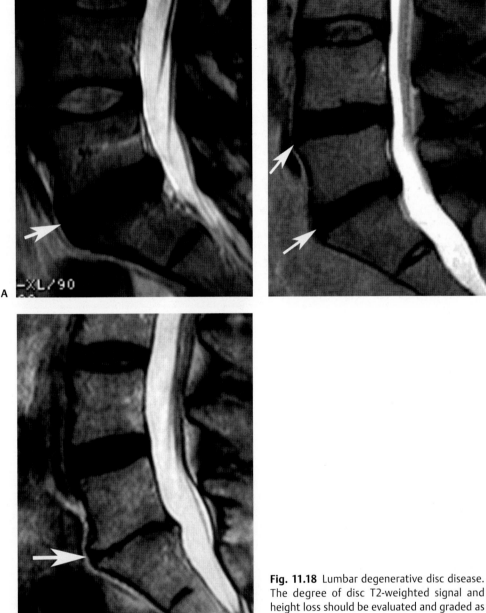

Fig. 11.18 Lumbar degenerative disc disease. The degree of disc T2-weighted signal and height loss should be evaluated and graded as mild **(A)**, moderate **(B)**, or severe **(C)** lumbar degenerative disc disease (*arrow[s] on each*).

- Normal
- Bulge (**Fig. 11.19**)
- Protrusion (**Fig. 11.20**)
- Extrusion (**Fig. 11.21**)

The status of the annulus provides insight into the status of a herniated disc. A disc protrusion is a herniation with an intact annulus, confined by the posterior longitudinal ligament. Extrusions occur when the nuclear material breaches the outer annular fibers. If a herniated disc becomes detached from the parent disc, it is termed *sequestrated*. The sequestrated fragment can migrate superiorly, inferiorly, or

occasionally, posterior to the thecal sac. Intradural disc herniation is very rare.[33]

It often is difficult to differentiate protrusion from extrusion. Several MRI signs may be used to aid this differentiation, including the following:

- If the AP diameter of the herniated disc is >50% of the spinal canal diameter, then an extrusion is present in >90% of cases.[33,41]
- Examination of the base of the disc shows that a protrusion usually has a broad base against the parent disc, broader than any other part of the hernia; an

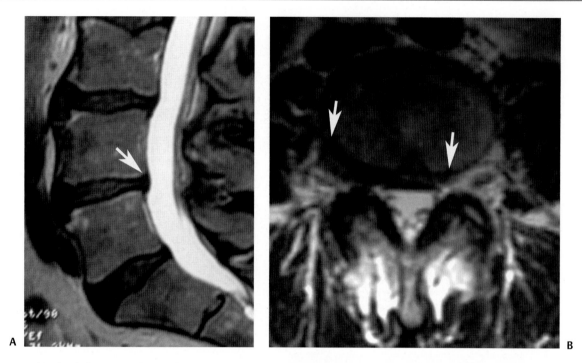

Fig. 11.19 Lumbar disc bulge. Sagittal **(A)** and axial **(B)** T2-weighted images showing a right paracentral disc bulge at the L4-L5 level (*at arrow on* **A** *and between arrows on* **B**).

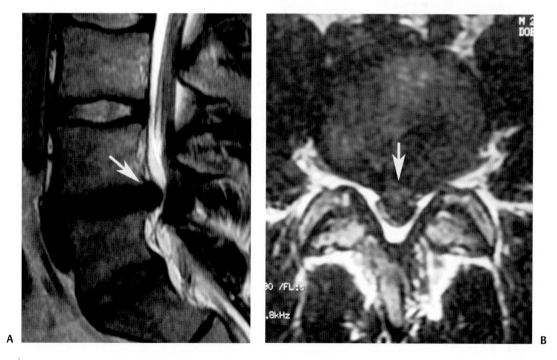

Fig. 11.20 Lumbar disc protrusion. Sagittal **(A)** and axial **(B)** T2-weighted images showing a central disc protrusion at the L4-L5 level (*arrow on each*).

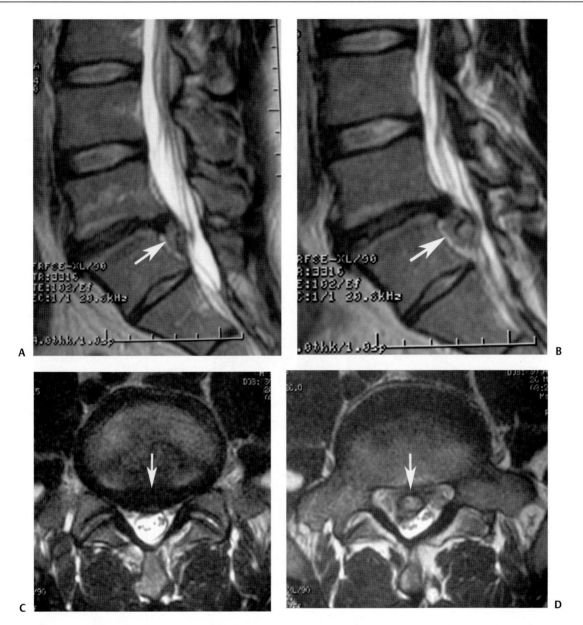

Fig. 11.21 Lumbar disc extrusion. Midline sagittal **(A)** and parasagittal **(B)** T2-weighted images showing a large disc extrusion at the L4-L5 level and distal migration of the disc fragment (*arrow on each*) to behind the L5 vertebral body in a patient with transitional lumbosacral anatomy. Note the advanced degenerative disc disease at this level. **(C)** An axial T2-weighted image at the level of the L4-L5 disc showing what appears to be a central disc bulge (*arrow*). **(D)** However, an axial T2-weighted image at the L5 vertebral body level shows the disc extrusion (*arrow*).

extrusion has a base that is more narrow than the extruded material.

- Protrusions and extrusions can also be distinguished by their outlines. Protrusions are limited by the outer annular fibers and tend to have a smooth outline; in contrast, extrusions have a poorly defined outer margin.[33,42]

When reviewing an MRI study that shows lumbar disc displacement, the clinician or radiologist should use the appropriate term to describe the morphology of the disc

(bulge, protrusion, extrusion, sequestration) and should also describe several additional key characteristics of the disc pathology, including the following (see **Figs. 11.19** through **11.21** for examples of such descriptions):

- Level of the disc pathology
- Precise location relative to the disc space
- Size and degree of neural compression

With regard to location of the disc pathology, the axial and sagittal T2-weighted images should be carefully evaluated

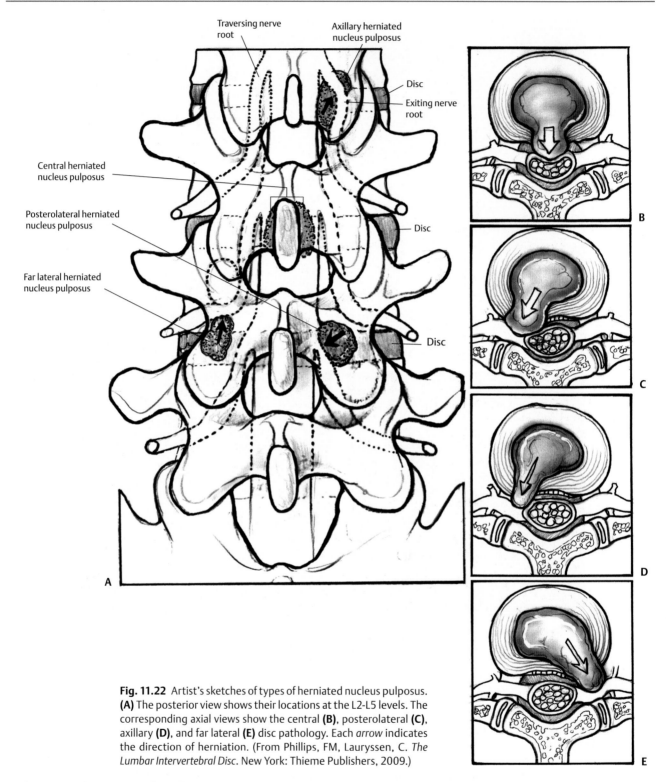

Fig. 11.22 Artist's sketches of types of herniated nucleus pulposus. **(A)** The posterior view shows their locations at the L2-L5 levels. The corresponding axial views show the central **(B)**, posterolateral **(C)**, axillary **(D)**, and far lateral **(E)** disc pathology. Each *arrow* indicates the direction of herniation. (From Phillips, FM, Lauryssen, C. *The Lumbar Intervertebral Disc*. New York: Thieme Publishers, 2009.)

to determine the location of the disc protrusion or other pathology. The following terms should be used to describe the location of the protrusion (primarily based on the appearance of the axial T2-weighted image) (**Figs. 11.22** and **11.23**):

- *Central* (**Fig. 11.24**)
- *Posterolateral* or *lateral recess* (**Fig. 11.25**)
- *Foraminal* (**Fig. 11.26**)
- *Far lateral* (**Fig. 11.27**)

Of all lumbar disc herniations, 90% are central or paracentral (5% are foraminal and 5% are far lateral).[43] It should be noted that a typical posterolateral disc protrusion compresses the traversing nerve root, whereas a far lateral disc

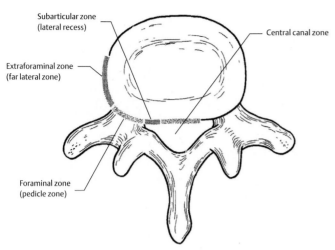

Fig. 11.23 Schematic representation of the anatomic "zones" identified on axial images. (From Wiltse LL, Berger PE, McCulloch JA. A system for reporting the size and location of lesions of the spine. Spine 1997;22:1534–1537. Reprinted with permission.)

protrusion compresses the exiting nerve root. Thus, for example, a posterolateral disc protrusion at the L4-L5 level will likely produce an L5 radiculopathy, whereas a far lateral disc protrusion at the same level will likely produce an L4 radiculopathy.

Another characteristic of the disc pathology that should be evaluated is its expected consistency at surgery. Specifically, the spine surgeon will benefit from knowing if the disc can be expected to be "soft" or "hard." A soft disc protrusion consists primarily of nucleus pulposus, whereas hard disc pathology may consist of a chronic and desiccated disc protrusion or a posterior or posterolateral osteophyte (**Fig. 11.28**). T2-weighted images occasionally show increased signal within the disc protrusion, a finding that often correlates with a soft disc at surgery.

Thoracic Disc Herniation

Thoracic disc herniations are rare, comprising only 1% to 2% of all disc herniations.[44] When they do occur, they are seen most often in the lower thoracic spine, likely the result of the increased mobility and load in this region. They can also be seen in association with Scheuermann's disease. Sagittal T2-weighted images show thoracic disc herniations, and axial T2-weighted images allow for additional characterization of the size, location, and morphology of the lesion (**Fig. 11.29**).

Schmorl's Nodes

Schmorl's nodes represent herniations of the intervertebral disc through weak areas in the adjacent vertebral end plates

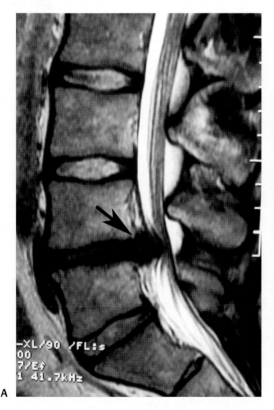

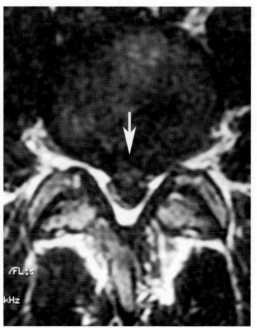

Fig. 11.24 Central disc protrusion. Sagittal **(A)** and axial **(B)** T2-weighted images showing a central disc protrusion (*arrow on each*) at the L4-L5 level.

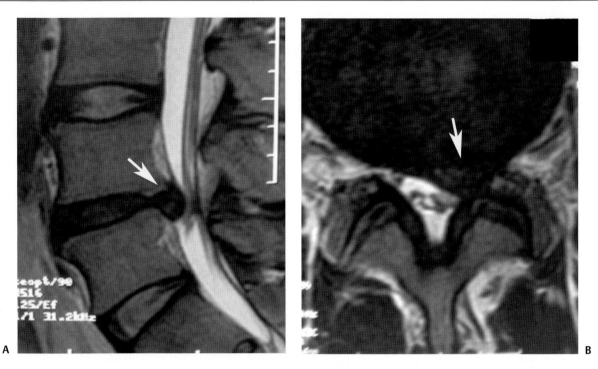

Fig. 11.25 Posterolateral disc protrusion. Sagittal **(A)** and axial **(B)** T2-weighted images showing a left posterolateral disc protrusion (*arrow on each*) at the L4-L5 level that is in the subarticular zone.

and into the vertebral body.[45] They are found most commonly in the thoracic and lumbar spine and occur in approximately 10% of the population, with no dependency on age or gender.[46] Scheuermann's kyphosis is one of several processes that is associated with Schmorl's nodes and premature disc degeneration. Patients may be asymptomatic or have nonspecific pain that may not be directly related to the presence of the Schmorl's node. When symptoms are the result of

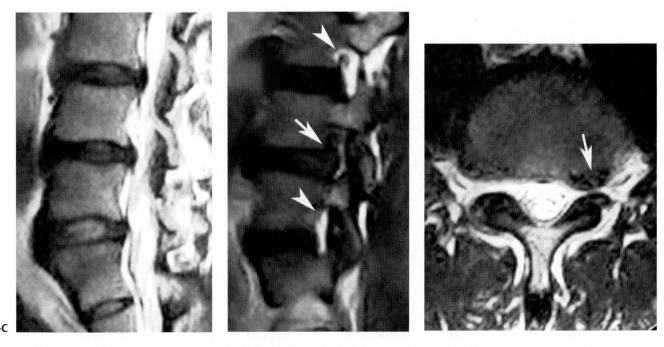

Fig. 11.26 Foraminal disc protrusion. **(A)** A sagittal T2-weighted image showing disc bulges at the L3-L4, L4-L5, and L5-S1 levels. **(B)** A parasagittal T2-weighted image at the level of the neural foramen shows disc material (*arrow*) within the left L4-L5 foramen with resultant compression of the exiting nerve root. Note the patency of the neural foramen at the L3-L4 and L5-S1 levels (*arrowheads*). **(C)** An axial T2-weighted image at the L4-L5 level showing a left-side disc protrusion (*arrow*) in the foraminal zone.

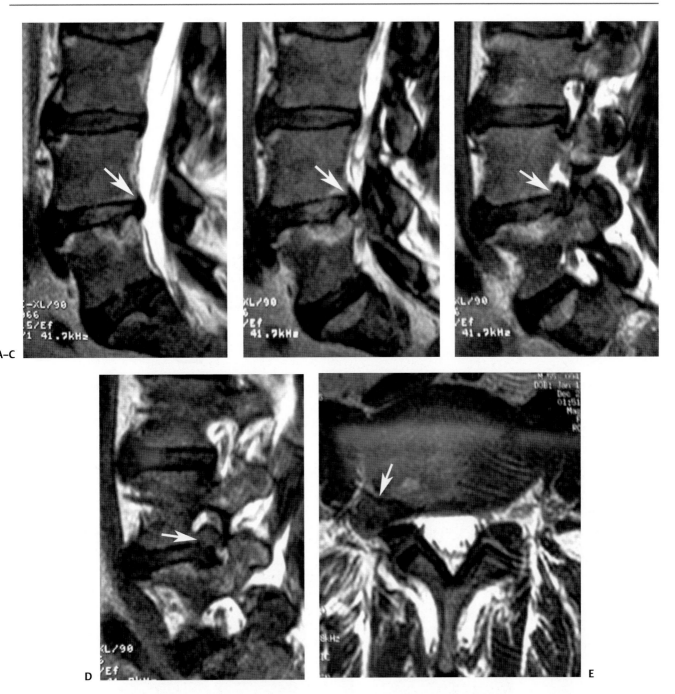

Fig. 11.27 Far lateral disc protrusion. Sagittal T2-weighted images obtained in the midline **(A)**, a few millimeters lateral to midline **(B)**, at the level of the pedicle **(C)**, and lateral to the pedicle and foramen **(D)** show a right-side far lateral disc herniation that is seen primarily on **D** (*arrow on each*) at the L4-L5 level. **(E)** The axial T2-weighted image confirms that the disc protrusion is in the far lateral zone (*arrow*).

the Schmorl's node(s), the patient may present with axial back pain. MRI allows for the optimal detection of Schmorl's nodes (**Fig. 11.29**); they appear as extensions of disc material (with direct continuity with the disc) into the vertebral body, surrounded by a rim of low signal intensity second-ary to reactive sclerosis.[33] Cases in which the Schmorl's node is associated with increased T2-weighted signal in the adjacent bone marrow are more commonly associated with back pain and may represent an acute or subacute Schmorl's node.[43,47]

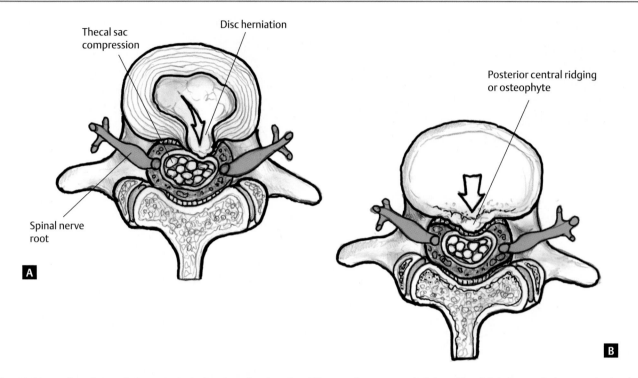

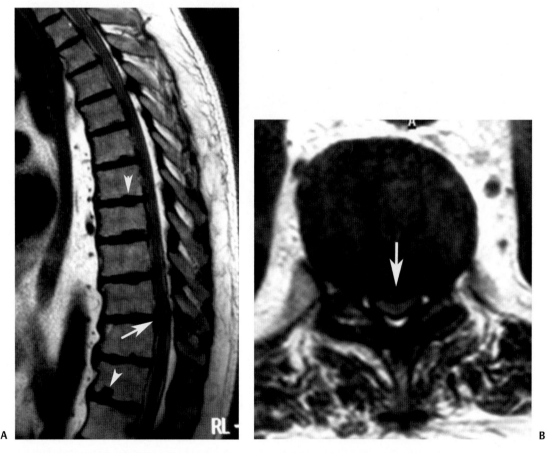

Fig. 11.28 Lumbar disc pathology. Artist's sketches showing the difference between soft **(A)** and hard **(B)** disc pathology in the lumbar spine. The *arrow* on each indicates the direction of herniation.

Fig. 11.29 Thoracic disc protrusion and stenosis. Sagittal **(A)** and axial **(B)** T2-weighted images showing moderate-severe stenosis at the T10-T11 level secondary to a moderate-sized central disc protru-sion (*arrows on each*) and underlying degenerative stenosis. Note the multilevel degenerative disc disease at other levels and the Schmorl's nodes (**A,** *arrowheads*).

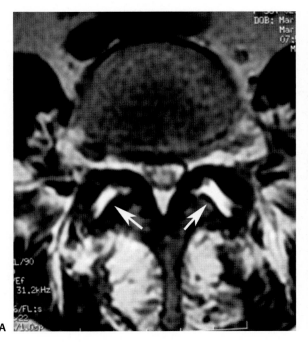
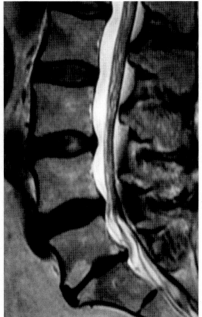

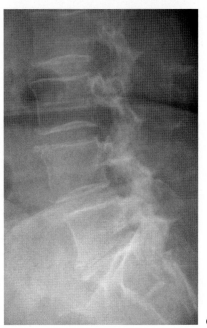

Fig. 11.30 Facet arthropathy and dynamic instability. **(A)** An axial T2-weighted image at the L4-L5 level showing bilateral facet arthropathy with fluid within and distending the L4-L5 facet joints (*arrows*). **(B)** A sagittal T2-weighted image (obtained with the patient in a supine position) shows evidence of stenosis at this level and also suggests the possibility of a subtle L4-L5 spondylolisthesis. Advanced degenerative disc disease is also seen at the L5-S1 level. **(C)** A standing lateral radiograph shows an obvious Meyerding grade 1 spondylolisthesis at the L4-L5 level. This series of images shows that degenerative changes and excessive fluid within the facet joints may be associated with instability; given that MRI is performed with the patient in the supine position, the spondylolisthesis may not be seen on the sagittal MR images.

Facets

Facet Arthropathy

Although it is now accepted that the facet joints may be a cause of pain in the degenerated spine, it is difficult to associate them with a particular clinical syndrome.[48–50] One of the earliest MRI findings of facet arthropathy is seen as fluid-like intraarticular signal intensity on sagittal or axial T2-weighted images (**Fig. 11.30**). Renfrew and Heithoff[22] described a practical and simple way to assess facet arthropathy:

- Mild: mild undulation of the margins with small (1- to 3-mm) osteophytes, minimal subchondral sclerosis,

mild narrowing of articular cartilage, and <25% increase in facet joint transverse dimension (**Fig. 11.31A**)
- Moderate: more pronounced changes, osteophytes up to 3 to 5 mm, and 25% to 50% increase in facet transverse dimension (**Fig. 11.31B**)
- Severe: additional progression of disease with near complete loss of cartilage, osteophytes >5 mm, and joint width >50% of expected transverse dimension (**Fig. 11.31C**)

Facet joint hypertrophy may cause canal, subarticular recess, or foraminal stenosis and neural compromise. Effusions may also be seen within facet joints, reflecting synovi-

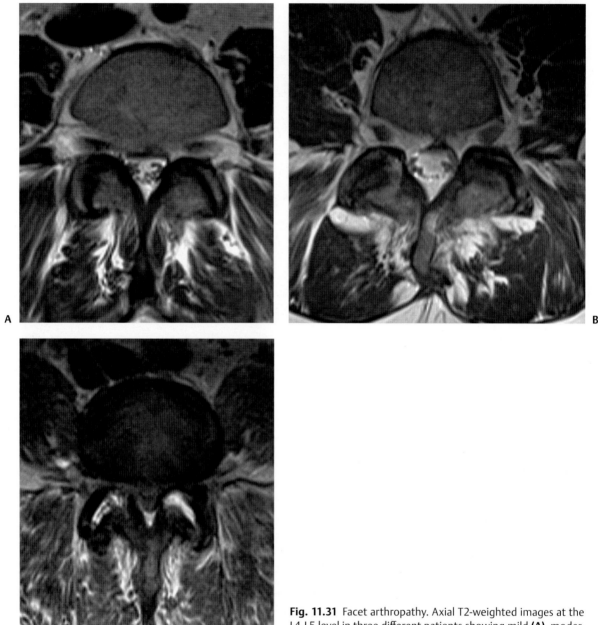

Fig. 11.31 Facet arthropathy. Axial T2-weighted images at the L4-L5 level in three different patients showing mild **(A)**, moderate **(B)**, and severe **(C)** facet arthropathy.

tis from osteoarthritis or a synovial proliferative process in an inflammatory arthritis. Finally, asymmetric facet disease may predispose to degenerative disc disease and eventual scoliosis.[51–53]

Synovial Cyst

A synovial cyst, which originates most commonly from lumbar facet joints, also may cause neural compression and may appear on a sagittal T2-weighted image as a hyperintense

cyst with a hypointense rim (**Fig. 11.32**). T2-weighted MR images in the axial plane show the degree of lateral recess stenosis. Neural foramen stenosis may arise from a reduction in the height of the neural foramen because of degenerative narrowing of the intervertebral disc space, facet-joint hypertrophy and osteophyte formation, or posterolateral encroachment from the disc in the form of bulges, protrusions, and extrusions. This compression is evaluated best on far lateral parasagittal T1-weighted and T2-weighted images that visualize the neural foramina in cross section.[54] On

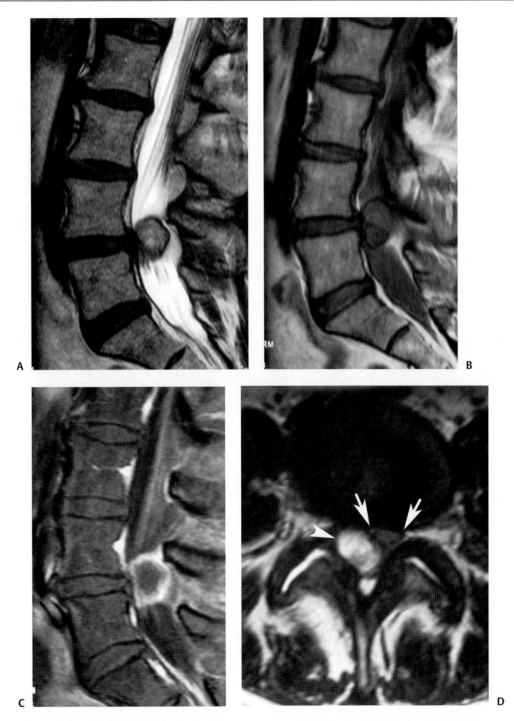

Fig. 11.32 Lumbar synovial cyst. Sagittal T2-weighted **(A)**, T1-weighted **(B)**, and postgadolinium fat-suppressed T1-weighted **(C)** images showing a large L4-L5 lesion compatible with a facet joint cyst when correlated with the axial T2-weighted image **(D)**. Note the intense peripheral enhancement of the lesion on **C**, the postgadolin-ium T1-weighted image. **(D)** The axial T2-weighted image shows that the cyst (*arrowhead*) likely originates from the right L4-L5 facet joint and that the thecal sac (*between arrows*) is severely compressed and shifted toward the left.

occasion, synovial cysts may contain air or may calcify, in which case they may not have the typical bright fluid signal on T2-weighted images and may appear gray or dark on all sequences.

Lumbar Spinal Stenosis

The term *spinal stenosis* describes the compression of the neural elements in the spinal canal, lateral recesses, or neural

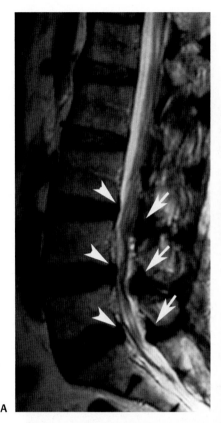

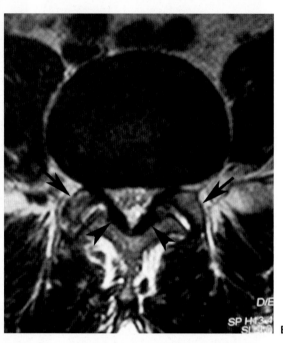

Fig. 11.33 Degenerative upon congenital lumbar stenosis. **(A)** A sagittal T2-weighted image showing multilevel degenerative disc disease at L3-L4, L4-L5, and L5-S1 with evidence of stenosis from disc bulges at these levels (*arrowheads*), ligamentum flavum hypertrophy (*arrows*), and a generalized narrow appearance of the spinal canal relative to the AP diameter of the vertebral bodies. **(B)** An axial T2-weighted image at the L4-L5 level shows minimal to moderate stenosis secondary to underlying congenital stenosis with superimposed degenerative changes, including ligamentum flavum hypertrophy (*arrowheads*) and facet arthropathy *(arrows).*

foramina. The evaluation of patients with known or suspected lumbar spinal stenosis is one of the primary indications for MRI of the lumbar spine. Patients with lumbar stenosis typically present with combinations of radicular leg pain or weakness, neurogenic claudication, and low back pain. After nonoperative management fails for such patients and conventional radiographs have been obtained, MRI can be considered. The MR images should be evaluated to determine the degree (i.e., mild to severe), level (i.e., L1 to S1), and type (e.g., degenerative, congenital) of lumbar spinal stenosis.

The authors' suggested method for the assessment of lumbar spinal stenosis begins with a systematic evaluation of the midsagittal T2-weighted images. These images show the conus medullaris in the patient without scoliosis. The clinician or radiologist should carefully trace the posterior margin of the vertebral bodies and intervening discs to ensure that there is no effacement of the CSF space. Next, the dorsal margin of the thecal sac should be evaluated on these images to evaluate for focal hypertrophy of the ligamentum flavum. This procedure should be repeated on the parasagittal T2-weighted images in each direction (left and right from center) to evaluate for lateral recess and foraminal stenosis. After the sagittal T2-weighted images have been evaluated, the axial T2-weighted images are sequentially evaluated from the sacrum toward the upper lumbar spine. Specifically, CSF should be seen ventral to the cauda equina, which is often displaced posteriorly within the spinal canal, given that most studies are obtained with the patient in a supine position. The lateral recess and foraminal region should be evaluated bilaterally at each level to rule out stenosis secondary to disc, facet, or ligamentum flavum pathology.

Spinal stenosis may involve the neural foramina, lateral recesses, or central canal of the lumbosacral spine and is usually developmental or acquired in nature. Developmental spinal stenosis, which constitutes approximately 15% of all cases of spinal stenosis, is hereditary-idiopathic or associated with disorders of skeletal growth.[54] MRI of the hereditary form shows minor hypoplasia of the posterior osseous

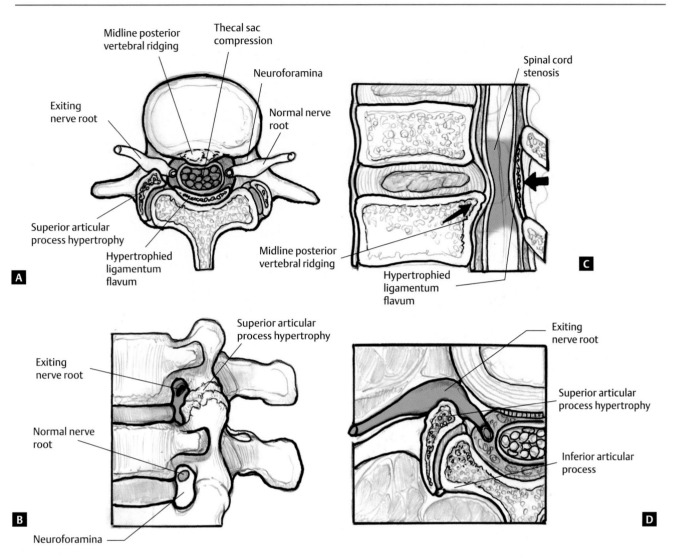

Fig. 11.34 Artist's sketches illustrating the anatomic changes that lead to lumbar stenosis. **(A)** An axial view. **(B)** A midline sagittal view. **(C)** A parasagittal view at the level of the neural foramina. **(D)** A magnified axial view showing the left lateral recess and foramen.

arch of the vertebrae, short pedicles, and narrowing of the cross-sectional area of the central spinal canal (**Fig. 11.33**). Sagittal images may show progressive narrowing of the AP dimension of the spine in the caudal direction, indicating developmental spinal stenosis.

Acquired central spinal canal stenosis may arise from hypertrophic or degenerative changes of the intervertebral discs, facet joints, or ligamentum flavum (**Fig. 11.34**). On MRI, central canal stenosis is characterized by compression of the thecal sac, best seen on sagittal and axial T2-weighted images. Fat-suppressed T2-weighted and STIR images provide a "myelographic effect," in which the CSF is seen as bright signal anterior and posterior to the neural elements on sagittal and axial images. Effacement, discontinuity, or displacement of this CSF space is seen in patients with focal and concentric spinal stenosis (**Fig. 11.35**).

There are several objective measures of lumbar spinal stenosis.[55,56] Hamanishi et al.[55] found that a cross-sectional area of <100 mm^2 at more than two of three lumbar intervertebral levels was highly associated with the presence of intermittent neurogenic claudication. Speciale et al.[56] evaluated observer variability in assessing lumbar spinal stenosis on MRI in relation to cross-sectional spinal canal area and found only a fair level of agreement among the observers; however, they found that the ability of the various readers to predict the degree of central stenosis was high.

Although such formal measurements of lumbar stenosis on MRI are well known, most clinicians and radiologists tend to grade the degree of spinal stenosis as mild, moderate, or severe. The authors use the following terms and definitions:

• Mild: stenosis in which the canal begins to assume a triangular shape, the thecal sac is not compressed, and

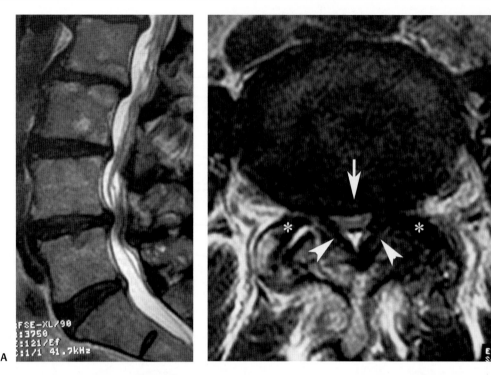

Fig. 11.35 Lumbar stenosis. **(A)** A sagittal T2-weighted image showing multilevel stenosis in the lumbar spine. **(B)** An axial T2-weighted image at the L4-L5 level shows moderate-severe stenosis secondary to contributions from a central disc bulge (*arrow*), ligamentum flavum hypertrophy (*arrowheads*), and facet arthropathy (*asterisks*).

there is only minimal (<2 mm) thickening of the ligamentum flavum. The AP canal diameter is >75% of expected normal without nerve root crowding.
- Moderate: findings similar to those of mild stenosis but with compression and minimal flattening and deformity of the thecal sac. The AP canal diameter is between 50% and 75% of expected normal.
- Severe: advanced stenosis with very pronounced flattening and deformity of the thecal sac that is obvious on both sagittal and axial T2-weighted images. The ligamentum flavum is often thickened to >4 mm. The AP canal diameter is <50% of expected normal.

It should be noted that in some cases, canal narrowing can be downgraded if there is ample CSF surrounding the neural structures and upgraded if the surrounding CSF is scant. Similar terminology can be applied to grading stenosis in the subarticular recesses or foramina.

In addition to evaluating the degree of central and canal stenosis, the lateral recess, foraminal, and extraforaminal zones should also be specifically assessed (**Fig. 11.23**). Lateral recess and foraminal stenosis are most often the result of a combination of pathology: facet arthropathy, ligamentum flavum hypertrophy, and disc bulge or protrusion. Specifically, hypertrophy of the superior articular process from the caudal level often leads to the development of foraminal stenosis. In

addition, degenerative disc disease with the associated loss of disc height and subsequent loss of foraminal height and volume can lead to the development or exacerbation of foraminal stenosis from other degenerative pathologies. Many clinicians and radiologists evaluate for the presence of foraminal stenosis in the axial plane. However, parasagittal images are also quite useful in confirming the presence of foraminal stenosis (**Figs. 11.26** and **11.27**). The normal foramen has an ovoid configuration on parasagittal images (see Chapter 2) where the superior aspect of the foramen contains the exiting nerve root and the inferior aspect of the foramen shows high signal intensity on both T1-weighted (from perineural fat) and T2-weighted (from CSF within the nerve root sleeve) images. On parasagittal images, patients with foraminal stenosis have progressive narrowing of the foramen, with resultant compression of the nerve root.

Cauda Equina Syndrome

Cauda equina syndrome is typically characterized by unilateral or bilateral sciatica, perianal or saddle anesthesia, bowel and bladder incontinence, and sensory and motor deficits in the lower extremities.[57] Often, it is caused by a space-occupying mass compressing against the cauda equina and/or conus terminale. There can be numerous etiologies, in-

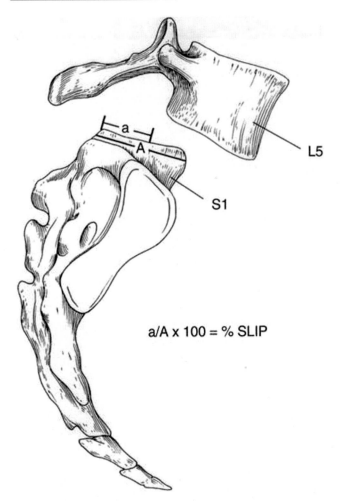

a/A x 100 = % SLIP

Fig. 11.36 Artist's sketch of the Meyerding classification, which is used to quantify the degree of spondylolisthesis. Grade 1 is 0% to 25% slip, grade 2 is 26% to 50% slip, grade 3 is 51% to 75% slip, and grade 4 is 76% to 99% slip. *A* = width of the superior end plate of S1, *a* = distance between the posterior edge of the inferior end plate of L5 and the posterior edge of the superior end plate of S1. (From Cavalier R, Herman MJ, Cheung EV, Pizzutillo PD. Spondylolysis and spondylolisthesis in children and adolescents. I. Diagnosis, natural history, and nonsurgical management. J Am Acad Orthop Surg 2006;14:417–424. This reprinted illustration was modified with permission from Herman MJ, Pizzutillo PD, Cavalier R. Spondylolysis and spondylolisthesis in the child and adolescent athlete. Orthop Clin North Am 2003;34:461–467. Reprinted with permission.)

cluding disc herniation, severe stenosis, trauma, tumor, or infection.[58,59]

MRI is the preferred imaging modality for the evaluation of the patient with suspected cauda equina syndrome. MRI allows visualization of space-occupying lesions within the spinal canal as well as identification of compression of neural structures. Lumbar myelography with CT of the lumbar spine is indicated in patients who are unable to undergo MRI. Given that the treatment of cauda equina syndrome is urgent decompression, one of these imaging studies should be obtained without delay.

Spondylolisthesis

Spondylolisthesis is defined as anterior displacement of a vertebral body relative to the one caudal to it. Retrolisthesis is seen when the superior vertebral body is displaced posterior to the one caudal to it. Wiltse et al.[60] classified lumbar spondylolisthesis on the basis of etiology: dysplastic, isthmic, degenerative, traumatic, iatrogenic, or pathologic. Meyerding[61] described the various degrees of forward slippage (from grade 1 to grade 4) based on a division of the superior surface of the lower vertebra into quarters (**Fig. 11.36**). According to this system, a complete slip of L5 on S1 is termed *spondyloptosis*. Each manifestation of spondylolisthesis has specific associated MRI findings.

The system of Wiltse et al.[60] details the features of spondylolisthesis as follows:

- *Dysplastic spondylolisthesis*: may present with degeneration and pseudobulging of the lumbosacral disc, with potential compression of the cauda equina between the neural arch of L4 and the superoposterior aspect of the sacrum (for a slip at L5). A parasagittal T1-weighted SE image may show severe compression of the exiting L5 nerve root.
- *Isthmic spondylolisthesis*: sagittal T2-weighted images often show obvious spondylolisthesis at the L5-S1 level (**Fig. 11.37**). Parasagittal images at the level of the pedicle may show compression of the exiting L5 nerve root between the bulging L5-S1 disc and the undersurface of the L5 pedicle, and reduction of foraminal height. The parasagittal images should also be scrutinized for the presence of a pars intraarticularis defect or reparative granulation tissue in that region; CT imaging may help confirm the presence of the pars defect.
- *Degenerative spondylolisthesis*: seen most commonly at the L4-L5 level. MRI can be used to evaluate narrowing of the central canal, lateral recesses, and neural foramina, and compression of the cauda equina and exiting nerve roots. Facet joint cysts are not uncommon in the presence of degenerative spondylisthesis. Sagittal and axial T2-weighted images delineate these entities clearly (**Fig. 11.38**).
- *Traumatic spondylolisthesis*: MRI shows the associated soft-tissue injury, which may include rupture of the intervertebral disc and posterior ligamentous complex, as seen with bilateral facet dislocation (**Fig. 11.9**).
- *Pathologic spondylolisthesis*: MRI shows very focal changes at the level of the pars intraarticularis based on the specific pathology involved.
- *Iatrogenic spondylolisthesis*: may occur after laminectomy, facetectomy, and extensive resection of the

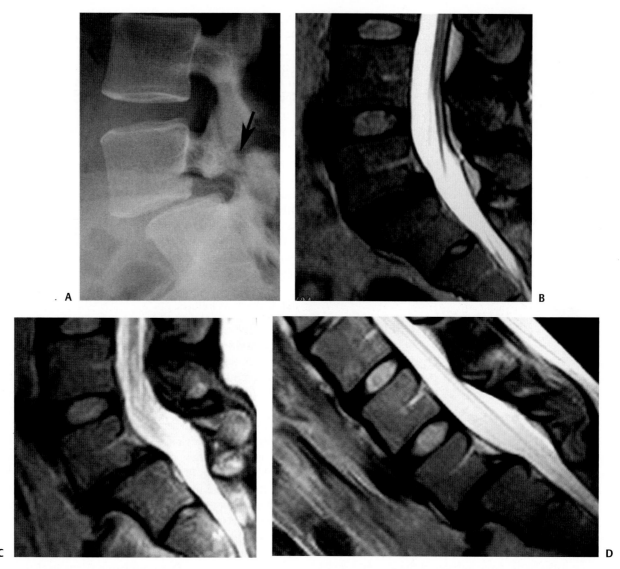

Fig. 11.37 Isthmic spondylolisthesis. **(A)** A lateral radiograph showing bilateral pars intraarticularis defects (*arrow*) at the L5-S1 level with Meyerding grade 2 spondylolisthesis. **(B)** A sagittal T2-weighted MR image obtained on a closed system with the same patient in a supine position showing grade 1 spondylolisthesis. **(C)** A sagittal T2-weighted MR image obtained on an open MRI system with the patient in a standing position shows that the spondylolisthesis progresses to grade 2. **(D)** A sagittal T2-weighted image obtained on an open MRI system with the patient in a flexed position shows that the grade 2 spondylolisthesis progresses compared with images in the neutral **(C)** and supine **(B)** positions.

facet joint and neural arch without fusion. MRI shows changes directly correlated to the specific areas altered during surgery.

Recently, the focus in spondylolisthesis has moved beyond the slippage of the vertebral bodies to include, among other issues, its etiologic factors and spinopelvic alignment. This change in focus has led to the development of more comprehensive classification systems that may be better at pre-dicting progression of the disease, especially in younger individuals.[62–64]

Scoliosis

Scoliosis is a lateral curvature of the vertebral column in the coronal plane involving lateral and rotational vectors, and it may be associated with spinal cord or other neuronal abnormalities that are best visualized with MRI before op-

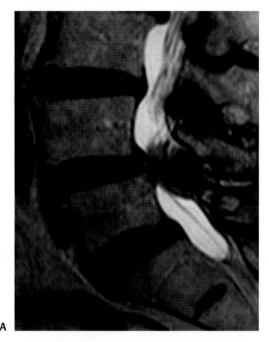

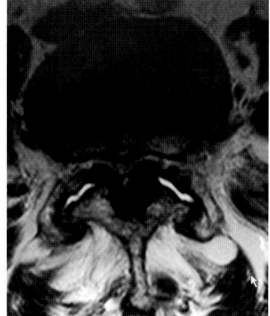

A   B

Fig. 11.38 Degenerative spondylolisthesis. **(A)** A sagittal T2-weighted image showing Meyerding grade 1 spondylolisthesis at the L4-L5 level with severe stenosis and evidence of a high-intensity zone at the posterior annulus of the L4-L5 disc. **(B)** An axial T2-weighted image showing severe stenosis from a central disc bulge, ligamentum flavum hypertrophy, and facet arthropathy.

erative intervention. The most common indication for MRI in patients with scoliosis is degenerative scoliosis. In this scenario, MRI is obtained to evaluate for the presence, degree, and levels of stenosis. Because of the unique challenge of obtaining contiguous visualization of the spinal canal content in the scoliotic spine, specific protocols should be followed to obtain the best views. Redla et al.[65] described the use of sagittal T1-weighted SE and T2-weighted FSE sequences, beginning from above the foramen magnum and including the brainstem down to the sacrum. However, for typical thoracolumbar scoliosis, MR images are obtained of the thoracic and lumbar spine only. When the curve is severe, sagittal sequences are obtained parallel to the two major portions of the curve and are planned from the coronal plane. Axial T1-weighted images are obtained through the apices of the curve, providing a second view of the cord. A coronal T1-weighted sequence also is obtained, especially to assess the vertebral bodies for congenital anomalies. In patients with degenerative stenosis, the sagittal and axial T2-weighted images should be evaluated in correlation with each other to determine the degree and type of stenosis at each level (**Fig. 11.39**). This information helps determine the levels for decompression in a patient who is being considered for surgical intervention.

Aside from the evaluation of the patient with lumbar degenerative scoliosis and suspected stenosis, the indications for MRI in patients with scoliosis have been the subject of debate (see Chapter 13). Although some studies have shown that routine MRI is not indicated for patients with adolescent idiopathic scoliosis who have a typical right thoracic curve and who are neurologically intact,[66-68] others have found a high incidence of spinal cord abnormalities (17.6% to 26%[65,69]) in patients with infantile and juvenile forms of scoliosis. Those studies stressed the importance of MRI in children younger than 11 years old. Spinal cord abnormality is suggested by several physical examination findings, including a left thoracic curve, absent abdominal reflexes, lower limb neurologic deficits, and cutaneous stigmata of occult spinal dysraphism.[65]

Specific MRI findings for abnormalities seen with scoliosis secondary to an underlying neurologic abnormality include the following:

- Tethered cord: thickened filum terminale and spinal lipoma seen on sagittal T1-weighted SE and T2-weighted FSE images
- Syringohydromyelia: dissection of CSF through the cord substance best seen on T2-weighted images with increased signal within the cord, sometimes associated with sacculation
- Diastematomyelia: a midline sagittal cleft of the spinal cord most commonly involving the lower thoracic and lumbar region, seen as two hemicords on MRI, with each having a single dorsal and ventral horn and a septum seen from the dorsal aspect of the vertebral body and extending into the cleft between the cords

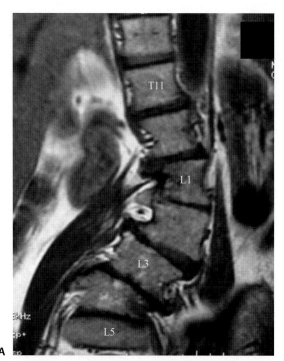

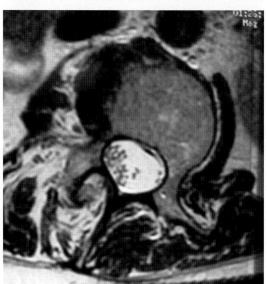

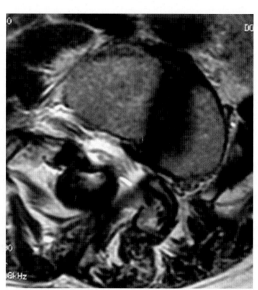

Fig. 11.39 Scoliosis. **(A)** A coronal T1-weighted image showing advanced thoracolumbar degenerative scoliosis that is primarily left convex with the apex of the curve at the L2 level. **(B)** An axial T2-weighted image at the L2 level showing rotation of the vertebral body but no substantial stenosis. **(C)** An axial T2-weighted image at the L3-L4 level showing rotation of the vertebral body level and moderate-severe stenosis secondary to degenerative changes.

- Neurofibromatosis: a congenital condition that may show dural ectasia, pseudomeningocele, and neurofibromas on MRI
- Pars defects: a common occurrence in patients with developmental scoliosis; may occur in up to 6.2% of patients with idiopathic scoliosis[70]

Epidural Lipomatosis

Epidural lipomatosis is a condition in which there is excessive deposition of fat in the epidural space that, in turn, leads to spinal stenosis and neural compression. The syndrome is primarily associated with excessive glucocorticoid levels, which may be exogenous or endogenous but also may be spontaneous or idiopathic.[71–73] In the lumbar spine, epidural fat surrounding and compressing the thecal sac is the key finding. In the thoracic spine, the presence of >6 mm of fat posterior to the cord is diagnostic. The characteristic feature of lumbar epidural lipomatosis is the presence of epidural tissue that follows the signal characteristics of subcutaneous fat on all pulse sequences, including fat-suppressed sequences (**Fig. 11.40**). The primary differential consideration includes an intraspinal lipoma, which is typically focal and is often located in the anterior

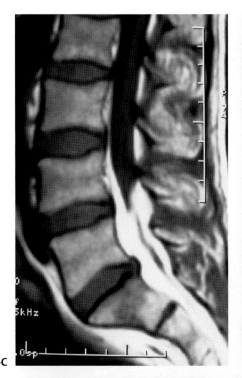
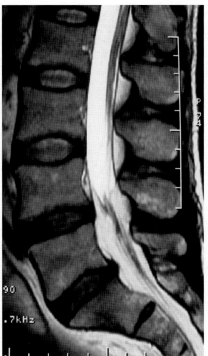
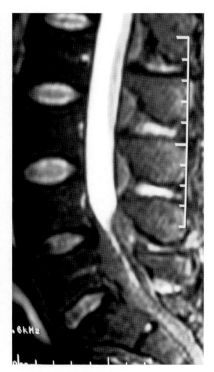

A–C

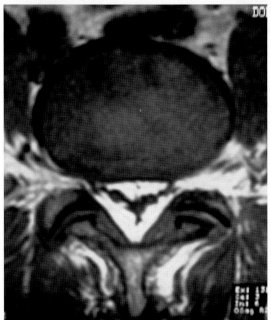

D

Fig. 11.40 Lumbar epidural lipomatosis. Sagittal T1-weighted **(A)**, T2-weighted **(B)**, and STIR **(C)** images showing advanced lumbar epidural lipomatosis extending from L4 to the sacrum with circumferential compression of the thecal sac. Note that the lipomatous tissue is most obvious on the T1-weighted image, blends in with the CSF on the T2-weighted image, and suppresses (becomes dark) on the STIR image. **(D)** An axial T1-weighted image at the L4-L5 level shows severe compression of the thecal sac by the extensive lumbar epidural lipomatosis.

thoracic spine.[74] Other epidural abnormalities tend to have a low T1-weighted signal and can be excluded.

■ Infectious Conditions

Vertebral Osteomyelitis

Cases of vertebral osteomyelitis comprise between 2% and 4% of all skeletal infections.[75,76] MRI is usually regarded as the imaging modality of choice for the detection of this process, with a sensitivity of >82% and a specificity of 53% to 94%.[77] Infection involving the vertebral body occurs through one of three primary routes[78]:

- Hematogenous (most common)
- Direct inoculation through surgery or penetrating trauma
- Contiguous spread from an adjacent soft-tissue infection

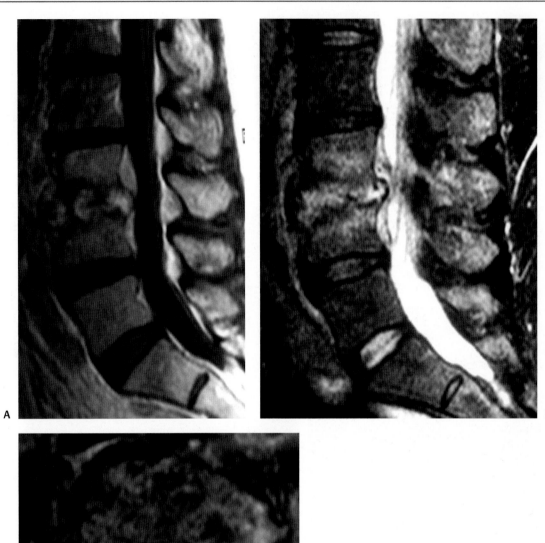

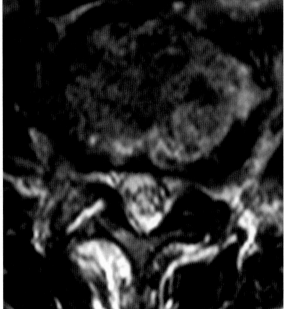

Fig. 11.41 Vertebral osteomyelitis and discitis. Sagittal postgadolinium T1-weighted **(A)** and STIR **(B)** images showing enhancement and increased signal within the L3-L4 disc space and edema within the adjacent vertebral bodies in a patient with infectious symptoms and findings. **(C)** An axial T2-weighted image at the L3-L4 disc level also shows heterogeneous and increased signal within the disc space compatible with discitis.

Hematogenous seeding occurs through nutrient arterioles of the vertebral bodies or by retrograde spread through the paravertebral venous plexus of Batson.[78–80] Infection then spreads from the vertebral body and marrow to the contiguous intervertebral disc and adjacent vertebral body, often sparing the central portion of the vertebral bodies.[78,80]

The general MRI signal changes in patients with osteomyelitis include the following:

- Decreased signal intensity of the intervertebral disc and adjacent vertebral bodies, with a discernible margin between the two on T1-weighted images
- Increased signal intensity of vertebral bodies adjacent to the involved disc on T2-weighted images
- An abnormal configuration and increased signal intensity of the intervertebral disc with loss of the nuclear cleft on T2-weighted images[76,81] (**Fig. 11.41**)

Gadolinium enhancement may be seen in adjacent vertebral bodies. However, gadolinium also may cause edematous marrow to blend in with the normal fatty marrow.[82] Combining fat-suppressed T1-weighted images with gadolinium contrast enhancement eliminates this problem.[81] STIR images may also be used for the MRI evaluation of osteomyelitis because they suppress the high signal intensity from fat and provide increased contrast.[83] STIR image are especially useful when combined with the anatomic detail from T1-weighted sequences.

The pattern of vertebral body involvement in vertebral osteomyelitis should be differentiated from that in patients with spinal tumors (see Chapter 12). Patients with vertebral osteomyelitis tend to have the epicenter of the pathologic change at the disc space, and those with tumors tend to have the epicenter at the vertebral body. In other words, infectious processes are based at and cross the disc space, whereas neoplastic processes are typically based in the vertebral body and do not cross the disc space.

Discitis

Disc infection often causes edema, which leads to hyperintensity of the disc and the end plate on T2-weighted images; it also causes loss of definition of the vertebral end plates, inflammatory changes in the adjacent vertebral marrow, and gadolinium enhancement within the disc.[33,84,85] In addition, it is not uncommon to have an associated paraspinal inflammatory mass.

Spondylodiscitis, which essentially is discitis with vertebral osteomyelitis, may be seen after lumbar disc surgery. It also may be seen after discography or myelography.[86] Postoperative spondylodiscitis is believed to occur in 0.1% to 3% of patients.[86] Intraoperative contamination usually is the most common mechanism for infection. The most common infecting organisms are *Staphylococcus epidermidis* and *Staphylococcus aureus*. MR images often show Modic type 1 changes at the level of the operated disc (vertebral end plate with decreased signal on T1-weighted images and increased signal intensity on T2-weighted images) and enhancement of the disc when contrast is used (**Fig. 11.42**). No enhancing tissue should be seen outside the intervertebral space. Normal vertebral bone marrow has low signal on T1-weighted images and high signal intensity on T2-weighted and contrast-enhanced images.[86] If a rim of soft tissue around the affected intervertebral space is noted to enhance, concern about septic spondylodiscitis arises, which can be ruled out with disc biopsy.

Epidural Abscess

An epidural abscess is a purulent epidural collection of material without involvement of the vertebral body or the disc space. Such collections are usually located anteriorly in the spinal canal and originate from the posterior aspect of the vertebral body and disc space. If the abscess originates from hematogenous sources, then it may be associated with a positive blood culture. MRI is very sensitive in the detection of these abscesses.[82] MRI also is useful in visualizing phlegmon and epidural abscesses, which usually are isointense or hypointense compared with the spinal cord on T1-weighted images and which usually have high signal intensity on T2-weighted images[83,86] (**Fig. 11.43**). The differentiation of epidural abscess and CSF may be difficult, necessitating gadolinium enhancement for better visualization. The high signal intensity of the enhancing mass can be distinguished easily from the lower signal intensity of the CSF and spine on T1-weighted images.[86] Sometimes fat suppression is necessary to differentiate an abscess from epidural fat.[86] Contrast enhancement also can aid in differentiating between epidural phlegmon and an abscess; dense homogeneous enhancement of the mass suggests phlegmon, whereas peripheral or ring enhancement of the mass suggests an abscess. Paraspinal abscesses, also well visualized with MRI, usually have low signal intensity on T1-weighted images and are commonly associated with swelling of the psoas on T1-weighted images and increased signal on T2-weighted images. Gadolinium-enhanced images provide additional abscess delineation.[86]

Tuberculosis

Tuberculosis has reappeared in the developed world because of the emergence of AIDS; 5% of all cases of tuberculosis affect the musculoskeletal system.[87]

Tuberculosis usually results from hematogenous seeding. The rich vascular supply of the vertebral bodies makes the spine susceptible to infection. A vertebral body receives its blood supply inferiorly from the ascending branch of the posterior spinal artery and superiorly from the descending

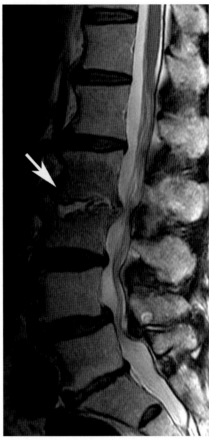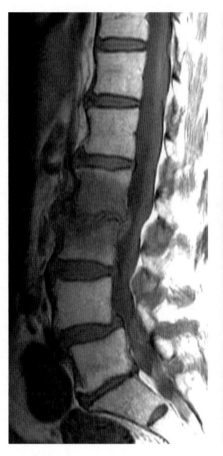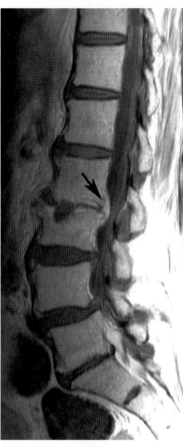

A–C

Fig. 11.42 Discitis. Sagittal T2-weighted **(A)**, T1-weighted **(B)**, and postgadolinium T1-weighted **(C)** images show the typical findings of discitis at the L2-L3 level (*arrows on* **A** *and* **C**). Note the increase in signal at the disc space on the T2-weighted image, the decrease in signal on the T1-weighted image, and the postgadolinium enhancement of the small epidural component (**C**, *arrow*).

branch of this artery. These two arteries anastomose and create a network of vessels in the anterior epidural space. The network then leads to three or four arteries that enter the vertebral body through the nutrient foramen. Children are at an increased risk for discitis because they still have an arterial anastomosis between the vertebral end plate and the disc.[87] The intervertebral disc becomes less vascularized in adolescence. Arteries end within the vertebral bodies, which result in increased rates of infection within the bodies.[87]

Tuberculous osteomyelitis usually involves the ventral trabecular bone marrow adjacent to the intervertebral disc, and it spreads via the anterior longitudinal ligament to adjacent vertebral bodies.[86] MRI signs of tuberculosis infection are hypointense signal on T1-weighted images and hyperintense signal on T2-weighted images seen in the subchondral tissue. There also may be a hyperintense signal within the disc on T2-weighted images (**Fig. 11.44**). As the disease progresses, it may lead to collapse of vertebral bodies, with an associated epidural abscess. Continuous destruction of the anterior cortices of single or contiguous vertebral bodies can lead to kyphotic deformity. Tuberculosis may also directly involve the spinal cord, a condition termed *tuberculosis myelitis*; it is usually seen in individuals younger than 30 years old. MRI with gadolinium is the best imaging modality for this phenomenon.[87]

It is not uncommon to see paraspinal involvement with abscess formation. Gadolinium enhancement usually is seen only in the periphery of abscesses, unlike granulation tissue, which enhances throughout. The observation of disc-space sparing and enhancement of granulation tissue is highly suggestive of tuberculosis.[77]

■ Postoperative MRI Findings

Previously, MRI had been considered to have limited use in evaluating the instrumented spine because of the resultant artifacts that were commonly seen. However, the introduction of titanium pedicle screws and specialized pulse se-

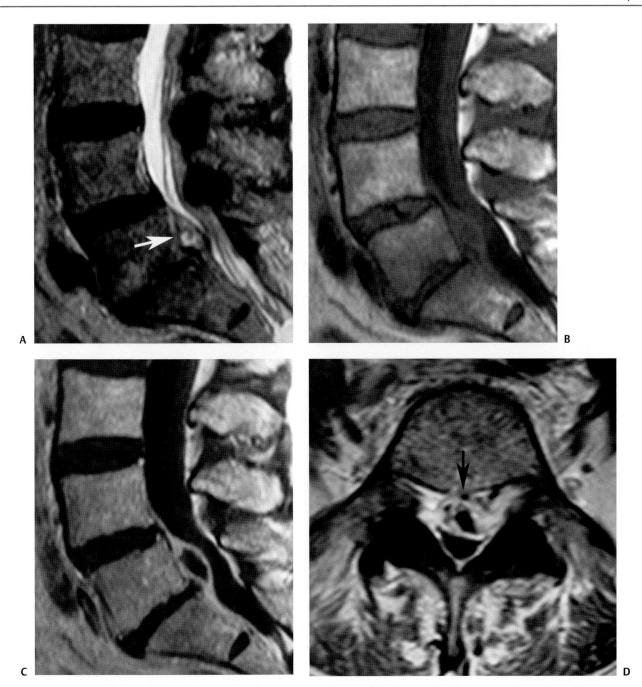

Fig. 11.43 Epidural abscess. **(A)** A sagittal T2-weighted image showing a ventral epidural collection (*arrow*) posterior to the L5 vertebral body in a patient with infectious symptoms and findings. **(B)** A sagittal T1-weighted image shows the same collection. **(C)** A sagittal postgadolinium T1-weighted image shows peripheral enhancement. **(D)** An axial postgadolinium T1-weighted image shows the ventral epidural collection (*arrow*), again with peripheral enhancement, which is producing moderate-severe stenosis.

quences has improved the MRI visualization of the central spinal contents[88–92] (see also Chapter 16). It is important to note that MRI may not always be the best imaging modality for the evaluation of the postoperative lumbar spine. Conventional radiographs are typically the starting point for the study of patients with an instrumented lumbar fusion, given that they allow for the evaluation of overall spinal alignment, position of instrumentation, and evidence of fusion. CT may be best for more precise determination of the presence or absence of fusion, infection, loosening, and

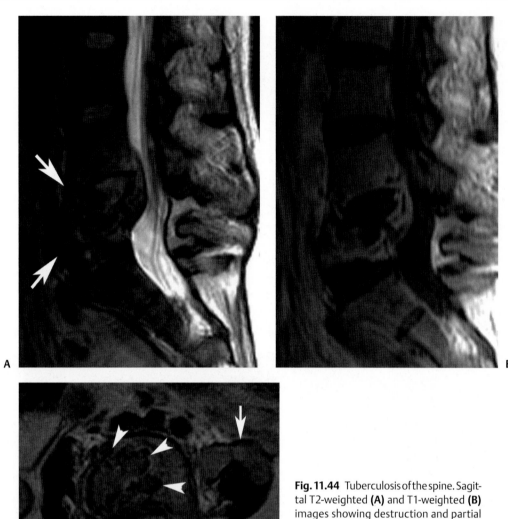

Fig. 11.44 Tuberculosis of the spine. Sagittal T2-weighted **(A)** and T1-weighted **(B)** images showing destruction and partial collapse of the L5 vertebral body (*between arrows on* **A**) with relative preservation of the intervertebral discs. **(C)** An axial T2-weighted image at the L5 level showing signal change within the anterior aspect of the left psoas muscle (*arrow*) compatible with an abscess and also heterogeneous signal within the vertebral body (*arrowheads*).

postoperative fluid collections. The addition of myelography to CT imaging provides excellent determination of the presence and degree of spinal stenosis, or its absence. MRI may be best for evaluating for the presence or absence of infection, postoperative fluid collection (such as hematoma or CSF), recurrent disc herniation, and residual or recurrent stenosis.

Surgical procedures in the spine are typically performed with the following goals in mind:

- Decompression of a stenotic spinal canal or neural foramen
- Removal of herniated disc material
- Stabilization and fusion of motion segments, for existing instability (such as spondylolisthesis, scoliosis, or posttraumatic injury) or after iatrogenic instability (such as with facetectomy or multilevel laminectomies)
- Excision of tumor or infection

Based on the type of surgery performed and the clinical scenario, the spine surgeon and radiologist can use MRI (and other imaging modalities) to evaluate for various postsurgical findings.

After Decompression without Instrumentation/Fusion

Almost all decompressive procedures in the lumbar spine are performed via a posterior approach. These procedures include a midline laminectomy and bilateral foraminotomies, hemilaminotomy with foraminotomy, and hemilaminotomy with discectomy. In most cases, careful review of the sagittal and axial images permits determination of the extent of bone removal during previous surgery(ies). Specifically, one should review the sagittal and axial T2-weighted images, follow the contour of the thecal sac, and look for focal areas of posterior expansion of the thecal sac or for regions of compression of the thecal sac by scar tissue or recurrent/residual disc fragments. The axial T1-weighted images (which show more osseous detail than do T2-weighted images) should be carefully reviewed for areas of postsurgical absence of the osseous structures. If additional information may benefit the surgeon for preoperative planning, CT imaging may be considered.

After discectomy, specific changes may be noted around the affected area, depending on the length of time between surgery and the imaging study. At the level of the disc, a high signal intensity band extending from the nucleus pulposus to the side of annular disruption may be appreciated on T2-weighted images up to 2 months after surgery. Annular enhancement may also be seen. There also may be a component of disc height loss, depending on the aggressiveness of the discectomy. T1-weighted images show increased soft tissue within the anterior epidural space immediately after surgery; an epidural mass effect is observed in 80% of patients.[93] Anterior epidural soft-tissue edema with disruption of the posterior annular margin secondary to disc curettage can mimic the appearance of disc herniation. It can take from 2 to 6 months after surgery for a normal signal to return.[94,95] One should use caution when evaluating MRI studies in the first 6 weeks after surgery because there may be a large amount of tissue disruption and edema, producing a mass effect on the anterior thecal sac.

Nerve root enhancement secondary to breakdown of the blood–nerve barrier is another common finding in the immediate postoperative period. This enhancement decreases by 3 months after surgery and is virtually gone by 6 months.[93,96] Posterior soft-tissue changes continue to be seen up to 3 months after surgery. These changes include disruption and edema of the paraspinal muscles with low signal intensity on T1-weighted images and high signal intensity on T2-weighted images. An enhancing subcutaneous track may be seen with gadolinium enhancement. After 6 months, all of the acute postoperative changes secondary to hemorrhage and edema usually have resolved.[93] The remaining scar tissue shows low to intermediate signal intensity on T1-weighted imaging and hypointensity on T2-weighted imaging.

Unfortunately, recurrent disc herniation is a relatively common occurrence after surgery for a lumbar disc herniation. The reported range for the incidence of recurrent disc herniation is from 2% to 18%, and a large recent meta-analysis has indicated the rate is 7% in patients who undergo limited discectomy and 3.5% in patients who undergo aggressive discectomy.[97] Another recent series found the incidence of recurrent lumbar disc herniation to be 7.1%.[98] MRI can be used to differentiate recurrent disc herniation from scar tissue.[99–103] The importance of making the differentiation between recurrent disc herniation and scar tissue or epidural fibrosis lies in the fact that outcomes for revision surgery for recurrent disc herniation are substantially better than surgery for patients with only scar tissue and no recurrent disc herniation.[104–108] MRI in patients with recurrent disc herniation shows a focal extradural lesion, typically in the posterolateral or lateral recess region, that has peripheral enhancement with a central area of nonenhancement on postgadolinium T1-weighted images (**Fig. 11.45**). Conversely, patients with epidural fibrosis show uniform enhancement of the epidural tissue.

After Instrumentation/Fusion

Stainless steel implants are considered superparamagnetic and produce the greatest degree of image degradation secondary to magnetic susceptibility artifacts.[104] Titanium and tantalum spinal implants, which are not superparamagnetic, produce less artifact than does stainless steel. Even with conventional T2-weighted and T1-weighted pulse sequences, the central canal can be adequately visualized in patients with titanium pedicle screws. These images can allow for the detection of postoperative fluid collections (such as hematoma, seroma, pseudomeningocele, and abscess) and can even accurately show the degree of thecal sac compression from these fluid collections. In addition, the degree of adjacent level stenosis at levels above and below an instrumented lumbar fusion can be seen well on sagittal and axial T2-weighted images (**Fig. 11.46**).

The position of interbody fusion devices (such as those placed for transforaminal lumbar interbody fusion, posterior lumbar interbody fusion, and anterior lumbar interbody fusion) can also be assessed by MRI. These devices should be located within the confines of the interbody space, and the posterior aspect of the interbody device after a transforaminal or posterior lumbar interbody fusion procedure should be positioned within the posterior

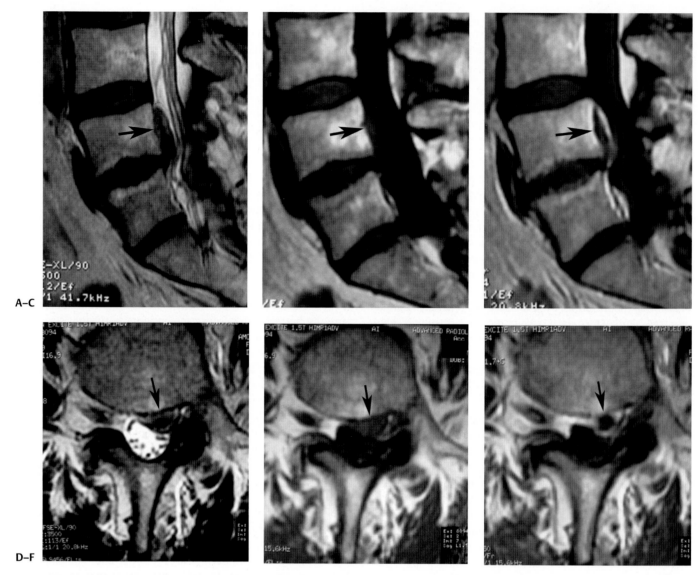

A–C

D–F

Fig. 11.45 Recurrent lumbar disc extrusion. Sagittal T2-weighted **(A)**, T1-weighted **(B)**, and postgadolinium T1-weighted **(C)** images in a patient with a history of previous L4-L5 discectomy showing a large disc extrusion (*arrow on each*) that has migrated proximally and is located behind the L4 vertebral body. Note that the disc is difficult to see on **B**, the T1-weighted image, and shows peripheral enhancement on **C**, the postgadolinium T1-weighted image. Axial T2-weighted **(D)**, T1-weighted **(E)**, and postgadolinium T1-weighted **(F)** images at the L4-L5 level showing the left paracentral extradural lesion (*arrows on each*) that appears to be disc material on **D**, the T2-weighted image, and shows peripheral enhancement on **F**, the postgadolinium T1-weighted image, compared with **E**, the pregadolinium T1-weighted image.

margin of the vertebral body. In cases of posterolateral graft extrusion into the spinal canal or neural foramen, patients often present with severe radicular pain and/or weakness. MR images show the contours of the interbody device compressing the thecal sac or nerve root and the associated inflammatory changes and epidural fibrosis (**Fig. 11.47**).

Hematoma

Postoperative epidural hematoma typically develops within a few days after a posterior lumbar surgery that includes decompression, and it can occur after "small" decompressive procedures, such as a microdiscectomy, as well as after larger procedures, such as multilevel laminectomy

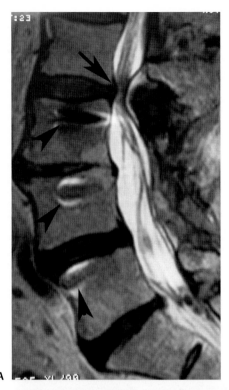

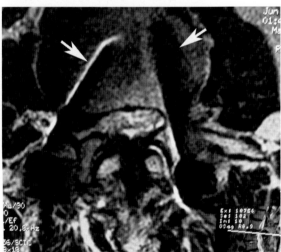

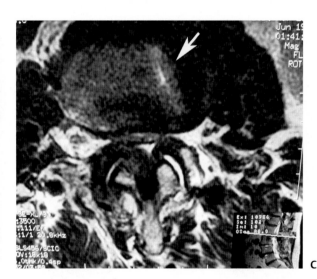

Fig. 11.46 Junctional lumbar stenosis above instrumented fusion. **(A)** A sagittal T2-weighted image showing junctional stenosis (*arrow*) at the L2-L3 level in a patient who has undergone L3-L5 laminectomy and instrumented fusion. Note the minimal artifact from the pedicle screws (*arrowheads*). **(B)** An axial T2-weighted image at the L3 pedicle screw level shows moderate-severe stenosis and also shows the pedicle screws (*arrows*). Note that the presence of the pedicle screws obscures the region of the lateral recess and foramen but does not prevent the evaluation of the status of the central canal. **(C)** An axial T2-weighted image at the L2-L3 level shows severe stenosis and only minimal residual artifact (*arrow*) from the pedicle screw below this level in the L3 vertebral body. Note the localizing sagittal image seen as an inset with each axial image **(B,C)**.

(**Fig. 11.48**) and posterior spinal fusion. Although CT is excellent for visualizing osseous detail and the precise location of spinal instrumentation relative to the spinal canal and neural foramen, MRI is superior for visualizing postoperative fluid collections such as an epidural hematoma and the size, location, and degree of compression of the thecal sac it produces.

Pseudomeningocele

A pseudomeningocele typically occurs in a patient who sustains a durotomy during an open surgical procedure or in a patient who undergoes resection of an intradural lesion. In both of these situations, there may be an incomplete closure of the dural opening, with resultant leakage of CSF into the

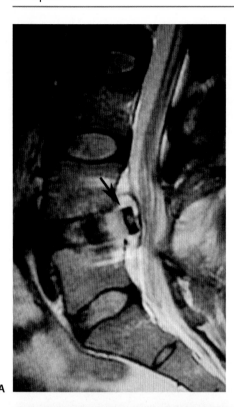

A

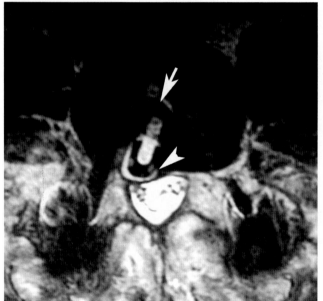

B

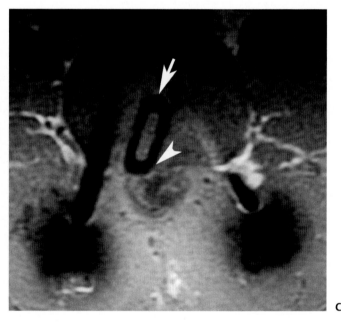

C

Fig. 11.47 Retropulsed interbody device. **(A)** A sagittal T2-weighted image showing retropulsion of an L4-L5 transforaminal interbody device (*arrow*) into the spinal canal. Axial T2-weighted **(B)** and T1-weighted **(C)** images showing that the interbody device (*arrows on each*) is retropulsed beyond the margin of the posterior vertebral body (*arrowhead on each*) and is producing right lateral recess stenosis.

operative site and posterior soft tissues. This collection of CSF is termed a *pseudomeningocele* because it is surrounded not by arachnoid and dura, but rather by a pseudomeninges of reactive fibrous tissue.[104] Pseudomeningoceles typically are well-circumscribed, communicate with the subarachnoid space, and contain fluid that matches the signal char-acteristics of CSF, which is homogeneous and has low signal intensity on T1-weighted images and high signal intensity on T2-weighted images (**Fig. 11.49**). Given that the pressure within a pseudomeningocele is often similar to that of the subarachnoid space, these collections often compress the thecal sac less than do postoperative epidural hematomas.

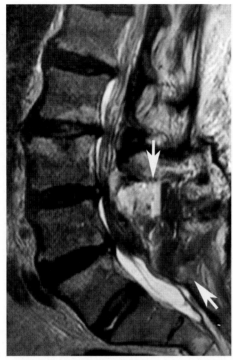

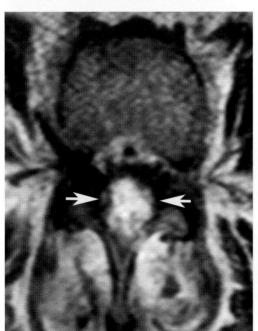

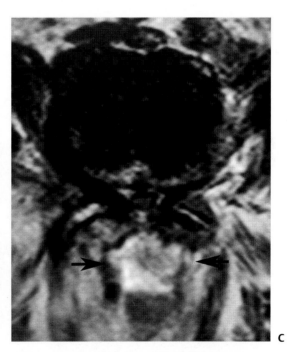

Fig. 11.48 Postoperative lumbar epidural hematoma. **(A)** A sagittal T2-weighted image showing a large and compressive fluid collection (*between large arrows*) at the L3-L5 level in a patient after revision L4-L5 laminectomies. Axial T2-weighted images at the L3-L4 **(B)** and L4-L5 **(C)** levels show the hematoma (*between arrows on each*) and the associated compression of the thecal sac.

Arachnoiditis

Signs of arachnoiditis include central adhesion of the nerve roots within the thecal sac into a central clump of soft-tissue signal (pseudocord) instead of their normal feathery appearance (**Fig. 11.50**), peripheral adh3esion of the nerve roots to the meninges (giving rise to an "empty" thecal sac sign), and an inflammatory mass that fills the thecal sac.[109] Various factors can lead to the development of arachnoiditis, including the trauma of the surgery itself, intradural blood after the repair of a durotomy, previous lumbar puncture, treated perioperative infection, and the previous use of myelographic contrast dye.[104]

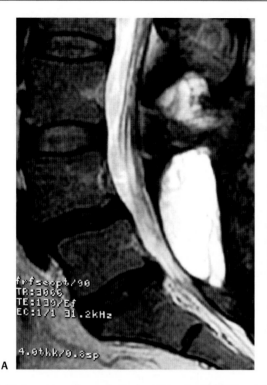
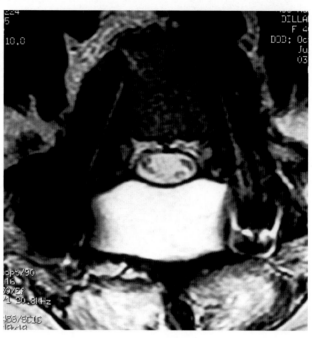

Fig. 11.49 Pseudomeningocele. Sagittal **(A)** and axial **(B)** T2-weighted images of a patient who sustained a durotomy during revision L4-S1 laminectomy and instrumented posterior fusion. The images show a well-circumscribed fluid collection that does not compress the thecal sac. Note that on the axial image **(B)** at the L5 level, the central canal can be well visualized in the presence of pedicle screws.

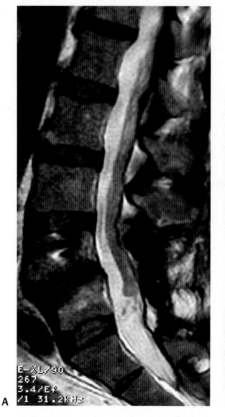
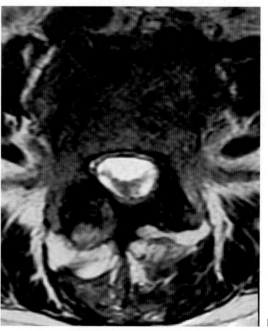

Fig. 11.50 Arachnoiditis. Sagittal **(A)** and axial **(B)** T2-weighted images of a patient after L4-L5 laminectomy and instrumented posterior fusion who had had several previous decompressive surgeries. Note the central adhesion of the nerve roots within the thecal sac into a central clump of soft-tissue signal (pseudocord) instead of their normal feathery appearance. **(B)** The axial image is at the L4-L5 level.

References

1. Melhem ER, Benson ML, Beauchamp NJ, Lee RR. Cervical spondylosis: three-dimensional gradient-echo MR with magnetization transfer. AJNR Am J Neuroradiol 1996;17:705–711

2. Magerl F, Aebi M, Gertzbein SD, Harms J, Nazarian S. A comprehensive classification of thoracic and lumbar injuries. Eur Spine J 1994;3:184–201

3. McCormack T, Karaikovic E, Gaines RW. The load sharing classification of spine fractures. Spine (Phila Pa 1976) 1994;19:1741–1744

4. Denis F. The three column spine and its significance in the classification of acute thoracolumbar spinal injuries. Spine (Phila Pa 1976) 1983;8:817–831

5. Vaccaro AR, Lehman RA Jr, Hurlbert RJ, et al. A new classification of thoracolumbar injuries: the importance of injury morphology, the integrity of the posterior ligamentous complex, and neurologic status. Spine (Phila Pa 1976) 2005;30:2325–2333

6. Blankenbaker DG, De Smet AA, Vanderby R, McCabe RP, Koplin SA. MRI of acute bone bruises: timing of the appearance of findings in a swine model. AJR Am J Roentgenol 2008;190:W1–W7

7. Brown DB, Glaiberman CB, Gilula LA, Shimony JS. Correlation between preprocedural MRI findings and clinical outcomes in the treatment of chronic symptomatic vertebral compression fractures with percutaneous vertebroplasty. AJR Am J Roentgenol 2005;184:1951–1955

8. Jung HS, Jee WH, McCauley TR, Ha KY, Choi KH. Discrimination of metastatic from acute osteoporotic compression spinal fractures with MR imaging. Radiographics 2003;23:179–187

9. Kaplan PA, Orton DF, Asleson RJ. Osteoporosis with vertebral compression fractures, retropulsed fragments, and neurologic compromise. Radiology 1987;165:533–535

10. Cuénod CA, Laredo JD, Chevret S, et al. Acute vertebral collapse due to osteoporosis or malignancy: appearance on unenhanced and gadolinium-enhanced MR images. Radiology 1996;199:541–549

11. Panjabi MM, Thibodeau LL, Crisco JJ III, White AA III. What constitutes spinal instability? Clin Neurosurg 1988;34:313–339

12. Wood KB, Khanna G, Vaccaro AR, Arnold PM, Harris MB, Mehbod AA. Assessment of two thoracolumbar fracture classification systems as used by multiple surgeons. J Bone Joint Surg Am 2005;87:1423–1429

13. Bono CM, Vaccaro AR, Hurlbert RJ, et al. Validating a newly proposed classification system for thoracolumbar spine trauma: looking to the future of the thoracolumbar injury classification and severity score. J Orthop Trauma 2006;20:567–572

14. Rihn JA, Anderson DT, Harris E, et al. A review of the TLICS system: a novel, user-friendly thoracolumbar trauma classification system. Acta Orthop 2008;79:461–466

15. Young PC, Petersilge CA. MR imaging of the traumatized lumbar spine. Magn Reson Imaging Clin N Am 1999;7:589–602

16. Mitra D, Cassar-Pullicino VN, McCall IW. Longitudinal study of high intensity zones on MR of lumbar intervertebral discs. Clin Radiol 2004;59:1002–1008

17. Peng B, Hou S, Wu W, Zhang C, Yang Y. The pathogenesis and clinical significance of a high-intensity zone (HIZ) of lumbar intervertebral disc on MR imaging in the patient with discogenic low back pain. Eur Spine J 2006;15:583–587

18. Carrino JA, Lurie JD, Tosteson ANA, et al. Lumbar spine: reliability of MR imaging findings. Radiology 2009;250:161–170

19. Mochida K, Komori H, Okawa A, Muneta T, Haro H, Shinomiya K. Regression of cervical disc herniation observed on magnetic resonance images. Spine (Phila Pa 1976) 1998;23:990–995, discussion 996–997

20. Watanabe N, Ogura T, Kimori K, Hase H, Hirasawa Y. Epidural hematoma of the lumbar spine, simulating extruded lumbar disc herniation: clinical, discographic, and enhanced magnetic resonance imaging features. A case report. Spine (Phila Pa 1976) 1997;22:105–109

21. Gundry CR, Heithoff KB. Epidural hematoma of the lumbar spine: 18 surgically confirmed cases. Radiology 1993;187:427–431

22. Renfrew DL, Heithoff KB. Degenerative disease. In: Renfrew DL, ed. Atlas of Spine Imaging. Philadelphia: Saunders; 2003:11–128

23. Schellinger D, Manz HJ, Vidic B, et al. Disc fragment migration. Radiology 1990;175:831–836

24. Flanders AE, Tartaglino LM, Friedman DP, Aquilone LF. Magnetic resonance imaging in acute spinal injury. Semin Roentgenol 1992;27:271–298

25. Fardon DF, Milette PC; Combined Task Forces of the North American Spine Society, American Society of Spine Radiology, and American Society of Neuroradiology. Nomenclature and classification of lumbar disc pathology. Recommendations of the Combined Task Forces of the North American Spine Society, American Society of Spine Radiology, and American Society of Neuroradiology. Spine (Phila Pa 1976) 2001;26:E93–E113

26. Modic MT, Ross JS. Lumbar degenerative disc disease. Radiology 2007;245:43–61

27. Modic MT. Degenerative disc disease and back pain. Magn Reson Imaging Clin N Am 1999;7:481–491

28. Modic MT, Steinberg PM, Ross JS, Masaryk TJ, Carter JR. Degenerative disc disease: assessment of changes in vertebral body marrow with MR imaging. Radiology 1988;166:193–199

29. Modic MT, Masaryk TJ, Ross JS, Carter JR. Imaging of degenerative disc disease. Radiology 1988;168:177–186

30. Alyas F, Turner M, Connell D. MRI findings in the lumbar spines of asymptomatic, adolescent, elite tennis players. Br J Sports Med 2007;41:836–841, discussion 841

31. Boden SD, Davis DO, Dina TS, Patronas NJ, Wiesel SW. Abnormal magnetic-resonance scans of the lumbar spine in asymptomatic subjects. A prospective investigation. J Bone Joint Surg Am 1990;72:403–408

32. Borenstein DG, O'Mara JW Jr, Boden SD, et al. The value of magnetic resonance imaging of the lumbar spine to predict low-back pain in asymptomatic subjects : a seven-year follow-up study. J Bone Joint Surg Am 2001;83:1306–1311

33. Morgan S, Saifuddin A. MRI of the lumbar intervertebral disc. Clin Radiol 1999;54:703–723

34. Pfirrmann CWA, Metzdorf A, Zanetti M, Hodler J, Boos N. Magnetic resonance classification of lumbar intervertebral disc degeneration. Spine (Phila Pa 1976) 2001;26:1873–1878

35. Toyone T, Takahashi K, Kitahara H, Yamagata M, Murakami M, Moriya H. Vertebral bone-marrow changes in degenerative lumbar disc disease. An MRI study of 74 patients with low back pain. J Bone Joint Surg Br 1994;76:757–764

36. Weishaupt D, Zanetti M, Hodler J, et al. Painful lumbar disc derangement: relevance of endplate abnormalities at MR imaging. Radiology 2001;218:420–427

37. Aprill C, Bogduk N. High-intensity zone: a diagnostic sign of painful lumbar disc on magnetic resonance imaging. Br J Radiol 1992;65:361–369

38. Gundry CR, Fritts HM. Magnetic resonance imaging of the musculoskeletal system. Part 8. The spine, section 1. Clin Orthop Relat Res 1997;338:275–287

39. Stadnik TW, Lee RR, Coen HL, Neirynck EC, Buisseret TS, Osteaux MJC. Annular tears and disc herniation: prevalence and contrast enhancement on MR images in the absence of low back pain or sciatica. Radiology 1998;206:49–55

40. Yoshida H, Fujiwara A, Tamai K, Kobayashi N, Saiki K, Saotome K. Diagnosis of symptomatic disc by magnetic resonance imaging: T2-weighted and gadolinium-DTPA-enhanced T1-weighted magnetic resonance imaging. J Spinal Disord Tech 2002;15:193–198

41. Herzog RJ. The radiologic assessment for a lumbar disc herniation. Spine (Phila Pa 1976) 1996;21(24, Suppl)19S–38S

42. Cassar-Pullicino VN. MRI of the ageing and herniating intervertebral disc. Eur J Radiol 1998;27:214–228

43. Malfair D, Beall DP. Imaging the degenerative diseases of the lumbar spine. Magn Reson Imaging Clin N Am 2007;15:221–238

44. Dietze DD Jr, Fessler RG. Thoracic disc herniations. Neurosurg Clin N Am 1993;4:75–90

45. Peng B, Wu W, Hou S, Shang W, Wang X, Yang Y. The pathogenesis of Schmorl's nodes. J Bone Joint Surg Br 2003;85:879–882

46. Hamanishi C, Kawabata T, Yosii T, Tanaka S. Schmorl's nodes on magnetic resonance imaging. Their incidence and clinical relevance. Spine (Phila Pa 1976) 1994;19:450–453

47. Wagner AL, Murtagh FR, Arrington JA, Stallworth D. Relationship of Schmorl's nodes to vertebral body endplate fractures and acute endplate disc extrusions. AJNR Am J Neuroradiol 2000;21:276–281

48. Jackson RP, Jacobs RR, Montesano PX. 1988 Volvo award in clinical sciences. Facet joint injection in low-back pain. A prospective statistical study. Spine (Phila Pa 1976) 1988;13:966–971

49. Revel M, Poiraudeau S, Auleley GR, et al. Capacity of the clinical picture to characterize low back pain relieved by facet joint anesthesia. Proposed criteria to identify patients with painful facet joints. Spine (Phila Pa 1976) 1998;23:1972–1976, discussion 1977

50. Schwarzer AC, Aprill CN, Derby R, Fortin J, Kine G, Bogduk N. Clinical features of patients with pain stemming from the lumbar zygapophysial joints. Is the lumbar facet syndrome a clinical entity? Spine (Phila Pa 1976) 1994;19:1132–1137

51. Farfan HF, Sullivan JD. The relation of facet orientation to intervertebral disc failure. Can J Surg 1967;10:179–185

52. Noren R, Trafimow J, Andersson GBJ, Huckman MS. The role of facet joint tropism and facet angle in disc degeneration. Spine (Phila Pa 1976) 1991;16:530–532

53. Boden SD, Riew KD, Yamaguchi K, Branch TP, Schellinger D, Wiesel SW. Orientation of the lumbar facet joints: association with degenerative disc disease. J Bone Joint Surg Am 1996;78:403–411

54. Jinkins JR. MR evaluation of stenosis involving the neural foramina, lateral recesses, and central canal of the lumbosacral spine. Magn Reson Imaging Clin N Am 1999;7:493–511

55. Hamanishi C, Matukura N, Fujita M, Tomihara M, Tanaka S. Cross-sectional area of the stenotic lumbar dural tube measured from the transverse views of magnetic resonance imaging. J Spinal Disord 1994;7:388–393

56. Speciale AC, Pietrobon R, Urban CW, et al. Observer variability in assessing lumbar spinal stenosis severity on magnetic resonance imaging and its relation to cross-sectional spinal canal area. Spine (Phila Pa 1976) 2002;27:1082–1086

57. Buchner M, Schiltenwolf M. Cauda equina syndrome caused by intervertebral lumbar disc prolapse: mid-term results of 22 patients and literature review. Orthopedics 2002;25:727–731

58. Bagley CA, Gokaslan ZL. Cauda equina syndrome caused by primary and metastatic neoplasms. Neurosurg Focus 2004;16:11–18

59. Harrop JS, Hunt GE Jr, Vaccaro AR. Conus medullaris and cauda equina syndrome as a result of traumatic injuries: management principles. Neurosurg Focus 2004;16:19–23

60. Wiltse LL, Newman PH, Macnab I. Classification of spondylolisis and spondylolisthesis. Clin Orthop Relat Res 1976;117:23–29

61. Meyerding HW. Spondylolisthesis. Surgical fusion of lumbosacral portion of spinal column and interarticular facets; use of autogenous bone grafts for relief of disabling backache. J Int Coll Surg 1956;26(5 Pt 1):566–591

62. Mac-Thiong JM, Labelle H. A proposal for a surgical classification of pediatric lumbosacral spondylolisthesis based on current literature. Eur Spine J 2006;15:1425–1435

63. Mac-Thiong JM, Labelle H, Parent S, Hresko MT, Deviren V, Weidenbaum M; members of the Spinal Deformity Study Group. Reliability and development of a new classification of lumbosacral spondylolisthesis. Scoliosis 2008;3:19

64. Hammerberg KW. New concepts on the pathogenesis and classification of spondylolisthesis. Spine (Phila Pa 1976) 2005;30(6, Suppl)S4–S11

65. Redla S, Sikdar T, Saifuddin A. Magnetic resonance imaging of scoliosis. Clin Radiol 2001;56:360–371

66. Slipman CW, Shin CH, Patel RK, et al. Etiologies of failed back surgery syndrome. Pain Med 2002;3:200–214, discussion 214–217

67. O'Brien MF, Lenke LG, Bridwell KH, Blanke K, Baldus C. Preoperative spinal canal investigation in adolescent idiopathic scoliosis curves > or = 70 degrees. Spine (Phila Pa 1976) 1994;19:1606–1610

68. Winter RB, Lonstein JE, Heithoff KB, Kirkham JA. Magnetic resonance imaging evaluation of the adolescent patient with idiopathic scoliosis before spinal instrumentation and fusion. A prospective, double-blinded study of 140 patients. Spine (Phila Pa 1976) 1997;22:855–858

69. Lewonowski K, King JD, Nelson MD. Routine use of magnetic resonance imaging in idiopathic scoliosis patients less than eleven years of age. Spine (Phila Pa 1976) 1992;17(6, Suppl)S109–S116

70. Fisk JR, Moe JH, Winter RB. Scoliosis, spondylolysis, and spondylolisthesis. Their relationship as reviewed in 539 patients. Spine (Phila Pa 1976) 1978;3:234–245

71. Badami JP, Hinck VC. Symptomatic deposition of epidural fat in a morbidly obese woman. AJNR Am J Neuroradiol 1982;3:664–665

72. Gero BT, Chynn KY. Symptomatic spinal epidural lipomatosis without exogenous steroid intake. Report of a case with magnetic resonance imaging. Neuroradiology 1989;31:190–192

73. Al-Khawaja D, Seex K, Eslick GD. Spinal epidural lipomatosis—a brief review. J Clin Neurosci 2008;15:1323–1326

74. St. Amour TE, Hodges SE, Laakman RW, Tamas DE. Epidural lipomas, angiolipomas, and epidural lipomatosis. In: St. Amour TE, Hodges SC, Laakman RW, Tamas DE, eds. MRI of the Spine. New York: Raven Press; 1994:501–507

75. Jaramillo-de la Torre JJ, Bohinski RJ, Kuntz C IV. Vertebral osteomyelitis. Neurosurg Clin N Am 2006;17:339–351

76. Modic MT, Feiglin DH, Piraino DW, et al. Vertebral osteomyelitis: assessment using MR. Radiology 1985;157:157–166

77. Vaccaro AR, Betz RR, Zeidman SM, eds. Principles and Practice of Spine Surgery. St. Louis: Mosby; 2003

78. Dagirmanjian A, Schils J, McHenry M, Modic MT. MR imaging of vertebral osteomyelitis revisited. AJR Am J Roentgenol 1996;167: 1539–1543

79. Batson OV. The vertebral vein system. Caldwell lecture, 1956. Am J Roentgenol Radium Ther Nucl Med 1957;78:195–212

80. Ratcliffe JF. Anatomic basis for the pathogenesis and radiologic features of vertebral osteomyelitis and its differentiation from childhood discitis. A microarteriographic investigation. Acta Radiol Diagn (Stockh) 1985;26:137–143

81. Dagirmanjian A, Schils J, McHenry MC. MR imaging of spinal infections. Magn Reson Imaging Clin N Am 1999;7:525–538

82. Post MJD, Quencer RM, Montalvo BM, Katz BH, Eismont FJ, Green BA. Spinal infection: evaluation with MR imaging and intraoperative US. Radiology 1988;169:765–771

83. Bertino RE, Porter BA, Stimac GK, Tepper SJ. Imaging spinal osteomyelitis and epidural abscess with short TI inversion recovery (STIR). AJNR Am J Neuroradiol 1988;9:563–564

84. Brown R, Hussain M, McHugh K, Novelli V, Jones D. Discitis in young children. J Bone Joint Surg Br 2001;83:106–111

85. Mahboubi S, Morris MC. Imaging of spinal infections in children. Radiol Clin North Am 2001;39:215–222

86. Van Goethem JWM, Parizel PM, van den Hauwe L, Van de Kelft E, Verlooy J, De Schepper AMA. The value of MRI in the diagnosis of postoperative spondylodiscitis. Neuroradiology 2000;42:580–585

87. Almeida A. Tuberculosis of the spine and spinal cord. Eur J Radiol 2005;55:193–201

88. Gundry CR, Fritts HM. Magnetic resonance imaging of the musculoskeletal system. Part 8. The spine, section 2. Clin Orthop Relat Res 1997;343:260–271

89. Berquist TH. Imaging of the postoperative spine. Radiol Clin North Am 2006;44:407–418

90. Malik AS, Boyko O, Aktar N, Young WF. A comparative study of MR imaging profile of titanium pedicle screws. Acta Radiol 2001;42: 291–293

91. Viano AM, Gronemeyer SA, Haliloglu M, Hoffer FA. Improved MR imaging for patients with metallic implants. Magn Reson Imaging 2000;18:287–295

92. Rupp RE, Ebraheim NA, Wong FF. The value of magnetic resonance imaging of the postoperative spine with titanium implants. J Spinal Disord 1996;9:342–346

93. Babar S, Saifuddin A. MRI of the post-discectomy lumbar spine. Clin Radiol 2002;57:969–981

94. Annertz M, Jönsson B, Strömqvist B, Holtås S. Serial MRI in the early postoperative period after lumbar discectomy. Neuroradiology 1995;37:177–182

95. Ross JS. Magnetic resonance imaging of the postoperative spine. Semin Musculoskelet Radiol 2000;4:281–291

96. Grand CM, Bank WO, Balériaux D, Matos C, Levivier M, Brotchi J. Gadolinium enhancement of vertebral endplates following lumbar disc surgery. Neuroradiology 1993;35:503–505

97. McGirt MJ, Ambrossi GLG, Datoo G, et al. Recurrent disc herniation and long-term back pain after primary lumbar discectomy: review of outcomes reported for limited versus aggressive disc removal. Neurosurgery 2009;64:338–344, discussion 344–345

98. Kim MS, Park KW, Hwang C, et al. Recurrence rate of lumbar disc herniation after open discectomy in active young men. Spine (Phila Pa 1976) 2009;34:24–29

99. Jinkins JR, Van Goethem JWM. The postsurgical lumbosacral spine. Magnetic resonance imaging evaluation following intervertebral disc surgery, surgical decompression, intervertebral bony fusion, and spinal instrumentation. Radiol Clin North Am 2001;39:1–29

100. Bradley WG. Use of contrast in MR imaging of the lumbar spine. Magn Reson Imaging Clin N Am 1999;7:439–457

101. Bundschuh CV, Modic MT, Ross JS, Masaryk TJ, Bohlman H. Epidural fibrosis and recurrent disc herniation in the lumbar spine: MR imaging assessment. AJR Am J Roentgenol 1988;150:923–932

102. Bundschuh CV, Stein L, Slusser JH, Schinco FP, Ladaga LE, Dillon JD. Distinguishing between scar and recurrent herniated disc in postoperative patients: value of contrast-enhanced CT and MR imaging. AJNR Am J Neuroradiol 1990;11:949–958

103. Sotiropoulos S, Chafetz NI, Lang P, et al. Differentiation between postoperative scar and recurrent disc herniation: prospective comparison of MR, CT, and contrast-enhanced CT. AJNR Am J Neuroradiol 1989;10:639–643

104. Van Goethem JWM, Parizel PM, Jinkins JR. Review article: MRI of the postoperative lumbar spine. Neuroradiology 2002;44: 723–739

105. Bernard TN Jr. Repeat lumbar spine surgery. Factors influencing outcome. Spine (Phila Pa 1976) 1993;18:2196–2200

106. Fandiño J, Botana C, Viladrich A, Gomez-Bueno J. Reoperation after lumbar disc surgery: results in 130 cases. Acta Neurochir (Wien) 1993;122:102–104

107. Herron L. Recurrent lumbar disc herniation: results of repeat laminectomy and discectomy. J Spinal Disord 1994;7:161–166

108. Jönsson B, Strömqvist B. Repeat decompression of lumbar nerve roots. A prospective two-year evaluation. J Bone Joint Surg Br 1993;75:894–897

109. Gundry CR, Fritts HM. Magnetic resonance imaging of the musculoskeletal system: the spine. Part 8, section 3. Clin Orthop Relat Res 1998;346:262–278

12 Tumors of the Spine

Daniel M. Sciubba, Bruce A. Wasserman, and Ziya L. Gokaslan

Spine tumors are traditionally classified by anatomic location into three compartments:[1-6]

- Extradural
- Intradural–extramedullary
- Intramedullary

The extradural compartment consists of all structures outside the dura, including the osseous structures, the paravertebral region (including the paraspinal musculature), and the epidural space. Although orthopaedic surgeons most commonly manage tumors of the extradural compartment, they must have an understanding of the other two compartments to provide comprehensive patient care and to communicate effectively with neurosurgical colleagues.

Spine tumors also are classified by type of origin as primary or metastatic. Although a large number of primary lesions may occur in the spinal cord, nerve roots, dura, and osseous spine, most lesions within the spine are metastatic tumors.[7] Such lesions occur primarily in the extradural compartment, especially in the osseous structures. As systemic therapies for metastatic disease have improved and the life expectancy of such patients has increased, the incidence of metastatic spread to the spine has also increased.

Up to 40% of patients with cancer develop visceral or osseous metastases, and the spinal column is the most common site of osseous metastases.[8] Prostate, lung, and breast cancer account for most of such lesions.[1,3] Metastases can occur in any compartment of the spinal column, but the vertebral body is the site most commonly affected (approximately 85%),[9] followed by the paravertebral region, epidural space, and intradural compartment. In addition, although all segments of the spine can be affected, such lesions occur most often in the thoracic spine (approximately 70%), followed by the lumbar spine (20%) and then the cervical spine and sacrum (10%).[9]

Epidemiologic data suggest that most patients with suspected spine tumors are eventually shown to have metastatic (rather than primary) disease in the vertebral body (rather than in other locations) and that metastatic and primary lesions (benign and malignant) can occur within any segment and compartment of the spine and in men or women of almost any age. Although most lesions have particular identifying characteristics, it is still imperative that, to arrive efficiently and effectively at the correct diagnosis of a spine tumor, the following steps are followed rigorously when reviewing imaging studies[4,6]:

1. The compartment location of the lesion in the spinal column (extradural, intradural–extramedullary, or intramedullary) must be identified. Such localization may provide a narrowed differential diagnosis.
2. The clinician generates a preimaging differential diagnosis based on patient demographics and clinical characteristics, such as patient age, sex, medical history, and neurologic signs and symptoms (**Table 12.1**). Such a meticulous evaluation not only guides the type and location of such imaging, but also provides substantial insight as to the true underlying pathology. In this way, imaging serves to corroborate or refute, rather than merely suggest, the previously hypothesized differential diagnosis.
3. The patient's demographic information and clinical presentation are used to narrow the differential diagnosis. For instance, tumors that present in pediatric patients often are extremely rare in adults and vice versa. In addition, in patients with a history of cancer, neck pain, or back pain should be assumed to be a symptomatic spinal metastasis until proven otherwise.
4. Various imaging modalities (conventional radiographs, CT, or MRI) can be used to narrow the differential to a working diagnosis. Although these steps often may lead the clinician to the correct diagnosis, it should be noted that the working diagnosis based on current imaging techniques is not always accurate. For this reason, image-guided or open biopsy often has a role in obtaining a definitive diagnosis before the initiation of a proposed treatment plan (surgery, radiation therapy, chemotherapy, etc.).

MRI is the preferred imaging modality for evaluating most disorders of the spine, including spine tumors.[10,11] MRI is more sensitive than conventional radiographs, CT, or bone scans in detecting primary malignant bone tumors and metastatic lesions in the spine.[12,13] This increased sensitivity results from the fact that MRI allows for superior resolution of soft-tissue structures, such as the intervertebral discs, spinal cord, nerve roots, meninges, and paraspinal musculature. In addition, MRI provides clarity at the osseous–soft-tissue interface, yielding precise anatomic detail of osseous compression or invasion of neural and paraspinal structures.

Table 12.1 Differential Diagnosis of Spine Lesion by Anatomic Compartment

Compartment	Malignant	Benign	Nontumorous Growths
Extradural	Metastases	Hemangioma	
	Myeloma	Aneurysmal bone cyst	
	Lymphoma	Giant cell tumor	
	Ewing sarcoma	Osteoid osteoma	
	Osteosarcoma	Osteoblastoma	
	Chordoma	Osteochondroma	
	Leukemia	Eosinophilic granuloma	
	Chondrosarcoma		
Intradural–extradural	Metastases	Nerve sheath tumors	Lipoma
	Malignant nerve sheath tumors	Schwannoma	Epidermoid
		Neurofibroma	Dermoid
		Meningioma	Arachnoid cyst
		Hemangiopericytoma	
		Paraganglioma	
Intramedullary	Astrocytoma	Astrocytoma	
	Metastases	Hemangioblastoma	
		Ependymoma	

Despite this excellent anatomic and soft-tissue depiction, however, MRI is limited in its detection of calcifications and small osseous fragments[3] and is subject to metal-induced artifact when used in the instrumented spine (usually with stainless steel or titanium), which may prohibit accurate assessment of neural compression and necessitate a fluoroscopic or CT myelogram for optimal evaluation. CT also provides superior osseous detail and permits resolution of calcification in areas within or around soft-tissue structures. Therefore, the ideal method of evaluating a patient with a suspected or known spinal mass involves a combination of conventional radiographs and/or CT imaging with MRI.

This chapter describes image interpretation techniques that permit identification of the compartment and the MRI appearance of the most common tumors in each location, facilitating the systematic and efficient creation of a differential diagnosis (**Table 12.1**) for any spine tumor evaluated with MRI.

■ Specialized Pulse Sequences and Imaging Protocols

MRI protocols vary widely among institutions and in relation to the spinal region involved. Despite such variation, the MRI protocol for any patient suspected of having a spine tumor should include T1-weighted and T2-weighted images and gadolinium-enhanced studies in the axial and sagittal planes.[4] Gadolinium enhancement often provides improved anatomic detail of spinal tumors and may supply signature clues to the underlying pathology. Because of the high signal intensity of fat within an adult's marrow on T1-weighted images, fat-suppression techniques are useful in evaluating osseous lesions that enhance with contrast.[4] Similarly, enhancing lesions in the epidural space are better seen with fat suppression, particularly in the lumbar spine in which the epidural space is composed primarily of fat. Gradient-echo sequences are not as useful in assessing spine tumors unless hemorrhage is suspected. On the other hand, diffusion-weighted imaging, which often reveals restricted diffusion in a vertebral body with a tumor, may be helpful in distinguishing benign and pathologic compression fractures.[14] Consultation with a neuroradiologist generally is advisable for the selection of the ideal imaging protocol.

■ Extradural Tumors

Extradural masses typically arise from the osseous spine, intervertebral discs, and adjacent soft tissues. With MRI, the hallmark of such lesions is focal displacement of the thecal sac away from the mass with an obliterated subarachnoid space and compressed spinal cord (**Fig. 12.1**). The dura often appears to be draped over the mass. The most common malignant extradural masses are metastases (**Fig. 12.2**), followed by primary malignant tumors of the spine.[5] The most common benign extradural masses are degenerative and traumatic lesions, such as disc herniations, osteophytes, and

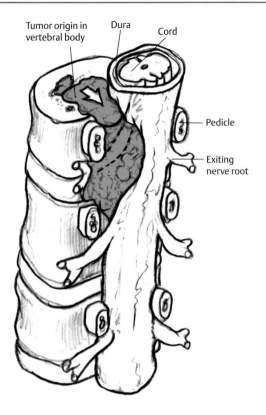

Fig. 12.1 Artist's sketch (posterior oblique view) depicting the characteristics of an extradural mass. The spinal cord and dura are displaced. The mass typically extends from the vertebral body (*arrow*) and into the extradural space.

fractures, followed by primary benign tumors of the spine.[5] In this chapter, such lesions pertain to *neoplastic* lesions of the spine, both malignant and benign.

Metastatic Disease

The spinal column is the most common site of osseous metastases, and the most common extradural malignant spine tumors in adults are metastatic lesions.[5] Autopsy studies reveal vertebral metastases in up to 40% of patients with systemic cancer, with 5% of adults presenting with epidural spinal cord compression.[7,8,15,16]

Most spine metastases in adults arise from lung, breast, and prostate cancer, followed less frequently by lymphoma, melanoma, renal cancer, sarcoma, and multiple myeloma.[17] Approximately 5% of children with solid malignant tumors develop spinal metastases with cord compression.[18] In such cases, spine metastases most often are caused by Ewing sarcoma and neuroblastoma, followed by osteogenic sarcoma, rhabdomyosarcoma, Hodgkin disease, soft-tissue sarcoma, and germ cell tumors.[18]

In adults, the initial site of metastatic tumor growth in the spine typically is the posterior vertebral body, followed by the epidural space and pedicle.[19] Conversely, metastatic tumors in children typically invade the spinal canal via the neural foramina, causing circumferential cord compression.[18] Spinal metastases in the adult can occur at any level, but they usually involve the lower thoracic and lumbar spine

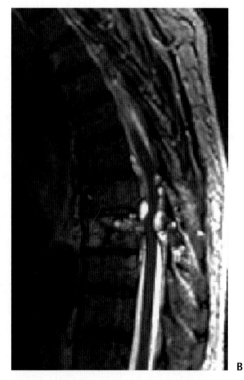

Fig. 12.2 Sagittal T2-weighted images of metastatic lesions, revealing compression and distortion of the underlying dura and cord. **(A)** Prostate metastasis in the thoracolumbar spine (*between arrows*).

(Other images confirmed that the lesion arose from the posterior elements.) **(B)** Non–small-cell lung cancer metastasis to the osseous thoracic spine with extradural extension.

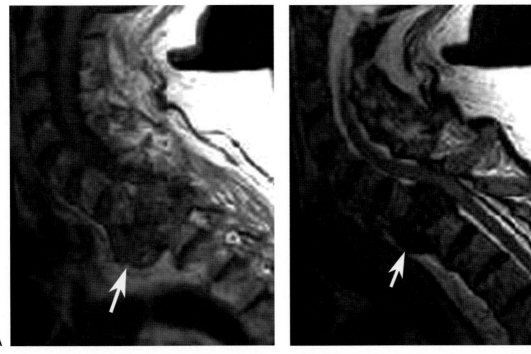

Fig. 12.3 Sagittal T1-weighted (**A**) and T2-weighted (**B**) images of a cervicothoracic metastasis from thyroid carcinoma. The expansile lesion is centered in the collapsed vertebral body (*arrow on each*) and compresses the spinal cord.

secondary to a higher proportion of red bone marrow in those locations.[12,19]

MRI is the method of choice for imaging metastatic spine disease because of its unparalleled ability to delineate epidural and paraspinous soft-tissue involvement. Imaging patterns of such lesions can reveal focal lytic, focal blastic/sclerotic, diffuse homogeneous, and diffuse inhomogeneous lesions.[5] The most common pattern seen is multifocal lytic lesions that are hypointense on T1-weighted images and hypo- to hyperintense on T2-weighted images (**Fig. 12.3**). Sclerotic lesions tend to be hypointense on T1-weighted images and T2-weighted images. Diffuse homogeneous and inhomogeneous lesions are hypointense on T1-weighted images and hyperintense on T2-weighted images, although the signal pattern can be variable and depends on the degree of fatty marrow. Contrast enhancement of such lesions also is extremely variable.

MRI also may be useful for distinguishing benign, osteoporotic fractures from pathologic, tumor-related fractures. Benign fractures typically have marrow signal intensity identical to that of neighboring normal vertebral bodies. Pathologic fractures are more hypointense on T1-weighted images and more hyperintense on T2-weighted images than are normal vertebral bodies.[20] Additionally, diffusion-weighted images, combined with apparent diffusion coefficient mapping, often shows more extensive restricted diffusion with pathologic fractures than with osteoporotic fractures.[4] The identification of epidural or paraspinal soft-tissue involvement also is helpful for confirming a pathologic etiology.

Primary Benign Tumors

Benign primary tumors of the extradural compartment of the spine have characteristic MRI findings and patient demographics (**Table 12.2**) that help differentiate them from malignant lesions.

Vertebral Hemangioma

Vertebral hemangioma is the most common spinal axis tumor.[21] This benign vascular tumor of the vertebral body, often discovered incidentally on imaging, can be associated with vertebral body collapse and epidural extension with spinal cord compression; on rare occasions, it may exhibit aggressive growth.[22] MRI sequences of the typical (fatty) hemangioma show lesions that are hyperintense on T1-weighted and T2-weighted images, with robust contrast enhancement[23] (**Fig. 12.4**). Vertebral hemangiomas are one of the very few spinal tumors that show increased signal intensity on T1-weighted images and T2-weighted images. Occasionally, such lesions are more vascular and may appear isointense or hypointense on T1-weighted images, making them difficult to distinguish from metastases. Although CT images show the typical "polka dot" appearance on axial images and the typical "corduroy" or "jailhouse striation" pattern on sagittal images, secondary to the thickened trabeculae, MRI is the best modality for characterizing the epidural extent and cord compromise of aggressive lesions. Although such lesions

Table 12.2 Benign Primary Tumors of the Extradural Compartment

Lesion	Location in Segment	Spinal Segment	Incidence	Age (years)	Imaging Clue
Hemangioma	Vertebral body	T, L > C	Most common	All	Bright on T1-weighted image
Osteoid osteoma	Neural arch	L, C > T	Common	10 to 20	Target lesion <2 cm
Osteoblastoma	Neural arch	C > L, T, S	Uncommon	<30	Expansile, lytic >2 cm
Giant cell tumor	Vertebral body	S >> C, T, L	Uncommon	20 to 50	Expansile, lytic, vascular
Osteochondroma	Spinous, transverse processes	C >> T, L	Rare in spine	5 to 30	Mushroom-shaped
Aneurysmal bone cyst	Neural arch	C, T > L, S	Rare	<20	Fluid–fluid levels, eggshell-like rims
Eosinophilic granuloma	Vertebral body	T > L, C	Rare	<15	Vertebra plana

Source: Adapted from Osborn AG. Cysts, tumors, and tumor-like lesions of the spine and spinal canal. In: Osborn AG, ed. Diagnostic Neuroradiology. St. Louis: Mosby; 1994:876–918.
Abbreviations: C, cervical; L, lumbar; S, sacral; T, thoracic.

primarily involve the vertebral body, 10% to 15% have concomitant involvement of the posterior elements.[21] Multiple lesions are seen in 25% to 30% of patients.[24]

Osteoid Osteoma

This benign, osteoid-producing tumor, usually <1.5 cm in size, is often surrounded by a ring of sclerotic bone. Almost all of these lesions involve the neural arch, and most occur within the lumbar spine, followed by the cervical, thoracic, and sacral regions. Bone scintigraphy and CT are gener-

ally more helpful for detecting and characterizing these lesions than is MRI. The nidus is hypo- or isointense on T1-weighted images and varies from hypo- to hyperintense on T2-weighted images, often with surrounding hyperintensity that likely is related to a local inflammatory response (**Fig. 12.5**).[25] The rapid enhancement pattern, typically located within the nidus, is best seen on dynamic sequences (e.g., serial postcontrast images). The surrounding reactive zone enhances more slowly with such imaging. Of note, up to 70% of patients may present with scoliosis, related to muscle spasm, with concavity on the side of the tumor.[26]

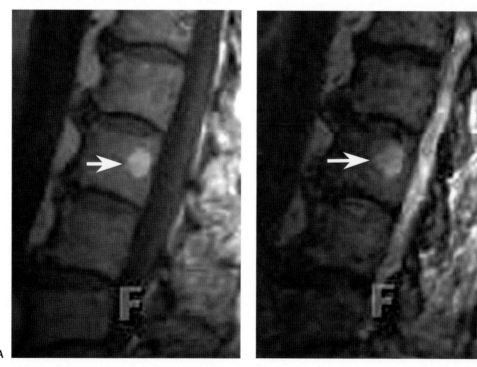

Fig. 12.4 Thoracolumbar vertebral hemangioma. This asymptomatic lesion (*arrow on each*) is centered in the vertebral body and appears hyperintense on T1-weighted **(A)** and T2-weighted **(B)** sagittal images.

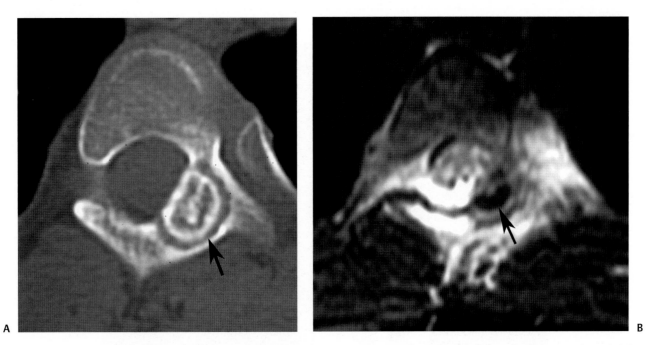

Fig. 12.5 Left-side thoracic osteoid osteoma. **(A)** An axial CT image shows characteristic hyperdense center with sclerotic rim (*arrow*). **(B)** An axial T2-weighted image reveals a hypointense center (*arrow*) corresponding to sclerotic bone surrounded by a region of high signal intensity corresponding to reactive edema.

Osteoblastoma

Osteoblastomas, also known as giant osteoid osteomas, are similar histologically to osteoid osteomas but are differentiated from them largely by size (>1.5 cm). Clinical symptoms also can help to distinguish these lesions: osteoblastomas cause a dull pain as opposed to the intense night pain caused by osteoid osteomas. Occasionally, osteoblastomas possess atypical features and behave aggressively. Like osteoid osteomas, these lesions originate in the neural arch but exhibit greater mass expansion.[5] Thus, they may be centered in the pedicle, lamina, transverse or spinous process, articular pillar, or pars interarticularis, with extension into the vertebral body. The lesion is hypo- or isointense on T1-weighted images and iso- or hyperintense on T2-weighted images with extensive peritumoral edema (flare phenomenon); fluid-fluid levels are often present within the lesion (**Fig. 12.6**). Contrast enhancement is variable.[27] Unlike osteoid osteomas, scoliosis may occur convex toward the side of the tumor.

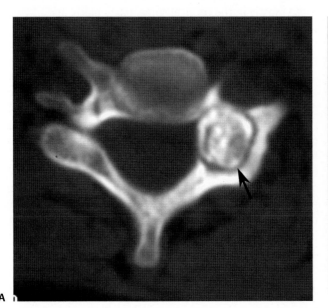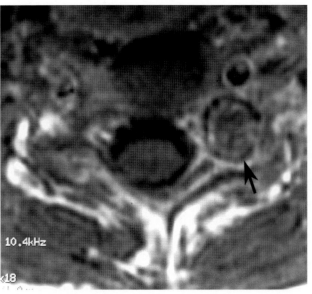

Fig. 12.6 Left-side cervical osteoblastoma. **(A)** An axial CT shows a lesion (*arrow*) similar to (but larger than) the osteoid osteoma shown in **Fig. 12.4A**. **(B)** An axial postgadolinium T1-weighted image shows the lesion (*arrow*).

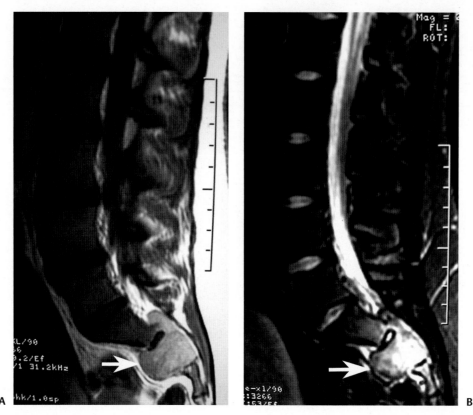

Fig. 12.7 Sacral giant cell tumor. This expansile lesion shows intermediate signal intensity on a sagittal T1-weighted image (*arrow*) **(A)** and high signal intensity on a sagittal fat-suppressed T2-weighted image (*arrow*) **(B)**.

Giant Cell Tumor

Giant cell tumors are locally aggressive, lytic tumors in the vertebral body and sacrum and are named for the osteoclast-like giant cells that are present on histology. Hemorrhage is common secondary to the hypervascular stroma of these lesions. MRI shows expansile lesions with hypo- to isointense signal on T1-weighted images and iso- to hyperintense signal on T2-weighted images (**Fig. 12.7**). Contrast enhancement often is heterogeneous, commonly surrounding areas of necrosis, blood, blood degradation products, and/or cystic cavities with fluid–fluid levels.[28] Such lesions can undergo sarcomatous transformation (10% of cases) to become malignant giant cell tumors,[29] and thus patients with these tumors must be monitored with MRI or CT because of the risk of recurrence. It is important to note that the differential diagnosis of midline tumors in the sacrum includes giant cell tumor, chordoma, aneurysmal bone cyst, plasmacytoma, and metastases in adults, and sacrococcygeal teratoma in children.[9]

Osteochondroma

Osteochondroma, also known as osteocartilaginous exostosis, consists of cartilage-covered osseous protuberances with a medullary cavity that is contiguous with the parent bone. These lesions grossly appear to be cauliflower- or mushroom-shaped lesions with cartilaginous caps. Only 5% of these growths occur within the spine (compared with 85% in long-bone metaphyses), but when they do, they are located mostly in the cervical spine, particularly at C2.[9] These lesions most commonly arise from the spinous and transverse processes, but they also may arise from the vertebral body. On T1-weighted and T2-weighted images, they appear as central hyperintense lesions surrounded by hypointense calcified cortex. The cartilaginous cap is hypo- to isointense on T1-weighted images and iso- to hyperintense on T2-weighted images and exhibits peripheral enhancement of cartilage (**Fig. 12.8**).[30] MRI is the preferred imaging modality for measuring the cartilaginous cap and determining the status of regional neural and musculoskeletal tissue. Thickening of the cap (>1 cm) should raise concern for malignant transformation to chondrosarcoma. CT may be used for evaluating the osseous structure of the lesion, confirming the contiguity of the medullary cavity with the parent bone, and evaluating for fractures.

Aneurysmal Bone Cyst

These lesions are expansile benign neoplasms containing thin-walled cavities filled with blood and blood products

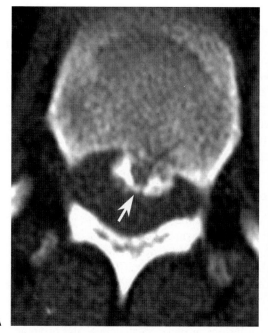
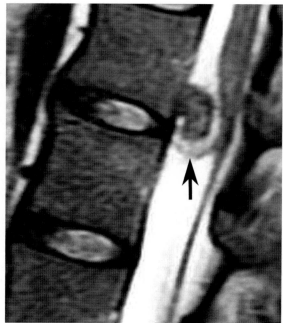

Fig. 12.8 Thoracic osteochondroma. **(A)** An axial CT image showing the characteristic "mushroom" appearance of the lesion (*arrow*) extending into the spinal canal. **(B)** A sagittal T2-weighted image show- ing a region of high signal intensity around the osteochondroma, which likely represents a cartilaginous cap (*arrow*).

that occur most commonly in patients less than 20 years old. A substantial proportion of aneurysmal bone cysts are associated with preexisting osseous lesions, such as an osteoblastoma, giant cell tumor, chondroblastoma, nonossifying fibroma, or fibrous dysplasia.[31] They arise in the neural arch, but most extend into the vertebral body. The classic presentation is a balloon-like expansile remodeling of bone, leaving a thinned "eggshell" cortex. On T1-weighted and T2-weighted images, the lesions appear as lobulated neural arch masses, commonly with extension into the vertebral body, epidural space, and adjacent vertebral bodies and ribs.[32] Intratumoral cysts contain fluid-fluid levels secondary to blood breakdown products (**Fig. 12.9**), although visualization of these levels often requires the patient to be motionless for

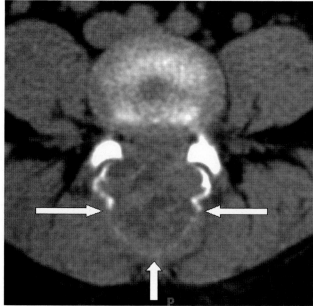
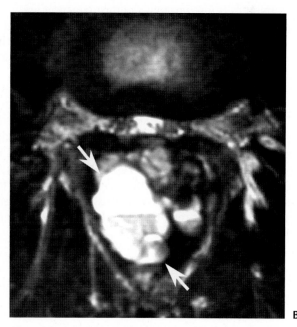

Fig. 12.9 Aneurysmal bone cyst. **(A)** An axial CT image of the lumbar spine shows a lytic lesion (*arrows*) expanding the posterior elements and surrounded by a thin rim of bone resembling an eggshell. **(B)** An axial T2-weighted image of the same patient shows a cystic lesion (*arrows*) within the posterior elements with fluid–fluid levels.

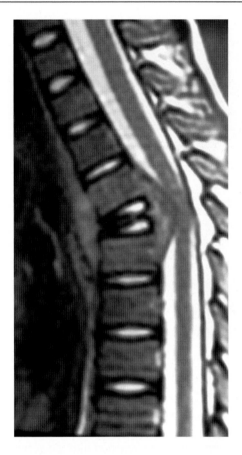

Fig. 12.10 A sagittal T2-weighted image of an eosinophilic granuloma showing the typical finding of a vertebra plana. In this case, there is also an epidural mass that displaces the spinal cord. Note the associated kyphotic deformity.

a few minutes before imaging. Contrast enhancement may be present at the periphery of the tumor and in the septations. Vertebral body collapse may occur secondary to the extensive vertebral body destruction associated with such lesions.

Eosinophilic Granuloma

This lytic lesion of the vertebral body classically presents with a single collapsed vertebral body (vertebra plana) in patients less than 10 years old (**Fig. 12.10**) and consists of a benign proliferation of Langerhans cell histiocytes. The lesions are hyperintense on T2-weighted images but present with variable intensity on T1-weighted images. Contrast enhancement is robust.[5]

Primary Malignant Tumors

Multiple Myeloma

Multiple myeloma is the multifocal, metastatic, and systemic presentation of a solitary bone plasmacytoma (see next paragraph). Like solitary bone plasmacytomas, focal lesions appear in the vertebral bodies with low to intermediate signal intensity on T1-weighted images compared with normal bone marrow, and they appear hyperintense on T2-weighted images. Postgadolinium enhancement is often present (**Fig. 12.11**). Multiple myeloma also is revealed on MRI by diffuse marrow involvement at multiple spinal levels.[33] Compared with other metastatic lesions that usually have early pedicle involvement, multiple myeloma usually involves the pedicle late in the course of disease.[9]

Solitary Bone Plasmacytoma

This tumor, a malignant tumor presenting as a mass of monoclonal plasma cells from bone or soft tissue, is the solitary form of multiple myeloma and may precede it by several years. Clinical differentiation from multiple myeloma requires a biopsy-proven solitary lesion, the absence of other such lesions in the skeleton, and the absence of anemia, hypercalcemia, and renal involvement suggesting systemic myeloma.[34] Such lesions are lytic, destructive, and often accompanied by compression fractures associated with soft-tissue masses and fractures that may lead to severe collapse (vertebra plana). T1-weighted images reveal a solitary lesion centered in the vertebral body that is hypo- or isointense compared with muscle and can show curvilinear low signal areas and/ or cortical infolding caused by end-plate fractures. In most cases, the posterior elements are involved and neural compression is varied. T2-weighted images reveal heterogeneous signal within the lesion with focal hyperintensities. Mild to moderate diffuse contrast enhancement is common and peripheral (rim) contrast enhancement is rare.[35] Scanning of the entire skeleton is mandatory to identify a secondary lesion, which occurs in the spine in one third of patients.[9]

Chordoma

These malignant tumors arising from notochord remnants typically present in one of two histologic patterns. The more common type, known as a *typical chordoma*, is composed of lobules and sheets of physaliphorous cells, which contain intracytoplasmic vacuoles and abundant mucin. The less common type contains cartilaginous foci and is termed *chondroid chordoma*.[5] Chordomas present as lytic, destructive lesions arising in the midline of the spinal column at any location from clivus to coccyx, but they are found more commonly at the sacrococcygeal (50%) and sphenooccipital (clival) (35%) areas and less commonly in the vertebral body (15%).[9] For lesions within the vertebral bodies, a cervical location (particularly at C2) is most common, followed by lumbar and thoracic areas. Chordomas often are several centimeters in size at discovery, usually involve two or more adjacent vertebrae, and extend into the intervertebral discs, surrounding paravertebral soft tissues, and spi-

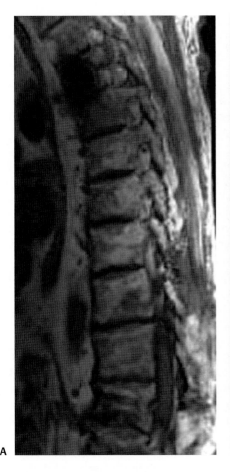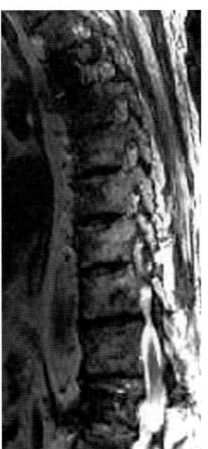

A   B

Fig. 12.11 Thoracic multiple myeloma. T1-weighted **(A)** and T2-weighted **(B)** images showing multiple lesions within the thoracic vertebral bodies at multiple spinal levels, centered about the posterior vertebral bodies and pedicles. The diagnosis can be confirmed by correlation with CT imaging and also with urine and serum protein electrophoresis.

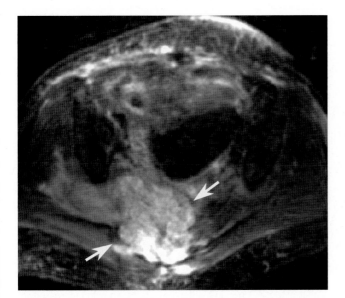

Fig. 12.12 An axial fat-suppressed T2-weighted image of a right-side sacral chordoma revealing a hyperintense lesion between the ilia that has extended into the pelvis and right gluteal muscles (between *arrows*).

nal canal. On T1-weighted images, the lesions are hypo- or isointense (compared with marrow). On T2-weighted images, lesions are hyperintense compared with intervertebral discs and CSF secondary to the high intratumoral mucin content, and are septated by low-signal fibrous bands (**Fig. 12.12**). STIR or fat-suppressed T2-weighted images can help in defining borders with neighboring soft tissues. Contrast-enhanced images range from contrast blush to robust enhancement.[36,37]

Sarcomas

Primary sarcomas include chondrosarcoma, osteosarcoma, and Ewing sarcoma, all of which involve the spine only occasionally. Primary fibrosarcomas of the spine are extremely rare.

Chondrosarcoma

These malignant, lytic tumors of chondrocytes are characterized by the formation of cartilaginous matrix, can occur as primary tumors or as malignant degeneration of

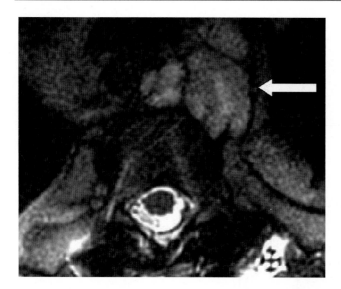

Fig. 12.13 An axial T2-weighted image of a hyperintense, exophytic, cauliflower-shaped lesion, found to be a chondrosarcoma, arising from the left anterior vertebral body (*arrow*).

osteochondromas and enchondromas, can cause cortical disruption, and can extend into surrounding soft tissues. Chondrosarcomas can occur wherever cartilage exists,[38] and approximately 5% occur in the spine.[39] T2-weighted images reveal high signal intensity in areas of hyaline cartilage and low intensity in areas of mineralized matrix. T1-weighted images are helpful in delineating soft-tissue invasion. Contrast-enhanced images show strong enhancement of the septa with "ring and arc" patterns that de-

lineate areas of hyaline cartilage, cystic mucoid tissue, and necrosis, all of which do not enhance with contrast (**Fig. 12.13**).[40]

Osteosarcoma/Osteogenic Sarcoma

Of all primary osteogenic sarcomas, 4% occur in the spine and sacrum, primarily in the posterior spinal elements.[41] These malignant, lytic tumors of osteoblasts are characterized by the formation of immature, woven osteoid and can occur as primary tumors or as malignant degeneration in individuals with Paget disease, irradiated bone, or bone infarcts. These tumors present primarily in the vertebral bodies, commonly with extension into the posterior elements, and typically have focal areas of low signal on all pulse sequences secondary to matrix mineralization (**Fig. 12.14**).[42] In the telangiectatic form, T2-weighted images may show fluid–fluid levels.

Ewing Sarcoma

The spine is a rare site for Ewing sarcoma. When it does occur, it usually represents a metastatic tumor from another site of origin.[26] Usually centered in the vertebral body or sacrum, Ewing sarcoma often causes a "moth-eaten" or permeative type of bone destruction rather than extensive bone loss. Fifty percent of these lesions have an extraosseous, noncalcified, soft-tissue mass.[43] On T1-weighted images, these lesions are hypo- to isointense compared with surrounding bone marrow, and the cortex usually is preserved despite extraosseous tumor spread. On T2-weighted images,

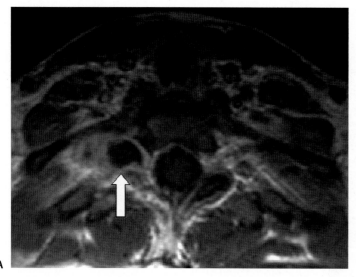
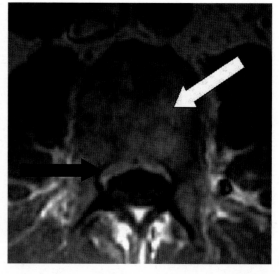

A   B

Fig. 12.14 Osteosarcoma. **(A)** An axial postgadolinium T1-weighted image of a right-side osteosarcoma at the cervicothoracic junction showing enhancement around a central hypointense cystic/necrotic area (*arrow*). **(B)** An axial postgadolinium T1-weighted image of a lumbar osteosarcoma, in a different patient, showing increased signal within the vertebral body (*white arrow*) and in the epidural space (*black arrow*). Both diagnoses were made via percutaneous biopsy.

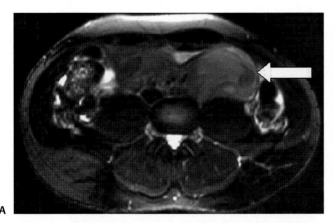

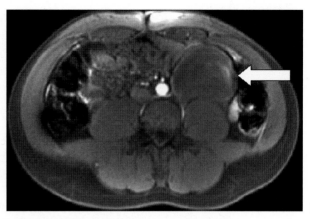

Fig. 12.15 Left-side paraspinal ganglioneuroma. **(A)** A T2-weighted image showing a lesion adjacent to the vertebral body and anterior to the psoas muscle. The lesion (*arrow*) is hyperintense compared with muscle. **(B)** A postgadolinium, T1-weighted image showing the lesion (*arrow*) to be isointense compared with muscle, with sparse intralesional and peripheral enhancement.

lesions are hyperintense. MRI is the ideal imaging study for delineating extension of soft-tissue mass. Because Ewing sarcoma is histologically a small, round cell tumor, it can be radiographically identical to primitive neuroectodermal tumors, Langerhans cell histiocytosis, lymphoma, leukemia, myeloma, and metastatic neuroblastoma. Ewing sarcoma may also have imaging characteristics similar to those of osteomyelitis. In addition, like patients with Langerhans cell histiocytosis, patients with Ewing sarcoma may present with vertebral body collapse.[44]

Other Tumors

Neuroblastic Tumors

These embryonal tumors, which are derived from neural crest cells, exist as a spectrum ranging from the most benign ganglioneuromas, to intermediate-differentiated ganglioneuroblastomas, to the most malignant neuroblastomas. These tumors present almost exclusively in patients less than 10 years old and almost exclusively as abdominal or thoracic paraspinal masses with intraspinal extension.[5] The lesions are typically large and extend through a widened neural foramen, creating dumbbell-shaped morphologies and compressing the spinal cord (**Fig. 12.15**). The lesions are hypo- to isointense on T1-weighted images and hypo- to hyperintense on T2-weighted images. Although classically they present as paraspinal masses, they may appear as metastatic lesions within vertebral bodies. Contrast enhancement varies but often surrounds areas of internal hemorrhage or necrosis.[45,46]

Angiolipoma

These benign lesions of adipose and vascular elements present in the spine primarily as epidural masses; they rarely

present in an intramedullary location. Because the lesions are composed of fat and vascular tissues, MRI shows heterogeneous signal intensity. On T1-weighted images, most lesions are hyperintense with iso- to hypointense areas around prominent vascular components. The lesion may appear heterogeneous on T2-weighted images, but it generally has high signal intensity. Thus, fat-suppressed T1-weighted images with contrast are most useful for defining this lesion and often show heterogeneous enhancement. Interestingly, these lesions do not show vascular flow voids. These lesions may destroy adjacent bone in the anterior epidural space, although only rarely in the posterior epidural space.[47]

Lymphoma

Lymphoreticular neoplasms present with variable imaging manifestations within the spine. All locations of the spine may be affected: epidural space (most common), osseous structures, lymphomatous meninges (within the subarachnoid space), and intramedullary (least common).[9] Lymphomas of the spine are usually metastatic lesions, not primary lesions arising in the spine.[48] Conversely, only 3% to 4% of all malignant bone tumors are primary osseous lymphoma. In the spine, non-Hodgkin lymphoma is far more common than Hodgkin disease, and more than 80% of such lesions are of B-cell origin.[49]

MRI is ideal for defining the spinal compartment within which the tumor resides. Epidural lesions are isointense on T1-weighted images and variable, but often isointense or hyperintense to spinal cord on T2-weighted images (**Fig. 12.16**). Osseous lesions are hypointense compared with normal marrow on T1-weighted images and iso- to hyperintense on T2-weighted images. Leptomeningitic lymphomas result in thickening of the nerve roots, occasionally with focal nodules, which are isointense compared with the spinal cord on T1-weighted and T2-weighted images.

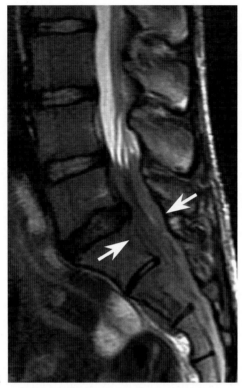
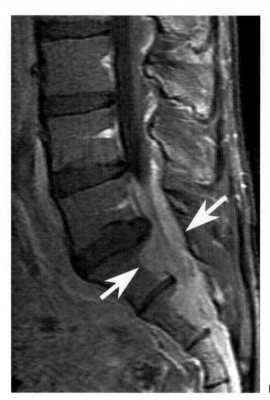

Fig. 12.16 Epidural B-cell lymphoma surrounding and compressing the thecal sac in the lumbar spine. **(A)** On a sagittal T2-weighted image, the lesion is isointense compared with the cord and fills the spinal canal with expansion of the canal at S1 (*arrows*). **(B)** On a sagittal postgadolinium T1-weighted image, the lesion shows robust enhancement.

Intramedullary masses show cord thickening that is isointense compared with the spinal cord on T1-weighted images and hyperintense with surrounding edema on T2-weighted images. Contrast-enhanced images show diffuse uniform enhancement regardless of the location, with a diagnostic accuracy of 99%.[9]

■ Intradural–Extramedullary Tumors

These lesions arise within the dura but not from within the spinal cord. Classic MRI findings include a widened ipsilateral subarachnoid space in which the cord and roots are displaced away from the mass (**Fig. 12.17**). Nerve sheath tumors (schwannomas and neurofibromas) and meningiomas account for more than 80% of such masses.[50]

Meningioma

Most of these tumors are slow growing, benign (>95%), and based on the dura mater.[51] CT imaging may provide added detail because these tumors can calcify; however, MRI is still the ideal imaging modality.[51] Classically, the lesions are isointense compared with the spinal cord on T1-weighted images and iso- to hyperintense on T2-weighted images (**Fig. 12.18**). Focal areas of hypointensity occur in the presence of calcifications or flow voids. Contrast-enhanced T1-weighted images show prominent enhancement, sometimes with a broad-based dural attachment (dural "tails"). Most lesions are solitary and occur most commonly in the thoracic spine (80%) followed by the cervical spine (16%) and lumbar spine (4%).[52,53] Compared with nerve sheath tumors, which are usually anterolateral, meningiomas are usually located dorsal to the cord.[52,53]

Schwannoma

These benign neoplasms of the peripheral nerve sheaths are the most common intradural–extramedullary masses and appear as well-circumscribed lesions that may be intradural–extramedullary (75%), completely extradural–paraspinal (15%), or intra- and extradural (dumbbell-shaped).[5] T1-

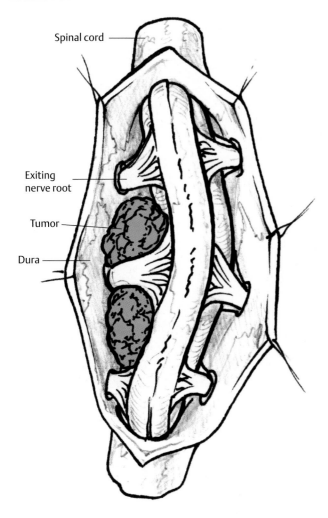

Spinal cord

Exiting
nerve root

Tumor

Dura

Fig. 12.17 Artist's sketch (dorsal view) depicting the imaging characteristics of an intradural–extramedullary mass.

weighted images often show an iso- to hypointense lesion relative to the spinal cord that may be associated with adjacent osseous erosion, such as widening of the neural foramen or vertebral scalloping.[54,55] In contrast to meningiomas, most schwannomas are hyperintense on T2-weighted images. Postgadolinium T1-weighted images show enhancement that may be homogeneous, heterogeneous, or rim-enhancing around cystic areas (**Fig. 12.19**). Hemorrhage and cystic degeneration are more common with schwannomas than with neurofibromas. Solitary lesions are usually sporadic, but when these lesions occur at multiple concurrent sites, the diagnosis of neurofibromatosis type 2 should be considered.

Neurofibroma

These benign neoplasms of the peripheral nerve sheaths can present as focal, diffuse, or plexiform lesions. They can undergo transformation to malignant tumors. Neurofibromas

have MRI characteristics similar to those of schwannomas (**Fig. 12.20**), but they often occur as multiple lesions in a patient with the stigmata, including the following:

- Vertebral anomalies
- Meningoceles
- Dural ectasia
- Intramedullary astrocytomas
- Short-segment thoracic scoliosis or kyphosis
- Axillary or inguinal freckling
- Café-au-lait spots
- Optic glioma
- Lisch nodules (hamartomas of the iris) of neurofibromatosis type 1

Therefore, if lesions that look like a schwannoma or neurofibroma on imaging occur in an individual with characteristics of neurofibromatosis type 1, the lesions are likely to be neurofibromas, not schwannomas. Even when isolated, these lesions are usually associated with neurofibromatosis type 1. Additionally, and unlike schwannomas, neurofibromas on T2-weighted images often have a peripheral area of high signal intensity surrounding a central area of low to intermediate signal intensity known as a *target sign*. Also unlike schwannomas, neurofibromas typically lack a cystic component.

Malignant Peripheral Nerve Sheath Tumor

These malignant spindle-cell sarcomas of neural origin involve the spinal roots, neural plexuses, peripheral nerves, and end organs and are divided into malignant schwannomas and neurofibrosarcomas. Approximately 50% to 60% are associated with neurofibromatosis type 1. They most commonly present as large (>5 cm), infiltrative, hemorrhagic, soft-tissue masses.[51] MRI is the preferred imaging modality. The lesions are hyperintense compared with surrounding fat on T2-weighted images and on STIR images, and isointense compared with muscle on T1-weighted images (**Fig. 12.21**). T1-weighted images with contrast show marked enhancement. Infiltration into surrounding soft tissue may lead to indistinct margins. Hemorrhage and necrosis within the mass may be seen, resulting in heterogeneous signal. Intradural–extramedullary masses often may show a dumbbell configuration with widening of the intervertebral foramina and erosion of the pedicles. Because of this characteristic, these lesions may be difficult to distinguish from benign spinal schwannomas. Thus, a malignant peripheral nerve sheath tumor should be suspected in the presence of sudden growth in a preexisting schwannoma or neurofibroma.

Hemangiopericytoma

Although these dural-based lesions appear, radiographically, very similar to meningiomas, they are hypervascular, more

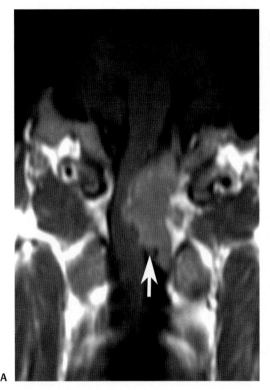
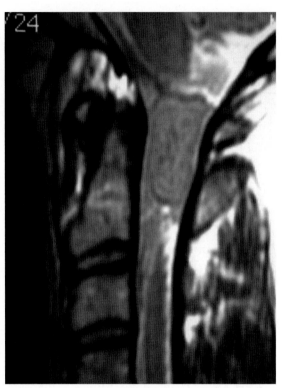

A

B

Fig. 12.18 Cervical meningioma. **(A)** A coronal postgadolinium T1-weighted image showing a widely dural-based lesion (*arrow*) that enhances and is hyperintense compared with the cord. **(B)** On a sagittal T2-weighted image, the lesion is slightly hyperintense compared with the cord, showing cord displacement and widening of the ipsilateral CSF space, characteristic of intradural–extramedullary lesions.

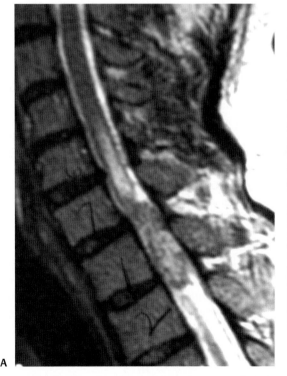
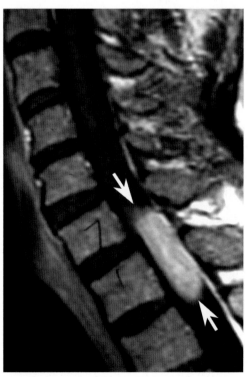

A

B

Fig. 12.19 A sagittal image of a schwannoma at the cervicothoracic junction. The dural-based lesion is slightly hyperintense compared with the cord on T2-weighted images **(A)** and shows strong homogeneous contrast enhancement with gadolinium on T1-weighted images (*arrows*) **(B)**.

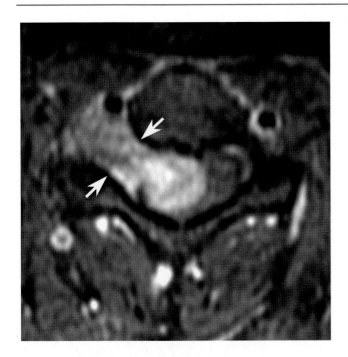

Fig. 12.20 An axial T2-weighted image of a cervical neurofibroma showing a dumbbell-shaped lesion that resides in both the intradural and extradural compartments. Note the neuroforaminal widening where the tumor exits the spinal canal (*arrows*).

locally aggressive, and more prone to metastasis. They often erode and replace adjacent bone and exhibit large soft-tissue components. MRI reveals multilobular masses hypointense on T1-weighted images and hyperintense on T2-weighted images.[56] T1-weighted images with contrast and fat suppression show robust, homogeneous enhancement. Malignant meningiomas may look similar to hemangiopericytomas,

but meningiomas often possess finger-like processes rather than the lobules of hemangiopericytomas.

◼ Intramedullary Tumors

These lesions of the spinal cord itself account for 5% to 10% of all central nervous system tumors, 20% of intraspinal neoplasms in adults, and 30% to 35% of intraspinal neoplasms in children.[9] More than 90% of these lesions are gliomas.[57] Of spinal cord gliomas, more than 95% are ependymomas and low-grade astrocytomas, with ependymomas being more common (60%) than astrocytomas (30%).[9,58] In children, however, astrocytomas are more common.[59] The remaining lesions include hemangioblastomas and metastases, but these lesions are very rare.

MRI is the diagnostic procedure of choice in evaluating possible spinal cord tumors and myelopathy in general. Classic MRI findings show a diffuse, multisegmental smoothly enlarged cord or filum terminale mass with gradual surrounding subarachnoid effacement. Many lesions are associated with syringomyelia, or cyst-like cavities within the cord, extending within the central canal of the cord or eccentric to the canal in a longitudinal orientation (**Fig. 12.22**).

Ependymoma and Low-Grade Astrocytoma

Ependymomas and low-grade astrocytomas appear nearly identical on MRI. Widening of the cord secondary to infiltration and syringomyelia are most obvious on T2-weighted images, in which the hyperintense CSF signal is contrasted against the less intense cord signal. Additionally, such lesions typically possess high signal intensity on T2-weighted images. T1-weighted images usually reveal lesions that are iso- or hypointense relative to the surrounding spinal cord (**Fig. 12.23**).[60,61]

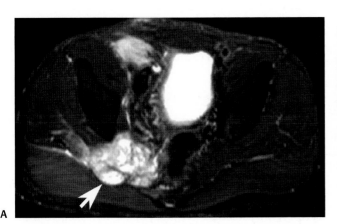
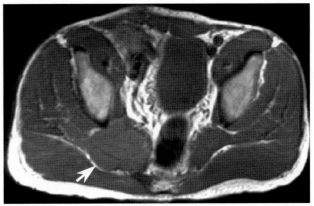

A **B**

Fig. 12.21 Right-side sacral malignant peripheral nerve sheath tumor. Compared with muscle, the lesion (*arrow on each*) is hyperintense on an axial fat-suppressed T2-weighted image (**A**) and isointense on an axial T1-weighted image (**B**).

Mixed signal lesions are seen if hemorrhage (more typical of ependymomas), tumor necrosis, or cyst formation has occurred. With the administration of contrast, intramedullary tumors generally show robust enhancement, often in a nodular, peripheral, or heterogeneous pattern (**Fig. 12.24**). Such lesions usually are located in the cervical and/or thoracic spinal cord.[62] Ependymomas more commonly have a "cap sign," referring to a focal hypointensity on T2-weighted images that appears in areas of hemosiderin at the cranial or caudal margin of the tumor. A helpful tool for learning to identify intramedullary spinal cord tumors, most specifically ependymomas, is recalling the five C's:

- Central within the cord
- Cervical in location
- Contrast-enhancing
- (Associated with) cysts
- Cap sign

Unlike cellular or mixed ependymomas, which most commonly occur in the cervical spine, myxopapillary ependymomas most often occur in the conus medullaris and filum terminale.[63] Because these lesions typically are slow growing, vertebral body scalloping is common with a large conus lesion that fills the entire lumbosacral thecal sac; the neural foramina also may be enlarged. Interestingly, although these lesions grow from ependymal cells of the conus and filum, making them intramedullary in origin, they most commonly appear like intradural–extramedullary masses because there is no widening of the cord at the level of the cauda equina. Thus, CSF signal on T2-weighted images creates a meniscus-like sign around the lesion (**Fig. 12.25**).

Paragangliomas are rare tumors that most commonly present in the cauda equina, where they often are indistinguishable from myxopapillary ependymomas. On MRI, these lesions are typically seen as well-defined areas of intense enhancement after contrast administration. Because of their high degree of vascularity, paragangliomas often show prominent foci of high-velocity signal loss ("flow voids"), corresponding to enlarged feeding arteries and/or draining veins.

Hemangioblastoma

Hemangioblastomas typically appear as highly vascular nodules within the *subpial* compartment; thus, they lie closer to the surface of the cord than do ependymomas and astrocytomas. They are associated with extensive cyst formation that diffusely enlarges the cord in up to 70% of patients.[64] Because of the highly vascular nature of such lesions, robust homogeneous contrast enhancement within the tumor nodule is the rule, and MRI almost always shows prominent flow voids (**Fig. 12.26**). Multiple lesions can occur in the presence of von Hippel–Lindau syndrome, with rare extensive involvement of the leptomeninges, referred to as *leptomeningeal*

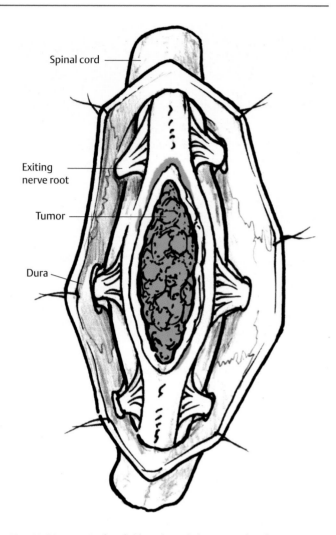

Fig. 12.22 Artist's sketch (dorsal view) depicting the characteristics of an intramedullary mass. The mass diffusely enlarges the cord over multiple spinal segments.

Spinal cord

Exiting nerve root

Tumor

Dura

hemangioblastomatosis.[65] When a spinal hemangioblastoma is suspected on MRI, it is advisable to image the entire central nervous system to exclude multiple lesions.

Intramedullary Metastases

Intramedullary metastases are rare, representing only 4% to 8.5% of all central nervous system metastases.[9] Most spinal cord metastases are localized to the pia mater in which they appear as a thin rim of enhancement along the cord surface on postcontrast T1-weighted images. In addition, edema out of proportion to a focal, small cord lesion suggests metastasis, even if isolated.[66] Primary malignancies accounting for such lesions are most commonly lung and breast carcinomas, lymphoma, leukemia, and melanoma.[67] In 20% of

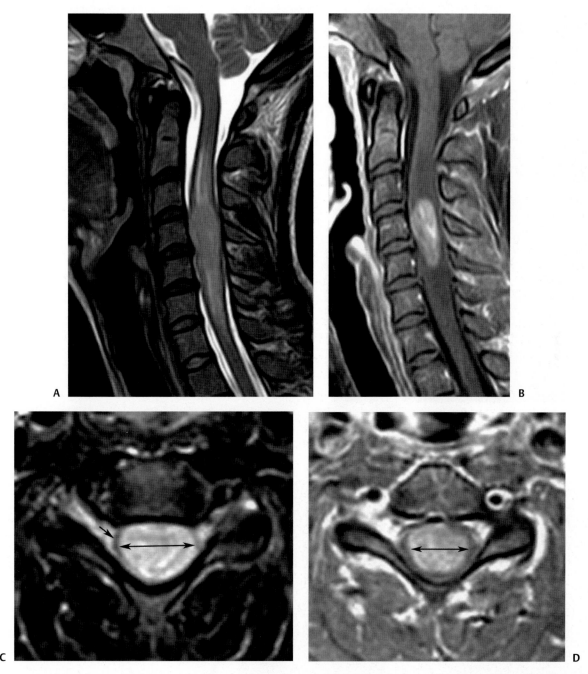

Fig. 12.23 Cervical ependymoma. **(A)** A sagittal T2-weighted image showing a large cervical ependymoma centered at C4-C5 but with cord signal change extending from C2 to C7. **(B)** A postgadolinium T1-weighted image showing that the tumor is located at C4-C5 and that the signal change extended from C2 to C7 shown in **A** represents edema proximal and distal to the lesion. **(C)** An axial T2-weighted im-age showing that the lesion (*between arrowheads*) is located within the spinal cord, which is seen as a thin sliver of low signal intensity surrounding the lesion (*arrow*). **(D)** A postgadolinium T1-weighted image showing similar findings with enhancement of the tumor (*between arrowheads*).

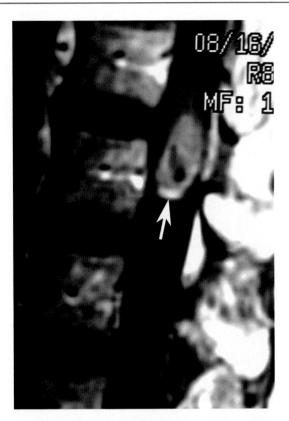

Fig. 12.24 A sagittal postgadolinium, T1-weighted image of a thoracolumbar ependymoma shows intrinsic enlargement of the cord, robust contrast enhancement, and an adjacent cyst inferiorly (*arrow*).

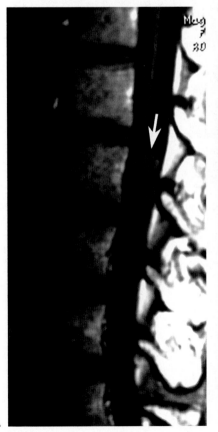

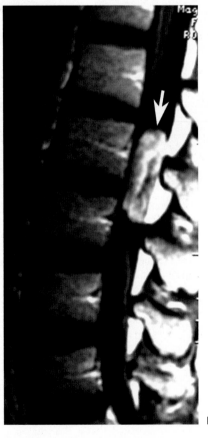

Fig. 12.25 Myxopapillary ependymoma of the lumbar region. Sagittal T1-weighted images revealing a hypointense lesion (*arrow on each*) on precontrast imaging **(A)** and robust enhancement with gadolinium **(B)**. Although derived from the filum, ependymomas in this segment of the spine reside in the intradural–extramedullary compartment.

A

B

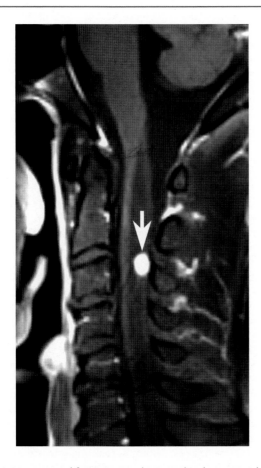

Fig. 12.26 A sagittal fat-suppressed T1-weighted image with gadolinium of a cervical hemangioblastoma, revealing a small, eccentrically located, robustly enhancing tumor nodule (*arrow*) associated with a large cervicothoracic syrinx.

patients, intramedullary metastasis is the first presentation of cancer for the patient.[9]

MRI with and without contrast can be quite helpful in distinguishing benign cysts or syrinxes from those associated with intramedullary tumors. Tumor cysts are smaller, more irregular, often eccentrically positioned within the cord, and almost always associated with an enhancing tumor, whereas benign cysts are rostral or caudal to the tumor, have smooth walls, cause symmetric cord expansion, and do not show contrast enhancement.[68]

Other lesions of the spinal cord that must be included in the differential diagnosis include autoimmune or inflammatory myelitis, cord ischemia or infarction, and arteriovenous malformations.[5]

References

1. Masaryk TJ. Neoplastic disease of the spine. Radiol Clin North Am 1991;29:829–845
2. Sevick RJ, Wallace CJ. MR imaging of neoplasms of the lumbar spine. Magn Reson Imaging Clin N Am 1999;7:539–553
3. Williams RS, Williams JP. Tumors. In: Rao KCVG, Williams JP, Lee BCP, Sherman JL, eds. MRI and CT of the Spine. Baltimore: Williams & Wilkins; 1994:347–426
4. Khanna AJ, Shindle MK, Wasserman BA, et al. Use of magnetic resonance imaging in differentiating compartmental location of spinal tumors. Am J Orthop 2005;34:472–476
5. Osborn AG. Cysts, tumors, and tumorlike lesions of the spine and spinal cord. In: Osborn AG, ed. Diagnostic Neuroradiology. St. Louis: Mosby; 1994:876–918
6. Gebauer GP, Farjoodi P, Sciubba DM, et al. Magnetic resonance imaging of spine tumors: classification, differential diagnosis, and spectrum of disease. J Bone Joint Surg Am 2008;90(Suppl 4):146–162
7. Perrin RG, Laxton AW. Metastatic spine disease: epidemiology, pathophysiology, and evaluation of patients. Neurosurg Clin N Am 2004;15:365–373
8. Kamholtz R, Sze G. Current imaging in spinal metastatic disease. Semin Oncol 1991;18:158–169
9. Ross JS. Neoplasms, pathways of spread. In: Ross JS, Brant-Zawadzki M, Moore KR, Crim J, Chen MZ, Katzman GL, eds. Diagnostic Imaging: Spine. Salt Lake City: Amirsys; 2004:IV-1-2–IV-1-5
10. Balériaux DLF. Spinal cord tumors. Eur Radiol 1999;9:1252–1258
11. Van Goethem JWM, van den Hauwe L, Ozsarlak O, De Schepper AMA, Parizel PM. Spinal tumors. Eur J Radiol 2004;50:159–176
12. Algra PR, Bloem JL, Tissing H, Falke TH, Arndt JW, Verboom LJ. Detection of vertebral metastases: comparison between MR imaging and bone scintigraphy. Radiographics 1991;11:219–232
13. Avrahami E, Tadmor R, Dally O, Hadar H. Early MR demonstration of spinal metastases in patients with normal radiographs and CT and radionuclide bone scans. J Comput Assist Tomogr 1989;13:598–602
14. Li KC, Poon PY. Sensitivity and specificity of MRI in detecting malignant spinal cord compression and in distinguishing malignant from benign compression fractures of vertebrae. Magn Reson Imaging 1988;6:547–556

15. Constans JP, de Divitiis E, Donzelli R, Spaziante R, Meder JF, Haye C. Spinal metastases with neurological manifestations. Review of 600 cases. J Neurosurg 1983;59:111–118

16. Tatsui H, Onomura T, Morishita S, Oketa M, Inoue T. Survival rates of patients with metastatic spinal cancer after scintigraphic detection of abnormal radioactive accumulation. Spine (Phila Pa 1976) 1996;21:2143–2148

17. Byrne TN. Spinal cord compression from epidural metastases. N Engl J Med 1992;327:614–619

18. Klein SL, Sanford RA, Muhlbauer MS. Pediatric spinal epidural metastases. J Neurosurg 1991;74:70–75

19. Algra PR, Heimans JJ, Valk J, Nauta JJ, Lachniet M, Van Kooten B. Do metastases in vertebrae begin in the body or the pedicles? Imaging study in 45 patients. AJR Am J Roentgenol 1992;158:1275–1279

20. Baker LL, Goodman SB, Perkash I, Lane B, Enzmann DR. Benign versus pathologic compression fractures of vertebral bodies: assessment with conventional spin-echo, chemical-shift, and STIR MR imaging. Radiology 1990;174:495–502

21. Yochum TR, Lile RL, Schultz GD, Mick TJ, Brown CW. Acquired spinal stenosis secondary to an expanding thoracic vertebral hemangioma. Spine (Phila Pa 1976) 1993;18:299–305

22. Bandiera S, Gasbarrini A, De Iure F, Cappuccio M, Picci P, Boriani S. Symptomatic vertebral hemangioma: the treatment of 23 cases and a review of the literature. Chir Organi Mov 2002;87:1–15

23. Baudrez V, Galant C, Vande Berg BC. Benign vertebral hemangioma: MR-histological correlation. Skeletal Radiol 2001;30:442–446

24. Djindjian M, Nguyen JP, Gaston A, Pavlovitch JM, Poirier J, Awad IA. Multiple vertebral hemangiomas with neurological signs. Case report. J Neurosurg 1992;76:1025–1028

25. Liu PT, Chivers FS, Roberts CC, Schultz CJ, Beauchamp CP. Imaging of osteoid osteoma with dynamic gadolinium-enhanced MR imaging. Radiology 2003;227:691–700

26. Dorwart RH, LaMasters DL, Watanabe TJ. Tumors. In: Newton T, Potts D, eds. Computed Tomography of the Spine and Spinal Cord. San Anselmo, CA: Clavadel Press; 1983:115–147

27. Boriani S, Capanna R, Donati D, Levine A, Picci P, Savini R. Osteoblastoma of the spine. Clin Orthop Relat Res 1992;278:37–45

28. Murphey MD, Nomikos GC, Flemming DJ, Gannon FH, Temple HT, Kransdorf MJ. From the archives of AFIP. Imaging of giant cell tumor and giant cell reparative granuloma of bone: radiologic-pathologic correlation. Radiographics 2001;21:1283–1309

29. Luther N, Bilsky MH, Härtl R. Giant cell tumor of the spine. Neurosurg Clin N Am 2008;19:49–55

30. Sharma MC, Arora R, Deol PS, Mahapatra AK, Mehta VS, Sarkar C. Osteochondroma of the spine: an enigmatic tumor of the spinal cord. A series of 10 cases. J Neurosurg Sci 2002;46:66–70, discussion 70

31. Manaster BJ. Skeletal Radiology. Chicago: Year Book Medical Publishers; 1989

32. Boriani S, De Iure F, Campanacci L, et al. Aneurysmal bone cyst of the mobile spine: report on 41 cases. Spine (Phila Pa 1976) 2001;26:27–35

33. Moulopoulos LA, Dimopoulos MA, Alexanian R, Leeds NE, Libshitz HI. Multiple myeloma: MR patterns of response to treatment. Radiology 1994;193:441–446

34. Ota K, Tsuda T, Katayama N, et al. A therapeutic strategy for isolated plasmacytoma of bone. J Int Med Res 2001;29:366–373

35. Shah BK, Saifuddin A, Price GJ. Magnetic resonance imaging of spinal plasmacytoma. Clin Radiol 2000;55:439–445

36. Boriani S, Weinstein JN, Biagini R. Primary bone tumors of the spine. Terminology and surgical staging. Spine (Phila Pa 1976) 1997;22:1036–1044

37. Soo MYS. Chordoma: review of clinicoradiological features and factors affecting survival. Australas Radiol 2001;45:427–434

38. Dorfman HD, Czerniak B. Bone Tumors. St. Louis: Mosby; 1998

39. Ross JS. Chondrosarcoma. In: Ross JS, Brant-Zawadzki M, Moore KR, Crim J, Chen MZ, Katzman GL, eds. Diagnostic Imaging: Spine. Salt Lake City: Amirsys; 2004:IV-1-38–IV-1-41

40. Aoki J, Sone S, Fujioka F, et al. MR of enchondroma and chondrosarcoma: rings and arcs of Gd-DTPA enhancement. J Comput Assist Tomogr 1991;15:1011–1016

41. Crim J. Osteosarcoma. In: Ross JS, Brant-Zawadzki M, Moore KR, Crim J, Chen MZ, Katzman GL, eds. Diagnostic Imaging: Spine. Salt Lake City: Amirsys; 2004:IV-1-42–IV-1-45

42. Bramwell VHC. Osteosarcomas and other cancers of bone. Curr Opin Oncol 2000;12:330–336

43. Crim J. Ewing sarcoma. In: Ross JS, Brant-Zawadzki M, Moore KR, Crim J, Chen MZ, Katzman GL, eds. Diagnostic Imaging: Spine. Salt Lake City: Amirsys; 2004:IV-1-50–IV-1-53

44. Boyko OB, Cory DA, Cohen MD, Provisor A, Mirkin D, DeRosa GP. MR imaging of osteogenic and Ewing's sarcoma. AJR Am J Roentgenol 1987;148:317–322

45. Lonergan GJ, Schwab CM, Suarez ES, Carlson CL. From the archives of the AFIP. Neuroblastoma, ganglioneuroblastoma, and ganglioneuroma: radiologic-pathologic correlation. Radiographics 2002;22:911–934

46. Sofka CM, Semelka RC, Kelekis NL, et al. Magnetic resonance imaging of neuroblastoma using current techniques. Magn Reson Imaging 1999;17:193–198

47. Oge HK, Söylemezoglu F, Rousan N, Ozcan OE. Spinal angiolipoma: case report and review of literature. J Spinal Disord 1999;12:353–356

48. Katzman GL. Lymphoma. In: Ross JS, Brant-Zawadzki M, Moore KR, Crim J, Chen MZ, Katzman GL, eds. Diagnostic Imaging: Spine. Salt Lake City: Amirsys; 2004:IV-1-54–IV-1-57

49. Koeller KK, Rosenblum RS, Morrison AL. Neoplasms of the spinal cord and filum terminale: radiologic-pathologic correlation. Radiographics 2000;20:1721–1749

50. Li MH, Holtås S, Larsson EM. MR imaging of intradural extramedullary tumors. Acta Radiol 1992;33:207–212

51. Burger PC, Shcheithauer BW, Vogel FS. Surgical Pathology of the Nervous System and Its Coverings. Philadelphia: Churchill Livingstone; 2002

52. Cohen-Gadol AA, Zikel OM, Koch CA, Scheithauer BW, Krauss WE. Spinal meningiomas in patients younger than 50 years of age: a 21-year experience. J Neurosurg 2003;98(Spine 3)258–263

53. Naderi S. Spinal meningiomas. Surg Neurol 2000;54:95

54. Conti P, Pansini G, Mouchaty H, Capuano C, Conti R. Spinal neurinomas: retrospective analysis and long-term outcome of 179 consecutively operated cases and review of the literature. Surg Neurol 2004;61:34–43, discussion 44

55. Murphey MD, Smith WS, Smith SE, Kransdorf MJ, Temple HT. From the archives of the AFIP. Imaging of musculoskeletal neurogenic tumors: radiologic-pathologic correlation. Radiographics 1999;19:1253–1280

56. Akhaddar A, Chakir N, Amarti A, et al. Thoracic epidural hemangiopericytoma. Case report. J Neurosurg Sci 2002;46:89–92, discussion 92

57. Brant-Zawadzki M. Astrocytoma, spinal cord. In: Ross JS, Brant-Zawadzki M, Moore KR, Crim J, Chen MZ, Katzman GL, eds. Diagnostic Imaging: Spine. Salt Lake City: Amirsys; 2004:IV-1-102–IV-1-105

58. Houten JK, Cooper PR. Spinal cord astrocytomas: presentation, management and outcome. J Neurooncol 2000;47:219–224

59. Houten JK, Weiner HL. Pediatric intramedullary spinal cord tumors: special considerations. J Neurooncol 2000;47:225–230

60. Lowe GM. Magnetic resonance imaging of intramedullary spinal cord tumors. J Neurooncol 2000;47:195–210

61. Sun B, Wang C, Wang J, Liu A. MRI features of intramedullary spinal cord ependymomas. J Neuroimaging 2003;13:346–351

62. McCormick PC, Torres R, Post KD, Stein BM. Intramedullary ependymoma of the spinal cord. J Neurosurg 1990;72:523–532

63. Bagley CA, Kothbauer KF, Wilson S, Bookland MJ, Epstein FJ, Jallo GI. Resection of myxopapillary ependymomas in children. J Neurosurg 2007;106(4, Suppl Pediatrics)261–267

64. Murota T, Symon L. Surgical management of hemangioblastoma of the spinal cord: a report of 18 cases. Neurosurgery 1989;25:699–707, discussion 708

65. Chu BC, Terae S, Hida K, Furukawa M, Abe S, Miyasaka K. MR findings in spinal hemangioblastoma: correlation with symptoms and with angiographic and surgical findings. AJNR Am J Neuroradiol 2001;22:206–217

66. Reddy P, Sathyanarayana S, Acharya R, Nanda A. Intramedullary spinal cord metastases: case report and review of literature. J La State Med Soc 2003;155:44–45

67. Chamberlain MC, Sandy AD, Press GA. Spinal cord tumors: gadolinium-DTPA-enhanced MR imaging. Neuroradiology 1991;33:469–474

68. Brunberg JA, DiPietro MA, Venes JL, et al. Intramedullary lesions of the pediatric spinal cord: correlation of findings from MR imaging, intraoperative sonography, surgery, and histologic study. Radiology 1991;181:573–579

13   The Pediatric Spine

A. Jay Khanna, Bruce A. Wasserman, and Paul D. Sponseller

■ Specialized Pulse Sequences and Imaging Protocols

Standard pulse sequences for spinal imaging include SE T1-weighted and FSE T2-weighted images. The FSE technique allows for the acquisition of T2-weighted images without prolonged imaging times. T1-weighted images allow for the evaluation of anatomic detail, including that of the osseous structures and soft tissues. T2-weighted images are primarily used to evaluate the spinal cord and enhance lesion conspicuity. Because CSF is bright on T2-weighted images and the spinal cord retains its intermediate signal, the T2-weighted images maximize the CSF to neural tissue contrast and therefore allow optimal delineation of the spinal cord and nerve roots. T2-weighted images are very sensitive to pathologic changes in tissue, including any processes in which cells and the extracellular matrix have increased water content. This pathologic change is usually shown as an increase in signal intensity on T2-weighted images, which increases the conspicuity of most pathologic processes affecting the spine.

Open MRI systems are becoming more frequently used, especially for pediatric imaging. Although these systems often have significantly lower field strengths than closed magnets and thus usually produce studies of inferior overall quality, the open environment provides young patients with access to their parents and makes the experience less intimidating for patients with claustrophobia. Open systems are also helpful for procedures that might benefit from MRI guidance. When possible, however, the authors recommend that MR imaging be performed using closed 1.5-T or 3-T MRI systems.

■ Pediatric Sedation Protocols

Formal sedation is often required for the successful MRI evaluation of the pediatric patient, and multiple studies and reviews have evaluated and recommended specific sedation protocols.[1,2] The American Academy of Pediatrics has published guidelines for the elective sedation of pediatric patients,[3,4] but compliance with these guidelines is not mandatory. The American Academy of Pediatrics has stated that careful medical screening and patient selection by knowl-edgeable medical personnel are needed to exclude patients at high risk for life-threatening hypoxia.[4] Also, monitoring using their guidelines is necessary for the early detection and management of life-threatening hypoxia.[3] The American Academy of Pediatrics recommends that, before examination in which sedation is to be used, children up to 3 years old should ingest nothing by mouth for 4 hours, and children 3 to 6 years old should ingest nothing by mouth for 6 hours.[4]

Although multiple protocols exist for the specific administration of various mediations for pediatric sedation and practices vary among institutions, a few agents are essential for most sedation protocols. Oral chloral hydrate is recommended for children less than 18 months old. However, the use of oral chloral hydrate is controversial because of its variable absorption, paradoxical effects, and nonstandardized dosing regimen. Older or larger children usually receive intravenous pentobarbital with or without fentanyl. Although several studies have reported the successful administration of sedation by trained nurses,[1,2] patients who may benefit from the expertise of an anesthesiologist include those with substantial comorbidities, such as the following:

- Cardiopulmonary disease
- Skeletal dysplasias
- Neuromuscular disease
- Abnormal airway anatomy

An important consideration after sedation for pediatric MRI is the need for strict adherence to established discharge criteria, including the following[5]:

- Return to baseline vital signs
- Level of consciousness close to baseline
- Ability to maintain a patent airway

Because of the potential risks associated with anesthesia and sedation in the young patient, there is a trend toward referring pediatric patients who require sedation to hospitals with pediatric anesthesiologists. Alternate techniques include sleep deprivation and rapid, segmental scanning; the latter permits the acquisition of high-quality images without the use of sedation. The surgeon referring pediatric patients for MR images of the spine should be familiar with the sedation protocols and level of expertise at the selected facilities. It is important to note that sedation protocols vary greatly from institution to institution and that no protocol is 100% safe, which emphasizes the need for monitoring, careful patient selection, and evaluation. The authors advise consultation with the pediatric anesthesiologists at the referring physician's institution when sedating patients for MRI studies.

■ Normal Pediatric MRI Anatomy

To better understand and predict the MRI appearance of pathologic processes involving the spine, one should have a basic understanding of the normal MRI anatomy.[6] Because most orthopaedic surgeons are more familiar with the normal anatomy of the adolescent (**Fig. 13.1**) and adult spines than with that of the pediatric spine, the salient points of the former two are presented first as a framework for understanding and differentiating the pediatric spine (for a full discussion of adult spine anatomy, see Chapter 2).

Adolescents and Adults

The lumbar spine is the most frequently imaged region in both children and adults. The lumbar spinal canal transitions from a round appearance in its proximal portion to a more triangular one distally. The lumbar facet joints are covered with 2 to 4 mm of hyaline cartilage. This cartilage can be nicely visualized on FSE pulse sequences and with gradient-echo pulse sequences. The epidural space and ligaments should also be carefully evaluated. The epidural fat is seen as high signal intensity on T1-weighted images; the ligamentum flavum shows minimally higher T1-weighted signal than do the other ligaments. The conus medullaris, usually located at the L1-L2 level, is best seen as a regional enlargement of the spinal cord on the sagittal images. The filum terminale extends from the conus medullaris to the distal thecal sac. The traversing nerve roots pass distally from the conus medullaris and extend anteriorly and laterally. These nerve roots exit laterally underneath the pedicle and into the neural foramen. The intervertebral disc, consisting of the cartilaginous end plates, annulus fibrosus, and the nucleus pulposus, normally shows increased T2 signal in its central portion. It is important to note that CSF pulsations often create artifacts that degrade the image of the lumbar spine; those artifacts must not be mistaken for a pathologic process.

Evaluation of the cervical spine begins with the vertebral bodies. A mild lordosis is noted on sagittal images. On axial images, the spinal canal is triangular, with the base located anteriorly. It is important to note the normal variant dark band at the base of the dens that represents a remnant of

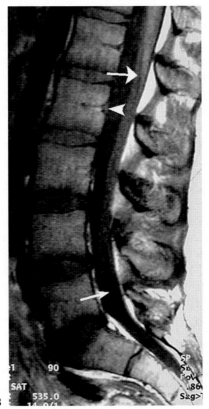
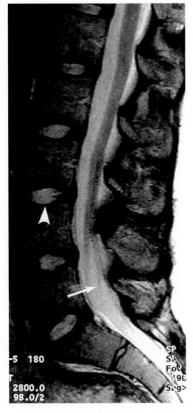

Fig. 13.1 Normal lumbar spine in a 16-year-old girl. **(A)** A sagittal T1-weighted image shows dark CSF (*arrow with small head*), the conus medullaris terminating at the L1-L2 level (*arrow with large head*), and the basivertebral channel (*arrowhead*). Note the normal rectangular appearance of the vertebral bodies and the lumbar lordosis. **(B)** A sagittal T2-weighted image shows bright CSF (*arrow*) and a bright nucleus pulposus (*arrowhead*).

A, B

the subdental synchondrosis; it should not be mistaken for a fracture. In adults, the facet joints are small and triangular, whereas in children they are relatively larger and flat. The spinal cord is elliptical in cross-section in the cervical spine. It is important to recognize that there is a difference in signal between the normal gray and white matter of the spinal cord. This signal heterogeneity should not be mistaken for intramedullary pathology. The intervertebral discs are similar in appearance to, but smaller than, those seen at the thoracic and lumbar levels. An important anatomic feature of the cervical spine is the prominent epidural venous plexus, which is not present in the thoracic or lumbar spine.

The thoracic vertebral bodies are relatively constant in size, and the spinal canal is relatively round. Abundant epidural fat is present posteriorly, but there is less anteriorly than in the lumbosacral region. The cord is more round than in the cervical or lumbar regions, and the cord segment lies between two and three levels above the corresponding vertebral body. The intervertebral discs are thinner than the discs in the lumbar spine. The appearance of the CSF is more variable in the thoracic spine than that in the lumbar region because of more prominent CSF pulsations, but it is most commonly seen as a region of low signal dorsal to the spinal cord on T1-weighted images. This artifact is often most severe at the apex of curves, including the thoracic kyphosis. Techniques are available for minimizing this artifact, including gating to the pulse or cardiac cycle.

Children

Differences Between the Pediatric and Adult Spine

Understanding the normal adult and adolescent spine leads to appreciation of the dynamic development of the pediatric spine. The MRI appearance of the growing spine is quite complex. Multiple substantial changes occur in the vertebral ossification center and the intervertebral discs that markedly alter the overall appearance of the spine, especially between infancy and 2 years of age.[7] In general, the vertebral ossification centers are incompletely ossified early in childhood, and the discs are thicker and have a higher water content than those in the adult. The spinal canal and neural foramina are larger, and there is less curvature. In addition, the overall signal intensity of the vertebral bodies is lower than that of the adult spine on T1-weighted images because of the abundance of red (hematopoietic) marrow relative to yellow (fat) marrow in the pediatric, adolescent, and young adult spine.

By understanding the MRI appearance of this development process, the clinician is better equipped to differentiate normal from pathologic states. Sze et al.[7] have characterized the MRI evolution of the pediatric spine between infancy and 2 years of age, and Goske et al.[6] have described this dynamic process through the age of 10 years (see details later).

Full-Term Infant

In the newborn, the overall size of the vertebral body is small relative to the spinal canal, and the spinal cord ends at approximately the L2 level. The lumbar spine does not show the usual lordosis and is straight. The vertebral bodies show markedly low signal intensity on T1-weighted images, with a thin central hyperintense band that likely represents the basivertebral plexus. The spongy bone of the ossification center is ellipsoidal rather than rectangular and is often mistaken for a disc. The intervertebral disc is relatively narrow and often contains a thin, bright central band on T2-weighted images that represents the notochordal remnants.

Age: 3 Months

At 3 months, the osseous component of the vertebral body has increased and the amount of hyaline cartilage has decreased, with a resultant rectangular appearance to the vertebral bodies. The ossification centers begin to increase in signal intensity, starting at the end plates and progressing centrally. The neural foramina have not substantially changed at this age, remaining relatively large and ovoid in shape.

Age: 2 Years

At 2 years, the spine has begun to show its normal curvature, most likely because of the effects of weight bearing (**Fig. 13.2**). The ossified portion of the vertebral body increases substantially in size and begins to assume its adult appearance, with near-complete ossification of the pedicles and the articular processes. The disc space and nucleus pulposus become longer and thinner. The cartilaginous end plate has decreased in size and is often difficult to identify. The neural foramen also begins to take its adult appearance as its inferior portion narrows.

Age: 10 Years

At 10 years, the spinal curvature resembles that of an adult (**Fig. 13.3**). The ossification of the vertebral bodies and posterior elements is nearly complete, with a resultant decrease in the spinal canal diameter. The vertebral bodies also develop concave superior and inferior contours. The nucleus pulposus becomes smaller at this age and spans approximately half of the disc space in the sagittal plane. The neural foramina continue to narrow inferiorly.

Conus Medullaris

The spinal cord extends to the inferior aspect of the osseous spinal column in early fetal life.[6] Because of the more rapid longitudinal growth of the vertebral bodies relative to

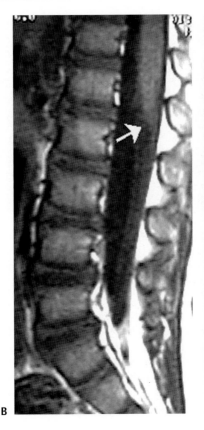 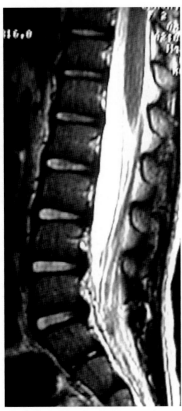

Fig. 13.2 Normal lumbar spine in a 2-year-old boy. **(A)** A sagittal T1-weighted image shows rectangular vertebral bodies and a wide, thin intervertebral disc. Note that the conus medullaris terminates at the L1-L2 level (*arrow*). **(B)** A T2-weighted image shows increased disc signal.

A, B

the spinal cord, the conus medullaris is repositioned in the upper lumbar spine by birth. It is important to note the location of the conus medullaris on every pediatric spine MRI study (**Figs. 13.1** and **13.2**). A conus level below the L2-L3 interspace in children more than 5 years old is abnormal and indicates possible tethering.[8,9] Saifuddin et al.[10] reviewed the MRI findings of 504 normal adult spines and found that the average conus position was the lower third of L1 (range, middle third of T12 to upper third of L3).

■ Pathologic Processes Involving the Pediatric Spine

Infection

Infectious processes involving the pediatric spine include osteomyelitis, discitis, epidural abscess, and paraspinal abscess.[11–13] In general, the MRI signal characteristics of infection include a region of low T1 signal intensity and high T2 signal intensity in bone and soft tissue.

MRI is more sensitive than conventional radiographs or CT and is more specific than nuclear scintigraphy in identifying vertebral osteomyelitis.[14,15] MRI provides the optimal means of imaging osteomyelitis (**Fig. 13.4**). Marrow edema can be detected on STIR images, and enhancement of the disc

and adjacent vertebral bodies on postcontrast fat-suppressed T1-weighted images helps to confirm the diagnosis. The specificity of MRI for infection is higher in children than in adults because one of the primary confounding findings, degenerative arthritis, can be removed from the differential diagnosis. A key concept in both children and adults is differentiating osteomyelitis from neoplastic disease. An important characteristic that may help make this differentiation is the fact that infectious processes are more likely to cross intervertebral discs than are neoplastic conditions (**Fig. 13.5**).

Discitis, seen as a disruption of the normally well-defined disc-vertebral borders on T1-weighted images and as an increase in signal of the disc on T2-weighted images,[12] may obliterate the normally seen horizontal cleft within the intervertebral disc on T2-weighted images (**Fig. 13.6**). The abnormal signal seen in infectious discitis is classically associated with surrounding soft-tissue inflammation and reactive end-plate changes. Compared with adult patients, pediatric patients are more likely to develop primary discitis because of increased blood supply to the disc. Adults are more likely to develop infectious discitis after surgery or from contiguous spread from primary end-plate osteomyelitis.

Epidural abscesses are rare, but when they do develop, it is usually after surgery or vertebral osteomyelitis. The diagnosis of epidural abscesses can be made in the patient who has

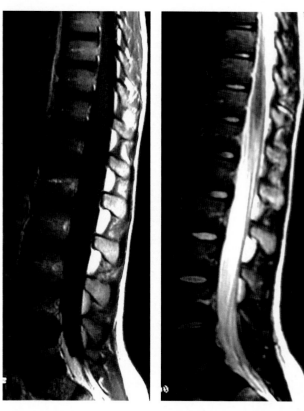

A, B

Fig. 13.3 This 10-year-old girl has a normal lumbar spine with normal lordosis. (**A**) A sagittal T1-weighted image. (**B**) A sagittal T2-weighted image. Note that the posterior elements are well formed, with a resultant decrease in the canal diameter.

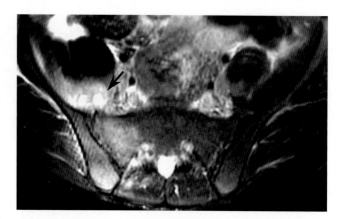

Fig. 13.4 This axial T2-weighted image in a 15-year-old boy with infectious symptoms and complaints of low back pain shows increased T2-weighted signal in the region of the right sacroiliac joint and an associated soft-tissue component at the anterior aspect of the joint (*arrow*), compatible with a sacroiliac joint infection.

radionuclide imaging can show increased radiotracer activity in the region of the defect.

With regard to acute disc herniation in the pediatric age group, it is important to note that this herniation represents more of a fracture with a hinge-like displacement of fibrocartilage and displacement of the entire disc and vertebral

a collection in the epidural space and a clinical history that supports infection.[11] Gadolinium-enhanced T1-weighted images often show a peripheral rim of enhancement that represents the abscess wall.

Trauma

An important role of MRI is to evaluate for the presence of neural injury in the pediatric patient who has sustained substantial trauma to the spine and who has an abnormal neurologic examination or is unresponsive. The initial evaluation is performed with conventional radiographs, which are often normal. MRI evaluation may then be performed to evaluate for osseous, ligamentous, intervertebral disc, cord, and nerve root injury. Although CT allows for better evaluation of osseous detail and displaced fractures, MRI allows for improved evaluation of nondisplaced fractures because of its ability to detect marrow signal abnormalities (**Fig. 13.6**). MRI is also useful in its ability to help determine the age of the fracture and to evaluate for posttraumatic myelopathy. MRI, however, is not the optimal method for the evaluation of spondylolysis. CT offers increased spatial resolution and the ability to define accurately the osseous defect, whereas

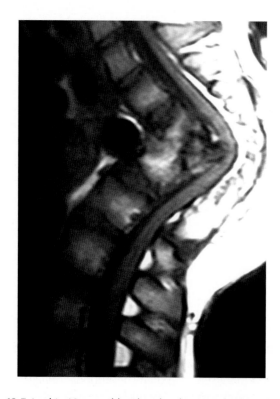

Fig. 13.5 In this 16-year-old girl with a history of tuberculosis, a sagittal T1-weighted image shows destruction of three consecutive mid-thoracic vertebral bodies with associated kyphosis and gibbus deformity, compatible with tuberculous osteomyelitis.

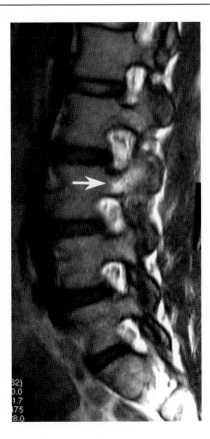

Fig. 13.6 In this 12-year-old boy with persistent low back pain and normal radiographs, a parasagittal T2-weighted image shows an area of increased signal (*arrow*) within the region of the pars intraarticularis, compatible with edema from an acute or subacute nondisplaced pars intraarticularis fracture.

end plate than extrusion of a disc fragment, as is seen in the adult population.[16] Such avulsion fractures are often occult on conventional radiographs and are better detected with CT and MRI.[16] Axial MR images show the fracture fragment as an area of low signal intensity protruding into the spinal canal, and the sagittal images show a low signal intensity region in the shape of a Y or 7 on all pulse sequences.[16]

Spinal cord injury without radiographic abnormality is an established entity seen after pediatric spine trauma.[17,18] The characteristic hypermobility and ligamentous laxity of the pediatric osseous cervical and thoracic spine predispose children to a spinal cord injury without radiographic abnormality-type injury.[17] The elasticity of the osseous pediatric spine as well as the relatively large size of the head allow for deformation of the musculoskeletal structures beyond physiologic limits, which results in cord trauma followed by spontaneous reduction of the spine.[17]

As with other types of spinal cord injuries, the most important predictor of outcome is the severity of neurologic injury. A patient with a complete neurologic deficit after spinal cord injury without radiographic abnormality has a poor prognosis for recovery of neurologic function. The role of MRI in the spinal cord injury without radiographic abnormality syndrome is to define the degree of neural injury, rule out occult fractures and subluxation that may require surgical intervention, and evaluate for the presence of ligamentous injury. The T2-weighted and STIR images should show increased signal in the cord or vertebral body. The increased T2 signal in the cord is compatible with edema and can range from a partial, reversible contusion to complete transsection of the cord.

■ Imaging of Spinal Dysraphism

Spinal dysraphism is a general term used to describe a wide range of anomalies resulting from incomplete fusion of the midline mesenchyme, bone, and neural elements. The osseous abnormalities consist of defects within the neural arch with partial or complete absence of the spinous processes, laminae, or other components of the posterior elements. MRI has been shown to be the best modality for the evaluation of spinal dysraphism.[19,20]

To better understand the MRI of spinal dysraphism, it is important to have a basic knowledge of its various types. A classification system has been proposed that permits the systematic evaluation of a patient with a suspected spinal dysraphism (**Table 13.1**).[20] By using this clinical classification system, the differential diagnosis can be rapidly narrowed to one of three categories: spinal dysraphism with a non–skin-covered back mass, spinal dysraphism with a skin-covered back mass, and spinal dysraphism with no back mass. The final diagnosis can then be selected from the identified category based on the lesion's MRI characteristics.

Table 13.1   Classification of Spinal Dysraphism

Category	Types
Spinal dysraphism with a non–skin-covered back mass	Myelomeningocele Myelocele
Spinal dysraphism with a skin-covered back mass	Lipomeningocele Myelocystocele Simple posterior meningocele
Spinal dysraphism without a back mass	Diastematomyelia Dorsal dermal sinus Intradural lipoma Tight filum terminale Anterior sacral meningocele Lateral thoracic meningocele Hydromyelia Split notochord syndrome Caudal regression syndrome

Source: From Byrd SE, Darling CF, McLone DG, Tomita T. MR imaging of the pediatric spine. Magn Reson Imaging Clin N Am 1996;4(4):797–833. Reprinted by permission.

Myelomeningoceles represent a common type of spina bifida, the most common form of spinal dysraphism (**Fig. 13.7**). It most often presents as a non–skin-covered back mass in the lumbosacral region, although it can also be seen at higher levels. This mass may or may not be covered by leptomeninges containing a variable amount of neural tissue. The sac herniates through a defect in the posterior elements of the spine. The spinal cord usually contains a dorsal cleft, is splayed open, and is often tethered within the sac.[20] Progressive scoliosis is seen in 66% of patients; Arnold-Chiari type II malformation, in 90% to 99%; diastematomyelia, in 30% to 40%; and syringohydromyelia, in 40% to 80%.[21] Scarring can occur at the surgical site after sac closure, and it is important to monitor these patients for the signs and symptoms of the tethered cord syndrome.

Of the entities presenting with a skin-covered back mass in the presence of spinal dysraphism, lipomeningocele is the most common. The lipomeningocele consists of lipomatous tissue that is continuous with the subcutaneous tissue of the back and also insinuates through the dysraphic defect and dura and into the spinal canal. The spinal cord often contains a dorsal defect at the level of the lipomatous tissue and may be tethered at this level. The essential MRI feature of this lesion is that the lipomatous tissue matches the signal characteristics of subcutaneous fat on all pulse sequences, including fat-suppressed pulse sequences.

Occult spinal dysraphism presents without a back mass and includes many entities (**Table 13.1**). Diastematomyelia is characterized by a sagittal splitting of the spinal cord, conus medullaris, or filum terminale into two segments, often in the thoracic or lumbar spine. The dural tube and arachnoid are undivided in approximately half of the patients; in such patients, clinical findings are rare, and surgery is not indicated. In the other half, the dural tube and arachnoid are completely or partially split at the level of the spinal cord cleft, which results in tethering of the cord and subsequent clinical symptoms. Coronal T1-weighted and T2-weighted images best define the sagittal split in the cord; the findings should be confirmed on axial images. The osseous spur or fibrous band that occurs between each hemicord appears dark on T1-weighted and T2-weighted images and can be better visualized on CT.

Another important entity often seen in patients with spinal dysraphism is syringohydromyelia, or syrinx (**Fig. 13.8**). A syrinx is a longitudinal cavity within the spinal cord that may or may not communicate with the central canal. Multiple theories exist to explain the etiology of a syrinx, including developmental and trauma-, inflammation-, ischemia-, and pressure-related causes. Sagittal MR images show

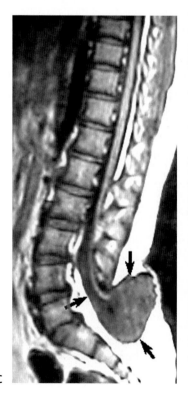
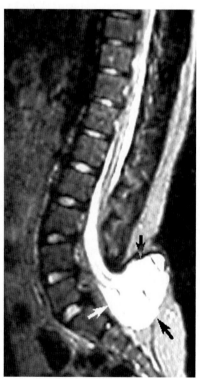
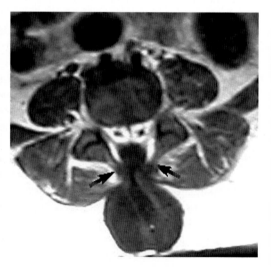

A–C

Fig. 13.7 A 6-year-old girl with a myelomeningocele. **(A)** The sagittal T1-weighted image shows a low back mass contiguous with the contents of the spinal canal (*arrows*). **(B)** The T2-weighted image shows that the mass is filled with high signal intensity fluid, compatible with CSF (*arrows*). **(C)** The axial T1-weighted image confirms the communication of the mass with the spinal canal through a defect in the posterior elements (*arrows*).

a linear low T1 signal intensity and high T2 signal intensity within the parenchyma of the spinal cord. Identification of a syrinx is sometimes an indication for contrast administration to exclude an underlying enhancing lesion.

Chiari Malformations

Chiari malformations are frequently seen in patients with spinal dysraphism. Chiari type I malformations consist of cerebellar tonsillar ectopia, in which the cerebellar tonsils extend below the level of the foramen magnum. The commonly quoted measurement for the degree of herniation of the tonsils below the foramen magnum is 5 mm. Mikulis et al.[22] reported a variation by age in the upper limit of normal: 6 mm in the first decade of life, 5 mm in the second and third

decades, and 3 mm by the ninth decade. In Chiari type I malformations, the brainstem is spared and the fourth ventricle remains in its normal location. Chiari type I malformations are associated with syringohydromyelia, CVJ anomalies, and basilar invagination. Chiari type II malformations are more advanced and consist of downward displacement of the brainstem and inferior cerebellum into the cervical spinal canal, with a decrease in size of the posterior fossa.

Tethered Cord Syndrome

The tethered cord syndrome, an important problem, is seen in a substantial number of patients with spinal dysraphism, especially those who have undergone surgical closure of the defect.[23,24] During fetal life, the spinal cord extends to the

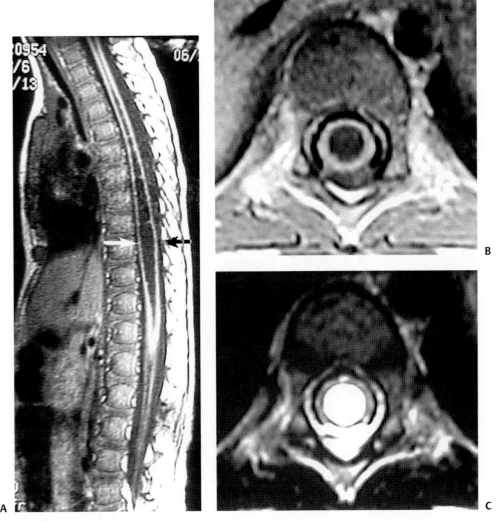

Fig. 13.8 A 2-year-old boy with a large syrinx involving the entire spinal cord. **(A)** The sagittal T1-weighted image shows the syrinx to be largest at the level of the lower thoracic spine (*arrows*). The axial T1-weighted **(B)** and T2-weighted **(C)** images confirm that the syrinx is located within the center of the spinal cord.

sacrococcygeal level. Because of the more rapid growth of the vertebral column after birth, the cord ascends to the L1-L2 level in the newborn. During the formation of a spinal dysraphic defect such as myelomeningocele, the open neural elements often attach to the peripheral ectoderm, resulting in spinal cord tethering. After surgical closure of the sac, there is a tendency for the spinal cord to become adherent at the repair site. As the child grows, this adherence may result in tethering of the cord and prevention of cephalad cord migration, with eventual symptoms. Thus, tethered cord should be ruled out as the potential cause of any deterioration in neurologic function in patients with spinal dysraphic and related conditions, including the following:

- Myelomeningoceles
- Myeloceles
- Lipomeningoceles
- Diastematomyelia

MRI has been proposed as the initial, and possibly the only, imaging modality for a patient with a suspected tethered spinal cord.[9] The sagittal images should be evaluated to determine the level of the conus medullaris (**Fig. 13.9**). A conus level below the L2-L3 interspace in children more than 5 years old is abnormal and an indication of possible tethering.[8,9] In addition, the tethered cord is often displaced posteriorly in the spinal canal. Other findings include lipoma or scar tissue within the epidural space and increased thickness of the filum terminale.[9]

It is important to note that although MRI can determine whether a spinal cord is anatomically tethered, these findings should be correlated with the patient's symptoms

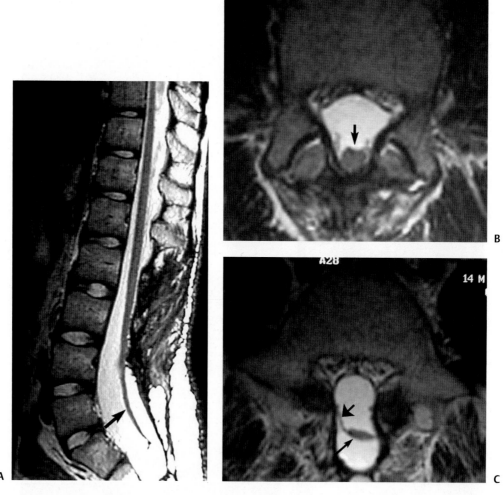

Fig. 13.9 This 14-year-old boy had a history of lipomeningocele. After surgical resection, he developed bowel and bladder dysfunction and new lower extremity paresthesias. **(A)** A sagittal T2-weighted image shows the cord to extend to approximately the L4 level and the filum terminale to extend to the S1 level (*arrow*), compatible with a tethered cord. **(B)** An axial T2-weighted image at the L4 level shows the cord to be located posteriorly within the thecal sac (*arrow*). **(C)** An axial T2-weighted image at the L5 level shows the placode (*arrow with small head*) with a right-side nerve root coursing anteriorly and laterally (*arrow with large head*).

and serial physical examinations before surgical release is considered.

◼ Controversies with MRI of the Pediatric Spine

As with any diagnostic test, there remain several areas for which the use of MRI of the pediatric spine is controversial, including the specific indications for the following:

- Imaging of scoliosis
- Imaging of tethered cord syndrome
- Imaging in the presence of spinal instrumentation

Scoliosis

Idiopathic scoliosis most often presents with a right-side lower thoracic curve. The purpose of MRI in the imaging of scoliosis is to detect intraspinal pathology, which is most frequently associated with left lower thoracic curves, an

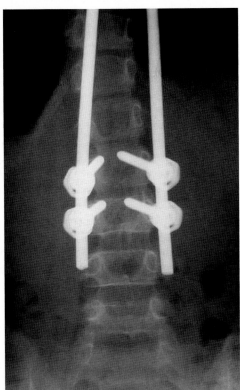
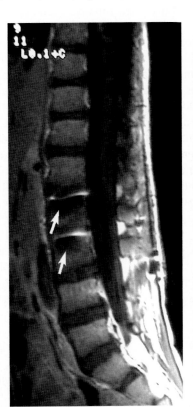
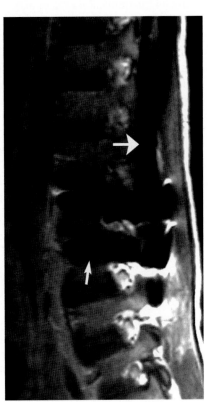
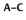
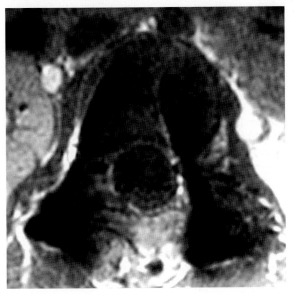

Fig. 13.10 A 6-year-old boy with a history of high-grade astrocytoma underwent resection, multilevel laminectomy, and posterior spinal arthrodesis from T4 to L3 with titanium pedicle screws, hooks, and rods. **(A)** An AP radiograph 6 weeks after surgery. **(B)** A midline sagittal postgadolinium T1-weighted image allows visualization of the canal contents with only minimal artifact from the pedicle screws (*arrows*). **(C)** A parasagittal postgadolinium T1-weighted image shows a rod (*arrow with large head*) and a pedicle screw (*arrow with small head*), neither of which substantially degrades the image. **(D)** An axial postgadolinium T1-weighted image also shows the pedicle screws and a patent spinal canal.

abnormal neurologic examination, and a young age at presentation.[25–29] Recently, Do et al.[25] concluded that MRI is not indicated before spinal arthrodesis in a patient with an adolescent idiopathic scoliosis curve pattern and normal physical and neurologic examinations.

One particular area of controversy is the pediatric patient with back pain in the presence of scoliosis. In the authors' experience, young patients with typical idiopathic scoliosis often complain of intermittent and vague back pain at some point during their clinical course. In a retrospective study of 2,442 patients, Ramirez et al.[30] found that a left thoracic curve or an abnormal neurologic examination was most predictive of an underlying pathologic condition. They found a significant association between back pain and an age of more than 15 years, skeletal maturity, postmenarchal status, and a history of injury. Their conclusion was that it is unnecessary to perform extensive diagnostic studies on every patient with scoliosis and back pain. Based on clinical experience and a review of the literature, the current authors recommend obtaining MRI in pediatric patients with scoliosis with a left lower thoracic curve, abnormal neurologic findings, infantile scoliosis, or juvenile scoliosis. Because coronal images are especially useful in evaluating patients with scoliosis, they should be a part of the routine imaging protocol.

Evaluation of the Tethered Cord Syndrome

As mentioned above, imaging of the tethered cord syndrome remains controversial. A dilemma arises when the MRI findings of tethered cord syndrome are noted and a decision with regard to nonoperative versus operative treatment has to be made. It is important to remember that although anatomic tethering of the cord can be easily identified by MRI, the determining factors for surgical intervention are the clinical history and examination, preferably obtained on a serial basis.

Imaging in the Presence of Implants

MRI of the spine in the presence of instrumentation is generally safe but limited because image artifacts produced by implants vary in degree based on the type of metal used and the pulse sequence used. Titanium produces less image degradation from artifact because it is less ferromagnetic than stainless steel.[31,32] However, with appropriate imaging techniques, clinically useful information can be safely obtained in the presence of both types of implants.[33] Specialized pulse sequences can help reduce the degree of tissue-obscuring artifact produced by spinal hardware and improve image quality compared with conventional T1-weighted SE pulse sequences.[34] For example, the metal-artifact-reduction pulse sequence has been shown to substantially reduce the amount of tissue-obscuring artifact produced by spinal hardware.[34] The current authors use MRI to evaluate pediatric spines with stainless steel or titanium implants (**Fig. 13.10**), but the fact that the latter produces substantially less artifact affects the implant choice for a patient who may require follow-up MRI evaluation.

References

1. Beebe DS, Tran P, Bragg M, Stillman A, Truwitt C, Belani KG. Trained nurses can provide safe and effective sedation for MRI in pediatric patients. Can J Anaesth 2000;47:205–210
2. Sury MR, Hatch DJ, Deeley T, Dicks-Mireaux C, Chong WK. Development of a nurse-led sedation service for paediatric magnetic resonance imaging. Lancet 1999;353:1667–1671
3. Vade A, Sukhani R, Dolenga M, Habisohn-Schuck C. Chloral hydrate sedation of children undergoing CT and MR imaging: safety as judged by American Academy of Pediatrics guidelines. AJR Am J Roentgenol 1995;165:905–909
4. American Academy of Pediatrics Committee on Drugs. Guidelines for monitoring and management of pediatric patients during and after sedation for diagnostic and therapeutic procedures. Pediatrics 1992;89(6 pt 1):1110–1115
5. Malviya S, Voepel-Lewis T, Prochaska G, Tait AR. Prolonged recovery and delayed side effects of sedation for diagnostic imaging studies in children. Pediatrics 2000;105:E42
6. Goske MJ, Modic MT, Yu S. Pediatric spine: normal anatomy and spinal dysraphism. In: Modic MT, Masaryk TJ, Ross JS, eds. Magnetic Resonance Imaging of the Spine. St. Louis: Mosby-Year Book; 1994:352–387
7. Sze G, Baierl P, Bravo S. Evolution of the infant spinal column: evaluation with MR imaging. Radiology 1991;181:819–827
8. Barson AJ. The vertebral level of termination of the spinal cord during normal and abnormal development. J Anat 1970;106(pt 3):489–497
9. Moufarrij NA, Palmer JM, Hahn JF, Weinstein MA. Correlation between magnetic resonance imaging and surgical findings in the tethered spinal cord. Neurosurgery 1989;25:341–346
10. Saifuddin A, Burnett SJD, White J. The variation of position of the conus medullaris in an adult population. A magnetic resonance imaging study. Spine (Phila Pa 1976) 1998;23:1452–1456
11. Auletta JJ, John CC. Spinal epidural abscesses in children: a 15-year experience and review of the literature. Clin Infect Dis 2001;32:9–16
12. du Lac P, Panuel M, Devred P, Bollini G, Padovani J. MRI of disc space infection in infants and children. Report of 12 cases. Pediatr Radiol 1990;20:175–178
13. Modic MT, Feiglin DH, Piraino DW, et al. Vertebral osteomyelitis: assessment using MR. Radiology 1985;157:157–166
14. Fernandez M, Carrol CL, Baker CJ. Discitis and vertebral osteomyelitis in children: an 18-year review. Pediatrics 2000;105:1299–1304
15. Miller GM, Forbes GS, Onofrio BM. Magnetic resonance imaging of the spine. Mayo Clin Proc 1989;64:986–1004
16. Banerian KG, Wang AM, Samberg LC, Kerr HH, Wesolowski DP. Association of vertebral end plate fracture with pediatric lumbar intervertebral disk herniation: value of CT and MR imaging. Radiology 1990;177:763–765

17. Kriss VM, Kriss TC. SCIWORA (spinal cord injury without radiographic abnormality) in infants and children. Clin Pediatr (Phila) 1996;35:119–124

18. Pang D, Pollack IF. Spinal cord injury without radiographic abnormality in children—the SCIWORA syndrome. J Trauma 1989;29:654–664

19. Altman NR, Altman DH. MR imaging of spinal dysraphism. AJNR Am J Neuroradiol 1987;8:533–538

20. Byrd SE, Darling CF, McLone DG, Tomita T. MR imaging of the pediatric spine. Magn Reson Imaging Clin N Am 1996;4:797–833

21. Modic MT, Yu S. Normal anatomy. In: Modic MT, Masaryk TJ, Ross JS, eds. Magnetic Resonance Imaging of the Spine. St. Louis: Mosby-Year Book; 1994:37–79

22. Mikulis DJ, Diaz O, Egglin TK, Sanchez R. Variance of the position of the cerebellar tonsils with age: preliminary report. Radiology 1992;183:725–728

23. Hall WA, Albright AL, Brunberg JA. Diagnosis of tethered cords by magnetic resonance imaging. Surg Neurol 1988;30:60–64

24. Heinz ER, Rosenbaum AE, Scarff TB, Reigel DH, Drayer BP. Tethered spinal cord following meningomyelocele repair. Radiology 1979;131:153–160

25. Do T, Fras C, Burke S, Widmann RF, Rawlins B, Boachie-Adjei O. Clinical value of routine preoperative magnetic resonance imaging in adolescent idiopathic scoliosis. A prospective study of three hundred and twenty-seven patients. J Bone Joint Surg Am 2001;83:577–579

26. Evans SC, Edgar MA, Hall-Craggs MA, Powell MP, Taylor BA, Noordeen HH. MRI of 'idiopathic' juvenile scoliosis. A prospective study. J Bone Joint Surg Br 1996;78:314–317

27. Gupta P, Lenke LG, Bridwell KH. Incidence of neural axis abnormalities in infantile and juvenile patients with spinal deformity. Is a magnetic resonance image screening necessary? Spine (Phila Pa 1976) 1998;23:206–210

28. Mejia EA, Hennrikus WL, Schwend RM, Emans JB. A prospective evaluation of idiopathic left thoracic scoliosis with magnetic resonance imaging. J Pediatr Orthop 1996;16:354–358

29. Schwend RM, Hennrikus W, Hall JE, Emans JB. Childhood scoliosis: clinical indications for magnetic resonance imaging. J Bone Joint Surg Am 1995;77:46–53

30. Ramirez N, Johnston CE II, Browne RH. The prevalence of back pain in children who have idiopathic scoliosis. J Bone Joint Surg Am 1997;79:364–368

31. Rudisch A, Kremser C, Peer S, Kathrein A, Judmaier W, Daniaux H. Metallic artifacts in magnetic resonance imaging of patients with spinal fusion. A comparison of implant materials and imaging sequences. Spine (Phila Pa 1976) 1998;23:692–699

32. Rupp R, Ebraheim NA, Savolaine ER, Jackson WT. Magnetic resonance imaging evaluation of the spine with metal implants. General safety and superior imaging with titanium. Spine (Phila Pa 1976) 1993;18:379–385

33. Lyons CJ, Betz RR, Mesgarzadeh M, Revesz G, Bonakdarpour A, Clancy M. The effect of magnetic resonance imaging on metal spine implants. Spine (Phila Pa 1976) 1989;14:670–672

34. Chang SD, Lee MJ, Munk PL, Janzen DL, MacKay A, Xiang QS. MRI of spinal hardware: comparison of conventional T1-weighted sequence with a new metal artifact reduction sequence. Skeletal Radiol 2001;30:213–218

V Special Considerations

14 Articular Cartilage

Michael K. Shindle, Li Foong Foo, Bryan T. Kelly, and Hollis G. Potter

■ Overview of Articular Cartilage

There have been considerable advances in the MRI of articular cartilage in recent years. Cartilage-sensitive pulse sequences should be included as a part of all joint-imaging protocols to provide a reproducible, noninvasive means of monitoring disease progression in inflammatory and degenerative arthritides, detecting traumatic cartilage injury, and evaluating surgically manipulated cartilage. Cartilage repair techniques such as autologous chondrocyte implantation, microfracture, and osteochondral autografting are being performed with increased frequency, and MRI offers a noninvasive method for evaluating the results of these procedures.

To differentiate the MR appearance of normal and abnormal cartilage morphology, it is important to understand the structure of articular cartilage, which is the basis for the development of new imaging techniques. Articular cartilage, a metabolically active tissue, has viscoelastic properties and is composed of chondrocytes (approximately 1%) and an extracellular matrix that consists mainly of water (65% to 80%), proteoglycan, and collagen.[1] Type II collagen is the most common type (95%), but other types have been identified (IV, VI, IX, X, and XI).[1] Collagen provides the tensile strength of articular cartilage. The proteoglycans consist mainly of chondroitin and keratin sulfates, which provide compressive strength to the cartilage.

Articular cartilage ranges in thickness from 2 to 5 mm, depending on the contact pressures that occur across a joint. Because of high peak pressures, the patellofemoral joint has the thickest articular cartilage in the body. Articular cartilage can be divided structurally and functionally into four zones (**Fig. 14.1**):

- Superficial
- Transitional or middle
- Deep or radial
- Calcified

The superficial zone accounts for 10% to 20% of the total thickness of cartilage, has the highest collagen content of all of the zones, and has highly organized collagen fibers that are oriented parallel to the articular surface.[2] This zone resists shear stress and has a low proteoglycan content. At

clinically relevant field strengths, this zone is typically not distinguishable from the transitional zone. The middle or transitional zone accounts for 40% to 60% of the cartilage thickness, has collagen fibers that are randomly oriented, and has a higher compressive modulus than the superficial zone because the inhomogeneity of fiber orientation distributes the stress more uniformly across the loaded tissue.[3] The deep or radial zone accounts for 30% of cartilage thickness and has highly organized collagen fibers that are oriented perpendicular to the cartilage surface. This zone also has the lowest water content and highest proteoglycan content. The collagen fibers have a radial orientation that crosses the tidemark, the interface between the articular cartilage and the calcified cartilage beneath it, which anchors the cartilage to the underlying bone.[4] The calcified cartilage layer is the final zone. This zone is separated from the radial zone by the tidemark, which also represents a potential shear plane for articular cartilage defects.[5] At clinically relevant field strengths, the tidemark cannot be differentiated from the subchondral plate.

The water, proteoglycan, and collagen content all account for the MR signal characteristics. However, the bulk of the signal comes from the free water present and not from the water that is electrostatically bound to proteoglycan or from the water that is associated with collagen. Depending on the pulse sequence used, cartilage will have a bilaminar or trilaminar appearance secondary to the highly ordered structure of the collagen of the deeper radial zone, which yields a shorter T2 relaxation time and corresponding lower signal intensity. Understanding the normal signal characteristics and anatomy of articular cartilage is imperative for detecting abnormal cartilage morphology.

■ Specialized Pulse Sequences and Imaging Protocols

Although MRI provides soft-tissue contrast that is superior to that of traditional imaging techniques, standardized conventional radiographs are also a valuable part of cartilage assessment. In particular, when planning for cartilage repair,

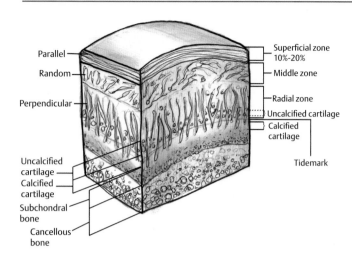

Parallel
Random
Perpendicular

Superficial zone 10%-20%
Middle zone
Radial zone
Uncalcified cartilage
Calcified cartilage

Tidemark

Uncalcified cartilage
Calcified cartilage
Subchondral bone
Cancellous bone

Fig. 14.1 Artist's depiction of cartilage zonal histology.

standing hip-to-ankle films are important for preoperative planning to determine the following:

- The mechanical axis of the limb, so that any preexisting deformity that may limit the clinical success of cartilage repair can be identified
- Whether concomitant procedures (such as a high tibial osteotomy) should be performed

The orthopedic surgeon should be aware that different pulse sequences are available for the evaluation of articular cartilage and should be included as a part of all joint-imaging protocols. Some institutions prefer using a T1-weighted 3D fat-suppressed gradient-echo sequence because it shows high contrast between the low signal intensity of the fat-suppressed bone and the high signal intensity of articular cartilage (**Fig. 14.2**). However, this sequence has several drawbacks: it requires a relatively long scan time, it is not suitable for meniscal or ligamentous evaluation, it is less sensitive to partial-thickness cartilage defects, and it undergoes image signal degradation in the presence of metal.[6-8]

For these reasons, the authors' institution prefers an intermediate TE, 2D non–fat-suppressed FSE sequence that provides good differential contrast between the intermediate signal intensity of articular cartilage, the high signal intensity of synovial fluid, and the low signal intensity of fibrocartilage[6,8] (**Fig. 14.3**). With proper technique, this sequence offers several advantages, including the following (**Table 14.1**):

- It has a relatively short scan time.
- It is effective in the presence of instrumentation.
- It can detect partial-thickness chondral lesions.
- It has very good differential contrast between the underlying bone, cartilage, ligaments, joint fluid, and menisci.

This pulse sequence shows cartilage as a laminar gray scale appearance that corresponds to the different orientations of collagen within the cartilage zones: a relatively hypointense radial zone and a higher signal intensity transitional zone[6] (**Fig. 14.4**).

Contrast agents, either intraarticular or intravenous, have been advocated by some authors for the evaluation of articular cartilage.[9-12] However, the use of such agents converts MRI into an invasive procedure and may be associated with longer imaging time and increased costs.

As mentioned above, the bulk of the MR signal derives from the free-water content of the cartilage. Novel approaches have been developed to supplement traditional MRI techniques by targeting additional "bound" components of the extracellular matrix, specifically collagen or proteoglycan. For example, with osteoarthritis and after traumatic cartilage injuries, there is a loss of negatively charged glycosaminoglycan, and MRI techniques such as positively charged sodium (^{23}Na) MRI,[13] T1 ρ, or delayed gadolinium-enhanced MRI of cartilage have been developed to detect these changes.[13-17] T2 mapping is an imaging technique that can be used to reflect the collagen component of the extracellular matrix. T2 relaxation time is a function of the free-water content of the tissue, and therefore it varies depending on the zone of articular cartilage.[18] For example, in the middle zone, collagen orientation is relatively random and water is

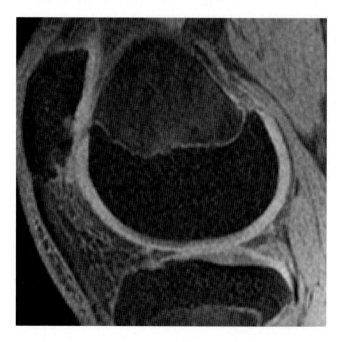

Fig. 14.2 A sagittal 3D fat-suppressed T1-weighted gradient-echo image of the knee, showing high contrast between hyperintense articular cartilage and hypointense bone. (From Shindle MK, Foo LF, Kelly BT, et al. Magnetic resonance imaging of cartilage in the athlete: current techniques and spectrum of disease. J Bone Joint Surg Am 2006;88:27–46. Reprinted by permission.)

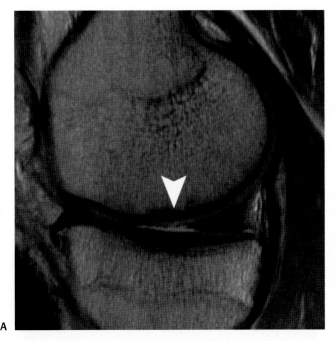

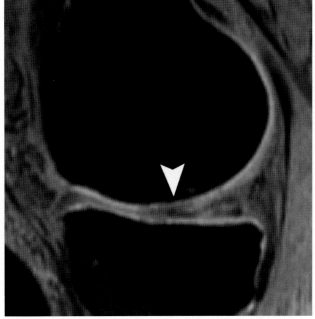

A   B

Fig. 14.3 Knee images. **(A)** A sagittal FSE sequence shows a focal partial-thickness cartilage defect overlying the medial femoral condyle (*arrowhead*). **(B)** A sagittal fat-suppressed T1–weighted gradient-echo sequence, in which the lesion is not as well appreciated. Obtaining this image took twice as long as the FSE image. (From Potter HG, Foo LF. Magnetic resonance imaging of articular cartilage: trauma, degeneration, and repair. Am J Sports Med 2006;34:661–677. Reprinted by permission.)

more mobile, corresponding to longer T2 values. In contrast, the deep zone has highly ordered collagen, and therefore T2 values are short because water is relatively immobilized (**Fig. 14.5**). Clinically, T2 mapping is important because of its ability to detect changes in cartilage structure before the substantial loss of cartilage thickness or the development of gross signal alterations in the cartilage gray scale. This early detection can help surgical decision-making by potentially optimizing the timing of operative procedures, such as meniscal transplantation or patellofemoral realignment.

Table 14.1   Comparison of Commonly Used Pulse Sequences in Cartilage Imaging

Parameter	2D Fat-Suppressed* Moderate TE FSE	2D Non–Fat-Suppressed Moderate TE FSE	3D Fat-Suppressed T1– Weighted Gradient Echo
Signal intensity characteristics			
Joint fluid	High	High	Low
Cartilage	Intermediate	Intermediate	High
Fat in subchondral bone marrow	Low	High	Very low
Ability to see meniscus and ligament	Good	Good	Poor
Scan time	+	+	++
Signal-to-noise ratio†	Good	Good	Fair
Subject to chemical shift misregistration	No	Yes§	No
Image quality in presence of instrumentation	Fair	Good	Poor

Source: From Potter HG, Foo LF. Articular cartilage. In: Stoller D, ed. Magnetic Resonance Imaging in Orthopaedics and Sports Medicine. Baltimore: Lippincott Williams & Wilkins; 2007:1099–1130. Reprinted by permission.
* Frequency selective fat suppression.
† These are general observations only. Actual measurements of signal to noise will depend on specific parameters, including segment thickness and spatial resolution.
§ May be minimized by the use of wider receiver bandwidth.

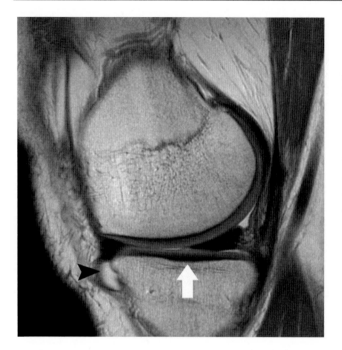

Fig. 14.4 Sagittal FSE image of the knee in a 50-year-old patient that shows gray-scale stratification of the tibial plateau articular cartilage (*arrow*). Note the differential contrast for the high signal intensity joint fluid within the meniscosynovial recess (*arrowhead*), the intermediate signal intensity of hyaline cartilage, and the low signal intensity of meniscal fibrocartilage. (From Potter HG, Foo LF. Articular cartilage. In: Stoller D, ed. Magnetic Resonance Imaging in Orthopaedics and Sports Medicine. Baltimore: Lippincott Williams & Wilkins; 2007:1099–1130. Reprinted by permission.)

■ Classification

Many scoring systems can be used to classify articular cartilage lesions.[19-22] The most common is the Outerbridge system, which is an arthroscopic system that divides lesions into five grades[22]:

- Grade 0: normal cartilage
- Grade I: cartilage with softening and swelling
- Grade II: a partial-thickness defect with fissures on the surface that do not reach subchondral bone or that are <1.5 cm in diameter
- Grade III: fissuring to the level of subchondral bone in an area with a diameter of more than 1.5 cm
- Grade IV: exposed subchondral bone

This classification system was originally used to classify chondromalacia patellae but has been extrapolated to classify chondral lesions throughout the body with moderate accuracy.[23] However, the limitation of this system is that it does not include a description of lesion depth for grade II or grade III lesions. The International Cartilage Repair Society has a validated standardization system for the evaluation

of cartilage injury and repair, and it may be applied to MRI (**Table 14.2**).[19,24]

■ Clinical Cartilage Imaging

Knee

MRI after injury allows for noninvasive evaluation of cartilage and can detect clinically relevant lesions such as a cartilage shear injury or a displaced cartilage flap, which can mimic other injuries such as a displaced meniscal tear[25] (**Fig. 14.6**). In the knee, articular cartilage injuries have been

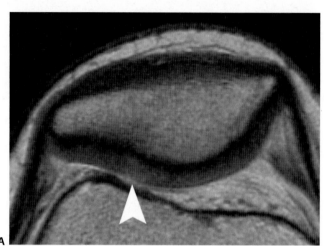

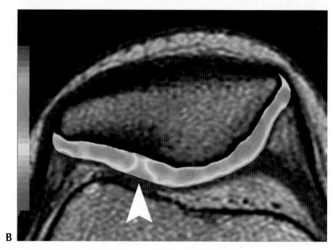

Fig. 14.5 Images of the knee in an avid marathon runner with anterior knee pain. **(A)** An axial FSE image shows focal increased signal (*arrowhead*) affecting normal-thickness cartilage in the lateral patella facet with subchondral sclerosis. **(B)** A corresponding quantitative T2 relaxation time map shows geographic loss of stratification and prolongation in T2 values (*arrowhead*) throughout the thickness of the cartilage at this site. (From Potter HG, Foo LF. Articular cartilage. In: Stoller D, ed. Magnetic Resonance Imaging in Orthopaedics and Sports Medicine. Baltimore: Lippincott Williams & Wilkins; 2007:1099–1130. Reprinted by permission.)

Table 14.2   Modified International Cartilage Repair Society Classification: MRI, Arthroscopic, and Anatomy Correlations

Grade*	Pathologic Change	Arthroscopic Findings	MRI Findings	MR Images	Anatomic Sketch
0	Normal articular cartilage	None	Normal cartilage with gray-scale stratification		
1	Superficial lesions: chondral softening	Softening to probe	Increased signal in articular cartilage		
2	Superficial lesions extending down to ≤50% of cartilage depth	Fissures/ fibrillation involving ≤50% thickness	Linear to ovoid foci of increased signal involving ≤50% thickness	Fibrillation ≤50% Fissure ≤50%	

(continued on next page)

Table 14.2 (continued)

Grade*	Pathologic Change	Arthroscopic Findings	MRI Findings	MR Images	Anatomic Sketch
3	Cartilage defects extending down >50% of depth but not through subchondral bone	Blisters/ fissures/ fibrillation involving >50% thickness	Linear to ovoid foci of increased signal involving >50% of cartilage thickness but not extending down to bone		
4	Ulceration to subchondral bone	Exposed subchondral bone	Complete loss of articular cartilage or surface flap		

Source: Adapted from Shindle MK, Foo LF, Kelly BT, et al. Magnetic resonance imaging of cartilage in the athlete: current techniques and spectrum of disease. J Bone Joint Surg Am 2006;88:27–46. Adapted by permission.

*Modified Outerbridge classification.[19,24]

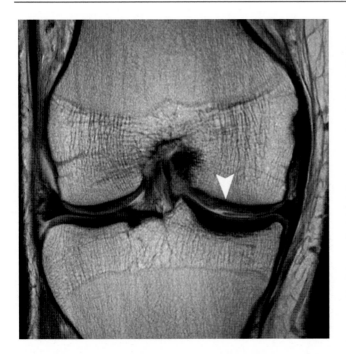

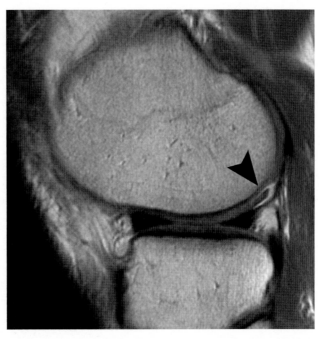

Fig. 14.6 A coronal cartilage-sensitive image of the knee in a 31-year-old man with a clinically suspected meniscal tear shows a focal chondral flap (*arrowhead*) over the right medial femoral condyle. (From Potter HG, Foo LF. Magnetic resonance imaging of articular cartilage: trauma, degeneration, and repair. Am J Sports Med 2006;34:661–677. Reprinted by permission.)

Fig. 14.7 Chondral delamination. This sagittal FSE image of the knee shows articular cartilage delaminating (*arrowhead*), with fluid signal intensity between the cartilage flap and the underlying subchondral bone. (From Shindle MK, Foo LF, Kelly BT, et al. Magnetic resonance imaging of cartilage in the athlete: current techniques and spectrum of disease. J Bone Joint Surg Am. 2006;88:27–46. Reprinted by permission.)

associated with poor clinical outcomes.[26–28] Thus, MRI before surgical intervention can aid in diagnosis, help predict prognosis, and identify patients who may benefit from cartilage repair techniques.[27]

Chondral delamination can occur when shear stresses cause separation of the articular cartilage from the underlying subchondral bone at the tidemark[29,30] (**Fig. 14.7**). Careful scrutiny of traumatic cartilage injury is necessary to distinguish an osteochondral fracture from an isolated cartilage shearing injury. Osteochondral injuries are recognized by the absence of the thin, low signal intensity subchondral plate and tidemark between the bone and cartilage or the presence of a hyperintense fatty marrow signal attached to the cartilage fragment[7] (**Fig. 14.8**).

OCD is the result of the separation of a portion of subchondral bone along the articular surface secondary to an acute shear injury or repetitive trauma. It most commonly occurs at the lateral aspect of the medial femoral condyle. In this setting, MRI is useful for assessing the stability of the lesion (**Fig. 14.9**). Signs of an unstable fragment include the following[31]:

- High signal intensity surrounding the fragment on water-sensitive pulse sequences (e.g., proton density) and T2-weighted images
- Size >5 mm

- High signal intensity defect in the overlying cartilage
- Prominent cystic changes of ≥5 mm between the fragment and host bone

Hip

Articular cartilage injuries of the hip are difficult to evaluate because of the deep ball-and-socket configuration. Traditionally, chondral damage to the hip has been associated with progressive generalized joint deterioration from such conditions as osteoarthritis or inflammatory arthritis. However, there are several other mechanisms that result in more focal chondral lesions, such as trauma, osteonecrosis, femoroacetabular impingement, and dysplastic conditions. Focal chondral injuries on the femoral side are relatively uncommon, but they may result from axial loading or a shear injury of the head within the socket. Cartilage injuries on the acetabular side are more common and typically present as localized cartilage delamination in the anterosuperior weight-bearing zone of the acetabular rim. Femoroacetabular impingement is the most common underlying condition resulting in these types of cartilage defects. The articular surfaces of the acetabulum and femoral head should be evaluated with the use of all three imaging planes. Although some authors advocate the use of MR arthrography to improve contrast between the articular cartilage and synovial fluid, this addition converts

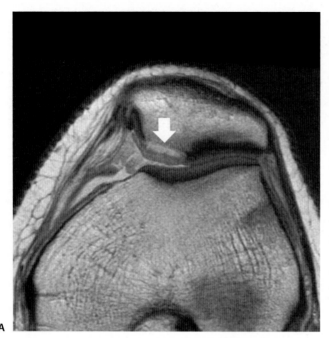

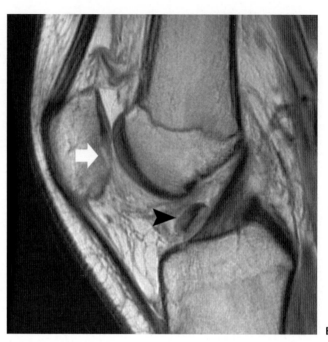

Fig. 14.8 Axial **(A)** and sagittal **(B)** FSE images after a left patellar dislocation in a 15-year-old boy show an osteochondral fracture of the medial facet (*arrow*). This injury can be distinguished from an isolated chondral shear injury because there is a displaced osteochondral fragment (*arrowhead*) with the presence of high signal intensity bone marrow, a low signal intensity subchondral plate, and intermediate signal intensity cartilage in the displaced fragment. (From Potter HG, Foo LF. Articular cartilage. In: Stoller D, ed. Magnetic Resonance Imaging in Orthopaedics and Sports Medicine. Baltimore: Lippincott Williams & Wilkins; 2007:1099–1130. Reprinted by permission.)

MRI to an invasive procedure.[32–34] Mintz et al.[35] evaluated 92 patients with noncontrast imaging before hip arthroscopy and concluded that an optimized protocol can identify labral and chondral abnormalities. The authors' protocol includes a screening examination of the whole pelvis, acquired with the use of coronal inversion recovery and axial proton-density sequences. This procedure is followed by the use of a surface coil over the hip joint, with high-resolution, cartilage-sensitive images acquired in three planes (sagittal, coronal, and oblique axial) with the use of an FSE pulse sequence and intermediate TE.

Acute isolated traumatic articular surface injuries most commonly occur from impact loading across the hip joint. The type and degree of injury vary depending on the amount and direction of the impact load. A posteriorly directed force can lead to hip subluxation, in which the femoral head is forced against the labrum and rim of the posterior wall. This subluxation can lead to shear injuries at the level of the articular cartilage and associated fractures of the subchondral bone (**Fig. 14.10**). Moorman et al.[36] described the pathognomonic MRI triad of posterior acetabular lip fracture, hemarthrosis, and iliofemoral ligament disruption. In addition, MRI is useful for monitoring for the detection of subsequent osteonecrosis that can help determine whether an athlete may return to play.

The concept of femoroacetabular impingement as a source of anterosuperior chondral and labral damage was introduced by Ganz et al.[37] Abnormal contact between the femoral head–neck junction and the anterior acetabulum during terminal hip flexion leads to a reproducible pattern of anterosuperior labral and chondral injury. Based on anatomic features, they classified femoroacetabular impingement into two distinct entities: cam and pincer. Cam impingement results from pathologic contact between an abnormally shaped femoral head and neck with a morphologically normal acetabulum. During hip flexion, this abnormal region engages the anterior acetabulum and results in the characteristic anterosuperior chondral injury with a relatively untouched labrum.[38] Pincer impingement is the result of contact between a typically normal femoral head–neck junction and an abnormal acetabular rim. This abnormal anterior acetabular "over-coverage" can be the consequence of different anatomic variants, including the following:

- Acetabular retroversion
- Coxa profunda (protrusio)
- Deformity after trauma or periacetabular osteotomies

This type of impingement can lead to degeneration, ossification, and tears of the anterosuperior labrum as well as a characteristic posteroinferior contre-coup pattern of cartilage loss over the femoral head and corresponding acetabulum. Despite the two types of distinct anatomic variants of femoroacetabular impingement, most cases involve a combination of femoral-side and acetabular-side lesions[38–40] (**Fig. 14.11**) (see Chapter 7 for additional details).

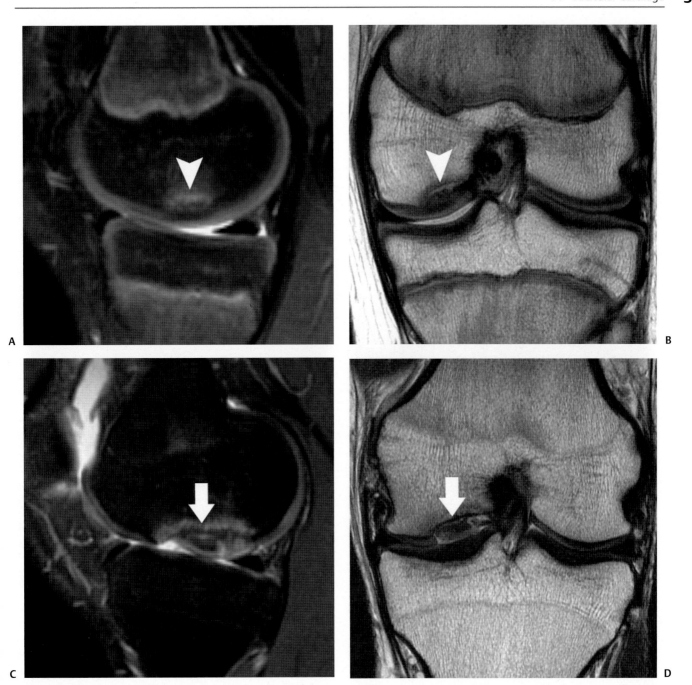

Fig. 14.9 Sagittal fat-suppressed **(A)** and coronal non–fat-suppressed **(B)** FSE images of the knee showing a small, stable OCD lesion (*arrowhead on each*). In comparison, sagittal fat-suppressed **(C)** and coronal non–fat-suppressed **(D)** FSE images show a large, unstable lesion (*arrow on each*), with low signal intensity sclerosis at the margins of the underlying bone, indicating the presence of a "mature" bed. (From Shindle MK, Foo LF, Kelly BT, et al. Magnetic resonance imaging of cartilage in the athlete: current techniques and spectrum of disease. J Bone Joint Surg Am 2006;88:27–46. Reprinted by permission.)

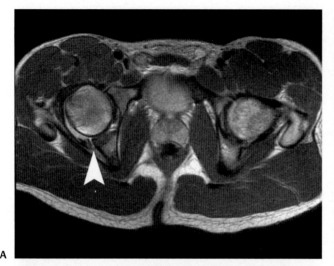

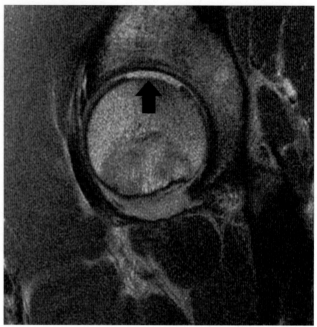

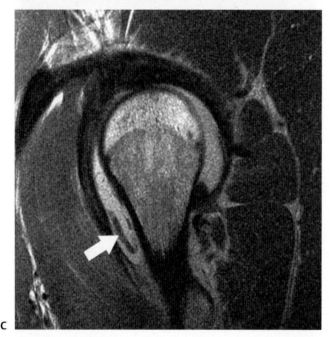

Fig. 14.10 Posterior hip subluxation sequelae in an 18-year-old patient. (**A**) Axial body coil FSE image shows an intact right posterior hip capsule (*arrowhead*) attached to a posterior wall fracture. (**B**) Sagittal surface coil FSE image shows a large full-thickness chondral shear injury (*black arrow*) of the femoral head. (**C**) Sagittal surface coil FSE image shows cartilaginous debris (*white arrow*) within the anteroinferior dependent recess of the joint. (From Shindle MK, Foo LF, Kelly BT, et al. Magnetic resonance imaging of cartilage in the athlete: current techniques and spectrum of disease. J Bone Joint Surg Am 2006;88:27–46. Reprinted by permission.)

Smaller Joints

Cartilage imaging in the elbow and smaller joints such as those in the hands and feet is also possible, but superior surface coil design and meticulous attention to pulse sequence parameters are necessary to have the ability to detect partial-thickness defects in the thinner cartilage lining these joints[6–8] (**Fig. 14.12**).

■ Osteoarthritis and Inflammatory Arthritis

In osteoarthritis, articular cartilage becomes thinner and degenerates, with fissuring, ulceration, and eventually full-

thickness loss of the joint surface. In chronic osteoarthritis, a bone marrow edema pattern may develop secondary to subchondral osseous remodeling in the presence of substantial cartilage loss. This pattern should not be misinterpreted as tumor infiltration of bone or osteonecrosis, especially in the absence of a segmental subchondral fracture or demarcation of a necrosis–viable bone interface. Associated findings of osteoarthritis may include the following:

• Subchondral sclerosis
• Osteophyte formation
• Subchondral cysts
• Bone marrow changes

However, the bone marrow edema pattern is a nonspecific MRI finding; it does not necessarily indicate a traumatic cartilage injury, but it may indicate that patients are at increased risk for additional cartilage degeneration.[6,7,41]

In contrast to osteoarthritis, cartilage thinning is uniform and diffuse in inflammatory arthritis and usually does not have focal chondral defects, except where the pannus erodes the cartilage and subchondral bone.[41] In a rheumatoid joint, conventional radiographs may remain normal for at least 6 to 12 months after the onset of symptoms.[42] MRI studies of the hand and wrist in patients with RA have shown that osseous erosions also develop much earlier than hypothesized from conventional radiographs.[43] MRI has clinical applications in the diagnosis of inflammatory arthritis and in the prediction of prognosis, which has the potential to influence management decisions in early disease.[44]

■ Cartilage Imaging After Repair

Articular cartilage injuries are common and difficult to treat because there is little to no inherent capacity for spontaneous

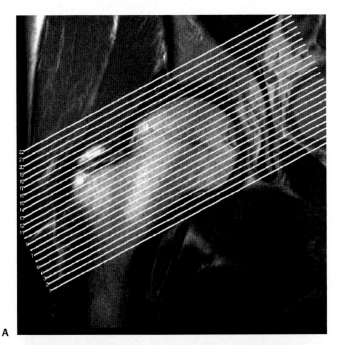

A

Fig. 14.11 FSE images and sketches of a 41-year-old patient with combined femoroacetabular impingement of the right hip. **(A)** The segment prescription (©2009 Hospital for Special Surgery, New York, NY). The coronal image (©2009 Hospital for Special Surgery, New York, NY) **(B)** and associated artist's sketch **(C)** show a torn superior labrum (*arrowhead on each*) and a cam lesion at the neck–shaft junction (*arrow on each*). (Adapted from Shindle MK, Foo LF, Kelly BT, et al. Magnetic resonance imaging of cartilage in the athlete: current techniques and spectrum of disease. J Bone Joint Surg Am 2006;88:27–46. Adapted by permission.) (Continued on page 364)

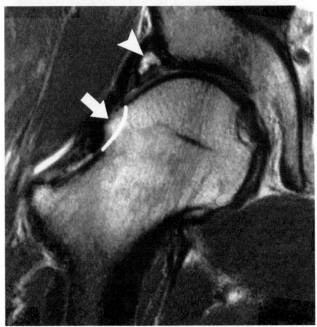

B

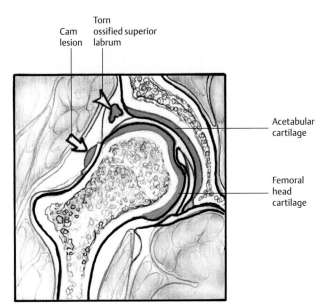

Cam lesion

Torn ossified superior labrum

Acetabular cartilage

Femoral head cartilage

C

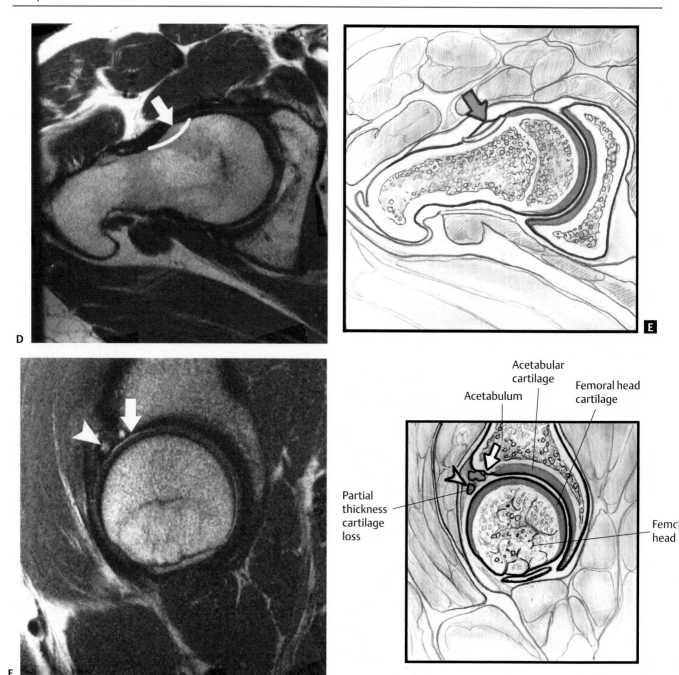

Fig. 14.11 (*Continued*) The oblique axial view (©2009 Hospital for Special Surgery, New York, NY) **(D)** and associated artist's sketch **(E)** (*arrow on each*) accentuate the osseous defect (cam lesion). The sagittal image (©2009 Hospital for Special Surgery, New York, NY) **(F)** and associated artist's sketch **(G)** show full-thickness cartilage loss over the anterior acetabular dome (*arrow on each*) and an ossified labral tear (*arrowhead on each*). (Adapted from Shindle MK, Foo LF, Kelly BT, et al. Magnetic resonance imaging of cartilage in the athlete: current techniques and spectrum of disease. J Bone Joint Surg Am 2006;88:27–46. Adapted by permission.)

repair secondary to the avascular nature of hyaline cartilage. Several techniques have been described for the repair of articular injuries, but the clinical outcomes and results have varied widely. To evaluate these techniques, most studies have relied on second-look surgery combined with biopsies.[45] However, with advances in imaging techniques, MRI has become a noninvasive alternative for the evaluation of the results of articular cartilage repair procedures.[7]

After a cartilage repair procedure, several variables should be assessed on MRI[46]:

- Degree of defect filling
- Relative signal intensity of the regenerated cartilage as compared with the surrounding native tissue
- Absence or presence of displacement
- Degree of peripheral integration to adjacent cartilage or underlying bone
- Surface geometry and morphology of the repaired tissue
- Presence of proud subchondral bone formation
- Presence of any reactive synovitis

One of the most popular articular cartilage repair techniques is microfracture, which entails creating perforations in the underlying subchondral bone using a drill or pick.[47,48] This procedure relies on the release of multipotential stem cells from the bone marrow that create a covering of largely

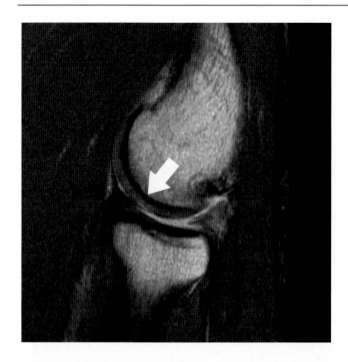

Fig. 14.12 Sagittal FSE image of the elbow in a professional baseball player, showing a partial-thickness cartilage injury overlying the capitellum (*arrow*). (From Shindle MK, Foo LF, Kelly BT, et al. Magnetic resonance imaging of cartilage in the athlete: current techniques and spectrum of disease. J Bone Joint Surg Am 2006;88:27–46. Reprinted by permission.)

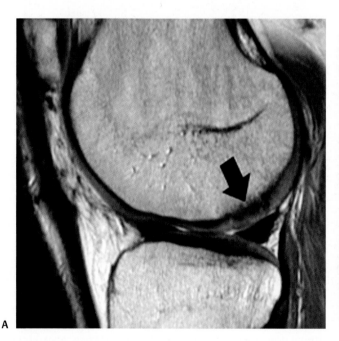

A

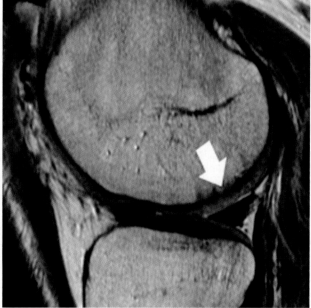

B

Fig. 14.13 Sagittal FSE images of the knee in a 32–year-old patient after microfracture. **(A)** At 5 months after surgery, there is irregularity of the subchondral plate (*black arrow*) adjacent to the repair cartilage that is hyperintense. **(B)** At 13 months after surgery, the mature reparative cartilage is now partially hypointense (*white arrow*) compared with the adjacent hyaline cartilage. Note the presence of subtle osseous overgrowth of the subchondral bone. (From Shindle MK, Foo LF, Kelly BT, et al. Magnetic resonance imaging of cartilage in the athlete: current techniques and spectrum of disease. J Bone Joint Surg Am 2006;88:27–46. Reprinted by permission.)

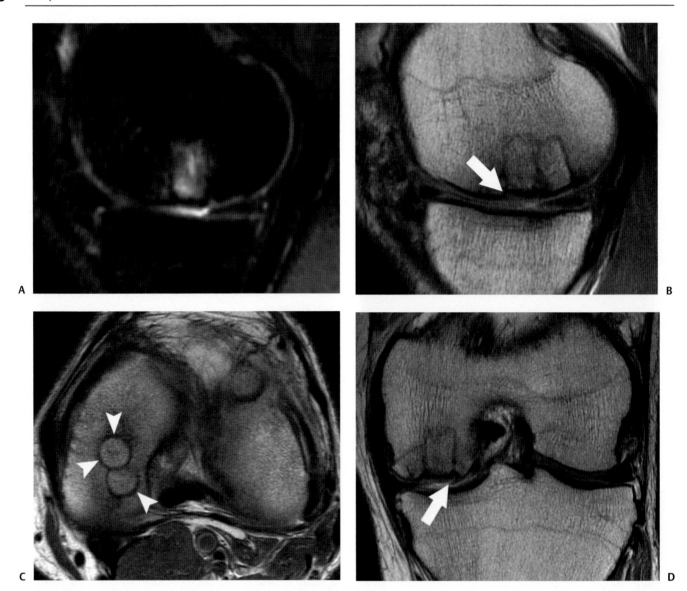

Fig. 14.14 Images of the knee in a 52–year-old patient after the transfer of two autologous osteochondral plugs. Sagittal fat-suppressed **(A)** and non–fat-suppressed **(B)** FSE images show osseous incorporation of the plugs. Although the cartilage surface remains flush over the anterior plug, there is slight depression of the subchondral bone (*black arrow* in **B**). **(C)** There is slight sclerosis in the side walls of the plugs in the axial plane (*white arrowheads*), reflecting the "press-fit" technique. **(D)** A fissure at the lateral interface with the native cartilage (*white arrow*) is shown on the coronal image. The medial tibial plateau has a degenerative pattern of partial-thickness cartilage loss. (From Shindle MK, Foo LF, Kelly BT, et al. Magnetic resonance imaging of cartilage in the athlete: current techniques and spectrum of disease. J Bone Joint Surg Am 2006;88:27–46. Reprinted by permission.)

reparative fibrocartilage (type I collagen). At short-term follow-up, this reparative tissue created from the microfracture technique appears hyperintense compared with native hyaline cartilage (type II collagen) because it is less organized and has a higher water content.[7,49] Over time, the signal intensity of reparative cartilage decreases as it matures (**Fig. 14.13**). Osseous overgrowth of the underlying subchondral bone has been reported after microfracture[50]; it may result in a thinner layer of reparative tissue, but it has not been shown to be a negative clinical prognostic factor.[50]

Another cartilage repair technique is the use of autologous or allograft osteochondral plugs.[51] The advantages of these plugs are that they can be used for a large defect and that they contain hyaline cartilage rather than a reparative fibrocartilage. Autologous osteochondral plugs are harvested from a non–weight-bearing portion of the knee, usually the side of the intercondylar notch or anterior margin of the femoral condyle. Allograft plugs are harvested from a cadaver and usually are inserted with use of a press-fit technique in which the plug and the recipient site are prepared to match-

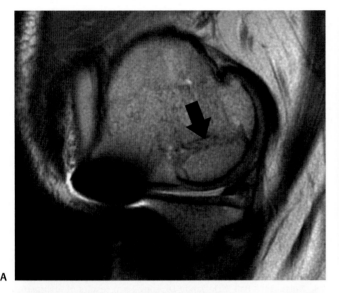

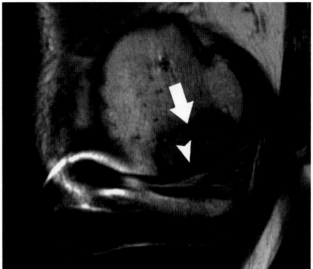

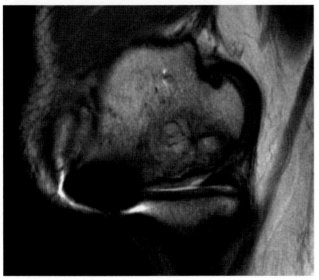

Fig. 14.15 Postoperative sagittal FSE images of the knee in a 46–year-old patient with progressive collapse of an allograft osteochondral transfer. (**A**) Incomplete osseous incorporation of the graft (*black arrow*) is seen at early follow-up. (**B**) Nine months after surgery, there is sclerosis of the bone at the graft–host bone interface (*white arrow*). The low-signal intensity subchondral bone (*white arrowhead*) indicates devitalized bone with partial collapse. (**C**) This scenario subsequently led to graft failure. (From Shindle MK, Foo LF, Kelly BT, et al. Magnetic resonance imaging of cartilage in the athlete: current techniques and spectrum of disease. J Bone Joint Surg Am 2006;88:27–46. Reprinted by permission)

ing sizes. Evaluation of these procedures on MRI should include assessment of the integration of the osseous portion of the plug and the accuracy of the restoration of the surface morphology and radius of curvature (**Fig. 14.14**). Because of the press-fit technique, there is usually a hypointense signal at the osseous interface. A hyperintense signal at the native bone–graft interface may indicate failure of integration[7] (**Fig. 14.15**). Although the osseous portion of the plug typically shows excellent incorporation, persistent gaps at the cartilaginous level have been reported between the graft and the native tissue.[52]

Autologous chondrocyte implantation is another cartilage restoration technique. In this procedure, a patient's native chondrocytes are harvested arthroscopically, grown in tissue culture for 3 to 5 weeks, and then, via an open arthrotomy, injected into a periosteum cover harvested from the patient.[19,53] Similar to microfracture, the reparative tissue remains disorganized, with increased water content and hyperintense signal on MRI. In contrast, the overlying periosteum appears hypointense and allows differentiation from the reparative tissue.[41] Complete integration may take up to 2 years, during which a decline in the signal intensity of the reparative tissue occurs as it becomes increasingly organized and incorporated. A hyperintense fluid signal between the reparative tissue and the underlying bone may indicate delamination of the reparative tissue because of incomplete integration.[41,54] Compared with microfracture, autologous chondrocyte implantation has been found to provide a better defect fill, but hypertrophy of the periosteum at early follow-up intervals has been problematic.

References

1. West RV, Fu FH. Soft-tissue physiology and repair. In: Vaccaro AR, ed. Orthopaedic Knowledge Update 8: Home Study Syllabus. Rosemont, IL: American Academy of Orthopaedic Surgeons; 2005:15–27

2. Mow VC, Proctor CS, Kelly MA. Biomechanics of articular cartilage. In: Nordin M, Frankel VH, eds. Basic Biomechanics of the Musculo-skeletal System. Philadelphia: Lea & Febiger; 1989:31–58

3. Askew MJ, Mow VC. The biomechanical function of the collagen ultrastructure of articular cartilage. J Biomech Eng 1978;100:105–115

4. Bullough PG, Jagannath A. The morphology of the calcification front in articular cartilage. Its significance in joint function. J Bone Joint Surg Br 1983;65:72–78

5. Bullough P, Goodfellow J. The significance of the fine structure of articular cartilage. J Bone Joint Surg Br 1968;50:852–857

6. Potter HG, Foo LF. Articular cartilage. In: Stoller D, ed. Magnetic Resonance Imaging in Orthopaedics and Sports Medicine. Baltimore: Lippincott Williams & Wilkins; 2007:1099–1130

7. Potter HG, Foo LF. Magnetic resonance imaging of articular cartilage: trauma, degeneration, and repair. Am J Sports Med 2006;34: 661–677

8. Shindle MK, Foo LF, Kelly BT, et al. Magnetic resonance imaging of cartilage in the athlete: current techniques and spectrum of disease. J Bone Joint Surg Am 2006;88(suppl 4):27–46

9. Kassarjian A, Yoon LS, Belzile E, Connolly SA, Millis MB, Palmer WE. Triad of MR arthrographic findings in patients with cam-type femoroacetabular impingement. Radiology 2005;236:588–592

10. Kramer J, Recht MP. MR arthrography of the lower extremity. Radiol Clin North Am 2002;40:1121–1132

11. Schmid MR, Nötzli HP, Zanetti M, Wyss TF, Hodler J. Cartilage lesions in the hip: diagnostic effectiveness of MR arthrography. Radiology 2003;226:382–386

12. Vahlensieck M, Peterfy CG, Wischer T, et al. Indirect MR arthrography: optimization and clinical applications. Radiology 1996;200: 249–254

13. Reddy R, Insko EK, Noyszewski EA, Dandora R, Kneeland JB, Leigh JS. Sodium MRI of human articular cartilage in vivo. Magn Reson Med 1998;39:697–701

14. Bashir A, Gray ML, Boutin RD, Burstein D. Glycosaminoglycan in articular cartilage: in vivo assessment with delayed Gd(DTPA)(2-)-enhanced MR imaging. Radiology 1997;205:551–558

15. Duvvuri U, Charagundla SR, Kudchodkar SB, et al. Human knee: in vivo T1(rho)-weighted MR imaging at 1.5 T—preliminary experience. Radiology 2001;220:822–826

16. Wheaton AJ, Dodge GR, Elliott DM, Nicoll SB, Reddy R. Quantification of cartilage biomechanical and biochemical properties via T1rho magnetic resonance imaging. Magn Reson Med 2005;54:1087–1093

17. Williams A, Gillis A, McKenzie C, et al. Glycosaminoglycan distribution in cartilage as determined by delayed gadolinium-enhanced MRI of cartilage (dGEMRIC): potential clinical applications. AJR Am J Roentgenol 2004;182:167–172

18. David-Vaudey E, Ghosh S, Ries M, Majumdar S. T2 relaxation time measurements in osteoarthritis. Magn Reson Imaging 2004;22: 673–682

19. Brittberg M, Winalski CS. Evaluation of cartilage injuries and repair. J Bone Joint Surg Am 2003;85(suppl 2):58–69

20. Dougados M, Ayral X, Listrat V, et al. The SFA system for assessing articular cartilage lesions at arthroscopy of the knee. Arthroscopy 1994;10:69–77

21. Noyes FR, Stabler CL. A system for grading articular cartilage lesions at arthroscopy. Am J Sports Med 1989;17:505–513

22. Outerbridge RE. The etiology of chondromalacia patellae. J Bone Joint Surg Br 1961;43:752–757

23. Cameron ML, Briggs KK, Steadman JR. Reproducibility and reliability of the Outerbridge classification for grading chondral lesions of the knee arthroscopically. Am J Sports Med 2003;31:83–86

24. Smith GD, Taylor J, Almqvist KF, et al. Arthroscopic assessment of cartilage repair: a validation study of 2 scoring systems. Arthroscopy 2005;21:1462–1467

25. Curl WW, Krome J, Gordon ES, Rushing J, Smith BP, Poehling GG. Cartilage injuries: a review of 31,516 knee arthroscopies. Arthroscopy 1997;13:456–460

26. McCauley TR, Disler DG. MR imaging of articular cartilage. Radiology 1998;209:629–640

27. McCauley TR, Disler DG. Magnetic resonance imaging of articular cartilage of the knee. J Am Acad Orthop Surg 2001;9:2–8

28. Northmore-Ball MD, Dandy DJ. Long-term results of arthroscopic partial meniscectomy. Clin Orthop Relat Res 1982;167:34–42

29. Kendell SD, Helms CA, Rampton JW, Garrett WE, Higgins LD. MRI appearance of chondral delamination injuries of the knee. AJR Am J Roentgenol 2005;184:1486–1489

30. Levy AS, Lohnes J, Sculley S, LeCroy M, Garrett W. Chondral delamination of the knee in soccer players. Am J Sports Med 1996;24: 634–639

31. De Smet AA, Ilahi OA, Graf BK. Reassessment of the MR criteria for stability of osteochondritis dissecans in the knee and ankle. Skeletal Radiol 1996;25:159–163

32. Chan YS, Lien LC, Hsu HL, et al. Evaluating hip labral tears using magnetic resonance arthrography: a prospective study comparing hip arthroscopy and magnetic resonance arthrography diagnosis. Arthroscopy 2005;21:1250e1–1250e8

33. Leunig M, Podeszwa D, Beck M, Werlen S, Ganz R. Magnetic resonance arthrography of labral disorders in hips with dysplasia and impingement. Clin Orthop Relat Res 2004;418:74–80

34. Werlen S, Leunig M, Ganz R. Magnetic resonance arthrography of the hip in femoroacetabular impingement: technique and findings. Oper Tech Orthop 2005;15:191–203

35. Mintz DN, Hooper T, Connell D, Buly R, Padgett DE, Potter HG. Magnetic resonance imaging of the hip: detection of labral and chondral abnormalities using noncontrast imaging. Arthroscopy 2005;21:385–393

36. Moorman CT III, Warren RF, Hershman EB, et al. Traumatic posterior hip subluxation in American football. J Bone Joint Surg Am 2003; 85:1190–1196

37. Ganz R, Parvizi J, Beck M, Leunig M, Nötzli H, Siebenrock KA. Femoroacetabular impingement: a cause for osteoarthritis of the hip. Clin Orthop Relat Res 2003;417:111–119

38. Beck M, Kalhor M, Leunig M, Ganz R. Hip morphology influences the pattern of damage to the acetabular cartilage: femoroacetabular impingement as a cause of early osteoarthritis of the hip. J Bone Joint Surg Br 2005;87:1012–1018

39. Bredella MA, Stoller DW. MR imaging of femoroacetabular impingement. Magn Reson Imaging Clin N Am 2005;13:653–664

40. Meislin R, Abeles A. Role of hip MR imaging in the management of sports-related injuries. Magn Reson Imaging Clin N Am 2005;13: 635–640

41. Verstraete KL, Almqvist F, Verdonk P, et al. Magnetic resonance imaging of cartilage and cartilage repair. Clin Radiol 2004;59:674–689

42. van der Heijde DMFM, van Leeuwen MA, van Riel PLCM, et al. Bi-annual radiographic assessments of hands and feet in a three-year prospective followup of patients with early rheumatoid arthritis. Arthritis Rheum 1992;35:26–34

43. Foley-Nolan D, Stack JP, Ryan M, et al. Magnetic resonance imaging in the assessment of rheumatoid arthritis—a comparison with plain film radiographs. Br J Rheumatol 1991;30:101–106

44. McQueen FM. Magnetic resonance imaging in early inflammatory arthritis: what is its role? Rheumatology (Oxford) 2000;39:700–706

45. Mainil-Varlet P, Aigner T, Brittberg M, et al. Histological assessment of cartilage repair: a report by the Histology Endpoint Committee of the International Cartilage Repair Society (ICRS). J Bone Joint Surg Am 2003;85(suppl 2):45–57

46. Brown WE, Potter HG, Marx RG, Wickiewicz TL, Warren RF. Magnetic resonance imaging appearance of cartilage repair in the knee. Clin Orthop Relat Res 2004;422:214–223

47. Steadman JR, Rodkey WG, Briggs KK, Rodrigo JJ. [The microfracture technic in the management of complete cartilage defects in the knee joint]. Orthopade 1999;28:26–32

48. Steadman JR, Rodkey WG, Rodrigo JJ. Microfracture: surgical technique and rehabilitation to treat chondral defects. Clin Orthop Relat Res 2001; 391(suppl):S362–S369

49. Knutsen G, Engebretsen L, Ludvigsen TC, et al. Autologous chondrocyte implantation compared with microfracture in the knee. A randomized trial. J Bone Joint Surg Am 2004;86:455–464

50. Mithoefer K, Williams RJ III, Warren RF, et al. The microfracture technique for the treatment of articular cartilage lesions in the knee. A prospective cohort study. J Bone Joint Surg Am 2005;87:1911–1920

51. Hangody L, Feczkó P, Bartha L, Bodó G, Kish G. Mosaicplasty for the treatment of articular defects of the knee and ankle. Clin Orthop Relat Res 2001;391(suppl):S328–S336

52. Glenn RE Jr, McCarty EC, Potter HG, Juliao SF, Gordon JD, Spindler KP. Comparison of fresh osteochondral autografts and allografts: a canine model. Am J Sports Med 2006;34:1084–1093

53. Brittberg M, Lindahl A, Nilsson A, Ohlsson C, Isaksson O, Peterson L. Treatment of deep cartilage defects in the knee with autologous chondrocyte transplantation. N Engl J Med 1994;331:889–895

54. Alparslan L, Winalski CS, Boutin RD, Minas T. Postoperative magnetic resonance imaging of articular cartilage repair. Semin Musculoskelet Radiol 2001;5:345–363

15 Soft-Tissue and Bone Tumors

Derek F. Papp, A. Jay Khanna, Edward F. McCarthy, Laura M. Fayad, Adam J. Farber, and Frank J. Frassica

■ Background

The management of soft-tissue masses presents an interesting quandary for physicians that has important implications. Although it has been suggested that 1 of 100 soft-tissue lesions seen by a physician is malignant, the precise overall number is unknown.[1] The incidence of soft-tissue sarcomas has been estimated to be approximately 8,100 cases per year in the United States.[2] In most cases, soft-tissue masses are benign. Indeed, many of these soft-tissue lesions have no potential for metastasis or local invasion and can simply be observed. The danger in simple observation occurs when the physician observes a lesion without having a firm diagnosis; this situation can lead to errors in management with resultant poor outcomes, including local invasion of neurovascular structures and metastatic disease. Similarly, excision of a lesion without a definitive diagnosis can also result in catastrophic outcomes. With an incorrect diagnosis, excision of a malignant lesion can lead to the contamination of unaffected tissues, recurrence, and, in some cases, eventual amputation of an affected limb.

For many years, the use of tissue biopsy was the only means of obtaining a definitive diagnosis. Today, the increased use of MRI has substantially improved the diagnosis and management of soft-tissue tumors. MRI provides excellent soft-tissue resolution and allows the physician to differentiate various soft-tissue types based on imaging characteristics via the use of various pulse sequences,[3,4] a feature not afforded by other imaging modalities such as conventional radiographs and CT. The excellent spatial resolution provided by MRI also provides sharp delineation of soft-tissue boundaries and highlights the boundaries between the soft-tissue tumor and the adjacent normal tissues. This information can help guide the determination of the diagnosis of a soft-tissue lesion, which can obviate tissue biopsy. Another advantage of MRI relates to its use in preoperative planning. With the guidance of multiplanar imaging provided by MRI, neurovascular structures can be avoided during the approach to the lesion, eliminating or decreasing the potential for contamination during planned biopsies or providing a means to ensure adequate margins when resection is planned. With all of its inherent capabilities, MRI has become a powerful tool in the diagnosis and management of soft-tissue tumors.

In addition to its value in diagnosing soft-tissue tumors, the diagnosis of bone tumors has been enhanced by the use of MRI in conjunction with conventional radiographs and CT. Although conventional radiographs often provide enough information to make a diagnosis of a given bone tumor, MRI can provide additional details that will help guide the management of the lesion. MRI also allows for the visualization of pathology that cannot be seen on conventional radiographs, such as fluid–fluid levels or the degree of invasion of the adjacent soft-tissue structures. A lesion's tissue composition also can be identified more easily with MRI than with conventional radiographs. This information can affect the surgeon's management decisions, such as the choice of neoadjuvant or postoperative chemotherapy.

The clinician must properly diagnose the soft-tissue lesion before planning any type of treatment, including simple observation. Understanding this point and the consequences of misdiagnosis, the surgeon must take a methodical, systematic approach to the diagnosis of these lesions. Therefore, a diagnostic and treatment algorithm directed toward soft-tissue and bone lesions depends on information from the history, physical examination, conventional radiographs, CT scans, and MRI studies. This chapter provides such an algorithm based on the concept of determinate versus indeterminate soft-tissue tumors, reviews common soft-tissue and bone lesions, and describes them and their characteristic MRI findings.

■ Soft-Tissue Tumors

As with any medical condition, the evaluation of a soft-tissue tumor begins with the history and physical examination. Although they are essential parts of the diagnostic process, these two items often do not provide a definitive diagnosis for soft-tissue lesions. Most soft-tissue tumors are slow-growing lesions. A history of trauma, although suggestive of a hematoma or heterotopic ossification, does not ensure that the lesion is a benign, posttraumatic process. The trauma may merely alert the patient to a soft-tissue tumor that had previously been present in the area. In addition, it is important to note that a history of pain is not a reliable indicator of the benign or malignant nature of a lesion and that only

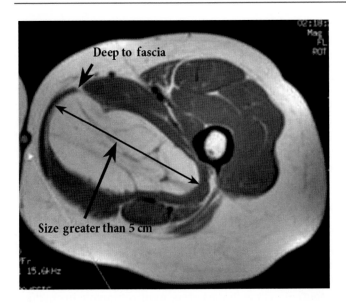

Fig. 15.1 An axial, postgadolinium, T1-weighted image of the left proximal thigh showing a lesion that displays two of the common signs of a malignant soft-tissue lesion: size >5 cm and location deep to the fascia.

half of all patients with a malignant soft-tissue mass complain of pain.[5] Systemic symptoms, such as fever, malaise, chills, or night sweats, are associated with the presence of malignant lesions, but the absence of systemic complaints does not necessarily indicate that the lesion is benign. Ultimately, the history may assist the physician in diagnosis, but the lack of consistency in soft-tissue tumor symptomatology often means that the history alone is seldom beneficial in definitively diagnosing soft-tissue lesions.

Similarly, the physical examination is frequently nonspecific in nature and often cannot be used to determine whether a lesion is benign or malignant. It is extremely helpful in some cases (e.g., periarticular ganglion cysts), but, for most soft-tissue masses, physical examination does not provide a definitive answer. For example, although a size of >5 cm, a location beneath the fascia, and a feeling of firm or matted material are associated more with malignant than with benign lesions, none of these criteria is pathognomonic for malignancy (**Fig. 15.1**).[6] At the same time, malignant lesions can present as small or nongrowing lesions. Sarcomas are typically large, but to characterize a small lesion as benign without having a definitive diagnosis is a mistake. Neurologic deficit can result from malignant or benign lesions. It has been reported that certain lesions have characteristic appearances on MRI and other imaging modalities, which allows the physician to diagnose the lesion with a high degree of confidence.[7] Lesions in this category are termed determinate. Lesions that cannot be diagnosed with certainty without biopsy are termed indeterminate.

Determinate Lesions

With determinate lesions, that is, those with a distinctive appearance on a radiograph or MRI or a very characteristic physical examination, the physician feels comfortable making a diagnosis without a tissue sample and can make the appropriate decision about treatment without gathering additional information. It is important to remember that, as with all tumors, good communication between the treating physician and physicians from other disciplines is essential to making the proper diagnosis. Discussions with an experienced musculoskeletal radiologist can help guide or confirm

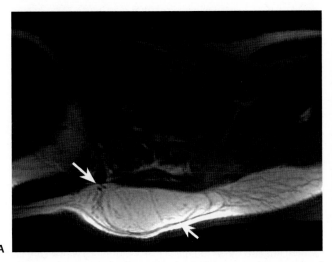

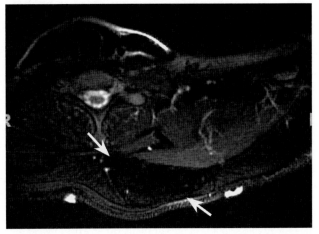

Fig. 15.2 Lipoma of the left upper back. **(A)** An axial T1-weighted image shows a high signal intensity lesion (*arrows*) with the same intensity of surrounding fat. The lesion itself is homogeneous and superficial. **(B)** An axial STIR image shows suppression of the signal within the lesion (*arrows*). Fiduciary markers on the skin delineate the lesion.

the physician's diagnosis, as can discussions with a pathologist, especially one with a special interest or advanced training in the evaluation of soft-tissue and bone tumors. A multidisciplinary approach reduces the risk of diagnostic errors.[7] Each physician will develop his or her own level of comfort in classifying such lesions.

Lipoma

Lipomas, the most common of all soft-tissue tumors, are composed of mature fatty tissue. Although typically asymptomatic, these lesions can cause pain and neurologic symptoms by compressing neurovascular structures. Lesions that cause such symptoms usually lie deep to the fascia. Because lipomas consist of mature fatty tissue, the signal intensity of a lipoma on MRI exactly matches the intensity of subcutaneous fat. On routine SE pulse sequences, this appearance translates to high signal intensity on T1-weighted images and moderate to high intensity on T2-weighted images. When lipomas are suspected, the use of a fat-suppression technique and STIR images can confirm the lipomatous nature of the lesion by suppressing the high signal intensity related to the adipose tissue.[7] The tissue seen in the lipoma should match the signal characteristics of subcutaneous fat on all pulse sequences, including fat-suppressed and STIR images (**Fig. 15.2**). Fibrous septations may appear as hypointense thin lines that may or may not enhance with contrast.[8]

Lipomas, especially those in superficial or subcutaneous locations, are well-demarcated lesions that do not invade surrounding structures. However, deep lipomas may surround vascular and neural structures. Lipomatous variants that contain other mesenchymal elements, such as fibrous or myxoid tissue, differ from the typical lipoma. The physician must evaluate atypical lipomas carefully. Differentiating them from low-grade liposarcomas without a tissue sample may be difficult, if not impossible. Areas of heterogeneity on MRI should alert the physician to possible malignancy. Broad septations or septations with nodules are characteristics of well-differentiated liposarcomas (**Fig. 15.3**).

Hemangioma

Hemangiomas are relatively common benign soft-tissue tumors composed of benign blood vessel elements. Estimates of female-to-male predominance range as high as 3:1,[9] although other investigators have not shown that same distribution.[7] These lesions occur most commonly in children, and cutaneous manifestations of the lesion usually spontaneously involute in the first decade of life. Other manifestations include the following:

- Cavernous subtype lesions
- Venous lesions
- Arteriovenous lesions
- Mixed-type lesions

Hemangiomas that prove more difficult to diagnose are those that lie deep in the soft tissues. Superficial blood vessel tumors can have a spongy or fluctuant quality, and, on

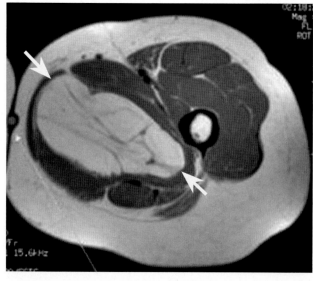
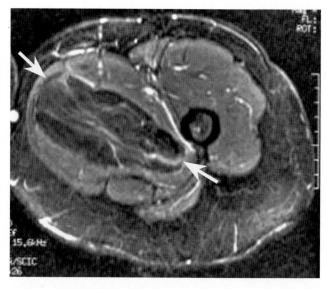

Fig. 15.3 Atypical lipoma in the left thigh. **(A)** An axial T1-weighted image shows a large, high signal intensity lesion (*arrows*) with multiple septations, suggestive of an atypical lipoma. **(B)** An axial STIR image shows suppression of most of the signal within the lesion (*arrows*) but also shows multiple fibrous septations with a complex, heterogeneous composition. Because of its large size and heterogeneous appearance, this lipoma was biopsied.

occasion, such lesions fill or swell when the limb is placed in a dependent position. In contrast, lesions that lie deep to the fascia may not have any unique findings on physical examination and can only be palpated; these lesions can increase in size during pregnancy.[10] Approximately half of these lesions cause pain after exertion, which may relate to a vascular steal phenomenon and the resultant tissue ischemia when the lesion absorbs blood flow or results in retrograde flow.[11]

Phleboliths may be seen on conventional radiographs in approximately 50% of patients with hemangiomas.[11] Phleboliths appear as small, round, mineralized soft-tissue densities that have a lucent center. A nondescript soft-tissue mass may be seen. The MRI is often diagnostic. A hemangioma is a heterogeneous mass that can contain varying degrees of thrombus, hemosiderin, vessel formation, fibrosis, and fat. The amount of fat can be substantial. With T1-weighted SE imaging, the areas corresponding to adipose tissue show high signal. The lipomatous portion usually involves the periphery of the lesion. Blood-filled cavernous or vessel components of the lesion also appear bright with T2-weighted and STIR imaging, and they enhance on postgadolinium T1-weighted images (**Fig. 15.4**). Depending on the nature of the vessel formation, a "serpentine" figure may be apparent; septations and lobules are easily recognized. If there is rapid flow within the lesion, flow voids or focal regions of low signal on T2-weighted or STIR images are seen.[12] On ultrasound, the lesions appear echogenic, and color-flow Doppler often shows obvious flow within the lesion.[13]

Ganglion Cyst

Another common determinate lesion, the ganglion cyst, arises from periarticular tissues and tendon sheaths. This lesion is composed of viscous mucinous fluid contained by a thick fibrous shell, but debate still exists over its etiology. Some believe that repeated stress causes mucoid degeneration,[14,15] whereas others hypothesize that lining cell hyperplasia with production of a hyaluronic acid-rich substance causes degeneration into a cystic lesion.[15,16] The most common locations for a ganglion cyst include the dorsal and volar aspects of the wrist. Because the lesion typically occurs in this location and has a characteristic appearance, the physician often can make the diagnosis without additional imaging.

Other common locations include the following:

- Foot and ankle
- Tendon sheaths
- Labra
- Joint capsules

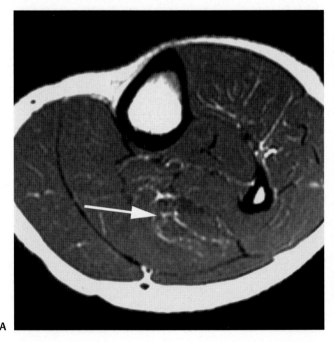
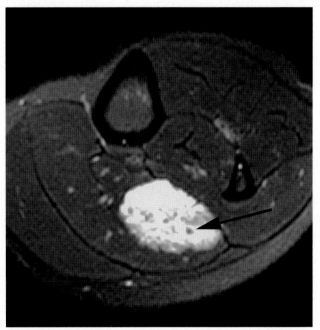

A   B

Fig. 15.4 Hemangioma. Axial T1-weighted **(A)** and axial fat-suppressed T2-weighted **(B)** images of the right calf show a mass (*arrow*) in the medial head of the gastrocnemius muscle. The mass is minimally high signal on the T1-weighted image and heterogeneous and serpentine high signal on the STIR image. (From Papp DF, Khanna AJ, McCarthy EF, Carrino JA, Farber AJ, Frassica FJ. Magnetic resonance imaging of soft tissue tumors: determinate and indeterminate lesions. J Bone Joint Surg Am 2007;89(suppl 3):103-115. Reprinted by permission.)

The ganglion cysts often do not communicate with a joint. When the lesion is located in other areas, additional imaging often is needed. On conventional radiographs, osseous erosion is occasionally seen as a result of pressure erosion. MRI delineates the cyst as a smooth, round, or ovular well-circumscribed structure that may have septations. These septations, or the peripheral rim of the lesion, may enhance with gadolinium, but the center of the lesion should not enhance with contrast. T1-weighted imaging shows decreased signal intensity, and lesions appear bright on T2-weighted or STIR imaging, with signal intensity similar to that of water (**Fig. 15.5**).[4,12,17-19]

Synovial Cyst (Baker Cyst)

Although a ganglion cyst rarely arises inside of a joint and does not communicate with the joint itself, the synovial (Baker) cyst is contiguous with the joint space. Classically described by Baker,[20] the lesion arises from synovial fluid by pushing its way from the joint into a communicating bursa (often under the medial head of the gastrocnemius at the knee) or by causing herniation of the synovial membrane itself. The lesion arises in the popliteal fossa and may cause posterior knee pain. Occasionally, these cysts can cause complications, such as the following[21,22]:

- Cyst leakage
- Thrombophlebitis
- Compartment syndrome
- Lower limb claudication

Meniscal tears have been described as the most common etiology of these lesions, although the cyst can form from other intraarticular processes, such as degenerative arthritis or ACL injury. The prevalence of this entity in adults ranges from 5% to 20%.[23,24] Approximately half of patients with osteoarthritis have a Baker cyst.[25] Excision of the cyst may not provide relief because the cysts commonly recur. Treatment of the underlying condition often results in resolution of the cyst.

Radiographs often show osteoarthritis, which (as described above) can cause the development of the disease. They do not show the process itself. Although ultrasound is another modality that can show synovial cyst formation, MRI is the standard for diagnosis because the underlying pathology, such as ACL or meniscal tears, also can be evaluated with this modality. MRI shows a well-circumscribed

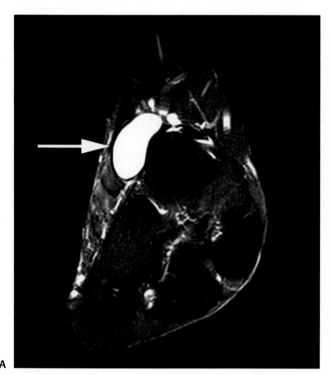

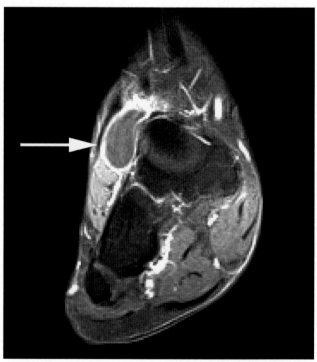

A

B

Fig. 15.5 Ganglion cyst. Coronal STIR **(A)** and coronal contrast-enhanced, fat-suppressed T1-weighted **(B)** images show the typical appearance of a ganglion cyst (*arrow*) along the dorsum of the midfoot. The lesion is round, well-circumscribed, and hyperintense compared with muscle on the STIR image with a thin rim of enhancement, which is compatible with the fluid-filled, cystic nature of a ganglion cyst. (From Papp DF, Khanna AJ, McCarthy EF, Carrino JA, Farber AJ, Frassica FJ. Magnetic resonance imaging of soft tissue tumors: determinate and indeterminate lesions. J Bone Joint Surg Am 2007;89(suppl 3):103-115. Reprinted by permission.)

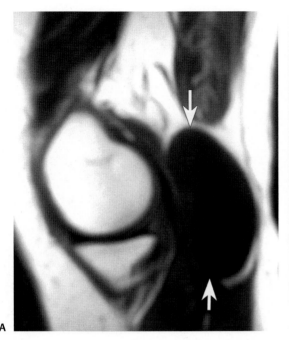
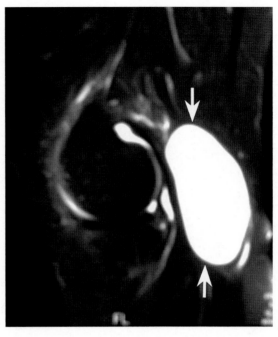

Fig. 15.6 Synovial cyst. **(A)** A sagittal T1-weighted image shows a large, low signal intensity mass (*arrows*) posterior to the knee joint. **(B)** A sagittal T2-weighted image shows the same lesion (*arrows*) to be of high signal intensity and well circumscribed, compatible with a cyst (in this case, a Baker cyst).

mass in the posterior fossa of the knee. T1-weighted and T2-weighted images show fluid with the same intensity as that of joint fluid (dark on T1-weighted images and bright on T2-weighted images) (**Fig. 15.6**). The addition of gadolinium contrast shows enhancement of only the rim.

Hematoma

The differentiation of a hematoma from hemorrhage within a sarcoma can be difficult. Although not definitive, a history of trauma favors the diagnosis of a hematoma. A history of bruising or ecchymosis noted on physical examination may help with the diagnosis. Most patients with a hematoma have a history of trauma or surgical intervention. The natural history of hematomas follows one of three pathways:

- Spontaneous involution
- Development of peripheral calcification and progression to myositis ossificans (see below)
- Chronic expansion of the hematoma

The clinical picture for the last presentation differs somewhat from that of the other two, as described by Reid et al.[26] Typically, a patient presents with a slow-growing soft-tissue mass that does not involute within a month of the initial injury. Some clinicians believe that the hemosiderin breakdown products do not allow the lesion to heal completely and that the persistent irritation caused by these products maintains patent capillary bleeding into the hematoma.[26-28] Systemic anticoagulation has been described as a cause of the formation of these lesions.[28] Often painless, these lesions can produce neurologic deficits via neurovascular compression. Radiographs may show pressure erosion of the surrounding bones.[27]

The MRI findings are characteristic. T1-weighted images usually show a well-defined mass. Centrally, the lesion is heterogeneous, with bright foci that correspond with areas of new or continuing hemorrhage. T2-weighted images also show heterogeneity, with areas of high and low signal intensity corresponding to granulation tissue and hemosiderin deposition, respectively. The presence of a low signal intensity pseudocapsule completes the picture (**Fig. 15.7**). Gradient-echo images may help isolate hemosiderin in the lesion.[27,28] When the lesion does not show any enhancement with gadolinium contrast, the diagnosis is most likely a hematoma.

Enhancement of the pseudocapsule has been described with gadolinium, but it is rare. Fluid–fluid levels also have been described.[29] Likewise, Liu et al.[28] described occasional internal patchy enhancement of the lesion. Given the increased likelihood of sarcoma with contrast enhancement, these lesions may then not be classified as determinate and must be biopsied.[28,30] If biopsy is considered, it is important to confirm that the lesion is not a vascular lesion, such as a pseudoaneurysm or arteriovenous malformation, and that the patient does not have an untreated coagulopathy. The

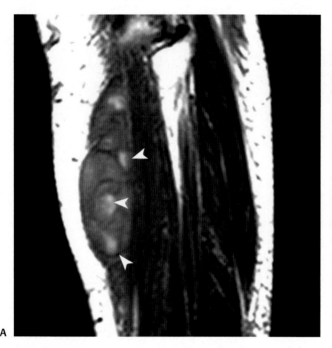

A

B

Fig. 15.7 Hematoma. Sagittal T1-weighted **(A)** and sagittal fat-suppressed T2-weighted **(B)** images of the leg show a mass lesion in the anterior compartment (*arrow* in **B**). The T1-weighted image shows areas of hyperintensity (*arrowheads*), reflecting methemoglobin. The high signal intensity areas on the fat-suppressed T2-weighted image are related to soft-tissue edema and hemorrhage. Clinical correlation is especially helpful for the diagnosis of hematoma, and attention should be given to the presence or absence of coagulopathy, history of surgery, or other trauma. (From Papp DF, Khanna AJ, McCarthy EF, Carrino JA, Farber AJ, Frassica FJ. Magnetic resonance imaging of soft tissue tumors: determinate and indeterminate lesions. J Bone Joint Surg Am 2007;89(suppl 3):103-115. Reprinted by permission.)

diagnoses of pseudoaneurysm and arteriovenous malformation can often be made via a duplex ultrasound examination.

Myositis Ossificans

Heterotopic ossification is the formation of extraskeletal, mature, lamellar bone. This process most often occurs after direct trauma, as a complication of orthopaedic procedures and spinal cord injury, and in the burn patient. In posttraumatic cases, the process is termed myositis ossificans. Myositis ossificans occurs at sites of previous hematoma formations, although the process by which a hematoma involutes or evolves into myositis ossificans or a chronically expanding hematoma is not fully understood. Most patients present in the third decade of life, and the most common locations include the quadriceps and the brachialis muscles.[31,32] The process is thought to arise after a direct impact to the affected muscle; the more severe the injury, the higher is the likelihood of hematoma formation.[33]

Radiographs show a well-circumscribed, calcified lesion in the pattern of mature, lamellar bone peripherally when the lesion has matured.[15] In such cases, a conventional radiograph may be sufficient for diagnosis. However, when the diagnosis is in doubt, MRI can be helpful. T1-weighted images often show a lesion in the belly of the muscle, with a signal intensity the same as or slightly higher than that of the adjacent muscle. At times, this similarity may lead to the recognition of the lesion on T1-weighted images solely by noting the distortion of fascial planes.[32] For lesions in patients who present early in their course, T2-weighted images show central high signal intensity with an external ring of low signal intensity. This configuration is pathognomonic and represents the zonal pattern of growth of myositis ossificans in which the external edges of the lesion ossify first. Surrounding edema may or may not be seen (**Fig. 15.8**).

Myonecrosis (Diabetic and Idiopathic)

The diagnosis of myonecrosis should be considered when a patient presents with a rapidly growing, painful mass that involves at least one extremity. Patients who present with myonecrosis most frequently have involvement of the lower extremities, especially the quadriceps and calf muscles. Diabetes is the most frequently associated cause, but myonecrosis also has been associated with alcohol abuse and other, less common, entities. Diabetic myonecrosis has been reported in a previously healthy woman as a presenting symptom of her diabetes,[34] although patients with diabetes more

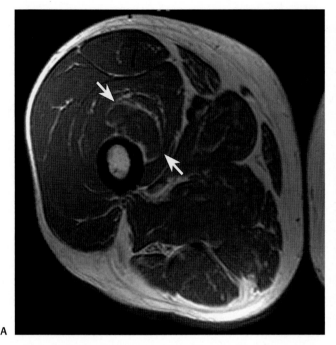
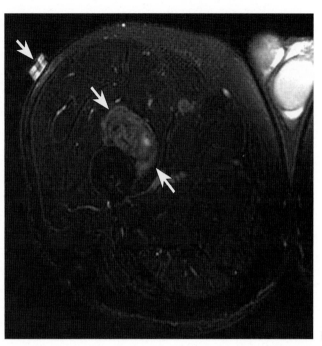

A   B

Fig. 15.8 Myositis ossificans. **(A)** An axial T1-weighted image of the right leg shows a lesion (*arrows*) with the same intensity as the surrounding muscle, making the lesion difficult to see. The disruption of fascial planes is the only indication of abnormality. **(B)** An axial STIR image shows that the lesion (*arrows*) has a higher signal intensity than the surrounding muscles. Absence of a low signal intensity ring identifies it as an early lesion. Conventional radiographs with a zonal pattern of calcification aid with the diagnosis.

often have other existing sequelae, such as nephropathy or other forms of end-organ damage.[35,36] Laboratory values are typically within normal limits, although elevated creatinine serum kinase levels have been reported.[34,36] The ultimate pathophysiology of the process is not fully understood; it is best presented as a mixture of activated coagulation factors, impaired fibrin degradation, and endothelial damage from diabetic microangiopathy.[37] These factors ultimately overcome the skeletal muscle's abundant blood supply, leading to necrosis.

The early recognition of myonecrosis, before tissue biopsy, can be important because patients with diabetes frequently have wound-healing problems. For this reason, nonsurgical management approaches are preferred.[38] Conventional radiographs and CT imaging provide little data about the nature of this entity; however, MRI provides valuable information that facilitates diagnosis. T1-weighted imaging shows swelling and disruption of the involved muscles along the fascial planes. The muscle fiber pattern persists after the necrosis occurs, and there is no infiltration of the fascia. Although the resultant loss of striations is seen grossly on MRI, the overall structure remains unchanged. T2-weighted imaging shows a diffuse increase in signal intensity in the muscle, indicative of edema, and areas of necrosis. The muscles show heterogeneous signal intensity on T2-weighted images, which likely corresponds to fiber regeneration. The findings with myo-

necrosis contrast with those seen with neoplasms, which often disrupt the surrounding anatomy. Contrast-enhanced images may show a mixture of enhancing linear or serpentine fibers within low signal intensity regions. The dark (low signal intensity) areas represent necrotic tissue, and the enhancing areas represent viable or inflamed tissue (**Fig. 15.9**). The lesions frequently show peripheral enhancement on postgadolinium T1-weighted images.[34,36,39]

Neurofibroma

Neurofibromatosis type 1, formerly known as von Recklinghausen disease, is an autosomal dominant disorder characterized by neurofibromas and other systemic complications, such as the following:

- Skeletal dysplasias
- Café-au-lait spots
- Lisch nodules
- Vascular malformations
- Learning disabilities
- Optic gliomas

In addition, these patients are at risk for other malignancies, such as nerve-sheath tumors and rhabdomyosarcoma, as well as for dedifferentiation of their neurofibromas into neurofibrosarcomas.[40] With an incidence of approximately

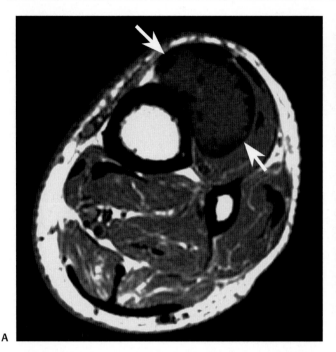
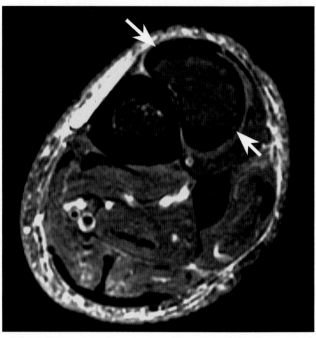

Fig. 15.9 Myonecrosis. Axial T1-weighted **(A)** and T2-weighted **(B)** images of the right leg show a well-defined area (*arrows*) of low signal within the muscles of the anterior compartment of the leg in a patient with a history of diabetes mellitus. Note that the surrounding fascia and tissue planes are well preserved.

1 in 3500, neurofibromatosis type 1 is more common than neurofibromatosis type 2 and is associated with the formation of true neurofibromas; the formation of schwannomas is more characteristic of neurofibromatosis type 2.[40]

On examination, the lesions can be superficial or deep and are not always painful. Despite their association with nerves, neurologic findings are uncommon. The MRI findings of neurofibromatosis are quite specific and therefore can help with diagnosis. The T1-weighted images show a lesion that is hyperintense relative to skeletal muscle. The appearance is fascicular or nodular. T2-weighted imaging classically shows a *target sign*, manifesting as an area of low signal centrally situated within a high signal intensity lesion. The myxoid nature of the neurofibroma accounts for the bright periphery, whereas the dark central region represents the compressed nerve fibers[41,42] (**Fig. 15.10**). This specific finding simplifies the diagnosis and allows for ease of continued follow-up of the multiple lesions, which can help monitor for conversion to a neurofibrosarcoma. Superficial lesions do not always present with a target sign, can appear homogeneous, and usually extend to the skin.[42]

Muscle Tear

The presentation of a muscle tear masquerading as a soft-tissue mass occurs often enough that the orthopaedic surgeon should consider this possibility when addressing unknown soft-tissue lesions. Muscle tears commonly have a specific inciting incident; patients often remember hearing a snapping sound or feeling that their strength is "giving way," followed by a period of muscle swelling, tenderness, ecchymosis, and/or edema. However, this scenario does not always occur. In fact, a study at the Walter Reed Army Medical Center showed that, in six of seven patients with rectus femoris muscle tears presenting as soft-tissue masses, there was no specific event; rather, the tear appeared insidiously, and only half of the lesions were painful.[43] As old muscle tears scar and retract, they can present in a manner similar to that of soft-tissue tumors.[44,45] The physician who understands this presentation can avoid unnecessary biopsy and its associated complications.

Radiographs are not helpful; however, as with other soft-tissue lesions, MRI facilitates diagnosis. T1-weighted imaging shows clear muscle or tendon deformity. T2-weighted images vary, depending on the time course of the process: acute injuries show increased signal intensity compatible with edema, whereas chronic injuries have low to intermediate intensity (**Fig. 15.11**).

PVNS

Most patients present with chronic pain and swelling about the involved joint, but other nonspecific symptoms, such as warmth and effusion, also occur.[46] PVNS usually

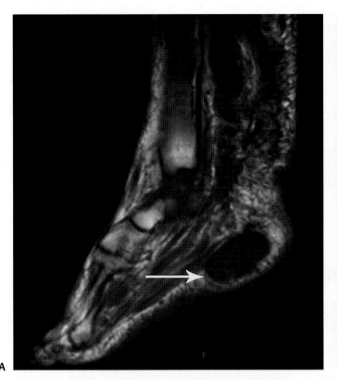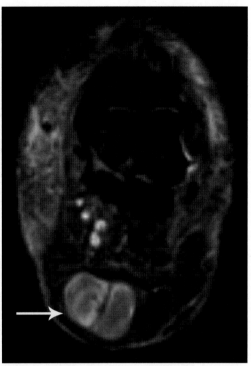

A   B

Fig. 15.10 Neurofibroma. Sagittal T1-weighted **(A)** and coronal STIR **(B)** images of the ankle show a well-circumscribed mass (*arrow*) in the plantar aspect of the foot that is hypointense compared with muscle on the T1-weighted image. The STIR image shows the typical "target" sign in which the periphery of the lesion is bright and the center is dark. (From Papp DF, Khanna AJ, McCarthy EF, Carrino JA, Farber AJ, Frassica FJ. Magnetic resonance imaging of soft tissue tumors: determinate and indeterminate lesions. J Bone Joint Surg Am 2007;89(suppl 3):103-115. Reprinted by permission.)

involves the large joints (e.g., the knee and hip), with the knee being affected most frequently. It presents as a nodular process or a diffuse disease involving the entire joint. This distinction determines the prognosis for surgical removal, with nodular disease being less likely to recur. If the disease is left untreated, progression to secondary arthritis may occur; therefore, surgical removal of the diseased tissue will likely improve the natural history and patient outcome.[47,48]

Conventional radiographs provide a good starting point for diagnosis, although characteristic findings are not always present. An effusion typically is seen. Over time, well-defined erosions occur with relative maintenance of the joint space. When joint space narrowing occurs, it is usually concentric. Although rare, with an incidence of approximately two per million cases, PVNS is readily identifiable on MRI because of its characteristic imaging findings.[45] MRI allows for a more thorough evaluation of the joint and disease process than does conventional radiographic imaging (**Fig. 15.12**). PVNS appears as a low signal intensity entity on both T1-weighted and T2-weighted images because of its high hemosiderin content. The mass often is nodular, with varying amounts of joint involvement and associated erosion. Gradient-echo sequences show the PVNS lesions as "blooming" from the joint capsule.[46] More recently, specific sequences, such as a "fast field" echo, show hemosiderin in a manner superior to that of the more conventional SE sequences.[49] It is important to remember, however, that if MRI is obtained early in the disease process, hemosiderin deposition may not have occurred, thus leaving the diagnosis uncertain.[47,50]

Bursitis

Patients presenting with a mass near a joint or tendon sheath should prompt the physician to consider bursitis, especially if the presentation is acute or subacute. It is important to keep in mind, however, that bursitis can also be a chronic process. Chronic bursitis and its associated growth have been reported to mimic a tumor.[51] The causes of bursitis include the following[51-53]:

- Infection
- A single traumatic event
- Repetitive trauma
- Gout
- RA

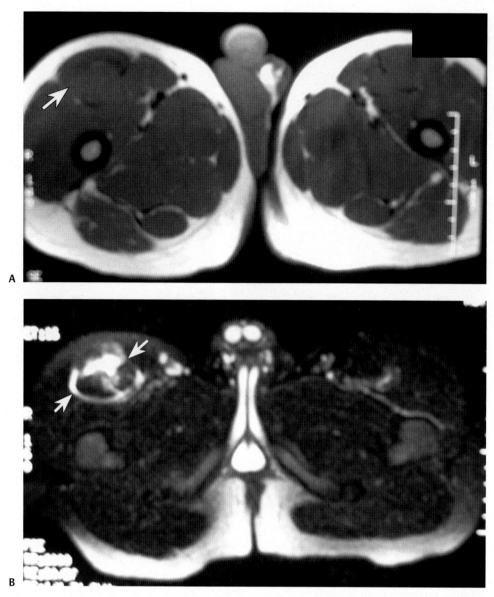

Fig. 15.11 Muscle tear. **(A)** An axial T1-weighted image of a muscle tear (*arrow*) of the right rectus femoris. The muscle belly appears expanded and asymmetric relative to the contralateral side. **(B)** An axial fat-suppressed T2-weighted image shows the surrounding edema (*arrows*).

These masses typically cause pain on palpation or motion of the involved joint or musculature, and they may or may not feel warm to the touch. Locations vary and can include almost any joint. More common locations include the prepatellar bursa and the trochanteric bursa; in such locations, advanced imaging usually does not aid in the diagnosis.

MRI can be useful in making the diagnosis of bursitis in locations other than the prepatellar and greater trochanteric regions, such as at the following[52-54]:

- Ankle
- Pes anserine insertion
- Olecranon

It is important to remember that the diagnoses of nonseptic, septic, and inflammatory bursitis share many of the same MRI findings, although septic bursitis differs in that postgadolinium images show enhancement of the infectious process.[52,53] Conventional radiographs add little to the diagnosis other than the exclusion of other conditions. T1-weighted images show a cystic structure that is isointense compared with muscle, and T2-weighted images show increased signal intensity within the lesion secondary to the fluid collection. The bursa margins enhance, as does edema, which commonly arises in surrounding tissues (**Fig. 15.13**). As stated above, it is important to note that inflammatory processes

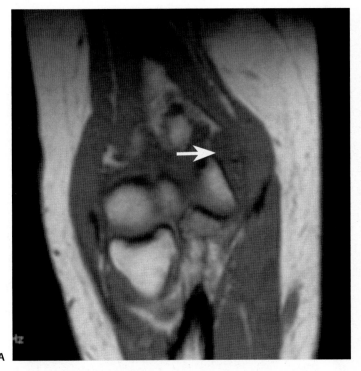 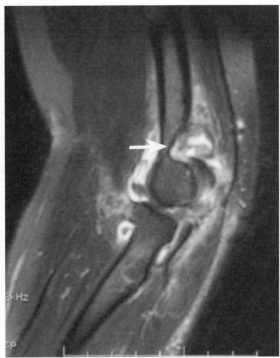

A   B

Fig. 15.12 PVNS of the right elbow. **(A)** A coronal T1-weighted image shows a lobular hypointense soft-tissue mass (*arrow*) with areas of signal dropout corresponding to hemosiderin deposition. **(B)** A sagittal STIR image shows several loci of the PVNS process (*arrow*) with high signal intensity, along with areas of signal dropout corresponding to hemosiderin deposition. (From Papp DF, Khanna AJ, McCarthy EF, Carrino JA, Farber AJ, Frassica FJ. Magnetic resonance imaging of soft tissue tumors: determinate and indeterminate lesions. J Bone Joint Surg Am 2007;89(suppl 3):103-115. Reprinted by permission.)

such as RA, gout, or infection show enhancement on postgadolinium images.[52,53,55]

Aneurysm

The formation of aneurysms in the extremities is rare, and the primary etiology is trauma. Other etiologies include the following:

- Atherosclerosis
- Mycosis
- Congenital disease
- Ehlers-Danlos syndrome

These lesions occur most commonly in the fifth or sixth decade of life and affect males more frequently than females. Extremity aneurysms are often false (pseudoaneurysms), and aneurysms below the knee occur infrequently.[56] In the lower extremity, an aneurysm occurs most frequently in the popliteal artery.[57] The location of the aneurysm dictates the symptomatology, and some reports have described the occlusion of tibial veins by the posterior tibial artery and the dysfunction of the peroneal nerve by an aneurysm of the anterior tibial artery.[58,59] In addition to compromising the function of surrounding neurovascular structures, aneurysms can present as painful or nonpainful masses; frequently, they are pulsatile. Ischemic consequences, such as claudication or even thrombosis, can occur. When these ischemic conditions are found, the evaluation should include investigation of the contralateral leg and imaging of the abdominal aorta. Up to 50% of patients with a popliteal artery aneurysm have concomitant abdominal aortic aneurysm.[60]

MRI of an aneurysm shows the diameter of the affected vessel to be at least 50% larger than that of the adjacent normal region. Mural thrombus may or may not exist in the lesion and does not enhance to the same degree with the administration of gadolinium as the vessel itself. MRI may be better suited than ultrasound for discerning the extent of thrombus, if present[60] (**Fig. 15.14**).

Indeterminate Lesions

When a diagnosis cannot be established based on the imaging features, the lesion is categorized as indeterminate. As

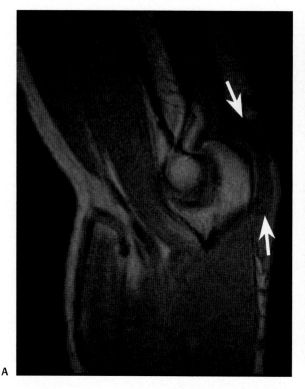
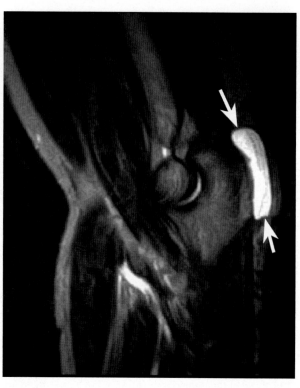

Fig. 15.13 Olecranon bursitis. **(A)** A sagittal T1-weighted image shows a hypointense lesion (*arrows*) posterior to the olecranon process, with a well-defined ovular shape. **(B)** A sagittal T2-weighted image shows the lesion (*arrows*) to be well-circumscribed and hyperintense, compatible with the fluid present in the olecranon bursa. Motion artifact is seen on the T2-weighted image.

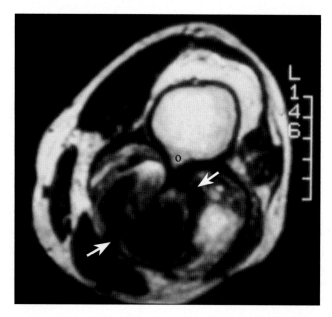

Fig. 15.14 An axial T1-weighted image of the right knee showing a pseudoaneurysm of the popliteal artery (*arrows*) with vessel dilatation of >50% of previous sections and signal dropout consistent with hemosiderin deposition. This particular lesion was associated with an osteochondroma (*O*) of the tibia.

discussed above, dialogue with a multidisciplinary team can help with diagnosis, although occasionally the MRI findings and physical examination do not provide enough information for diagnosis.[7] In this situation, the lesion must be biopsied for identification. However, excision of the lesion without previous biopsy, or excisional biopsy, should be avoided for indeterminate lesions. Although certain lesion characteristics (size >5 cm, firm mass, mass deep to the fascia, and lesion adherent to surrounding tissues) are indicative of a malignant process, such examination findings are not completely reliable in terms of reaching a diagnosis.[6] Similarly, MRI findings, such as low signal intensity on T1-weighted imaging and high signal intensity on T2, are nonspecific. The physician must investigate these types of lesions further.

Liposarcoma

Liposarcoma arises from primitive mesenchymal cells and differentiates into adipose tissue. Depending on the subtype, varying amounts of fat are found. Liposarcomas with little adipose formation are often categorized as indeterminate lesions, and their appearance is similar to that of most aggressive soft-tissue sarcomas. These types include the round-cell, dedifferentiated, and pleomorphic liposarcomas. For these lesions, MRI shows low signal on T1-weighted images and high signal on T2-weighted images. Varying degrees of necrosis or hemorrhage may exist in the lesion, as may heterogeneity.[8] One cannot diagnose these lesions with noninvasive methods; they must be biopsied.

Myxoid liposarcoma, the most common type of liposarcoma, also cannot be diagnosed definitively without a tissue sample, but its appearance on MRI differentiates it from more aggressive lesions. Myxoid liposarcoma tumors consist of a myxoid matrix of soft-tissue elements, including dedif-ferentiated lipoblasts and a plexiform formation of vessels.[61] The MRI appearance of this lesion varies, but it is typical to see scattered high-intensity centers on T1-weighted images within a low signal intensity lesion. The adipose tissue in these lesions has been described as "lacy" or amorphous in nature.[62] On T2-weighted images, these lesions often have high signal intensity, given the myxomatous nature of the lesion. In fact, differentiating these lesions from cystic masses can be difficult. With gadolinium, intense enhancement commonly occurs, which can help differentiate this lesion from others (**Fig. 15.15**).[8,62]

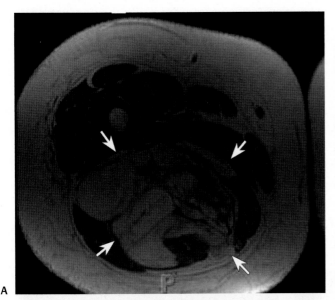

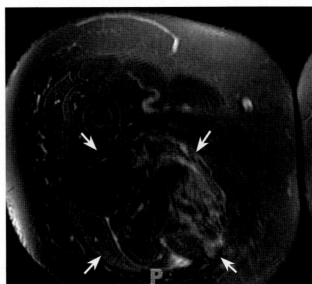

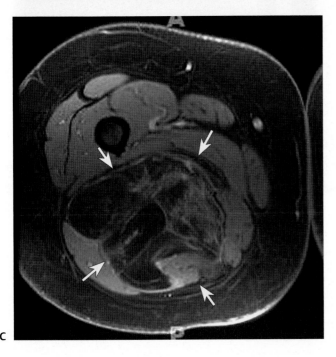

Fig. 15.15 Liposarcoma. **(A)** An axial T1-weighted image shows a large soft-tissue mass (*arrows*) with septations and heterogeneity in the posterior aspect of the right thigh. Much of the lesion appears bright, corresponding to fat, although other nonadipose tissues are clearly visible. **(B)** An axial T2-weighted image shows areas of increased intensity compatible with edema. **(C)** An axial fat-suppressed, postgadolinium, T1-weighted image shows enhancement of the lesion (*arrows*). This lesion was an indeterminate soft-tissue tumor, and the diagnosis of liposarcoma was made after biopsy. (*P*, posterior; *A*, anterior)

Synovial Sarcoma

Despite its name, synovial sarcoma is a malignant transformation of primitive mesenchymal, not synovial, cells. It typically involves periarticular regions, tendon sheaths, bursae, and fascial structures, most commonly around the knee. This tumor has a predilection for young adults and adolescents, although occurrences in infants and the elderly also have been reported.[63] There are approximately 800 cases per year in the United States.[63] Grossly, the tumor is usually well circumscribed with a heterogeneous appearance. Cystic, solid, and hemorrhagic components may be present. Histologically, the tumor resembles developing synovial tissue with large polygonal, epithelioid cells that secrete hyaluronic acid. Depending on the dominant cell type, the patient's sarcoma can be differentiated as a monophasic or biphasic type. Monophasic synovial sarcomas typically consist of spindle cells resembling fibrosarcoma, although monophasic epithelioid synovial sarcomas do occur. The lesion also may be calcified; one third of all lesions are visible radiographically.[64,65] Radiographs also may show pressure-related deformity and bone resorption, disuse osteopenia, or gross tumoral infiltration.[64,66] The MRI appearance is indeterminate. The mass most typically has a centripetal pattern of growth and shows as low intensity to isointense signal on T1-weighted images and as high signal intensity

on T2-weighted images (**Fig. 15.16**). Postgadolinium images show enhancement within the lesion, unlike that with cystic entities.[64,66]

For a diagnosis of synovial sarcoma, a tissue sample must be obtained. Immunohistochemistry is helpful in the diagnosis of synovial sarcoma because tumors show reactivity for markers such as cytokeratin (an antigen found in epithelial cells), vimentin (mesenchymal intermediate filament), epithelial membrane antigen, and cell adhesion molecules.[63] Moreover, the specific chromosomal abnormality in synovial sarcoma has been elucidated and the (X; 18)(p11.2; q11.2) translocation is uniquely present. A polymerase, chain-reaction-based diagnostic assay for this translocation has been reported to be useful in differentiating synovial sarcoma from other similar lesions, such as the following[67]:

- Spindle-cell sarcomas
- Round-cell sarcomas
- Myoepitheliomas
- Epithelioid fibrosarcomas

Although diagnosis of synovial sarcoma is accomplished most often with clinical, histologic, and immunologic markers, molecular testing for the chromosomal translocation can be valuable considering the rarity of the lesion.[63,67]

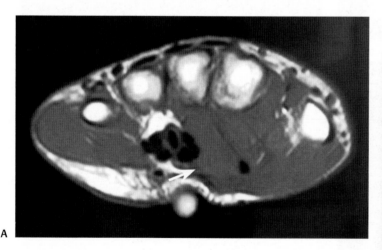

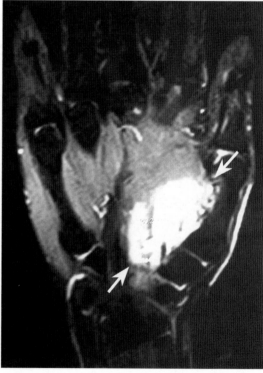

Fig. 15.16 Synovial sarcoma. **(A)** An axial T1-weighted image shows ulnar deviation of the flexor tendons by a mass (*arrow*) that appears isointense compared with muscle. A fiduciary marker was placed at the skin surface to help locate the potential mass. **(B)** A coronal T2-weighted image shows high signal intensity within the lesion (*arrows*). The signal pattern of hypointensity on T1-weighted images and hyperintensity on T2-weighted images is compatible with an indeterminate lesion; the diagnosis was made with biopsy.

MFH

MFH arises from soft tissue and from bone, although soft-tissue origination occurs more commonly. Males are at a slightly higher risk than females, and the peak prevalence is in the fourth or fifth decade of life.[68,69] It is the most common soft-tissue sarcoma in adults, accounting for approximately 20% to 30% of sarcomas.[68] With bone lesions, MFH makes up 5% of all malignancies.[68,69] In the soft tissues, MFH presents with visible swelling and an associated soft-tissue mass. This malignant lesion also can develop secondary to dedifferentiation from benign osseous lesions (such as Paget disease, bone infarcts, enchondromas, and giant cell tumor) or from previously irradiated areas.[70,71] Histologically, MFH shows a pleomorphic or storiform pattern with scattered giant cells.

Conventional radiographs show a destructive, aggressive lesion with diffuse cortical involvement when the bone is involved.[68] Approximately one in five patients presents with a pathologic fracture.[72] MRI does little to elucidate the diagnosis for this lesion, but it can show features common to indeterminate malignant lesions. The lesion has a low to isointense signal compared with muscle on T1-weighted images and has high signal intensity on T2-weighted images. Heterogeneity is often seen, corresponding to areas of hemorrhage (and regions of high signal intensity on T1-weighted images).[68,69] MRI does not allow for definitive diagnosis of osseous lesions because MFH mimics other malignancies, but MRI does allow for preoperative planning by showing the extent of the disease and important adjacent neurovascular structures. MFH is a high-grade sarcoma in bone and soft tissue and has a >50% risk of metastasis.[68]

Epithelioid Sarcoma

This rare sarcoma presents most often in the upper extremity (especially in the hand) in young adults, but it can be found anywhere in the body, including the following:

- Lower extremities
- Trunk
- Head/neck
- Penis

Because these tumors are found in superficial and deep locations, it is important to avoid incorrectly identifying a lesion close to the skin as being benign. Intraarticular processes have also been described.[73,74] The tumor most commonly presents in the subcutaneous tissues and has a nodular growth pattern along the aponeuroses, tendon sheaths, and fascia. As for most malignant processes, predictors of outcome include the following:

- Size
- Recurrence
- Metastasis
- Age at diagnosis
- Stage
- Vascular invasion

Males are affected more commonly than females and have a worse prognosis.[73,75] Histologically, the tumor has random nests of epithelioid cells that stain immunohistologically for epithelial membrane antigen and cytokeratins.

A nodular growth pattern is seen on MRI. The lesion is hypointense or isointense compared with muscle on T1-weighted images and has high signal intensity on T2-weighted images. This lack of definitive MRI identification makes tissue biopsy required for definitive diagnosis. Wide resection is recommended; irradiation and chemotherapy are often used as adjuncts to surgery.[73]

■ Bone Tumors

The clinical presentation of bone tumors often mimics the more common causes of musculoskeletal pain, such as the following:

- Arthritis
- Tendinitis/bursitis
- Sports-related injuries

A history of pain that awakens the patient during rest must prompt concern about a potential neoplasm or malignancy. The clinical history may not always be helpful for the diagnosis of a neoplasm, but, when one is suspected, taking the patient's age into account often helps to narrow the differential diagnosis. The common malignant bone tumors in patients more than 40 years old are the following:

- Metastatic bone disease
- Multiple myeloma
- Lymphoma
- Chondrosarcoma
- MFH

In contrast, osteosarcoma and Ewing tumor are common malignant tumors in patients less than 40 years old. As always, the initial evaluation includes conventional radiographs in two planes. Technetium bone scans are excellent for evaluating for metastases and occult lesions.

MRI is likely less useful for diagnosing bone tumors than for soft-tissue lesions.[76] In many cases, conventional radiographs alone will provide the orthopaedic surgeon with enough information to establish a diagnosis; however, the increasing use of MRI in clinical practice makes knowledge of the appearance of the various bone tumors useful. In the presence of bone tumors, MRI is used primarily for staging and preoperative planning. MRI offers several advantages over other imaging modalities:

- Visualization of intratumoral necrosis or hemorrhage
- Optimal visualization of articular involvement or spread[77,78]
- Earlier visualization of periosteal reaction than with conventional radiography[79]
- Superior visualization of intramedullary involvement and soft-tissue invasion
- Periosteal reaction appearing as a high-signal region immediately adjacent to the bone

Nevertheless, it must be emphasized that diagnosis should not be based on MRI findings alone. A diagnosis should be made based on a combination of history, physical examination, all appropriate imaging modalities, and discussion with a musculoskeletal radiologist and pathologist. This section focuses on MRI of osseous lesions in the extremities.

Benign Tumors

Osteoid Osteoma

This lesion most commonly presents in young patients and is seen more commonly in males than in females.[80] Classically, this benign lesion presents with progressively worsening pain that can disappear completely with the administration of nonsteroidal antiinflammatory medications. The lesion itself is termed the nidus, and reactive intense bone formation occurs around the lesion. Although the lesion can be diagnosed with conventional radiographs or CT, MRI allows for definitive diagnosis in many cases. However, one should note that the literature describes several cases of incorrect diagnosis of more aggressive lesions based on MRI findings without other imaging modalities.[28] Ideally, one should see the nidus, which should not be >15 mm in diameter. On T1-weighted images, the nidus has low to intermediate signal intensity. T2-weighted images often show high signal intensity. Gadolinium causes enhancement of the lesion that can be better identified when combined with fat suppression techniques.[81] When an osteoid osteoma is suspected, T1-weighted imaging with gadolinium can provide superior results, showing osteoid osteoma 82% of the time on the arterial phase and with conspicuity equal to that of thin-segment CT.[28] Associated bone marrow edema, synovitis of associated joints, and associated soft-tissue involvement with increased vascularity and inflammatory cell infiltration have also been associated with osteoid osteoma. These findings may confuse the diagnosis and lead to impressions of infection or malignancy. Ultimately, T1-weighted imaging with gadolinium enhancement provides the best sensitivity for MRI-based evaluation, but correlation with conventional radiography or CT provides definitive diagnosis.

The diagnosis of osteoid osteoma highlights the fact that MRI is not always the ideal imaging modality for all lesions.

In the case of osteoid osteoma, where the lesion is often small and consists of an osseous abnormality, the excellent spatial resolution and osseous detail provided by CT makes it a better imaging modality than MRI.

Osteoblastoma

Osteoblastomas are commonly located in the spine, ankle, proximal humerus, and femur, and they can become large lesions. Males are affected more commonly than females (2:1) and the lesion tends to occur in the second and third decades of life.[43,77,82] On T1-weighted MR images, this lesion is isointense compared with muscle; on T2-weighted images, it has high signal intensity. Areas of low signal intensity also occur and likely correspond to regions of osteoid formation.[77,82] Soft tissues surrounding the lesion often show edema on T2-weighted images (see Chapter 12 for more details).

Chondroblastoma

Chondroblastomas, which occur most commonly in the first through third decades of life and which occur with a slight predominance in males, originate in the epiphysis and extend to the metaphysis in two thirds of patients.[29] The femur, tibia, and humerus are most commonly affected. As with other osseous lesions, pain and swelling are the most common clinical features, although an effusion occurs in up to 30% of cases.[29] MRI shows a lesion with low signal intensity on T1-weighted images and a heterogeneous appearance on T2-weighted images (**Fig. 15.17**). The rim of the tumor is of low signal intensity, and associated bone marrow edema is common.[29,83] A fluid–fluid level within the tumor is seen in approximately one of five cases, although it may occur in up to 50% of chondroblastomas in the foot.[29] Although chondroblastomas are often benign, these tumors have the capacity to metastasize. In addition, if not excised properly, they recur locally in approximately 2% of patients.[84]

Periosteal Chondroma

Although a rare lesion, periosteal chondroma has a characteristic appearance on conventional radiographs and MRI that can make diagnosis relatively simple without biopsy. The lesion most commonly appears in patients during the third and fourth decades of life on the metaphysis of long bones or at the insertion sites of tendons or ligaments. All lesions abut the cortex of the affected bone, with lobules of cartilage and a minimal amount of pressure erosion of the involved cortex. The periosteum appears intact on T2-weighted images. On T1-weighted images, the lesion is hypointense to isointense compared with muscle and shows a sharp demarcation. As with other cartilaginous lesions, it appears bright

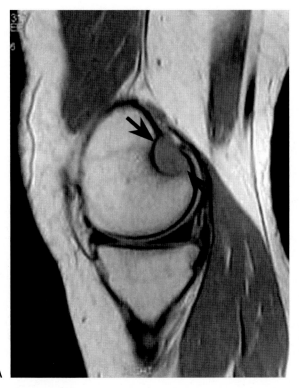

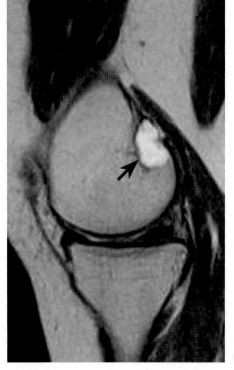

A   B

Fig. 15.17 Chondroblastoma. **(A)** A sagittal T1-weighted image shows a low signal intensity lesion (*arrows*) at the posterior aspect of the medial femoral condyle. **(B)** A sagittal T2-weighted image shows a primarily high signal intensity lesion (*arrow*) with heterogeneity and a slight lobular pattern. Conventional radiographic findings would also aid in the diagnosis of this lesion.

on T2-weighted or STIR images. If enhancement occurs with gadolinium, it commonly occurs at the periphery, where the vascular supply for the lesion is located.[76]

Enchondroma

This common benign bone lesion appears in the metaphysis of long bones, although it also often arises in the bones of the hands and feet. On conventional radiographs, the lesion appears lucent, often with characteristic rings and stipples common to cartilage lesions that have calcified; however, this lesion can appear without these findings if the cartilaginous components of the lesion have not calcified. MRI displays the cartilage better, with low signal intensity on T1-weighted images and high signal intensity on T2-weighted images and with a pattern similar to that of articular cartilage (**Fig. 15.18**). These lesions enhance with gadolinium. When diagnosed with certainty, there is no reason to biopsy them if they are asymptomatic. However, a painful lesion should be monitored with follow-up examinations because it may be a slow-growing, low-grade chondrosarcoma.[85,86]

Osteochondroma

Osteochondromas, the most common benign bone tumor, are thought to arise from a region of the growth plate that grows diagonally or perpendicularly to the surface of the bone. One study indicated that the prevalence of osteochondroma in the general population is as high as 2%.[87] Although the lesion is commonly asymptomatic, patients may complain of pain with range of motion (mechanical irritation), or they may have decreased range of motion. Neurologic or vascular sequelae rarely occur.[76,87] Conventional radiographs are often diagnostic. The lesion extends from the involved bone and is contiguous with the medullary cavity. MRI (especially T1-weighted images) has the advantage of showing the tumor's relationship with the affected bone's medullary canal. T2-weighted images show high signal intensity in the cartilage cap, secondary to the high water content (**Fig. 15.19**). Moreover, MRI can be used to assess the malignant transformation of an osteochondroma to a chondrosarcoma. If the cartilage cap exceeds 2 cm in adults and 3 cm in children, malignant transformation is considered to be more likely.[84]

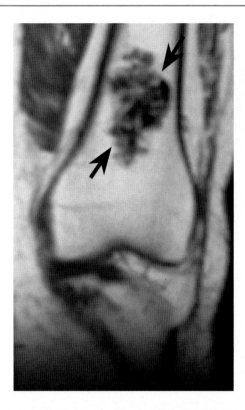

Fig. 15.18 A coronal T1-weighted image of the right knee shows a lesion in the distal femur (*arrows*) with a hypointense signal compatible with the calcification seen in enchondromas. The conventional radiographic findings also confirmed the diagnosis of enchondroma.

Giant Cell Tumor

Giant cell tumors of bone most commonly affect young adults and are found in a metaphyseal-epiphyseal location. The most common sites include the femur, tibia, and distal radius. Although benign (approximately 2% metastasize[88]), the lesion can cause destruction of affected bones. Given its predilection for the periarticular region, the subchondral bone may be specifically affected. Conventional radiographs show a poorly marginated lytic lesion with no sclerotic rim. The multiplanar images provided by MRI can be useful for detailing soft-tissue involvement. Approximately 60% of all giant cell tumors appear dark on all pulse sequences because of hemosiderin deposition.[89] The remaining 40% appear dark on T1-weighted and bright on T2-weighted images.[89] T1-weighted images show the destructive nature of the lesion best and can detail any soft-tissue extension, which is usually contained by a reactive osseous rim.[89,90]

Aneurysmal Bone Cyst

Aneurysmal bone cysts occur most commonly in young adults, and pain and swelling are the most common symp-

toms. The formation of an aneurysmal bone cyst occurs secondary to preexisting lesions in up to one third of cases and affects females more than males.[91] The primary lesions that may predispose to the development of an aneurysmal bone cyst include the following:

- Chondroblastoma
- Nonossifying fibroma
- Giant cell tumor
- Fibrous dysplasia

Other lesions can also predispose to the development of an aneurysmal bone cyst.[29,91]

Conventional radiographs show an expansile, lytic lesion that expands the cortex into the surrounding soft tissues. MRI shows a rim of low signal intensity, with multiple lobules and septations (**Fig. 15.20**). Overall, the lesion is heterogeneous, with each loculated collection having different signal characteristics. These lesions commonly show fluid–fluid levels. Telangiectatic osteosarcoma (see below), which presents in a similar fashion, shows nodularity in its septations along the rim, which correspond to nests of tumor cells. Similarly, an associated soft-tissue mass occurs in telangiectatic osteosarcoma in 89% of cases.[10,29,92]

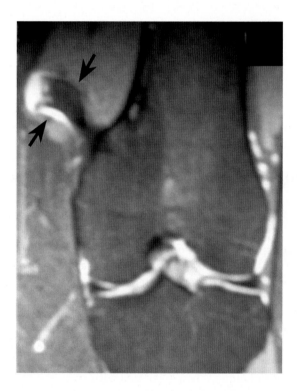

Fig. 15.19 A coronal T2-weighted image of the right knee shows an osteochondroma (*arrows*) of the distal femur. Note the continuity with the normal cortex. The cartilage cap of the lesion shows high signal intensity.

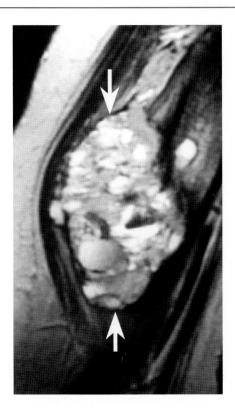

Fig. 15.20 A coronal T2-weighted image of the distal femur shows an aneurysmal bone cyst with multiple fluid–fluid levels (*arrows*). The lesion is expansile, destroying the cortex.

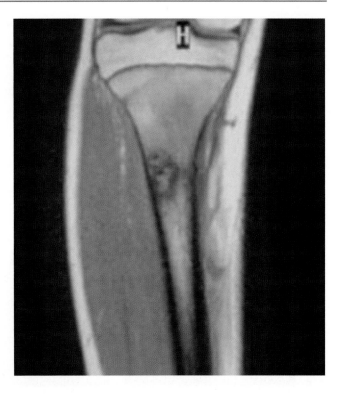

Fig. 15.21 A coronal T1-weighted image shows a metaphyseal lesion at the posterior aspect of the proximal right tibia, which is isointense compared with muscle. The conventional radiographic findings help confirm the diagnosis of nonossifying fibroma.

Nonossifying Fibroma

This cortically based lesion occurs in the metaphysis of long bones (most commonly, the femur and tibia) and slowly migrates into the diaphysis. Conventional radiographs show a sclerotic rim, with scalloped margins.[93] As with other fibrous lesions, the MRI findings can be variable and depend on the amount of fibrous tissue relative to other tissue content within the lesion, including hemorrhage, collagen, and osseous trabeculae. All nonossifying fibromas present as low signal intensity lesions on T1-weighted images (**Fig. 15.21**). Most nonossifying fibromas are hypointense compared with muscle on T2-weighted images, with clear evidence of septations.[88] However, not all lesions present in this manner, and it is important to compare the MR images with conventional radiographs. Unless these lesions cause pathologic fracture, they typically need no therapy.

Fibrous Dysplasia

Fibrous dysplasia is a developmental disorder in which there is a failure to form normal lamellar bone. It is typically asymptomatic.[29,93] One in five patients present with polyostotic disease, and in such cases fibrous dysplasia has an association with McCune-Albright syndrome and other endocrine abnormalities.[91] Conventional radiographs are often diagnostic, with lesions having a "ground glass" appearance and affected bones often showing gross deformity and narrowing of the cortex.[93] As with other sclerotic lesions, the lesion appears dark on T1-weighted images.[85] T2-weighted imaging does not always present a consistent picture: in one series, 79% of all lesions were hypointense and 21% were hyperintense compared with muscle (**Fig. 15.22**).[94] Gadolinium enhancement occurs in approximately 70% of cases.[94] Given this mixed picture on MRI, correlation with conventional radiographs is recommended.

Malignant Tumors

Osteosarcoma

Osteosarcoma, the most common primary malignant mesenchymal bone tumor, develops most frequently in young adults or adolescents. There are varying patterns of growth,

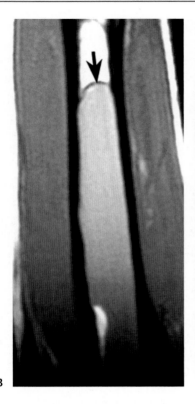 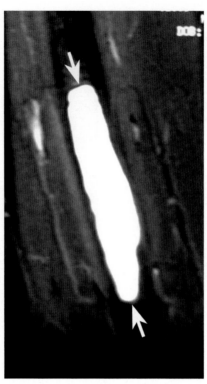

A, B

Fig. 15.22 Fibrous dysplasia. (A) A coronal T1-weighted image of the midshaft femur shows a well-circumscribed hypointense lesion (*arrow*). (B) A coronal T2-weighted image shows the same lesion (*arrows*) as hyperintense. The lack of surrounding soft-tissue edema or inflammation makes it more likely that this lesion is benign. The conventional radiographic findings help confirm the diagnosis of fibrous dysplasia.

but the trait shared by all osteosarcomas relates to the formation of osteoid by malignant cells. The general patterns (**Fig. 15.23**) seen include the following:

- Conventional osteosarcoma
- Parosteal osteosarcoma
- Periosteal osteosarcoma
- Telangiectatic osteosarcoma
- Well-differentiated intramedullary variant

The most common features of a high-grade intramedullary osteosarcoma are the following:

- Replacement of the metaphyseal bone marrow
- Cortical disruption
- Extension into the soft tissues

Much like soft-tissue sarcomas, osteosarcoma appears dark on T1-weighted images and has high signal intensity on T2-weighted or STIR images (**Fig. 15.24**). Areas of increased bone formation (bone sclerosis) appear dark on T1-weighted and T2-weighted images. Bone marrow and associated soft-tissue edema appear bright on T2-weighted and STIR images; this characteristic makes T1-weighted images better for assessing the extent of tumor burden.[85,92,95] Periosteal osteosarcomas show cortical thickening, scalloping, and extension into the soft tissue. Parosteal osteosarcomas arise directly from the cortex, which is shown well on T1-weighted

images. The high signal intensity on T2-weighted images of periosteal osteosarcomas relates to the large amount of cartilage-based tissue produced and the associated water content.[96] Telangiectatic osteosarcoma can be difficult to diagnose because this tumor mimics an aneurysmal bone cyst in its imaging appearance: multiple septations with fluid–fluid levels and heterogeneous enhancement. However, telangiectatic osteosarcoma shows the growth of nests of tumor cells along the septations, which appear on MRI as nodules along the rim septations. Also, associated soft-tissue masses occur with telangiectatic osteosarcoma in 89% of cases and do not occur with aneurysmal bone cysts.[29,92,97]

Ewing Sarcoma

This highly malignant tumor arises primarily in children in the first or, more commonly, second decade of life. Patients typically present with the following:

- Pain
- Swelling
- Other systemic symptoms (e.g., fever, fatigue, weight loss, and leukocytosis)

Ewing sarcoma commonly presents in the long bones, including the femur, humerus, tibia, and fibula, although the axial skeleton and pelvis can also be affected. Radiographs

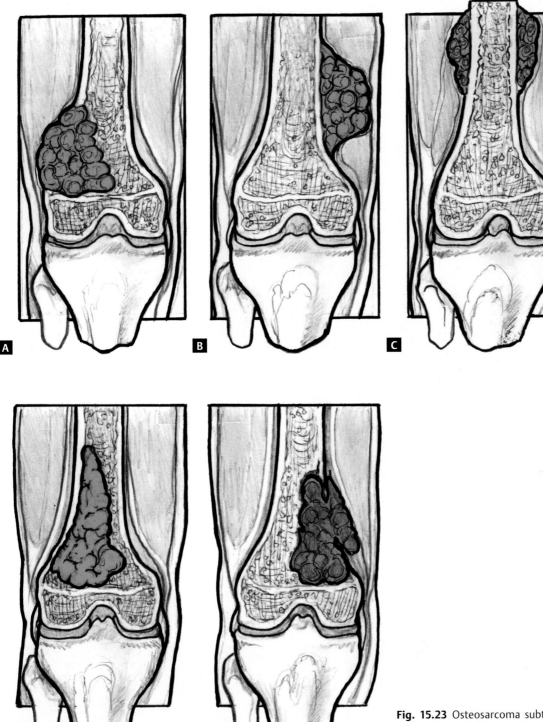

Fig. 15.23 Osteosarcoma subtypes. **(A)** Conventional. **(B)** Parosteal. **(C)** Periosteal. **(D)** Well-differentiated. **(E)** Telangiectatic.

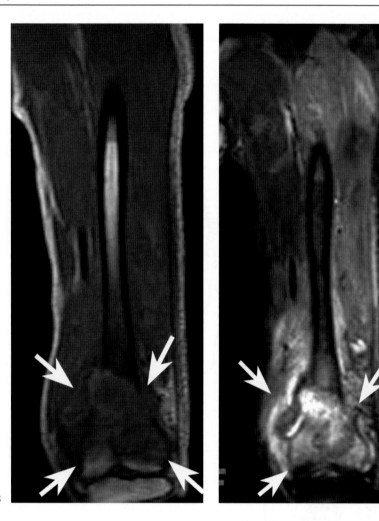

A, B

Fig. 15.24 Osteosarcoma. **(A)** A coronal T1-weighted image shows a large lesion based at the distal left femur (*arrows*) with low signal intensity and extensive cortical destruction. **(B)** A coronal STIR image of the same lesion (*arrows*) shows extensive surrounding edema in the soft tissues and the bone. Correlation with the conventional radiographs and eventual biopsy led to the definitive diagnosis of osteosarcoma.

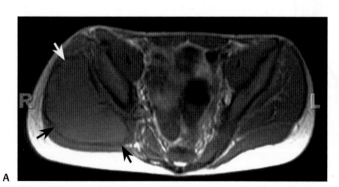

A

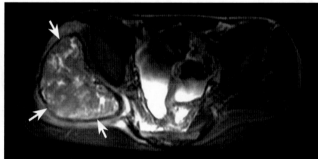

B

Fig. 15.25 Ewing sarcoma. **(A)** An axial T1-weighted image shows a large low signal intensity soft-tissue mass originating from the right gluteal muscles (*arrows*). **(B)** An axial T2-weighted image shows ex- tensive soft-tissue edema and a high signal intensity soft-tissue mass (*arrows*). The conventional radiographic findings and biopsy were conclusive for a diagnosis of Ewing sarcoma.

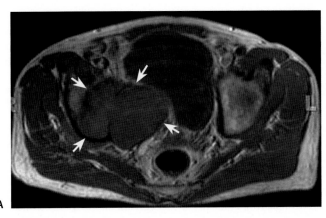
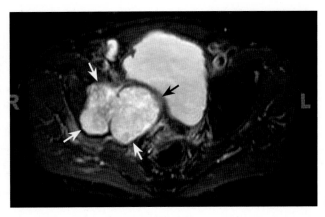

A   B

Fig. 15.26 Chondrosarcoma. **(A)** An axial T1-weighted image shows an aggressive, destructive lesion invading the right hemipelvis (*arrows*) and displacing the bladder. **(B)** An axial T2-weighted image shows a lobular pattern of growth by the chondrosarcoma (*arrows*), along with associated soft-tissue edema.

show a permeative, aggressive pattern of lytic destruction. The lesion has been described as occurring more commonly in the diaphysis.[85,92]

In most cases, an associated soft-tissue mass appears on MRI, which is seen best on T2-weighted, STIR, or contrast-enhanced T1-weighted images.[98] Bone destruction can be seen best on T1-weighted images, on which the lesion appears dark. Substantial surrounding edema can be seen on T2-weighted images and can suggest osteomyelitis (**Fig. 15.25**).[85,99]

Despite the aggressive nature of this disease, neoadjuvant chemotherapy has proved to be an effective treatment adjunct. Given that this round-cell sarcoma is very sensitive to chemotherapy, large soft-tissue masses often involute after induction chemotherapy. As with osteosarcoma, MRI can assess the effect of therapy on the lesion. With successful treatment, the lesion involutes and often has higher signal intensity on T2-weighted images, corresponding to necrosis.[85,99,100]

Chondrosarcoma

Chondrosarcoma, the second most common mesenchymal bone tumor, occurs most commonly in patients more than 40 years old. Chondrosarcoma occurs both as a primary lesion and as secondary lesion arising from other benign cartilage tumors such as enchondromas or osteochondromas. Chondrosarcomas can also occur as intramedullary and surface lesions, with growth rates varying from slow to aggressive. Radiographs show cortical destruction and the characteristic rings and stipples of cartilage calcification.

MRI assists with the evaluation of these tumors. Cartilaginous tumors, such as chondrosarcoma, have low signal intensity on T1-weighted images and high signal intensity on T2-weighted images. One can often recognize a lobular growth pattern within the cartilage, with nodules separated by fibrous tissue (**Fig. 15.26**). Dynamic MRI is a new technique in which gadolinium contrast agent is administered and serial MR images of a given region are obtained over time to visualize the enhancement pattern. This method can differentiate a low-grade chondrosarcoma from an enchondroma. The postgadolinium enhancement curve of a chondrosarcoma shows rapid enhancement and perfusion, whereas less active lesions (such as an endochondroma) show slower enhancement. As with other lesions, T1-weighted images show the anatomic detail of the lesion: cortical destruction and soft-tissue involvement. T2-weighted images show the cartilaginous nature of the lesion, as described above.[101] Treatment of these lesions includes wide resection with or without irradiation. Chondrosarcoma has proved resistant to chemotherapy and adjuvant radiation treatment.[102-104]

References

1. Weiss SW, Goldblum JR. General considerations. In: Weiss SW, Goldblum JR, eds. Enzinger and Weiss's Soft Tissue Tumors. St. Louis: Mosby; 2001:1–19

2. Yasko AW, Shreyaskumar RP, Pollack A, Pollock RE. Sarcomas of soft tissue and bone. In: Lenhard RE Jr, Osteen RT, Gansler T, eds. Clinical Oncology. Atlanta: American Cancer Society; 2001:611–631

3. Hanna SL, Fletcher BD. MR imaging of malignant soft-tissue tumors. Magn Reson Imaging Clin N Am 1995;3:629–650

4. Woertler K. Soft tissue masses in the foot and ankle: characteristics on MR Imaging. Semin Musculoskelet Radiol 2005;9:227–242

5. Hussein R, Smith MA. Soft tissue sarcomas: are current referral guidelines sufficient? Ann R Coll Surg Engl 2005;87:171–173

6. Sim FH, Frassica FJ, Frassica DA. Soft-tissue tumors: diagnosis, evaluation, and management. J Am Acad Orthop Surg 1994;2:202–211

7. Frassica FJ, Khanna JA, McCarthy EF. The role of MR imaging in soft tissue tumor evaluation: perspective of the orthopedic oncologist

and musculoskeletal pathologist. Magn Reson Imaging Clin N Am 2000;8:915–927

8. Drevelegas A, Pilavaki M, Chourmouzi D. Lipomatous tumors of soft tissue: MR appearance with histological correlation. Eur J Radiol 2004;50:257–267

9. Bauland CG, van Steensel MAM, Steijlen PM, Rieu PNMA, Spauwen PHM. The pathogenesis of hemangiomas: a review. Plast Reconstr Surg 2006;117:29e–35e

10. Murphey MD, Fairbairn KJ, Parman LM, Baxter KG, Parsa MB, Smith WS. From the archives of the AFIP. Musculoskeletal angiomatous lesions: radiologic-pathologic correlation. Radiographics 1995;15:893–917

11. Olsen KI, Stacy GS, Montag A. Soft-tissue cavernous hemangioma. Radiographics 2004;24:849–854

12. Frassica FJ, Thompson RC Jr. Evaluation, diagnosis, and classification of benign soft tissue tumors (Instructional Course Lectures, the American Academy of Orthopaedic Surgeons). J Bone Joint Surg Am 1996;78:126–140

13. Ostlere S, Graham R. Imaging of soft tissue masses. Imaging 2005;17:268–284

14. Feldman F, Johnston A. Intraosseous ganglion. Am J Roentgenol Radium Ther Nucl Med 1973;118:328–343

15. McCarthy CL, McNally EG. The MRI appearance of cystic lesions around the knee. Skeletal Radiol 2004;33:187–209

16. Bui-Mansfield LT, Youngberg RA. Intraarticular ganglia of the knee: prevalence, presentation, etiology, and management. AJR Am J Roentgenol 1997;168:123–127

17. Yilmaz E, Karakurt L, Ozercan I, Ozdemir H. A ganglion cyst that developed from the infrapatellar fat pad of the knee. Arthroscopy 2004;20:e65–e68

18. Tang P, Hornicek FJ, Gebhardt MC, Cates J, Mankin HJ. Surgical treatment of hemangiomas of soft tissue. Clin Orthop Relat Res 2002;399:205–210

19. Wahrman JE, Honig PJ. Hemangiomas. Pediatr Rev 1994;15:266–271

20. Baker WM. On the formation of the synovial cysts in the leg in connection with disease of the knee joint. St Bartholomew Hosp Rep. 1877;13:245–261

21. Fritschy D, Fasel J, Imbert JC, Bianchi S, Verdonk R, Wirth CJ. The popliteal cyst. Knee Surg Sports Traumatol Arthrosc 2006;14: 623–628

22. Zhang WW, Lukan JK, Dryjski ML. Nonoperative management of lower extremity claudication caused by a Baker's cyst: case report and review of the literature. Vascular 2005;13:244–247

23. Miller TT, Staron RB, Koenigsberg T, Levin TL, Feldman F. MR imaging of Baker cysts: association with internal derangement, effusion, and degenerative arthropathy. Radiology 1996;201:247–250

24. Sansone V, De Ponti A. Arthroscopic treatment of popliteal cyst and associated intra-articular knee disorders in adults. Arthroscopy 1999;15:368–372

25. Kornaat PR, Bloem JL, Ceulemans RYT, et al. Osteoarthritis of the knee: association between clinical features and MR imaging findings. Radiology 2006;239:811–817

26. Reid JD, Kommareddi S, Lankerani M, Park MC. Chronic expanding hematomas. A clinicopathologic entity. JAMA 1980;244:2441–2442

27. Aoki T, Nakata H, Watanabe H, et al. The radiological findings in chronic expanding hematoma. Skeletal Radiol 1999;28:396–401

28. Liu PT, Leslie KO, Beauchamp CP, Cherian SF. Chronic expanding hematoma of the thigh simulating neoplasm on gadolinium-enhanced MRI. Skeletal Radiol 2006;35:254–257

29. Keenan S, Bui-Mansfield LT. Musculoskeletal lesions with fluid-fluid level: a pictorial essay. J Comput Assist Tomogr 2006;30:517–524

30. Imaizumi S, Morita T, Ogose A, et al. Soft tissue sarcoma mimicking chronic hematoma: value of magnetic resonance imaging in differential diagnosis. J Orthop Sci 2002;7:33–37

31. Hait G, Boswick JA Jr, Stone NH. Heterotopic bone formation secondary to trauma (myositis ossificans traumatica). J Trauma 1970;10:405–411

32. Parikh J, Hyare H, Saifuddin A. The imaging features of posttraumatic myositis ossificans, with emphasis on MRI. Clin Radiol 2002;57:1058–1066

33. Beiner JM, Jokl P. Muscle contusion injury and myositis ossificans traumatica. Clin Orthop Relat Res 2002; 403(suppl):S110–S119

34. Khoury NJ, El-Khoury GY, Kathol MH. MRI diagnosis of diabetic muscle infarction: report of two cases. Skeletal Radiol 1997;26:122–127

35. Bunch TJ, Birskovich LM, Eiken PW. Diabetic myonecrosis in a previously healthy woman and review of a 25-year Mayo Clinic experience. Endocr Pract 2002;8:343–346

36. Kattapuram TM, Suri R, Rosol MS, Rosenberg AE, Kattapuram SV. Idiopathic and diabetic skeletal muscle necrosis: evaluation by magnetic resonance imaging. Skeletal Radiol 2005;34:203–209

37. Bjornskov EK, Carry MR, Katz FH, Lefkowitz J, Ringel SP. Diabetic muscle infarction: a new perspective on pathogenesis and management. Neuromuscul Disord 1995;5:39–45

38. Keller DR, Erpelding M, Grist T. Diabetic muscular infarction. Preventing morbidity by avoiding excisional biopsy. Arch Intern Med 1997;157:1611–1612

39. Jelinek JS, Murphey MD, Aboulafia AJ, Dussault RG, Kaplan PA, Snearly WN. Muscle infarction in patients with diabetes mellitus: MR imaging findings. Radiology 1999;211:241–247

40. Theos A, Korf BR. Pathophysiology of neurofibromatosis type 1. Ann Intern Med 2006;144:842–849

41. Kostelic JK, Haughton VM, Sether LA. Lumbar spinal nerves in the neural foramen: MR appearance. Radiology 1991;178:837–839

42. Lim R, Jaramillo D, Poussaint TY, Chang Y, Korf B. Superficial neurofibroma: a lesion with unique MRI characteristics in patients with neurofibromatosis type 1. AJR Am J Roentgenol 2005;184:962–968

43. Temple HT, Mizel MS, Murphey MD, Sweet DE. Osteoblastoma of the foot and ankle. Foot Ankle Int 1998;19:698–704

44. Peterson L, Stener B. Old total rupture of the adductor longus muscle. A report of seven cases. Acta Orthop Scand 1976;47:653–657

45. Rubin SJ, Feldman F, Staron RB, Zwass A, Totterman S, Meyers SP. Magnetic resonance imaging of muscle injury. Clin Imaging 1995;19:263–269

46. Al-Nakshabandi NA, Ryan AG, Choudur H, et al. Pigmented villonodular synovitis. Clin Radiol 2004;59:414–420

47. Tyler WK, Vidal AF, Williams RJ, Healey JH. Pigmented villonodular synovitis. J Am Acad Orthop Surg 2006;14:376–385

48. Stubbs AJ, Higgins LD. Pigmented villonodular synovitis of the knee: disease of the popliteus tendon and posterolateral compartment. Arthroscopy 2005;21:893.e1–893.e5

49. Cheng XG, You YH, Liu W, Zhao T, Qu H. MRI features of pigmented villonodular synovitis (PVNS). Clin Rheumatol 2004;23:31–34

50. Bouali H, Deppert EJ, Leventhal LJ, Reeves B, Pope T. Pigmented villonodular synovitis: a disease in evolution. J Rheumatol 2004;31: 1659–1662

51. García-Porrúa C, González-Gay MA, Vázquez-Caruncho M. Tophaceous gout mimicking tumoral growth. J Rheumatol 1999;26:508–509

52. Floemer F, Morrison WB, Bongartz G, Ledermann HP. MRI characteristics of olecranon bursitis. AJR Am J Roentgenol 2004;183: 29–34

53. Mutlu H, Sildiroglu H, Pekkafali Z, Kizilkaya E, Cermik H. MRI appearance of retrocalcaneal bursitis and rheumatoid nodule in a patient with rheumatoid arthritis. Clin Rheumatol 2006;25:734–736

54. Rennie WJ, Saifuddin A. Pes anserine bursitis: incidence in symptomatic knees and clinical presentation. Skeletal Radiol 2005;34: 395–398

55. Dawn B, Williams JK, Walker SE. Prepatellar bursitis: a unique presentation of tophaceous gout in an normouricemic patient. J Rheumatol 1997;24:976–978

56. Kato T, Takagi H, Sekino S, et al. Dorsalis pedis artery true aneurysm due to atherosclerosis: case report and literature review. J Vasc Surg 2004;40:1044–1048

57. Tatli S, Lipton MJ, Davison BD, Skorstad RB, Yucel EK. From the RSNA refresher courses: MR imaging of aortic and peripheral vascular disease. Radiographics 2003;23:S59–S78

58. Kars HZ, Topaktas S, Dogan K. Aneurysmal peroneal nerve compression. Neurosurgery 1992;30:930–931

59. Katz SG, Kohl RD, Razack N. Bilateral infrapopliteal artery aneurysms. Ann Vasc Surg 1992;6:168–170

60. Wright LB, Matchett WJ, Cruz CP, et al. Popliteal artery disease: diagnosis and treatment. Radiographics 2004;24:467–479

61. Weiss SW, Goldblum JR. Liposarcoma. In: Weiss SW, Goldblum JR, eds. Enzinger and Weiss's Soft Tissue Tumors. St. Louis: Mosby; 2001:641–693

62. Sung MS, Kang HS, Suh JS, et al. Myxoid liposarcoma: appearance at MR imaging with histologic correlation. Radiographics 2000;20:1007–1019

63. Spillane AJ, A'Hern R, Judson IR, Fisher C, Thomas JM. Synovial sarcoma: a clinicopathologic, staging, and prognostic assessment. J Clin Oncol 2000;18:3794–3803

64. Olsen KM, Chew FS. Tumoral calcinosis: pearls, polemics, and alternative possibilities. Radiographics 2006;26:871–885

65. Cadman NL, Soule EH, Kelly PJ. Synovial sarcoma: an analysis of 134 tumors. Cancer 1965;18:613–627

66. Abboud JA, Beredjiklian PK, Donthineni-Rao R. Forearm mass in an adolescent. Clin Orthop Relat Res 2004;428:302–307

67. Coindre JM, Pelmus M, Hostein I, Lussan C, Bui BN, Guillou L. Should molecular testing be required for diagnosing synovial sarcoma? A prospective study of 204 cases. Cancer 2003;98:2700–2707

68. Link TM, Haeussler MD, Poppek S, et al. Malignant fibrous histiocytoma of bone: conventional X-ray and MR imaging features. Skeletal Radiol 1998;27:552–558

69. Munk PL, Sallomi DF, Janzen DL, et al. Malignant fibrous histiocytoma of soft tissue imaging with emphasis on MRI. J Comput Assist Tomogr 1998;22:819–826

70. Grote HJ, Braun M, Kalinski T, et al. Spontaneous malignant transformation of conventional giant cell tumor. Skeletal Radiol 2004;33:169–175

71. Sheppard DG, Libshitz HI. Post-radiation sarcomas: a review of the clinical and imaging features in 63 cases. Clin Radiol 2001;56: 22–29

72. Capanna R, Bertoni F, Bacchini P, Bacci G, Guerra A, Campanacci M. Malignant fibrous histiocytoma of bone. The experience at the Rizzoli Institute: report of 90 cases. Cancer 1984;54:177–187

73. Herr MJ, Harmsen WS, Amadio PC, Scully SP. Epithelioid sarcoma of the hand. Clin Orthop Relat Res 2005;431:193–200

74. Hurtado RM, McCarthy E, Frassica F, Holt PA. Intraarticular epithelioid sarcoma. Skeletal Radiol 1998;27:453–456

75. Chase DR, Enzinger FM. Epithelioid sarcoma. Diagnosis, prognostic indicators, and treatment. Am J Surg Pathol 1985;9:241–263

76. Woertler K, Blasius S, Brinkschmidt C, Hillmann A, Link TM, Heindel W. Periosteal chondroma: MR characteristics. J Comput Assist Tomogr 2001;25:425–430

77. Nomikos GC, Murphey MD, Kransdorf MJ, Bancroft LW, Peterson JJ. Primary bone tumors of the lower extremities. Radiol Clin North Am 2002;40:971–990

78. Pettersson H, Gillespy T III, Hamlin DJ, et al. Primary musculoskeletal tumors: examination with MR imaging compared with conventional modalities. Radiology 1987;164:237–241

79. Wenaden AET, Szyszko TA, Saifuddin A. Imaging of periosteal reactions associated with focal lesions of bone. Clin Radiol 2005;60: 439–456

80. Hosalkar HS, Garg S, Moroz L, Pollack A, Dormans JP. The diagnostic accuracy of MRI versus CT imaging for osteoid osteoma in children. Clin Orthop Relat Res 2005;433:171–177

81. Gaeta M, Minutoli F, Pandolfo I, Vinci S, D'Andrea L, Blandino A. Magnetic resonance imaging findings of osteoid osteoma of the proximal femur. Eur Radiol 2004;14:1582–1589

82. Nakatani T, Yamamoto T, Akisue T, et al. Periosteal osteoblastoma of the distal femur. Skeletal Radiol 2004;33:107–111

83. Oxtoby JW, Davies AM. MRI characteristics of chondroblastoma. Clin Radiol 1996;51:22–26

84. Lin PP, Thenappan A, Deavers MT, Lewis VO, Yasko AW. Treatment and prognosis of chondroblastoma. Clin Orthop Relat Res 2005;438:103–109

85. Miller SL, Hoffer FA. Malignant and benign bone tumors. Radiol Clin North Am 2001;39:673–699

86. Woertler K. Benign bone tumors and tumor-like lesions: value of cross-sectional imaging. Eur Radiol 2003;13:1820–1835

87. Antonio ZP, Alejandro RM, Luis MRJ, José GR. Femur ostochondroma and secondary pseudoaneurysm of the popliteal artery. Arch Orthop Trauma Surg 2006;126:127–130

88. Jee WH, Choi KH, Choe BY, Park JM, Shinn KS. Fibrous dysplasia: MR imaging characteristics with radiopathologic correlation. AJR Am J Roentgenol 1996;167:1523–1527

89. James SLJ, Davies AM. Giant-cell tumours of bone of the hand and wrist: a review of imaging findings and differential diagnoses. Eur Radiol 2005;15:1855–1866

90. Vidyadhara S, Rao SK. Techniques in the management of juxta-articular aggressive and recurrent giant cell tumors around the knee. Eur J Surg Oncol 2007;33:243–251

91. Mendenhall WM, Zlotecki RA, Gibbs CP, Reith JD, Scarborough MT, Mendenhall NP. Aneurysmal bone cyst. Am J Clin Oncol 2006;29:311–315

92. Hoffer FA. Primary skeletal neoplasms: osteosarcoma and Ewing sarcoma. Top Magn Reson Imaging 2002;13:231–239

93. McCarthy EF, Frassica FJ. Pathology of Bone and Joint Disorders: With Clinical and Radiographic Correlation. Philadelphia: WB Saunders; 1998

94. Jee WH, Choe BY, Kang HS, et al. Nonossifying fibroma: characteristics at MR imaging with pathologic correlation. Radiology 1998;209:197–202

95. Onikul E, Fletcher BD, Parham DM, Chen G. Accuracy of MR imaging for estimating intraosseous extent of osteosarcoma. AJR Am J Roentgenol 1996;167:1211–1215

96. Murphey MD, Jelinek JS, Temple HT, Flemming DJ, Gannon FH. Imaging of periosteal osteosarcoma: radiologic-pathologic comparison. Radiology 2004;233:129–138

97. Murphey MD, wan Jaovisidha S, Temple HT, Gannon FH, Jelinek JS, Malawer MM. Telangiectatic osteosarcoma: radiologic-pathologic comparison. Radiology 2003;229:545–553

98. van der Woude HJ, Bloem JL, Hogendoorn PCW. Preoperative evaluation and monitoring chemotherapy in patients with high-grade osteogenic and Ewing's sarcoma: review of current imaging modalities. Skeletal Radiol 1998;27:57–71

99. Grier HE. The Ewing family of tumors. Ewing's sarcoma and primitive neuroectodermal tumors. Pediatr Clin North Am 1997;44:991–1004

100. Kauffman WM, Fletcher BD, Hanna SL, Meyer WH. MR imaging findings in recurrent primary osseous Ewing sarcoma. Magn Reson Imaging 1994;12:1147–1153

101. Verstraete KL, Lang P. Bone and soft tissue tumors: the role of contrast agents for MR imaging. Eur J Radiol 2000;34:229–246

102. Lee FY, Mankin HJ, Fondren G, et al. Chondrosarcoma of bone: an assessment of outcome. J Bone Joint Surg Am 1999;81:326–338

103. Rizzo M, Ghert MA, Harrelson JM, Scully SP. Chondrosarcoma of bone: analysis of 108 cases and evaluation for predictors of outcome. Clin Orthop Relat Res 2001;391:224–233

104. Terek RM. Recent advances in the basic science of chondrosarcoma. Orthop Clin North Am 2006;37:9–14

16 Advanced Techniques in Musculoskeletal MRI

Douglas E. Ramsey, Rick W. Obray, Priya D. Prabhakar, and John A. Carrino

Imaging of the musculoskeletal system typically begins with radiographs, CT, or conventional MRI. Several advanced MRI techniques have proven useful for the evaluation of subtle and complex pathology, such as early manifestations of disease, preoperative planning, and postoperative analysis. In addition, advanced MRI techniques may be helpful in narrowing a differential diagnosis, addressing a specific clinical question, or evaluating a finding detected on another imaging study. This chapter addresses techniques in musculoskeletal MRI that are increasingly used to assist clinical problem-solving.

■ MR Arthrography

Although conventional MRI often detects complex joint pathology with high sensitivity, MR arthrography is useful for the depiction of intraarticular structures that may be subtle or incompletely seen on a routine study. MR arthrography is especially useful for postoperative patients and for the evaluation of suspected ligamentous, cartilaginous, or labral injury. Arthrography relies on distention or enhancement of the joint with contrast medium to separate or enhance structures effectively, thereby defining joint pathology with increased clarity.[1] Direct and indirect methods of MR arthrography are commonly used.

Direct Arthrography

This technique is a sterile, minimally invasive procedure in which dilute gadolinium or saline is directly injected into the joint of interest under fluoroscopic guidance, followed by immediate MRI. Although gadolinium-based contrast agents have not been approved by the FDA for intraarticular injection, they are commonly used clinically under the doctrine of the practice of medicine. The optimal gadolinium concentration for adequate signal intensity is 2 mmol/L, which is achieved by dilution with normal saline; this solution then is combined with iodinated contrast material and 1% lidocaine before joint injection.[2] The total amount of dilute gadolinium injected varies by joint and patient size (**Table 16.1**).[3] To prevent suboptimal joint distention and additional dilution of gadolinium, imaging of the joint should be performed no later than 30 minutes after injection.

Although conventional MRI is often useful, direct arthrography offers improved sensitivity for the detection of many OCDs and other ligamentous, articular, and synovial defects. In the shoulder, partial-thickness rotator cuff tears are seen more clearly when there is filling of focal cuff defects with gadolinium solution. Anatomic variants of the shoulder that may otherwise be mistaken for pathology are often better defined with arthrography. Labral tears of the glenoid and hip are sometimes difficult to differentiate from normal anatomic structures (**Fig. 16.1**) and may be more clearly seen when contrast extends into the labral substance (**Fig. 16.2**). Recurrent or residual meniscal tears in the knee may be seen more clearly with arthrography because a normal postoperative meniscus has an abnormal configuration that may exhibit abnormal signal.[4] Arthrography offers additional detail in the evaluation of injury to the lateral ligaments of the ankle, especially the calcaneofibular ligament. Partial undersurface tears of the UCL and RCL in the elbow may not be clearly seen without arthrography (**Fig. 16.3**). TFCC and intrinsic intercarpal ligamentous abnormalities may be more conspicuous with MR arthrography. Direct arthrography is particularly useful for the detection of intraarticular loose bodies and OCDs.

Indirect Arthrography

This technique requires the uptake of intravenous gadolinium by highly vascular synovial membranes, which diffuses

Table 16.1 Recommended Volume of Dilute Contrast per Joint for Direct MR Arthrography

Joint	Minimum to Maximum Volume to Inject (mL)
Shoulder	10 to 20
Elbow	9 to 10
Wrist	3 to 6
Hip	8 to 20
Knee	20 to 40
Ankle	8 to 15

Source: Adapted from Sahin G, Demirtas M. An overview of MR arthrography with emphasis on the current technique and applicational hints and tips. Eur J Radiol 2006;58:416–430. Adapted by permission.

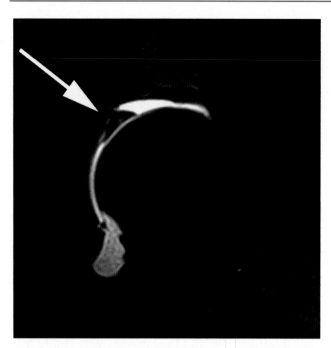

Fig. 16.1 This coronal oblique fat-suppressed T1-weighted image of a SLAP lesion in the left shoulder was obtained after the intraarticular injection of a dilute gadolinium solution posterior to the biceps attachment to the glenoid. This direct MR arthrogram shows an irregular collection of contrast material (*arrow*) extending into the superior labrum with partial detachment.

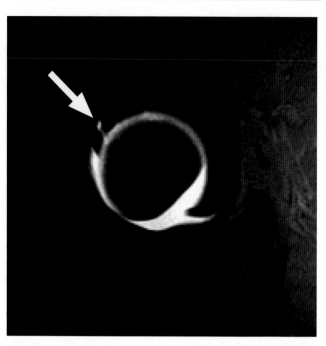

Fig. 16.2 This sagittal fat-suppressed T1-weighted image of the hip obtained after the intraarticular injection of a dilute gadolinium solution (direct MR arthrography) depicts contrast material through the anterior labral substance (*arrow*), reflecting a tear. Overall, the labrum maintains its triangular shape.

into existing joint fluid, creating the "arthrographic effect." The main benefit of this method is that intraarticular structures may be visualized without percutaneous access to a joint, which may be traumatic, time-consuming, or logistically difficult. Once gadolinium (0.1 mmol/kg) is injected intravenously, the patient must gently exercise the joint in question for approximately 10 to 15 minutes to increase vascular perfusion and joint pressure, improving the gadolinium's diffusion. Imaging is performed 5 to 30 minutes after contrast injection, depending on the joint.

The success of indirect arthrography is limited for noninflamed joints because noninflamed synovium does not enhance well. Additionally, indirect enhancement may not be helpful for large joints that require a greater amount of distention or for patients with tense joint effusions. Indirect arthrography is therefore best suited for smaller joints. Subtle cartilage defects, loose bodies, and hyperemic tendons and sheaths in the wrist, elbow, ankle, and knee may also be seen more clearly with contrast compared with conventional MRI techniques (**Fig. 16.4**). For example, recurrent tears in a postoperative knee may exhibit synovial hyperemia with joint fluid infiltrating a tear. Unfortunately, many normal and postoperative structures enhance with gadolinium, so enhancement does not necessarily reflect an abnormality. Indirect arthrography offers a better depiction of extraarticular osseous and soft-tissue abnormalities than does direct arthrography.[5]

■ Magnets and Imaging Equipment

3.0-T Magnets

High field strength MRI systems are becoming widely available in the clinical setting, typically with magnetic field strengths of 3.0 T. The higher intrinsic signal-to-noise ratio of high field strength MRI can be used to improve imaging speed or resolution, but there are changes in relaxation time at 3.0 T and increased artifacts to consider. Nevertheless, 3.0-T MRI offers the opportunity to explore physiologic imaging of joints and anatomy with greater definition.

Intrinsic signal-to-noise ratio is a function of the strength of the magnetic field, the volume of the tissue being imaged, and the RF coils used. All else being equal, 3.0 T should provide twice the intrinsic signal-to-noise ratio of 1.5 T, but this goal is not achieved clinically for several reasons. The FDA and manufacturers have mandated the use of power-monitoring systems for 3.0-T MRI systems because of the increased risk of RF burns. The more problematic sequences are FSE/turbospin and short TR SE (T1-weighted) sequences. Because motion, chemical shift, and susceptibility artifacts from metallic implants are increased at 3.0 T, postoperative imaging may be more problematic at higher field strengths.

Imaging speed is improved with higher field strength; therefore, it is theoretically possible to acquire images up

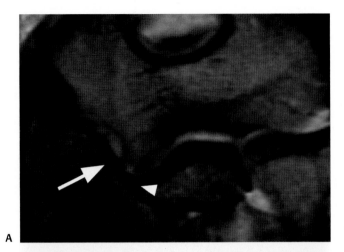

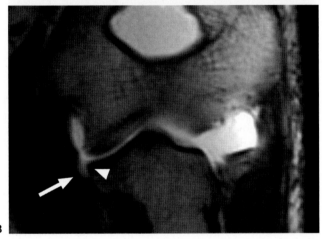

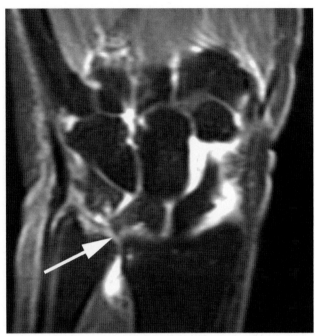

Fig. 16.4 This T1-weighted coronal oblique image of the wrist (indirect MR arthrography) shows multicompartment enhancement of the carpus and distal radioulnar joint. Findings of ulnocarpal abutment with a TFCC tear (*arrow*) are present.

Fig. 16.3 Direct MR arthrography of the elbow. The T1-weighted coronal oblique (prescribed as a plane bisecting the humeral condyles) images obtained after the intraarticular injection of a dilute gadolinium solution show **(A)** the normal intact anterior bundle of the UCL (*arrow*), which is firmly affixed to the medial margin of the ulna (*arrowhead*), and **(B)** a partial articular surface tear as detachment (*arrow*) of the deep portion of the distal anterior bundle of the UCL from the medial margin of the ulna (*arrowhead*). Note that the contrast remains contained by the intact superficial layer of the UCL without extraarticular extravasation. This finding has been described as the "T" sign.

Parallel Imaging

Parallel imaging is a relatively new class of techniques capable of substantially increasing the imaging speed of MRI. Parallel imaging involves using spatial information inherent in the elements of an RF coil array to allow a reduction in the number of time-consuming, phase-encoded steps required during a scan. Parallel imaging, therefore, imposes particular hardware requirements. Coil arrays must be used with separate preamplifiers and receivers for each individual element and with appropriate decoupling networks to decrease cross-talk between elements. Although these techniques may be used to some degree with existing coil arrays, many tailored array geometries have been designed specifically for parallel imaging. Parallel imaging techniques may be applied to any existing pulse sequence to reduce imaging time or increase spatial resolution. Resultant time savings can then be used to add modifications that would otherwise prohibitively lengthen a pulse sequence. Recent technical advances and increased availability have placed parallel imaging in widespread clinical use.

Increased imaging speeds do come with a well-defined signal-to-noise ratio penalty, which must be taken into account when developing protocols. Nevertheless, for sequences with sufficient baseline signal-to-noise ratio, parallel imaging can offer substantial benefits. There is great synergy with 3D volumetric acquisitions and high field

to four times faster at 3.0 T than at 1.5 T while maintaining a comparable signal-to-noise ratio. In actuality, given the number of different considerations, it is typical to image only twice as fast with 3.0 T as with 1.5 T. Image acquisition time at 3.0 T may be optimized by minimizing the number of signal averages, increasing TR to account for longer T1 relaxation, use of a higher receiver bandwidth for non-FSE sequences, and use of small echo spacing for FSE/turbo-spin sequences. As mentioned above, the increase in signal-to-noise ratio at 3.0 T may be used to improve spatial resolution of images acquired by producing thinner and more numerous sections (**Fig. 16.5**).[6–8]

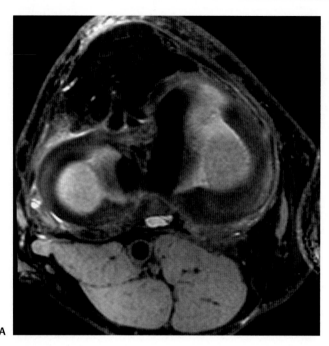
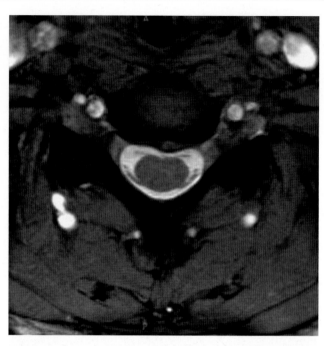

A

B

Fig. 16.5 3.0-T MRI. **(A)** An axial oblique multiplanar reconstruction image of the knee from a 3D isotropic image data set superbly shows the medial and lateral meniscal anatomy. **(B)** An axial T2*-weighted image (a T2-like image [bright fluid] created with a gradient-echo rather than an SE technique) at the C4-C5 level of the spine shows a high signal-to-noise ratio with high spatial resolution, providing excellent visualization of the ventral and dorsal roots in addition to a small central disc protrusion.

strength MRI systems (higher signal-to-noise ratio), which facilitates a shift toward rapid, volumetric image acquisitions. Recently, major vendors of MRI scanners have implemented versions of parallel imaging in several commercial systems.[9]

High-Resolution Imaging: MR Microscopy

MRI with microscopy coils offer much higher signal-to-noise ratio, higher contrast-to-noise ratio, and higher spatial resolution than does a conventional small surface coil. For example, resolution of conventional MRI has not permitted detailed evaluation of the entire TFCC, but primarily the triangular fibrocartilage proper (disc). However, the triangular ligament (upper and lower lamina), meniscus homologue, and ulnotriquetral ligament are clearly seen with microscopy coils. High-resolution MRI with a microscopy coil is a promising method with which to diagnose TFCC abnormalities and other ligamentous lesions (**Fig. 16.6**).

Microscopy coils are limited by inadequate depiction of deeper structures. This issue may be addressed by combined positioning with a larger surface coil or a flexible coil. In addition, the limited sensitivity of microscopy coils may make accurate coil setting over a targeted structure or lesion difficult. Superconducting coils have also been used for small joint imaging. Overall, it is likely that advanced coil develop-

ment will lead to improved diagnostic performance of MRI because high-resolution imaging is paramount for the depiction of infrastructural features of the wrist and elbow when evaluating internal derangements.

Extremity Scanners

Low field strength open MR scanners and extremity scanners have been used for several years. Recently, a higher field 1.5-T extremity scanner (ORTHONE, ONI, Inc., Wilmington, MA) has become available clinically.[10] This device can image the elbow, hand, wrist, knee, foot, and ankle, but it cannot acquire images of the shoulder, hip, or spine. Therefore, it is not considered as a stand-alone unit, but it may be useful as a supplement to a whole body scanner for a high-volume site with a backlog of musculoskeletal patients. Because there are fewer site requirements for this device than for a conventional high field strength system, an extremity scanner is often an economical imaging option. Additionally, extremity scanners may prove useful for imaging claustrophobic patients because the image quality of a 1.5-T extremity scanner is much better than that of a typical low field strength open MRI or a very low field strength extremity scanner. This type of device will likely fulfill a niche role, providing high-quality clinical images for designated body parts (**Fig. 16.7**).

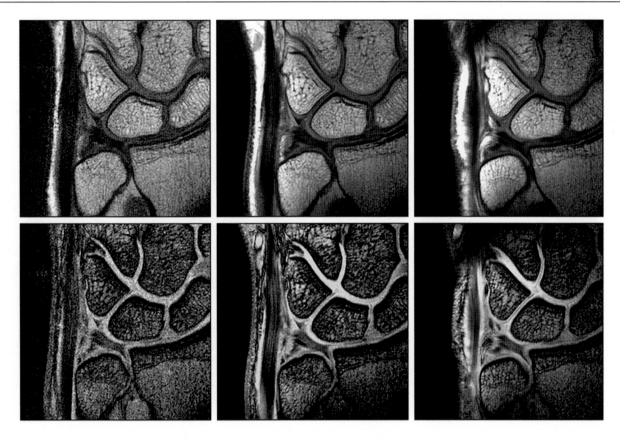

Fig. 16.6 These FSE proton-density images (top row) and coronal T2*-weighted images (T2-like images [bright fluid] created with a gradient-echo rather than a SE technique) (bottom row) of the TFCC were obtained with a 1.5-T MRI scanner and a conventional 80-mm diameter surface coil (left column), a 47-mm diameter microscopy surface coil (middle column), and a 23-mm diameter microscopy sur-face coil (right column). MRI with microscopy coils provided higher signal-to-noise ratios, higher contrast, and improved spatial resolution and depiction of the infrastructural details of the TFCC. (Courtesy of Hiroshi Yoshioka, MD, Department of Radiology, University of Tsukuba, Tsukuba, Japan, and Harvard Medical School, Brigham and Women's Hospital, Boston, MA.)

RF coils for extremity scanners are available in two sizes. Both are quadrature types of volume transmit-receive coils, which yield improved image quality compared with that of traditional surface coils. Extremity scanners offer several advantages compared with high field strength closed MRI systems:[11]

- Images are high quality despite lower field strength.
- Artifacts from off-isocenter imaging and signal-to-noise ratio loss are minimized.
- Most pulse sequences (including spectral fat suppression) are available.

Intraoperative MRI

New operating suites have been designed that incorporate MRI scanners, which allow a patient undergoing surgery to be imaged intraoperatively. Careful architectural planning and MRI-compatible surgical and anesthesia equipment allow for this new technique, which has been primarily used in neurosurgery. The value of such information has been shown to outweigh the cost of time necessary for image acquisition.[12] Low field strength open MRI units are common because of their lower cost and more flexible integration into the operative suite.[13] However, image quality is improved with high field strength closed magnets; such systems have been mounted on ceilings of neurosurgical operating rooms to image the brain.[13] Intraoperative MRI has the capacity to detect residual tumor during a difficult resection, define complex anatomy during orthopaedic procedures, and assess for complications. Although the potential for this technique is great, additional studies are needed to define the role of this technology in an orthopedic setting.

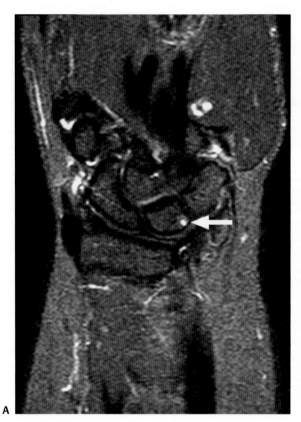

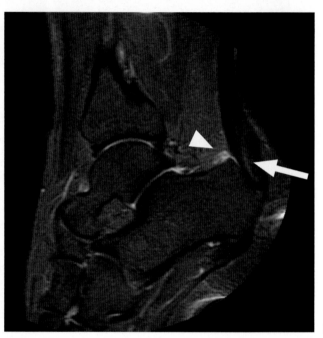

Fig. 16.7 Images obtained with an open high field strength extremity scanner. **(A)** This coronal oblique STIR image shows a characteristic focal signal abnormality along the ulnar aspect of the lunate, round fluid region (reflecting cystic change), and surrounding marrow edema (*arrow*), consistent with a wrist ulnolunate abutment. **(B)** This sagittal T2-weighted image with spectral fat suppression shows tendinosis, intrasubstance linear fluid signal (*arrow*) (reflect-ing interstitial tearing), and associated retrocalcaneal bursitis (*arrowhead*), consistent with Achilles tendinopathy. These images show high signal-to-noise ratio, good contrast resolution, and spatial resolution similar to that of high field strength closed systems. Adequate and uniform fat suppression is obtained because the region of interest is located at the magnet's isocenter, avoiding inadvertent water suppression.

■ Positional, Load-Bearing, or Dynamic (Functional) Imaging

Positional, load-bearing, or dynamic (functional) imaging of the spine has proven useful because imaging in the supine position may not fully reveal relevant pathology. Available options for imaging the spine include the supine, supine with axial loading (simulated weight bearing), seated, and standing upright positions.

Simulated weight bearing is performed by applying an axial load during supine imaging, which may be accomplished by having the patient wear a hardened plastic vest (DynaWell L-Spine, DynaWell, Billdal, Sweden).[14] This device, which is free of material that would disturb the magnetic field in the MRI scanner, is strapped over the patient's shoulders and upper chest. The patient's feet are placed against the footplate of a compression device, which is attached to two adjustable cords, one on each side of the vest. By tightening the cords to a desired measured load (up to 50% of body weight), it is pos-sible to provide compression that is similar to that of upright posture. This axially loaded position may reveal pathologies such as spondylolisthesis (see **Fig. 13.42**), kyphosis, and disc herniations that are otherwise not seen in a supine position (**Fig. 16.8**).

MRI in the seated position is possible in a specially designed vertically open intraoperative 0.5-T magnet (Signa SP, General Electric Medical Systems, Milwaukee, WI) configured as a double bore with a 60-cm gap, which has been likened to a "double donut."[15] A seat for the patient may be placed between the "donuts" in the center of the bore, allowing imaging of the lumbar spine in neutral, flexion, and extension positions for a seated patient, providing a form of dynamic imaging. The seated position provides an axial load that may reproduce back pain symptoms for some patients. This type of imaging has shown physiologic changes of the spinal canal; for example, the cross-sectional area of the spinal canal and neural foramina is smallest in the extended position (**Fig. 16.9**). Conventional MRI may show abnormalities that may take on greater importance because

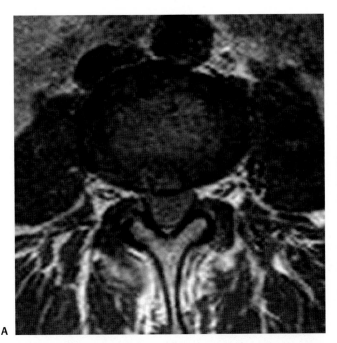
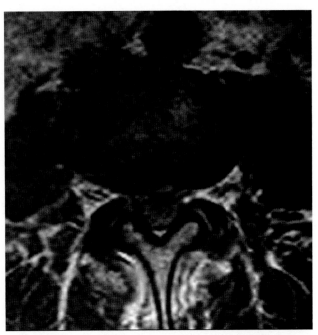

A

B

Fig. 16.8 Load-bearing spine imaging: simulated weight-bearing paradigm. These axial T1-weighted images were obtained at the level of the intervertebral disc in a conventional horizontal-bore 1.5-T MRI scanner with the use of a specially designed compression device (DynaWell Corp.) in a patient with neurogenic claudication. **(A)** A view without axial loading shows a mild disc bulge without substantial stenosis. **(B)** A view with axial loading shows a focal protrusion type disc herniation and increasing stenosis. (Courtesy of Per Lennart Westesson, MD, PhD, DDS, University of Rochester Medical Center, Rochester, NY.)

of encroachment or neural impingement on dynamic load-bearing (seated) sequences.

Another option for functional musculoskeletal imaging is upright, weight-bearing, dynamic-kinetic MRI of the spine. A specially designed 0.6-T magnet (Stand-Up MRI, Fonar Corporation, Melville, NY)[16] allows imaging of the standing patient. This system is applicable for imaging of the cervical, thoracic, and lumbar spine. This scanner is useful for normal positional and kinetic images, for showing position-related disc protrusions in the spine worsening with extension, and for showing fluctuating positional foraminal and central spinal stenosis in the spine between recumbent and upright neutral positions. This type of imaging has led to a concept of fluctuating kinetic central spinal stenosis (fluctuating fluid disc herniation) that can be shown only by imaging in various upright positions (**Fig. 16.10**). Although a cervical spine MRI in the recumbent position may show posterior osteophytes, an upright MRI with cervical extension may reveal cord compression.

Back pain often occurs in weight-bearing situations, so positional imaging has great potential for showing pathology that may be subtle or inconspicuous on conventional supine MRI. However, the role of imaging the hip, knee, and ankle under an axial load has not been fully investigated. If supine-simulated weight-bearing techniques become validated, traditional magnets can be used without having to

deploy new, costly, space-occupying devices.[17] Additional studies comparing simulated weight-bearing and upright imaging are needed to determine if new magnets are required for this purpose. Load-bearing and dynamic imaging may not be necessary to show relevant pathology for all patients; patient selection criteria need to be developed so that this technology can be applied appropriately.

■ Novel Pulse Sequences

Although often useful, conventional musculoskeletal MRI pulse sequences may yield nonspecific findings. Several new imaging techniques may help narrow a differential diagnosis and further characterize a disease entity. For example, in- and out-of-phase chemical-shift imaging uses an MR artifact to determine if there is a loss of normal marrow fat by an infiltrative process. Normal marrow and benign entities (such as vertebral fractures, hemangiomas, or Schmorl nodes) show loss of signal on out-of-phase images, which is not seen in neoplastic processes (**Fig. 16.11**). Chemical-shift sequences are therefore useful for determining whether heterogeneous marrow signal on T1-weighted images reflects tumor involvement or benign processes in the axial skeleton.[18,19]

Diffusion-weighted imaging is based on Brownian motion of water molecules in tissues. Pathologic processes typically

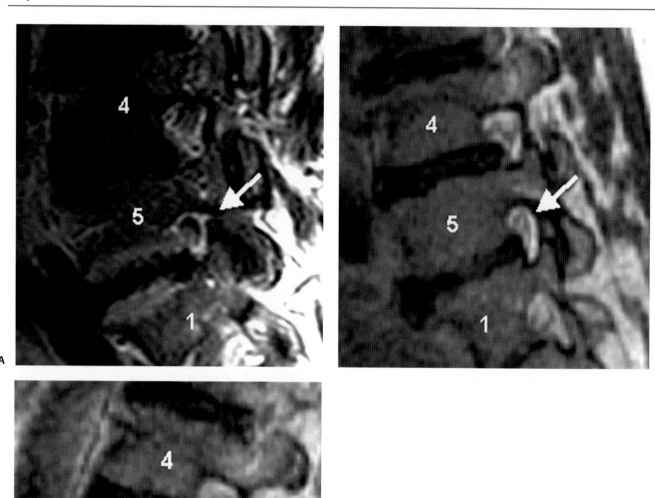

Fig. 16.9 Load-bearing spine imaging: seated positional paradigm. These sagittal **(A–C)** and axial **(D–F)** T2-weighted images were obtained in a specially designed vertically open 0.5-T MRI scanner (General Electric Medical Systems). The patient was seated and images were acquired in neutral **(A,D)**, flexion **(B,E)**, and extension **(C,F)** positions. **(A)** The L5-S1 foramen shows a slight foraminal stenosis with deformity of the epidural fat (*arrow*) on the conventional image. **(B)** This image obtained with the patient in seated flexion shows improvement with increased epidural fat surrounding the exiting nerve (*arrow*). **(C)** This image obtained with the patient in seated extension shows a marked foraminal stenosis at the L5-S1 foramen with epidural fat only partially surrounding the nerve root present (*arrow*). (Continued on page 405)

restrict spontaneous diffusion of water; the degree of diffusion can then be imaged to differentiate benign from malignant processes in the musculoskeletal system. This technique can show the extent of tumor necrosis and is used to differentiate tumor recurrence from posttreatment signal changes. Diffusion-weighted imaging is especially helpful for characterizing soft-tissue tumors because of the inherent contrast from high water diffusion in muscle. Diffusion-weighted imaging can also differentiate malignant from benign vertebral compression fractures because a benign fracture exhibits greater diffusion and bone marrow edema.[20]

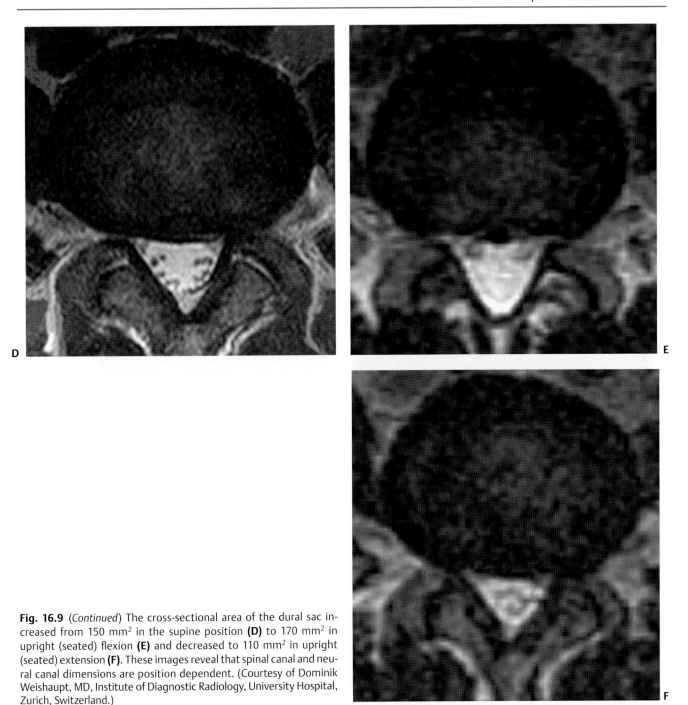

Fig. 16.9 (*Continued*) The cross-sectional area of the dural sac increased from 150 mm² in the supine position **(D)** to 170 mm² in upright (seated) flexion **(E)** and decreased to 110 mm² in upright (seated) extension **(F)**. These images reveal that spinal canal and neural canal dimensions are position dependent. (Courtesy of Dominik Weishaupt, MD, Institute of Diagnostic Radiology, University Hospital, Zurich, Switzerland.)

MR spectroscopy can assess the malignant potential of a lesion by evaluating its metabolic constituents. Because it represents an element of cell membranes, choline is present to a greater degree in malignant lesions, serving as a marker for increased cell turnover.[21] MR spectroscopy can be used to measure relative quantities of choline, which requires selecting a volumetric region of interest. Each region of interest can be located with dynamic gadolinium-enhanced imag-ing by defining regions of a tumor with early enhancement. Commercially available software then provides spectro-scopic data, whereby the relative amount of choline within a region of interest is measured at a peak of 3.2 ppm. MR-spectroscopy-based studies have shown that pathologically proven malignant lesions contain a significantly greater amount of choline than adjacent tissue.[22,23] MR spectros-copy, therefore, has the potential to provide a noninvasive

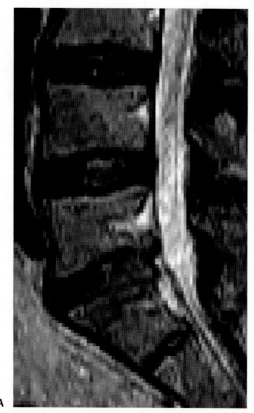
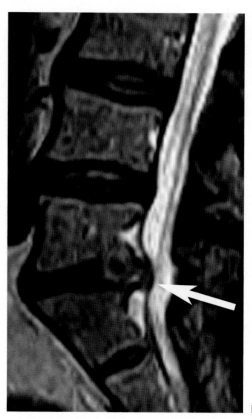

Fig. 16.10 Load-bearing spine imaging: standing positional paradigm. These sagittal T2-weighted views were obtained in a specially designed open 0.6-T magnet that allows for horizontal (recumbent) and vertical (upright) imaging (Fonar Corp.). This patient had recurrent radiculopathy 8 months after partial discectomy, with symptoms only when upright. **(A)** A supine image shows no focal contour abnormality at L5-S1. **(B)** An upright-neutral image reveals a posterior disc herniation at the L5-S1 level elevating the posterior longitudinal ligament (*arrow*), which was not visible on the supine image. (Courtesy of J. Randy Jinkins, MD, FACR, FEC, Downstate Medical Center, State University of New York, Brooklyn, NY.)

method for evaluating the malignant potential of tumors (**Fig. 16.12**).

■ MRI in the Presence of Metallic Implants

Susceptibility artifacts from metallic orthopaedic implants have historically limited the usefulness of MRI in the postoperative setting. Although radiography, conventional arthrography, and nuclear medicine studies are accessible and cost-effective, these imaging modalities have limited sensitivity and specificity for common postoperative clinical questions. With minor adjustments to routine pulse sequences, MRI can be a highly accurate tool for the evaluation of postoperative conditions, with excellent visualization of periprosthetic tissues.

Metallic objects cause local magnetic field distortions, which lead to varying degrees of misregistration and characteristic artifacts that are worsened at higher magnetic field strengths. Titanium and tantalum implants create sub-

stantially less artifact than does stainless steel,[24,25] and such artifacts are reduced when the long axis of a metallic object is parallel to the long axis of the magnet. Appropriate patient positioning and imaging protocols can dramatically reduce such artifacts. Metallic interference with the local magnetic field limits the usefulness of fat-suppression techniques; STIR sequences avoid this problem and are preferred for generating T2-weighted images.[26] Additionally, FSE/turbo-spin sequences are typically less susceptible to metallic artifacts than are conventional SE techniques.[27] Smaller fields of view also help to limit the influence of metallic objects.[28]

The diagnostic accuracy of metallic artifact reduction sequences compared with that of conventional MRI techniques is well established. Artifact reduction sequences are particularly important for imaging the spine, where key findings are routinely missed without appropriate imaging protocols.[29,30] MRI of hip, knee, and shoulder arthroplasties can be of more diagnostic value than CT, conventional radiography, or nuclear scintigraphy, particularly for the evaluation of common pathology (such as mechanical loosening, infection,

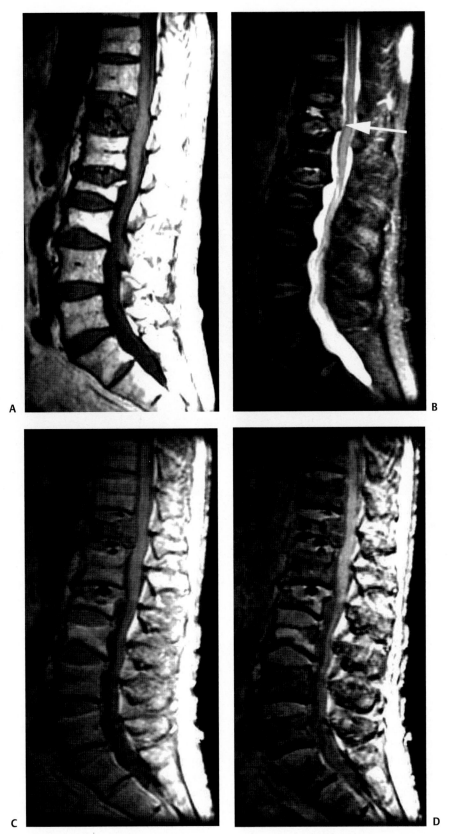

Fig. 16.11 Chemical-shift imaging: biopsy-proven benign vertebral compression. These lumbar spine images were obtained with a 1.5-T system. **(A)** A sagittal T1-weighted SE image. **(B)** A sagittal STIR image. **(C)** A sagittal gradient-echo in-phase (TE = 4.2 ms) image. **(D)** A sagittal gradient-echo out-of-phase (TE = 2.1 ms) image. The T11 vertebra shows a diffuse compression deformity and bone marrow edema (*arrow on* **B**). There is also a compression deformity at L1 with only minimal superior end-plate edema. The T11 vertebra signal intensity measured 185 on the in-phase image and 132 on the out-of-phase image, corresponding to a proportional decrease of –29.8%.

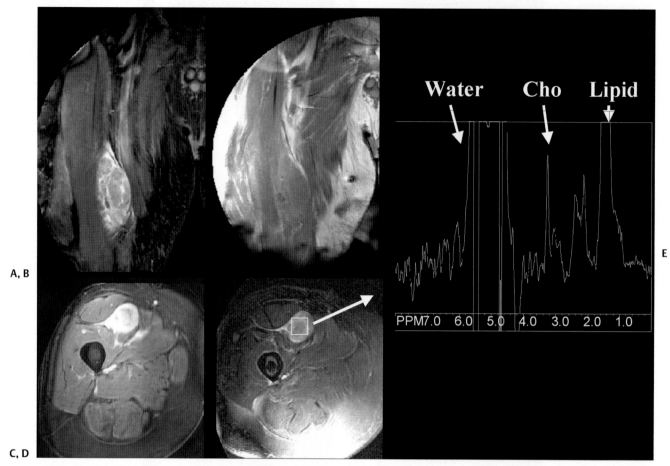

Fig. 16.12 For this 58-year-old man presenting with a palpable right-thigh soft-tissue mass, imaging-guided percutaneous biopsy with needle aspiration and core biopsies revealed a myofibroblastic lesion of uncertain malignant potential, possibly representing fibromatosis, schwannoma, or a low-grade sarcoma. Histology favored a diagnosis of low-grade sarcoma; MR spectroscopy results highly favored malignancy. **(A)** A coronal inversion recovery STIR image (TR/TE, 2462/100 ms; inversion time, 200 ms) of the right thigh shows an ovoid heterogeneous mass. **(B)** A coronal SE T1-weighted image (690/15 ms) of the same mass for comparison. **(C)** An axial gradient-echo contrast-enhanced T1-weighted image (8.7/4.3 ms; flip angle, 90 degrees) shows that the mass enhanced after contrast administration. **(D)** An axial FS gradient-echo T2-weighted image (2886/100 ms) shows mass with placement of 2 × 2 × 2 mL voxel over lesion. **(E)** A corresponding single-voxel point-resolved MR spectroscopy (2000/144 ms) shows a discrete choline (*Cho*) peak in the lesion, with a choline signal-to-noise ratio of 18.6, indicating malignancy. Final pathology after resection showed a low-grade sarcoma. (From Fayad LM, Barker PB, Jacobs MA, Eng J, Weber KL, Kulesza P, Bluemke DA. Characterization of musculoskeletal lesions on 3-T proton MR spectroscopy. AJR Am J Roentgenol 2007;188:1513-1520. Reprinted by permission.)

fracture, and osteonecrosis), and for the assessment of malignancy,[31,32] and it offers superior image quality, given minor modifications to conventional pulse sequences. MRI serves as an extremely useful problem-solving technique in the presence of metallic hardware, particularly when clinical suspicion is high and radiography is negative or equivocal (**Fig. 16.13**).

■ MR Angiography and Venography

MR angiography is a useful technique for defining vascular anatomy throughout the musculoskeletal system without ionizing radiation. Although initially difficult to perform because of the large fields of view, technical advances, including high magnetic field strengths, have made MR angiography practical for a variety of clinical uses.

With MR angiography, feeding arteries and draining veins can be clearly seen for vascular malformations, aiding surgical or endovascular planning. Additionally, MR angiography can reliably define tumor vascularity and vessel invasion,[33] and it is also useful for the detection of arterial dissection and pseudoaneurysms, particularly in the setting of craniocervical trauma. MR angiography is especially helpful for the evaluation of the peripheral vascular system and has replaced conventional diagnostic angiography of

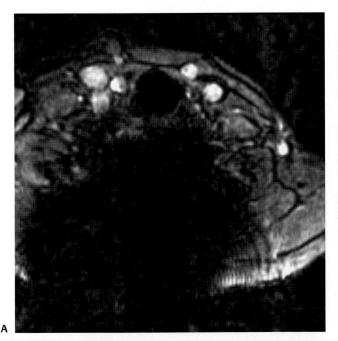

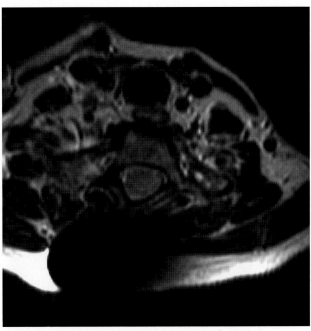

A   B

Fig. 16.13 MRI in the presence of metallic implants. This patient had posterior spinal fixation at the T1 vertebral level. **(A)** An axial gradient-echo T2*-weighted image (a T2-like image [bright fluid] created with a gradient-echo rather than a SE technique) shows a large signal void obscuring the spinal canal. **(B)** An axial T2-weighted image with FSE/turbo-spin technique at the same level in the same patient during the same imaging examination minimizes the susceptibility artifact from the metallic implants and substantially reduces the signal void so that the spinal canal contents are visible.

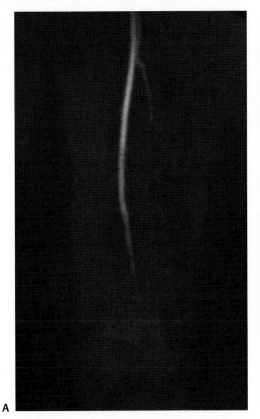

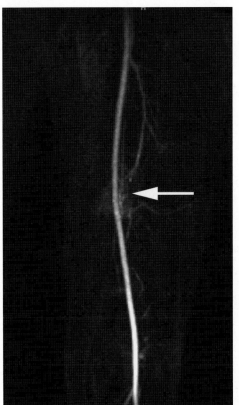

A   B

Fig. 16.14 MR angiography: vascular malformation. Frontal projection views of a left-thigh MR angiogram shows **(A)** filling of the superficial femoral artery to the level of the popliteal fossa accompanied by early filling of the profunda femoris artery and **(B)** an enhancing vascular malformation (*arrow*) only after the profunda femoris artery is filled, thus establishing it as the feeding vessel.

the upper and lower extremities in some centers for certain situations.[34] However, the widespread availability of CT angiography and rapid 3D postprocessing techniques have limited the use of MR angiography in the acute setting. MR angiography provides excellent definition of complex vascular anatomy, which can be helpful for preoperative planning.

Gadolinium-enhanced MR angiography offers clear definition of vasculature with short image acquisition times. Intravenous gadolinium shortens intravascular T1

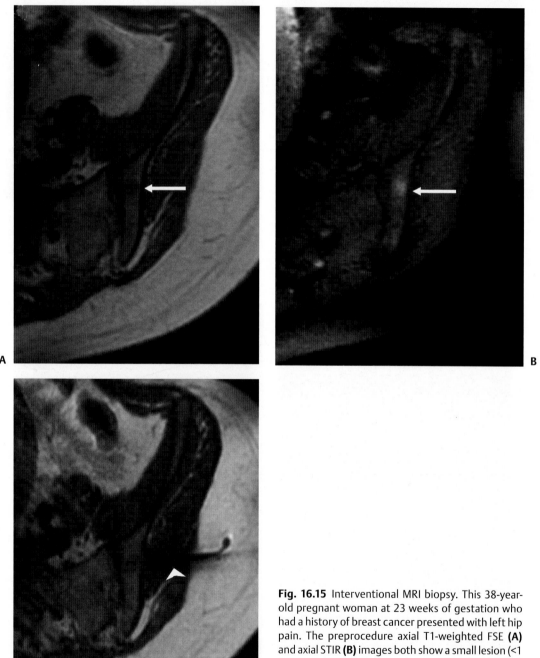

Fig. 16.15 Interventional MRI biopsy. This 38-year-old pregnant woman at 23 weeks of gestation who had a history of breast cancer presented with left hip pain. The preprocedure axial T1-weighted FSE **(A)** and axial STIR **(B)** images both show a small lesion (<1 cm) in the left ilium (*arrow*). **(C)** An intraprocedural axial T1-weighted FSE image with the patient in the right lateral decubitus position shows the trephine needle (*arrowhead*) positioned on the cortex at the level of the lesion. The specimen showed metastatic breast cancer.

relaxation time, providing excellent contrast with adjacent tissues. Dynamic imaging of a region of interest can be obtained to visualize arterial and venous phases of enhancement. Unlike a conventional angiogram, real-time data are superimposed on high soft-tissue contrast afforded by MRI, yielding a wealth of information. Although noncontrast MR angiographic techniques have been developed, they are of limited use in the musculoskeletal system, given the need for high spatial resolution and often-unpredictable orientation of blood vessels. Images can be acquired in a 2D format (i.e., segment by segment) or as a 3D volume, facilitating multiplanar reconstructions (**Fig. 16.14**).

MR venography has been used to detect deep venous thromboses with excellent overall sensitivity and specificity (91.5% and 94.8%, respectively, in a recent meta-analysis[35]). These values are comparable to Doppler ultrasound and conventional venography. However, sensitivity for distal venous thromboses is considerably lower (62.1%[35]). MR venography may serve as a useful adjunct when ultrasound is equivocal or falsely negative.

■ MRI-Guided Interventions

The use of MRI for image-guided musculoskeletal interventions has increased in popularity over the past several years.

The number and types of MRI-guided interventions have increased and likely will continue to do so.[36–39] Current applications include the following:

- Musculoskeletal lesion biopsy procedures[38]
- Cryoablation procedures[39]
- Pain management techniques, such as sacroiliac joint injections, discography, transforaminal epidural injection, selective nerve block, sympathetic block, celiac plexus block, and facet joint cryotherapy neurotomies[36,37]

Musculoskeletal Biopsy

MRI is a useful imaging technique for musculoskeletal lesion biopsy because of its excellent depiction of bone and soft-tissue pathology.[38,39] It is particularly helpful for the following:

- Lesions adjacent to critical structures best seen with MRI (**Fig. 16.15**)
- Lesions for which characterization of its internal composition, such as region of necrosis, is important in terms of obtaining a diagnostic specimen[38,39]

In many respects, open interventional MRI systems offer many of the advantages of ultrasound and CT, such as ultrasound's real-time visualization of tissue and CT's excellent visualization of bone.[40]

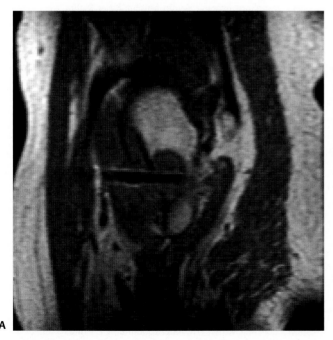
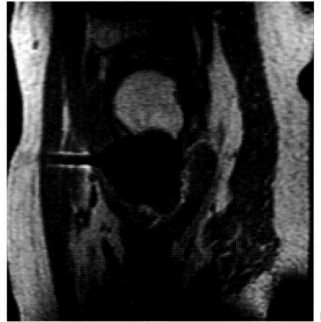

A   B

Fig. 16.16 Interventional MRI: cryotherapy. This 50-year-old man had renal cell carcinoma metastatic to the proximal right femur. **(A)** Sagittal T1-weighted image shows a cryotherapy needle in the hypointense metastasis in the region of the right lesser trochanter.

(B) Sagittal T1-weighted image shows an elliptical signal void of the ice ball, representing the treatment zone. Critical structures avoided were the femoral nerve, femoral vessels, and iliopsoas tendon attachment.

Cryotherapy

MR-guided cryotherapy of soft-tissue and bone metastases has been shown to be a safe and effective technique, and it can provide excellent local tumor control and pain relief in the appropriate clinical setting.[39] The efficacy of MR-guided cryotherapy is based on the fact that MRI is sensitive to temperature changes within tissue and that cryoablated tissue is easily recognized (and approximates tissue death) on standard MRI pulse sequences. Cryoablated tissue produces a signal void on standard pulse sequences and has been referred to as an *ice ball*[39] (**Fig. 16.16**). MRI-guided percutaneous cryotherapy reduces morbidity by using a percutaneous approach, and it offers the advantage of estimating the volume of tissue ablation during the procedure.[39]

Pain Management

MR-guided interventions have also been shown to be safe and effective when used for numerous pain management techniques, including the following:

- Sacroiliac joint injections
- Discography
- Transforaminal epidural injection
- Selective nerve block
- Sympathetic block
- Celiac plexus block
- Facet joint cryotherapy neurotomies[36,37]

The excellent depiction of soft-tissue structures provides a distinct advantage when isolating nerves and facet joints for injections. MR is also useful for recognizing reactive edema adjacent to arthritic joints.

References

1. Morrison WB. Indirect MR arthrography: concepts and controversies. Semin Musculoskelet Radiol 2005;9:125–134

2. Elentuck D, Palmer WE. Direct magnetic resonance arthrography. Eur Radiol 2004;14:1956–1967

3. Sahin G, Demirtaş M. An overview of MR arthrography with emphasis on the current technique and applicational hints and tips. Eur J Radiol 2006;58:416–430

4. Sciulli RL, Boutin RD, Brown RR, et al. Evaluation of the postoperative meniscus of the knee: a study comparing conventional arthrography, conventional MR imaging, MR arthrography with iodinated contrast material, and MR arthrography with gadolinium-based contrast material. Skeletal Radiol 1999;28:508–514

5. Bergin D, Schweitzer ME. Indirect magnetic resonance arthrography. Skeletal Radiol 2003;32:551–558

6. Ramnath RR. 3T MR imaging of the musculoskeletal system (Part I): considerations, coils, and challenges. Magn Reson Imaging Clin N Am 2006;14:27–40

7. Takahashi M, Uematsu H, Hatabu H. MR imaging at high magnetic fields. Eur J Radiol 2003;46:45–52

8. Tanenbaum LN. Clinical 3T MR imaging: mastering the challenges. Magn Reson Imaging Clin N Am 2006;14:1–15

9. Wiesinger F, Van de Moortele PF, Adriany G, De Zanche N, Ugurbil K, Pruessmann KP. Potential and feasibility of parallel MRI at high field. NMR Biomed 2006;19:368–378

10. Oni Medical Systems. The ONI MSK extreme with v-SPEC. http://www.onicorp.com/radiologists.html. Accessed on March 28, 2007.

11. American College of Rheumatology Extremity Magnetic Resonance Imaging Task Force. Extremity magnetic resonance imaging in rheumatoid arthritis: report of the American College of Rheumatology Extremity Magnetic Resonance Imaging Task Force. Arthritis Rheum 2006;54:1034–1047

12. Lewin JS, Nour SG, Meyers ML, et al. Intraoperative MRI with a rotating, tiltable surgical table: a time-use study and clinical results in 122 patients. AJR Am J Roentgenol 2007;189:1096–1103

13. Jolesz FA. Future perspectives for intraoperative MRI. Neurosurg Clin N Am 2005;16:201–213

14. DynaWell. Simulate upright position in CT and MRI using the DynaWell L-spine compression device. http://www.dynawell.biz. Accessed on March 28, 2007

15. Wipro GE. Healthcare. Signa SP/i 0.5T. http://www.gehealthcare.com/inen/rad/mri/products/spi/index.html. Accessed on March 28, 2007

16. Fonar Corporation. The upright MRI. http://www.fonar.com/standup.htm. Accessed on March 28, 2007

17. Shellock FG. Functional assessment of the joints using kinematic magnetic resonance imaging. Semin Musculoskelet Radiol 2003;7:249–276

18. Maas M, van Kuijk C, Stoker J, et al. Quantification of bone involvement in Gaucher disease: MR imaging bone marrow burden score as an alternative to Dixon quantitative chemical shift MR imaging—initial experience. Radiology 2003;229:554–561

19. Maas M, Akkerman EM, Venema HW, Stoker J, Den Heeten GJ. Dixon quantitative chemical shift MRI for bone marrow evaluation in the lumbar spine: a reproducibility study in healthy volunteers. J Comput Assist Tomogr 2001;25:691–697

20. Baur A, Stäbler A, Brüning R, et al. Diffusion-weighted MR imaging of bone marrow: differentiation of benign versus pathologic compression fractures. Radiology 1998;207:349–356

21. Aboagye EO, Bhujwalla ZM. Malignant transformation alters membrane choline phospholipid metabolism of human mammary epithelial cells. Cancer Res 1999;59:80–84

22. Fayad LM, Bluemke DA, McCarthy EF, Weber KL, Barker PB, Jacobs MA. Musculoskeletal tumors: use of proton MR spectroscopic imaging for characterization. J Magn Reson Imaging 2006;23:23–28

23. Wang CK, Li CW, Hsieh TJ, Chien SH, Liu GC, Tsai KB. Characterization of bone and soft-tissue tumors with in vivo 1H MR spectroscopy: initial results. Radiology 2004;232:599–605

24. Burtscher IM, Owman T, Romner B, Ståhlberg F, Holtås S. Aneurysm clip MR artifacts. Titanium versus stainless steel and influence of imaging parameters. Acta Radiol 1998;39:70–76

25. Wang JC, Yu WD, Sandhu HS, Tam V, Delamarter RB. A comparison of magnetic resonance and computed tomographic image quality after

the implantation of tantalum and titanium spinal instrumentation. Spine (Phila Pa 1976) 1998;23:1684–1688

26. Viano AM, Gronemeyer SA, Haliloglu M, Hoffer FA. Improved MR imaging for patients with metallic implants. Magn Reson Imaging 2000;18:287–295

27. Guermazi A, Miaux Y, Zaim S, Peterfy CG, White D, Genant HK. Metallic artefacts in MR imaging: effects of main field orientation and strength. Clin Radiol 2003;58:322–328

28. Lee MJ, Kim S, Lee SA, et al. Overcoming artifacts from metallic orthopedic implants at high-field-strength MR imaging and multi-detector CT. Radiographics 2007;27:791–803

29. Rudisch A, Kremser C, Peer S, Kathrein A, Judmaier W, Daniaux H. Metallic artifacts in magnetic resonance imaging of patients with spinal fusion. A comparison of implant materials and imaging sequences. Spine (Phila Pa 1976) 1998;23:692–699

30. Tartaglino LM, Flanders AE, Vinitski S, Friedman DP. Metallic artifacts on MR images of the postoperative spine: reduction with fast spin-echo techniques. Radiology 1994;190:565–569

31. Harris CA, White LM. Metal artifact reduction in musculoskeletal magnetic resonance imaging. Orthop Clin North Am 2006;37:349–359

32. Sofka CM, Potter HG. MR imaging of joint arthroplasty. Semin Musculoskelet Radiol 2002;6:79–85

33. Feydy A, Anract P, Tomeno B, Chevrot A, Drapé JL. Assessment of vascular invasion by musculoskeletal tumors of the limbs: use of contrast-enhanced MR angiography. Radiology 2006;238:611–621

34. Leiner T. Magnetic resonance angiography of abdominal and lower extremity vasculature. Top Magn Reson Imaging 2005;16:21–66

35. Sampson FC, Goodacre SW, Thomas SM, van Beek EJR. The accuracy of MRI in diagnosis of suspected deep vein thrombosis: systematic review and meta-analysis. Eur Radiol 2007;17:175–181

36. Carrino JA, Jolesz FA. MRI-Guided interventions. Acad Radiol 2005;12:1063–1064

37. Carrino JA, Blanco R. Magnetic resonance–guided musculoskeletal interventional radiology. Semin Musculoskelet Radiol 2006;10:159–173

38. Carrino JA, Khurana B, Ready JE, Silverman SG, Winalski CS. Magnetic resonance imaging-guided percutaneous biopsy of musculoskeletal lesions. J Bone Joint Surg Am 2007;89:2179–2187

39. Tuncali K, Morrison PR, Winalski CS, et al. MRI-guided percutaneous cryotherapy for soft-tissue and bone metastases: initial experience. AJR Am J Roentgenol 2007;189:232–239

40. Silverman SG, Collick BD, Figueira MR, et al. Interactive MR-guided biopsy in an open-configuration MR imaging system. Radiology 1995;197:175–181

17 Correlation of MRI with Other Imaging Studies

Uma Srikumaran, Laura M. Fayad, and A. Jay Khanna

Although the preceding chapters have focused on MRI of the musculoskeletal system, it is important for the clinician to recognize that other imaging modalities play an important role in the evaluation of patients with musculoskeletal disorders. These other commonly used imaging modalities include conventional radiography, CT, nuclear scintigraphy studies, and positron emission tomography. When the clinician is evaluating the patient for a particular disease process, a basic understanding of the strengths and weaknesses of these modalities is important in deciding which imaging study to request and evaluate for the patient. For many patients, one or more imaging modalities will be superior to MRI alone. In addition, after the patient has been evaluated with an MRI study, the other imaging modalities may provide additional anatomic or physiologic information that can help narrow the differential diagnosis and guide treatment.

◼ MRI

MRI provides excellent visualization of the tissues in the musculoskeletal system in multiple planes because of its high contrast resolution compared with other modalities. One of its major advantages is that the multiple pulse sequences (see Chapter 1) enable the detection of soft-tissue and bone-marrow pathology with great sensitivity (**Fig. 17.1**). In general terms, an MRI study is often obtained to evaluate the water content of tissues because most acute and subacute pathology results in free extracellular fluid. MR pulse sequences use the magnetization and relaxation properties of protons to assess and differentiate various tissue types. Tissues that contain larger amounts of water (e.g., CSF or joint fluid) are bright on fluid-sensitive sequences, and tissues that contain lesser amounts of water (e.g., cortical bone or physeal scar) are dark on all pulse sequences. Structures that contain little or no water are not well assessed by MRI. For example, the lungs have a large amount of air; therefore, although MRI is an advanced technique, it is rarely, if ever, used for the evaluation of tumors and other pathology of the lung parenchyma. Cortical bone also has a low water content, and therefore MRI is relatively limited (compared with CT, for example) for the evaluation of cortical osseous structures. The preceding chapters discuss specific indications for

MRI and the conditions that can be effectively evaluated using this imaging modality.

◼ Conventional Radiography

As most clinicians have learned throughout their training, conventional radiographs are often the initial step in the evaluation of a patient who has (or is suspected of having) a musculoskeletal disorder. Conventional radiographs are obtained via the use of ionizing irradiation. The radiation beam is attenuated by structures between the image intensifier and the cassette. Structures with high density (e.g., cortical bone, metallic implants) block a larger amount of the radiation and thus leave a white region on the film. Structures with lower density (e.g., air, subcutaneous tissues) block less radiation and thus leave a dark or gray region on the film.

Conventional radiographs are easily available and are good for the evaluation of osseous detail. This modality is also exceptionally time- and cost-effective, and the large field of view it affords allows for the study of global deformities, for example, in a patient with a spine deformity such as scoliosis or deformity or malalignment of the lower extremities. For these reasons, conventional radiography is frequently used in musculoskeletal imaging to evaluate the joints and spine (**Fig. 17.2**). On the other hand, conventional radiographs do not provide optimal visualization of the soft-tissue structures such as ligaments, menisci, and the spinal cord. Radiographs are also less sensitive than CT or MRI for the evaluation of osseous destruction and involvement of the bone marrow. As an example, a 30% decrease in bone mass is often required before osteoporosis can be appreciated on radiographs.[1,2] Conventional radiography is the study of choice for the initial evaluation of a patient with a traumatic injury to a joint, a long bone, or the spine. Radiography is also required as an adjunct to MRI in the evaluation of skeletal masses (**Fig. 17.3**) and of arthritis. However, conventional radiographs are less valuable in the evaluation of a patient with low back pain, neck pain, or spinal stenosis.

As a first-line imaging modality, conventional radiographs help the clinician determine the need for radiographic studies in other anatomic locations or for more advanced imaging studies of the local region. For example, a patient

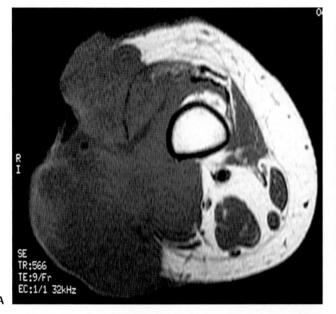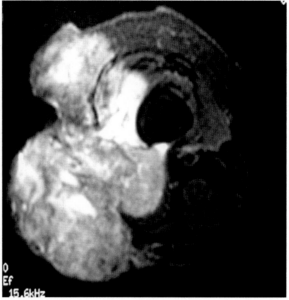

Fig. 17.1 MRI: excellent soft-tissue contrast. Axial T1-weighted **(A)** and fat-suppressed T2-weighted **(B)** images of the left distal femur show a large mass involving the bone marrow and adjacent soft tis- sues. Note the exquisite contrast between the soft tissues provided by MRI that allows for an accurate and detailed assessment of the extracompartmental involvement of the tissues.

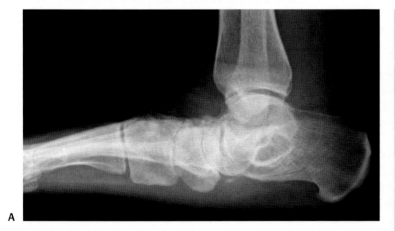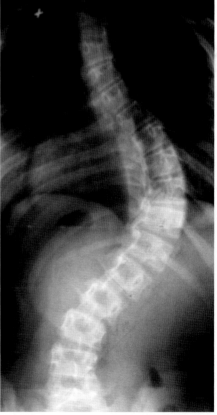

Fig. 17.2 Conventional radiographs: visualization of local and global deformity. **(A)** A lateral view of the foot shows a pes planus deformity and midfoot fault in an elderly woman. This deformity may indicate the presence of posterior tibial dys- function, although assessment of the actual posterior tibial tendon is not possible by conventional radiography alone. **(B)** A posteroanterior radiograph of the spine shows a large right thoracic scoliosis.

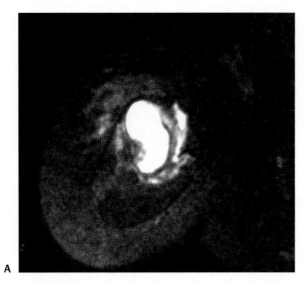

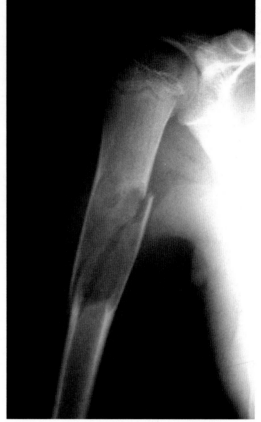

Fig. 17.3 Pathologic fracture through a unicameral bone cyst. **(A)** An axial fat-suppressed T2-weighted MR image of the right mid-humerus of a young woman shows a nodule at the periphery of a lesion occupying the humerus. The lesion is indeterminate by MRI. The diagnosis of a unicameral bone cyst with a pathologic fracture would not be possible with MRI alone; that diagnosis requires **(B)** a radiograph showing the specific features.

complaining of arm pain after trauma may be initially evaluated with humerus and elbow radiographs. Findings of an elbow fracture would then necessitate imaging of the forearm with conventional radiography to rule out associated injuries. If the fracture appeared to be intraarticular and comminuted, CT imaging may be used to study the elbow further, to delineate the fracture pattern, and to assist with preoperative planning. In another example, a patient presenting with a history of thigh pain may undergo conventional radiography to evaluate the hip, femur, and knee. If a lytic lesion were found in the proximal femur, CT would then be required to determine, more precisely, the degree of osseous destruction and to aid in characterizing the mass. MRI would also be indicated to evaluate the extent of marrow and soft-tissue involvement.

Conventional radiographs are also extremely useful for the preoperative evaluation of patients undergoing orthopedic surgery. For example, in spine surgery, preoperative radiographs facilitate evaluation of spinal alignment and localization of the level of pathology. This information can then be used intraoperatively and correlated with intraoperative radiographs or fluoroscopy to confirm the operative level.

■ CT

CT images, which are acquired based on principles similar to those used for conventional radiography, can be considered multiplanar high-resolution conventional radiography because the radiation is transmitted through the patient in multiple planes, which permits the acquisition of a large-volume data set. Unlike conventional radiography, in which the images are acquired in one plane, this data set can be manipulated using computer software algorithms to provide images in any plane. In addition, current-generation multidetector CT-scanning devices allow for the acquisition of very large volumes of data in incredibly small amounts of time. For example, with the development of multidetector CT, most studies can be completed in 10 seconds or less, a particularly valuable asset in the pediatric and trauma patient populations.[3]

With regard to its use in orthopedic surgery, CT is most valuable in the assessment of osseous detail where radiography is limited (**Fig. 17.4**). CT is also used secondarily to assist in characterizing disease processes in areas where the use of conventional radiography is limited, such as the sacrum and pelvic structures. Although CT does not provide physiologic

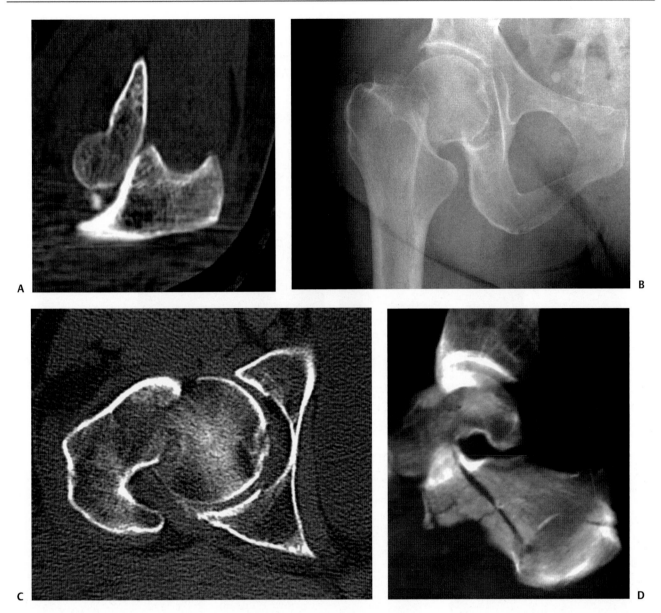

Fig. 17.4 CT: excellent osseous detail. **(A)** A sagittal CT image of the elbow shows a posterior elbow dislocation and fracture fragment in the joint. **(B)** An AP radiograph of the right femur shows a varus deformity at the femoral neck that was noted on all views. **(C)** Given this deformity, CT was requested and more clearly showed a femoral neck fracture. **(D)** A 3D sagittal reconstructed CT image of the foot and ankle shows a complex calcaneal fracture.

information about the status of the various tissues (except for limited cases in which an intravenous contrast is used), it does provide excellent spatial resolution. This modality is particularly useful for imaging the axial skeleton and for evaluating the extent of osseous lesions.[4–6] With the development of multiplanar 3D reconstructions, CT imaging provides additional guidance in preoperative planning, fracture assessment and classification, and the evaluation of complex deformities.[7,8] Although CT images provide excellent osseous detail and can precisely localize fracture extent and

fragmentation (information that can guide operative intervention), as a general rule, they do not provide high enough contrast resolution for optimal evaluation of the soft tissues, such as menisci and ligaments.[9] With the recent introduction of 16 and 64 multidetector CT and the advent of isotropic data sets, 3D CT evaluation of the tendons has emerged as a new indication for CT imaging (in patients in whom MRI is not possible).

CT can also assist in preoperative planning for orthopaedic surgical procedures. For example, a patient who presented with knee pain after direct trauma had normal-appearing conventional radiographs (**Fig. 17.5A,B**). Because the patient had a large knee effusion associated with severe pain, suspicion was high for a ligamentous injury or an occult fracture. Coronal and sagittal CT images confirmed a lateral anterior femoral condyle comminuted fracture and an avulsion fracture of the inferior pole of the patella (**Fig. 17.5C–E**). MR images showed osseous edema of the lat-

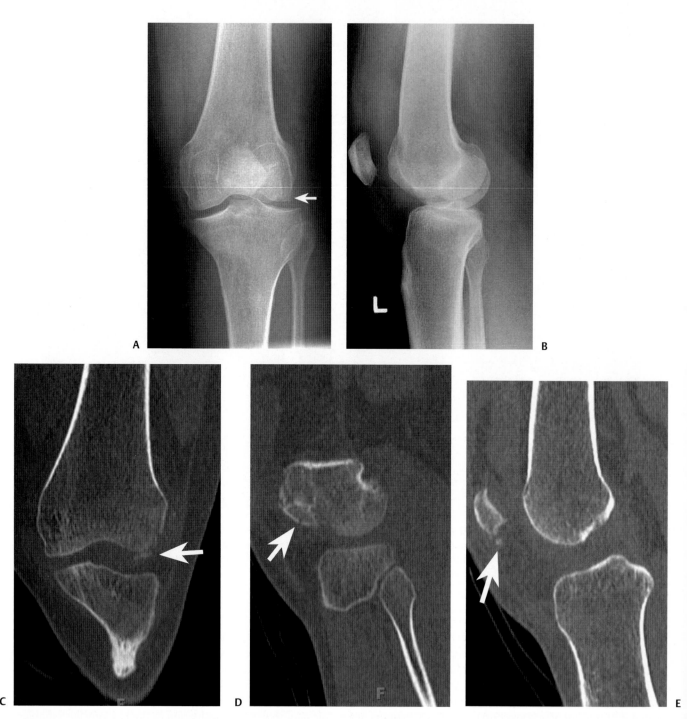

Fig. 17.5 Value of multimodality imaging. Posteroanterior **(A)** and lateral **(B)** radiographs of a young female involved in a motor vehicle accident show a mild cortical irregularity at the left lateral femoral condyle (*arrow on* **A**). **(C)** A coronal reconstructed CT image toward the anterior aspect of the knee better shows a small fracture frag-ment adjacent to the anterolateral femoral condyle (*arrow*). **(D)** A sagittal reconstructed CT image also shows the fracture (*arrow*) at the anterior aspect of the lateral femoral condyle. **(E)** A midline sagit-tal CT reconstructed image shows a small avulsion fracture at the inferior pole of the patella (*arrow*). (Continued on page 419)

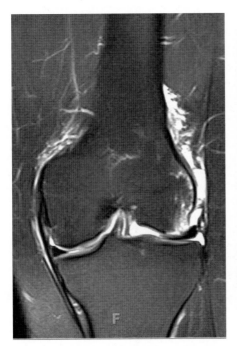

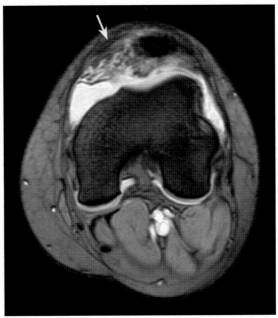

F

G

Fig. 17.5 (*Continued*) **(F)** A coronal STIR image shows a region of edema at the anterolateral aspect of the lateral femoral condyle but also shows disruption of lateral ligamentous structures. **(G)** An axial T2-weighted image better depicts disruption of the medial retinaculum (*arrow*).

eral anterior femoral condyle and the inferior pole of the patella, and disruption of the medial retinaculum (**Fig. 17.5F,G**).

■ Nuclear Scintigraphy

Although the imaging studies described above all provide excellent anatomic information, they are relatively limited in their abilities to provide high-quality physiologic information, specifically information related to bone turnover. In this regard, the imaging modality of choice is three-phase bone scintigraphy. For a bone scan, the patient is injected with technetium-99m phosphate or another radiopharmaceutical agent that emits gamma rays. Subsequently, the patient is placed under a scintillation camera to detect the presence and distribution of the radiotracer activity. The typical "three-phase" bone scan acquires the radiotracer activity information in the following phases:

- Blood-flow phase
- Soft-tissue phase
- Delayed or bone phase

Each one of these phases provides different information. In the blood-flow phase, increased uptake is found in areas of mature blood vessels. The second (soft-tissue) phase shows areas of neovascularity, such as with acute inflammation or vascular neoplasms. In the delayed or bone phase, the radio-

tracer has had time to adsorb newly formed crystals at sites of bone turnover.[10,11]

The advantages of bone scans are that they provide physiologic information regarding bone (more specifically, mineral turnover) and have the capability of surveying the entire body and detecting lesions early in their course. Their disadvantages are that the images are nonspecific and provide very poor spatial and anatomic resolution. Thus, the general thought is that with a bone scan, one is trading the anatomic detail provided by other imaging studies for physiologic information regarding the metabolic activity in the bone. Fortunately, in this era, systems have been developed that, in combination with CT scanning, allow scintigraphy and anatomic location to occur simultaneously. The indications for scintigraphy include evaluation of osseous lesions, usually metastatic disease, benign and malignant primary tumors, metabolic disorders, infection, and stress fractures.[10,12–14] Specifically, different findings in the phases of a three-phase bone scan can help differentiate a patient with osteomyelitis from one with soft-tissue infection without osseous involvement[15,16] (**Fig. 17.6**).

In the setting of osteomyelitis, conventional radiographs are the initial study of choice, but additional imaging modalities are often required for a definitive diagnosis because osteomyelitis is not detectable by radiography until approximately 40% bone destruction has occurred. MRI and nuclear scintigraphy can provide greater diagnostic sensitivity and

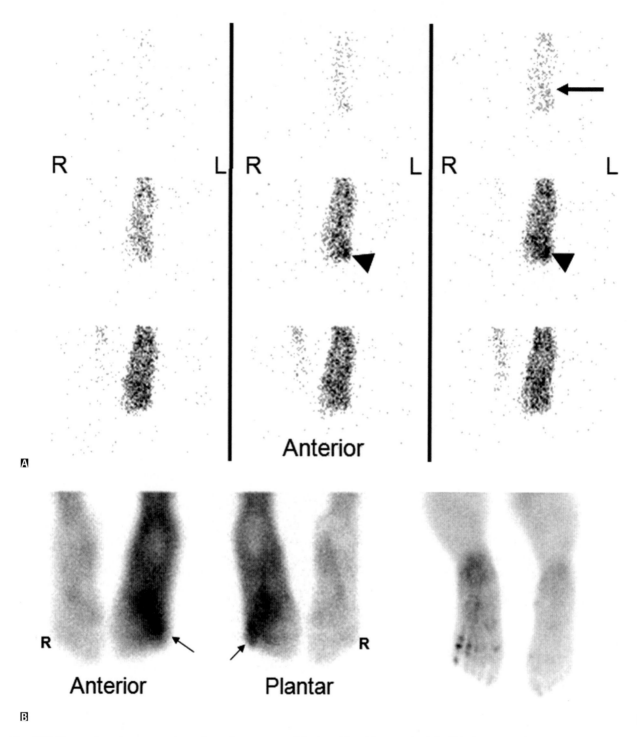

Fig. 17.6 Three-phase bone scan: to evaluate for osteomyelitis. In this 30-year-old female with a history of diabetes mellitus, left fifth metatarsal injury, overlying ulcer, and infection with clinical suspicion of osteomyelitis, conventional radiographs of the foot were negative for osteomyelitis or fracture. **(A)** The anterior blood flow image of the distal lower extremity shows asymmetrically increased blood flow to the entire left foot (*arrow*) with more focally increased blood flow to the left fifth digit (*arrowheads*). **(B)** A blood pool image shows increased blood pool diffusely in the left foot and more focally in the left fifth digit (*arrows*). **(C)** The delayed bone phase image shows focal, increased tracer uptake in the left fifth proximal and distal phalanx (*arrows*). Both sites are three-phase positive on bone scan, consistent with osteomyelitis. (Courtesy of Heather Jacene, MD.)

specificity: MRI is exquisitely sensitive to the presence of bone marrow edema and can show associated soft-tissue involvement. MRI is considered the imaging modality of choice for the early detection of osteomyelitis. Nuclear scintigraphy has an advantage in that it can quickly reveal other areas of involvement, which is a particularly important advantage for the pediatric patient who may have multiple sites of infec-tion.[17] It is important to note that when bone turnover is exceptionally high, such as in a patient with multiple myeloma and other lytic processes, conventional bone scan techniques may result in false-negative findings.[18,19]

Nuclear scintigraphy can also be used to help determine the age or physiologic activity of vertebral compression and other fractures[20–22] (**Fig. 17.7**). In such cases, nuclear

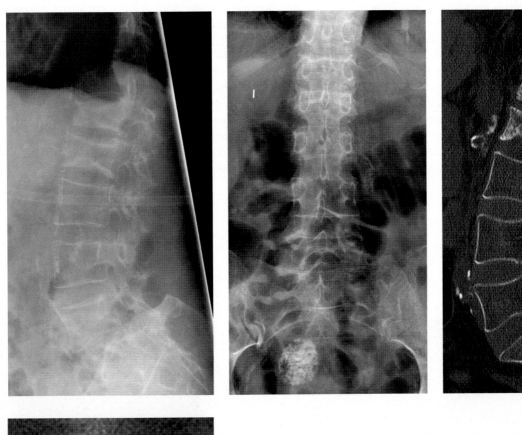
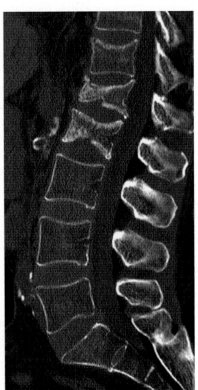

A–C

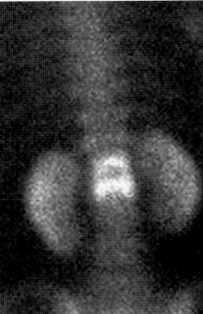

D

Fig. 17.7 Three-phase bone scan: to evaluate age and activity of vertebral compression fractures. Lateral **(A)** and posteroanterior **(B)** radiographs of an elderly woman with osteoporosis showing L2 and L3 vertebral compression fractures. **(C)** A sagittal reconstructed CT image better shows the osseous detail and configuration of the fractures, but it does not allow for accurate assessment of the relative age or physiologic activity of the fracture. **(D)** A posteroanterior delayed bone-phase image from a three-phase bone scan shows intense radiotracer uptake within the L2 and L3 vertebral bodies, suggestive of an acute or subacute fracture that is physiologically active.

scintigraphy may be indicated in patients for whom MRI is contraindicated, such as those with claustrophobia or non–MRI-compatible pacemakers and defibrillators.

■ Positron Emission Tomography

As does nuclear scintigraphy, positron emission tomography facilitates the evaluation of the physiologic activity in the tissues, in this case, glucose metabolism. Specifically, the patient is injected with a marker, 18-F-labeled 2-fluoro-2-deoxyglucose, which emits gamma rays based on the rate of glucose metabolism. A limited number of centers throughout North America provide this imaging modality, and therefore access to positron emission scanning may be somewhat difficult to obtain.

The most common indication for positron emission scanning is for the evaluation of malignant metastases or tumor recurrence (**Fig. 17.8**); positron emission tomography has shown limited promise in differentiating benign and malignant lesions.[23–26] In one study of 45 heterogeneous lesions, positron emission scanning provided high sensitivity and specificity for the differentiation of malignant and benign lesions (91% and 100%, respectively[24]), but positron emission tomography remains to be validated with larger studies.

Novel applications of positron emission tomography continue to be developed. Preliminary studies have shown that it can effectively determine whether vertebral compression fractures are pathologic in nature or secondary to osteoporosis alone.[27,28] Recent work has shown a potential role for positron emission tomography in patients with arthroplasty in terms of evaluating osteolysis and determining whether the prosthetic loosening is aseptic or infectious in nature.[29–31] The combined technique of positron emission tomography and CT has recently been advocated for use in diagnostically difficult cases of adolescent back pain.[32] The strength of this technique lies in the combination and correlation of functional data with the detailed anatomic findings of CT.

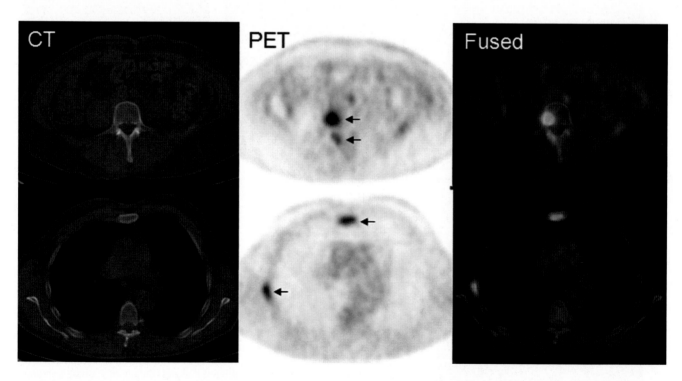

Fig. 17.8 A 50-year-old male with bladder transitional cell carcinoma. A proton emission tomography/CT image shows foci of intense fluorodeoxyglucose activity fusing a lumbar vertebra and pedicle, the sternum, and a right rib (*arrows*). Despite the lack of abnormality on the corresponding CT image, these findings are most consistent with bony metastases. *PET*, positron emission tomography. (Courtesy of Heather Jacene, MD.)

■ Summary

For the appropriate evaluation of a patient with musculoskeletal disease, it is important for clinicians to use all of the imaging tools and modalities in their armamentarium. Efficacy, cost, availability, and patient limitations all play roles in imaging modality selection. In most cases, most of the clinically important information can be obtained with conventional radiographs and MRI. However, for selected patients, the clinician must make the decision to request other imaging studies, such as CT, nuclear scintigraphy, and positron emission tomography, as they are indicated. With time, one can expect improvements in technology and the development of new imaging modalities that can be integrated into diagnosis and treatment algorithms.

References

1. Steinbach HL. The roentgen appearance of osteoporosis. Radiol Clin North Am 1964;2:191–207

2. Kamholtz R, Sze G. Current imaging in spinal metastatic disease. Semin Oncol 1991;18:158–169

3. Fayad LM, Johnson P, Fishman EK. Multidetector CT of musculoskeletal disease in the pediatric patient: principles, techniques, and clinical applications. Radiographics 2005;25:603–618

4. Fayad LM, Bluemke DA, Fishman EK. Musculoskeletal imaging with computed tomography and magnetic resonance imaging: when is computed tomography the study of choice? Curr Probl Diagn Radiol 2005;34:220–237

5. Genant HK, Wilson JS, Bovill EG, Brunelle FO, Murray WR, Rodrigo JJ. Computed tomography of the musculoskeletal system. J Bone Joint Surg Am 1980;62:1088–1101

6. Wilson JS, Korobkin M, Genant HK, Bovill EG Jr. Computed tomography of musculoskeletal disorders. AJR Am J Roentgenol 1978;131:55–61

7. Geijer M, El-Khoury GY. MDCT in the evaluation of skeletal trauma: principles, protocols, and clinical applications. Emerg Radiol 2006;13:7–18

8. Newton PO, Hahn GW, Fricka KB, Wenger DR. Utility of three-dimensional and multiplanar reformatted computed tomography for evaluation of pediatric congenital spine abnormalities. Spine (Phila Pa 1976) 2002;27:844–850

9. Mui LW, Engelsohn E, Umans H. Comparison of CT and MRI in patients with tibial plateau fracture: can CT findings predict ligament tear or meniscal injury? Skeletal Radiol 2007;36:145–151

10. Lee E, Worsley DF. Role of radionuclide imaging in the orthopedic patient. Orthop Clin North Am 2006;37:485–501

11. McCarthy EF, Frassica FJ. Diagnosing bone disease. In: McCarthy EF, Frassica FJ, eds. Pathology of Bone and Joint Disorders: With Clinical and Radiographic Correlation. Philadelphia: WB Saunders; 1998:1–24

12. Abdel-Dayem HM. The role of nuclear medicine in primary bone and soft tissue tumors. Semin Nucl Med 1997;27:355–363

13. Deutsch AL, Coel MN, Mink JH. Imaging of stress injuries to bone. Radiography, scintigraphy, and MR imaging. Clin Sports Med 1997;16:275–290

14. Greenspan A, Stadalnik RC. A musculoskeletal radiologist's view of nuclear medicine. Semin Nucl Med 1997;27:372–385

15. Alazraki NP. Radionuclide imaging in the evaluation of infections and inflammatory disease. Radiol Clin North Am 1993;31:783–794

16. El-Maghraby TAF, Moustafa HM, Pauwels EKJ. Nuclear medicine methods for evaluation of skeletal infection among other diagnostic modalities. Q J Nucl Med Mol Imaging 2006;50:167–192

17. Santiago Restrepo C, Giménez CR, McCarthy K. Imaging of osteomyelitis and musculoskeletal soft tissue infections: current concepts. Rheum Dis Clin North Am 2003;29:89–109

18. Ghanem N, Lohrmann C, Engelhardt M, et al. Whole-body MRI in the detection of bone marrow infiltration in patients with plasma cell neoplasms in comparison to the radiological skeletal survey. Eur Radiol 2006;16:1005–1014

19. Mulligan ME. Myeloma update. Semin Musculoskelet Radiol 2007;11:231–239

20. Masala S, Schillaci O, Massari F, et al. MRI and bone scan imaging in the preoperative evaluation of painful vertebral fractures treated with vertebroplasty and kyphoplasty. In Vivo 2005;19:1055–1060

21. Maynard AS, Jensen ME, Schweickert PA, Marx WF, Short JG, Kallmes DF. Value of bone scan imaging in predicting pain relief from percutaneous vertebroplasty in osteoporotic vertebral fractures. AJNR Am J Neuroradiol 2000;21:1807–1812

22. Fernandez-Ulloa M, Klostermeier TT, Lancaster KT. Orthopaedic nuclear medicine: the pelvis and hip. Semin Nucl Med 1998;28:25–40

23. Bastiaannet E, Groen H, Jager PL, et al. The value of FDG-PET in the detection, grading and response to therapy of soft tissue and bone sarcomas; a systematic review and meta-analysis. Cancer Treat Rev 2004;30:83–101

24. Feldman F, van Heertum R, Manos C. 18FDG PET scanning of benign and malignant musculoskeletal lesions. Skeletal Radiol 2003;32:201–208

25. Lodge MA, Lucas JD, Marsden PK, Cronin BF, O'Doherty MJ, Smith MA. A PET study of 18FDG uptake in soft tissue masses. Eur J Nucl Med 1999;26:22–30

26. Schwarzbach MHM, Dimitrakopoulou-Strauss A, Willeke F, et al. Clinical value of [18-F] fluorodeoxyglucose positron emission tomography imaging in soft tissue sarcomas. Ann Surg 2000;231:380–386

27. Schmitz A, Risse JH, Textor J, et al. FDG-PET findings of vertebral compression fractures in osteoporosis: preliminary results. Osteoporos Int 2002;13:755–761

28. Shin DS, Shon OJ, Byun SJ, Choi JH, Chun KA, Cho IH. Differentiation between malignant and benign pathologic fractures with F-18-fluoro-2-deoxy-D-glucose positron emission tomography/computed tomography. Skeletal Radiol 2008;37:415–421

29. Delank KS, Schmidt M, Michael JWP, Dietlein M, Schicha H, Eysel P. The implications of 18F-FDG PET for the diagnosis of endoprosthetic loosening and infection in hip and knee arthroplasty: results from a prospective, blinded study. BMC Musculoskelet Disord 2006;7:20–28

30. Manthey N, Reinhard P, Moog F, Knesewitsch P, Hahn K, Tatsch K. The use of [18 F] fluorodeoxyglucose positron emission tomography to differentiate between synovitis, loosening and infection of hip and knee prostheses. Nucl Med Commun 2002;23:645–653

31. Mumme T, Reinartz P, Alfer J, Müller-Rath R, Buell U, Wirtz DC. Diagnostic values of positron emission tomography versus triple-phase bone scan in hip arthroplasty loosening. Arch Orthop Trauma Surg 2005;125:322–329

32. Ovadia D, Metser U, Lievshitz G, Yaniv M, Wientroub S, Even-Sapir E. Back pain in adolescents: assessment with integrated 18F-fluoride positron-emission tomography-computed tomography. J Pediatr Orthop 2007;27:90–93

18 MRI Safety

Monica D. Watkins and Bruce A. Wasserman

As with any procedure, maintaining the safety of the patient and health care team during an MRI examination is of utmost importance, and patient safety considerations begin with the referring clinician. A sound understanding of MRI safety issues not only ensures minimal risk to the patient but also can avoid needless expenses and delays in examinations. Although the MRI center is generally responsible for safety screening, the referring physician can minimize even further the chance of an adverse effect by being aware of important contraindications to MRI and of safety concerns that might put an individual at risk. It can be very comforting to a patient to have the clinician alleviate safety concerns and answer preliminary questions that might otherwise contribute to a growing anxiety in the days leading up to the examination. This chapter reviews these issues and provides guidelines for maximizing safety.

■ Physiologic Effects of the Magnetic Field

In an MRI scanner, the patient's body is subjected to the baseline static magnetic field and the time-varying magnetic fields created by RF fields and receiver coils. The strength of these magnetic fields is measured in gauss or tesla (T) units; 1 T equals 10,000 gauss. For comparison, the strength of the earth's magnetic field is 0.6 gauss; the strength of clinical MRI scanners generally ranges from 0.5 to 3.0 T.[1] The FDA has guidelines for the exposure of patients to both static and time-varying magnetic fields.[2]

Static Magnetic Fields

Currently, the FDA approves clinical imaging using a static magnetic field strength of up to 4.0 T for patients <1 month old and up to 8.0 T for older patients.[2] Many studies have evaluated the potential biologic effects of a static magnetic field, and there has been no clear evidence of deleterious effects.[3] Although there have been concerns about an elevation of skin and core body temperatures induced by the magnetic field, investigators have concluded that harmful heating does not occur in human subjects.[4,5] Reversible electrocardiogram changes (e.g., an increase in the amplitude of the T wave or

a nonspecific wave form) secondary to the conductive nature of blood have been noted.[6] However, this "magnetohydrodynamic effect" has not been associated with a clinically adverse effect.

At strengths of 4 T, patients may experience transient reversible biologic effects, such as nausea (that may be caused by stimulation of the vestibulolabryrinthine complex) or a flashing light sensation (magnetophosphenes, thought to be caused by direct excitation of the optic nerves or retina, by changing magnetic fields, or by rapid eye movements).[7]

Time-Varying Magnetic Fields

Time-varying magnetic fields or gradient magnetic fields can induce current in the body, which can have two possible biologic effects: heating and neuromuscular stimulation. Even in the absence of metal implants, body temperatures have been shown to rise during MRI, although temperature changes were minor (i.e., <0.6°C).[8] The FDA has suggested guidelines to limit the risk of these effects by restricting the strength of time-varying magnetic fields.[2] The intensity of the RF energy absorbed by tissue is termed the specific absorption rate and is measured in watts per kilogram. The FDA reports that specific absorption rates of ≤3 W/kg for the head, ≤4 W/kg (averaged) for the rest of the body, and ≤8.0 W/kg for any 1 g of tissue pose no substantial risk.[2] Usually, higher specific absorption rate exposures are a concern with faster pulse sequences.

■ Metallic Substances

Field Distortion

Image quality depends on the ability to maintain homogeneity of the magnetic field surrounding the patient. Metallic artifacts can result in misregistered spatial information or signal loss, leading to image distortion. Three types of magnetic materials may cause artifacts because of their inherent abilities to disturb the uniformity of magnetic fields used for imaging: ferromagnetic, paramagnetic, and diamagnetic materials. Of these three, ferromagnetic materials (e.g., iron, nickel, and martensitic stainless steel) concentrate and retain magnetism the most, resulting in severe distortion of the images. Paramagnetic or weakly ferromagnetic materials (e.g., platinum) have a minimal effect on magnetic field homogeneity and result in less image distortion. Diamagnetic materials (e.g., zinc, gold, and copper) do not affect or affect only minimally the static or local magnetic fields.

Metallic Objects in Magnetic Fields

The clinical value of an MRI examination in a patient with metallic hardware depends on the proximity of the hardware to the site of interest. For example, one can anticipate a limited evaluation of neural foramina adjacent to an anterior cervical fusion or an inability to detect an epidural abscess adjacent to pedicle screw instrumentation. Newer pulse sequences have been developed that allow for imaging in the presence of metallic implants (see Chapter 16). Myelography remains a viable alternative for the postoperative spine. CT also is a valuable alternative in postoperative patients, particularly in conjunction with myelography.

In addition to causing distortion of images, some metallic foreign bodies or surgical implants can move or generate heat in the presence of a magnetic field, possibly leading to injury or death.[9,10] For this reason, each patient must be screened for metallic objects within the body, usually with a verbal interview and a written checklist.

Of particular concern are metallic foreign bodies within the orbit that may dislodge and rupture the globe or damage the optic nerve. To our knowledge, there is only one reported case of a patient who suffered a vitreous hemorrhage, caused by a dislodged metal fragment (2.0 × 3.5 mm), that led to blindness.[11] Although it is standard for MRI facilities to prescreen for metallic orbital foreign bodies, methods of accomplishing this screening vary. Conventional radiographs of the orbits are said to detect metallic fragments as small as 0.1 × 0.1 × 0.1 mm. However, there is debate over which patients should be referred for conventional radiographs. Many MRI centers obtain orbital radiographs of patients with an occupational history of welding, but some experts advocate obtaining films only if the patient is aware of a previous orbital exposure to metal without removal of the fragment by an ophthalmologist.[12] At the authors' institution, patients with a history of working with metal undergo screening orbital conventional radiographs. Alternatively, review of a previous CT scan, including the entirety of the orbits, is often considered sufficient.

In addition to assessing for orbital foreign bodies, the clinician should question the patient regarding any history of metallic foreign bodies near other vital structures, such as the lungs or spinal cord. For example, bullet fragments in the spinal canal contraindicate MRI because they may be ferromagnetic.

Implant Safety Profiles

The FDA requires testing of all implants to evaluate their safety profiles and classify them as MRI safe, conditionally safe, or unsafe. The list of these devices is extensive and constantly changing, especially as more objects are tested at 3 T and higher, precluding a complete review of these devices in this chapter. A regularly updated list of reviewed implants and devices is available online at http://www.MRIsafety.com. It is important to be aware of devices that absolutely contraindicate MRI scanning, including the following:

- Implantable cardiac defibrillators
- Cardiac pacemakers
- Implantable medication infusion pumps
- Ferromagnetic aneurysm clips (e.g., stainless steel)
- Poppen-Blaylock carotid artery clamps
- Spinal/bone fusion stimulators
- Cochlear implants
- Tissue expanders
- Gastric electrical stimulation devices

Certain models of some devices (e.g., implantable cardiac defibrillators, cardiac pacemakers, spinal/bone fusion stimulators, and cochlear implants) may be scanned under strict criteria. However, many MRI centers still consider as absolute contraindications the presence of such devices or of devices that do not meet the required technical conditions (see below). Of note, the Starr-Edwards Model Pre-6000 heart valve prosthesis (Baxter Healthcare, Santa Ana, CA) is now designated as conditionally MRI safe, although previously it was thought to be an absolute contraindication to an MRI examination.[13] In recent years, multiple in vitro and in vivo controlled studies have shown increasing evidence that some patients with cardiac pacemakers can be scanned safely under specific conditions, despite the potential for arrhythmia and death.[14–18] However, in most situations, a pacemaker remains an absolute contraindication for MRI unless the procedure is an orchestrated effort between cardiology and radiology, with informed consent of the patient.[19,20]

Similar caution is warranted for patients with neurostimulation systems for deep brain stimulation of the thalamus, globus pallidus, and subthalamic nucleus as a treatment for movement disorders. Although many patients have been scanned successfully without incident, there are specific guidelines regarding the technique.[21,22] Currently, the Pulsar Cochlear Implant (MED-EL Corp., Durham, NC) can be scanned, but only under specific conditions on a 0.2-T machine. The Nucleus 24 Auditory Brainstem Implant System (Cochlear Corp., Englewood, CO) has a removable magnet and may be scanned up to 1.5 T, again under specific conditions. It is suggested that the manufacturer of these cochlear devices be contacted before imaging.[23] In general, imaging of deep-brain stimulators and this specific implant should be performed only after discussion with a neurologist and radiologist. There are six specific requirements that also must be met to obtain an MRI study of a patient with a spinal/bone fusion stimulator[24,25]:

- Cathodes of the implantable spinal fusion stimulator should be a minimum of 1 cm from nerve roots.
- Conventional radiographs should be obtained before MRI to verify that there are no broken leads for the implantable spinal fusion stimulator.
- The study should be obtained on an MRI system with static fields of 1.5 T or less, avoiding pulse sequences that expose patient to high levels of RF energy.
- The patient should be observed continuously.
- To reduce artifact, the implantable spinal fusion stimulator should be placed as far from the spinal canal and bone graft as possible.
- Selected imaging techniques, such as the use of FSE pulse sequences, should be used to reduce artifact.

In the past, residual pacing wires also were considered to be a contraindication to MRI. However, the current consensus is that such patients may undergo MRI if the wires are cut short (flush with skin) and there are no loops of wire outside the patient. Again, consultation with the patient's cardiologist may be necessary.[26]

Devices that are conditionally safe for MRI are implants that may be scanned if certain guidelines are satisfied. These devices include weakly magnetic intravascular filters, stents, and coils. MRI of patients with such devices may require a waiting period of 6 to 8 weeks after implantation to ensure that movement of the device caused by the magnetic field does not disturb its implantation onto the vessel wall.[27,28] The evolving list of all such devices is beyond the scope of this chapter, but in general, one should acquire additional information (e.g., brand name of the device and date of implantation) for patients who have undergone recent placement of such devices. Many MRI centers require documentation of this information before scanning is allowed.

Devices that are safe for MRI are those known to produce no clinically significant hazard in the MRI environment. In general, these devices have no electronically or magnetically activated component, are made from a nonferromagnetic material (such as titanium or nitinol), and may undergo MRI scanning at ≤1.5 T immediately after implantation.[29,30] Many of these devices have been tested in the 3-T environment. It is important to obtain the brand name of the device from patients (who may have the package insert) or from their records. Safe devices also include orthopaedic implants firmly placed within the bone because, although they may be weakly magnetic, they do not dislodge or generate substantial heat.

Superficial Metal

There are safety concerns not only with internal metallic devices but also with skin surface metal, such as medicine patches containing a metal foil, surgical staples, tattoos, or permanent cosmetics. It is standard practice to remove transdermal medicine patches containing metallic foil at the time of an MRI. Tope and Shellock[31] reviewed the results of a questionnaire given to 1032 patients with cosmetic tattoos. Only two patients experienced any sensory consequences (i.e., "slight tingling" or a "burning" sensation). These sensations are thought to be caused by heating from iron oxide or other metal-based pigment. The FDA Center for Food Safety and Applied Nutrition, Office of Cosmetics and Colors fact sheet states, "The risks of avoiding an MRI when your doctor has recommended one are likely to be much greater than the risk of complications from the interaction between the MRI and tattoo or permanent makeup."[32] Most practices agree that an ice pack or cold compress can be applied during scanning to the site of the tattoo, permanent cosmetics, or surgical staples to reduce the chance of thermal injury.

External Metallic Objects

In addition to precautions about internal foreign bodies, MRI centers screen for external metallic devices that may become projectiles in the MRI suite. Injuries and death have occurred when large metallic objects, such as a ferrous oxygen tank, have been brought into the MRI suite.[33–35] Even small objects that may not seem dangerous to many patients, such as jewelry or hairpins, can become projectiles and cause injury. It is standard procedure to ask patients to remove such objects and to empty their pockets.

■ Pregnancy

Although there are no known deleterious effects of an MRI examination during pregnancy, concerns about potential side effects remain. One such concern is that electromagnetic fields could disrupt cell division. Because cell division is more rapid in the first trimester, it usually is acceptable to delay MRI until after the first trimester.

Because of such potential complications, MRI during pregnancy is obtained on a case-by-case basis, weighing the risk and benefit for each examination; this procedure is the accepted standard of care advocated by the American College of Radiology.[36] Shellock and Kanal[37] have suggested that "MR imaging may be used in pregnant women if other nonionizing forms of diagnostic imaging are inadequate or if the examination provides important information that would otherwise require exposure to ionizing radiation." In almost all institutions, written, informed consent is obtained.

■ Contrast

MRI contrast agents are often used in the postoperative patient to evaluate for infection or scar tissue, in patients with known or suspected musculoskeletal tumors, and for MR angiography of the carotid and peripheral arteries. The gadolinium ion contains seven unpaired electrons in the outer shell, providing a large magnetic moment. This paramagnetic property enhances the relaxation rates of nearby water protons. Although gadolinium itself is toxic, chelation with other substances makes it nontoxic and usable as a contrast agent. Over time, within the body, the free gadolinium ion can dissociate from its chelate. Normally, the amount of free ions is low because of rapid clearance through the kidney.

In addition to screening for the specific populations listed below, it is important to obtain a patient's allergy history, especially with regard to whether the patient had a reaction to gadolinium contrast previously and, if so, the nature of that reaction. A history of a mild reaction (such as hives) to gadolinium generally requires premedication with prednisone and diphenhydramine. A history of reactions as severe as respiratory or circulatory compromise is a contraindication to the use of MRI contrast. An adverse reaction to MRI contrast is rare and generally expected to occur in less than 1% of patients.[38] Reactions range from headache to weakness and, very rarely, anaphylaxis.[38]

For patients with renal failure, there is concern that decreased renal clearance may result in accumulating free ion levels and toxicity. Clinicians usually recommend that a patient undergo dialysis within 24 hours after contrast administration. The FDA recently issued an alert for the use of gadolinium intravenous contrast in patients with advanced renal failure (i.e., those currently requiring dialysis or with an estimated glomerular filtration rate of <30 mL/min/1.73m^2) because of the risk of inducing nephrogenic systemic fibrosis/nephrogenic fibrosing dermopathy.[39]

Nephrogenic systemic fibrosis/nephrogenic fibrosing dermopathy is a progressive and sometimes fatal disease seen in patients with reduced renal function, and it causes fibrosis of the skin and connective tissues throughout the body, including muscles of the extremities or abdomen, the diaphragm, and pulmonary vessels. Gadolinium has been detected in the soft tissues of several patients with nephrogenic systemic fibrosis who were exposed to it as a radiographic contrast agent, supporting its association with this disease.[40] Deo et al[41] studied a population of end-stage renal disease patients for 18 months and found that each radiologic study that used a gadolinium-based contrast agent presented a 2.4% risk for nephrogenic systemic fibrosis. Broome et al[42] reported an odds ratio of 22.3 (95% confidence interval; range, 1.3 to 378.9) for the development of nephrogenic systemic fibrosis after gadolinium exposure in 168 dialysis patients. An important observation in that study was that 10 of the 12 patients who developed nephrogenic systemic fibrosis underwent dialysis within 2 days of gadolinium administration. The timing of dialysis relative to gadolinium administration may be critical for the prevention of this disease, but thus far little is known regarding the effectiveness of dialysis in reducing the risk of nephrogenic systemic fibrosis.[43] At the authors' institution, a creatinine/estimated glomerular filtration rate measurement is currently obtained for patients at risk for renal dysfunction, including those ≥65 years old or with a history of diabetes, those with renal disease or transplantation, and those with liver disease or hepatorenal syndrome.

In pregnant patients, contrast agents cross the placenta, enter the fetal collecting system, and then are excreted into the amniotic fluid. To the authors' knowledge, no studies show the clearance rate of MRI contrast agents in the fetus, but it is possible that a chelated gadolinium agent could stay within the amniotic fluid long enough to allow toxic free ions to accumulate. Gadolinium-based intravenous MR contrast is labeled by the FDA as a category C medication; that is, there is a lack of controlled studies with which to evaluate the effects. Contrast is generally not administered to pregnant patients unless the potential benefit outweighs its risks and unless written, informed consent has been obtained.[20,44] The theoretic risk of free ion accumulation is smaller if the agent is administered toward the end of gestation in the third trimester, leaving less time for dissociation and accumulation of free ions before fetus delivery.

When a breast-feeding mother receives contrast, it is expected that most of the contrast will have cleared by 24 hours, leaving minimal residual contrast (<0.04%) to be excreted into the breast milk.[20,45] However, a breast-feeding woman should be given the option to abstain from breast-feeding for 24 hours and to pump and discard breast milk for this time period.

Other patient populations have a theoretic risk of toxicity from gadolinium, although no direct clinical evidence has been established. For example, patients with elevated levels of copper (such as those with Wilson disease) or zinc may have increased free ion accumulation after contrast administration because these metals may compete with gadolinium for the chelate. In vivo studies suggest that gadolinium administration can lead to vasoocclusive complications in patients with sickle cell disease because deoxygenated sickle erythrocytes align perpendicularly to a magnetic field.[46,47] However, no clinical evidence suggests that these agents precipitate a sickle cell crisis. Some facilities consider sickle cell disease to be a contraindication to the administration of gadolinium.

Physicians, both clinicians and radiologists, are often faced with the decision to give gadolinium contrast to a patient with a history of an allergy to ionic contrast agents, such as those used for CT. Studies have shown that patients with a history of an ionic contrast allergy are at a higher risk for a reaction, as are those with asthma and multiple medication allergies.[38,48] Often, MRI centers will require consent from such patients before giving contrast, and some centers may require that the patient be premedicated.

■ Claustrophobia

The key to obtaining an informative MRI study is a cooperative patient who is able to remain still for the duration of the examination. Scanning an uncooperative patient often leads to poor image quality with motion artifact, and it increases the anxiety level of the individual for future examinations. It is important to identify claustrophobic patients who may be unable to tolerate the examination and to determine if sedation is needed. In some cases, patients' fears and anxiety may be alleviated by being told they can communicate with the technicians via an intercom and can stop the examination if needed. A benzodiazepine, such as diazepam, may be used to sedate a nervous patient, with additional monitoring provided by the nursing staff. Occasionally, a patient may be unable to tolerate imaging, even with sedation. In such cases, an open (unenclosed) MRI examination might be the best

alternative. However, image quality may be sacrificed in this procedure because of the lower field strength of some open MRI systems.

■ Summary

Although MRI facilities are mandated to present patients with a prescreening checklist, the referring physician can prevent the need to reschedule the patient or abort the procedure by beginning the screening process and alleviating some of the concerns or fears the patient may have regarding the examination. It is imperative that the physician be familiar with the few absolute contraindications to MRI and identify patients for whom additional information is needed. Furthermore, brief questions to screen for claustrophobia, pregnancy, and known gadolinium contrast allergy, combined with identifying potential safety hazards via knowledge of the patient's history that might put the patient at risk during an examination, can facilitate obtaining the most informative and the safest study possible.

References

1. Roth CK. Patient care and safety for magnetic resonance imaging. In: Rad Tech's Guide to MRI: Imaging Procedures, Patient Care, and Safety. Williston, VT: Blackwell Science Publishers; 2002:1–38
2. United States Department of Health and Human Services. Criteria for Significant Risk Investigations of Magnetic Resonance Diagnostic Devices. Rockville, MD: U.S. Department of Health and Human Services, Office of the Surgeon General; 2003
3. Schenck JF. Health effects and safety of static magnetic fields. In: Shellock FG, ed. Magnetic Resonance Procedures: Health Effects and Safety. Boca Raton, FL: CRC Press; 2001:1–29
4. Shellock FG, Schaefer DJ, Crues JV. Exposure to a 1.5-T static magnetic field does not alter body and skin temperatures in man. Magn Reson Med 1989;11:371–375
5. Shellock FG, Schaefer DJ, Gordon CJ. Effect of a 1.5 T static magnetic field on body temperature of man. Magn Reson Med 1986;3:644–647
6. Chakeres DW, Kangarlu A, Boudoulas H, Young DC. Effect of static magnetic field exposure of up to 8 Tesla on sequential human vital sign measurements. J Magn Reson Imaging 2003;18:346–352
7. Schenck JF, Dumoulin CL, Redington RW, Kressel HY, Elliott RT, McDougall IL. Human exposure to 4.0-Tesla magnetic fields in a whole-body scanner. Med Phys 1992;19:1089–1098
8. Shellock FG, Crues JV. MR procedures: biologic effects, safety, and patient care. Radiology 2004;232:635–652
9. Boutin RD, Briggs JE, Williamson MR. Injuries associated with MR imaging: survey of safety records and methods used to screen patients for metallic foreign bodies before imaging. AJR Am J Roentgenol 1994;162:189–194
10. Klucznik RP, Carrier DA, Pyka R, Haid RW. Placement of a ferromagnetic intracerebral aneurysm clip in a magnetic field with a fatal outcome. Radiology 1993;187:855–856

11. Kelly WM, Paglen PG, Pearson JA, San Diego AG, Soloman MA. Ferromagnetism of intraocular foreign body causes unilateral blindness after MR study. AJNR Am J Neuroradiol 1986;7:243–245
12. Seidenwurm DJ, McDonnell CH III, Raghavan N, Breslau J. Cost utility analysis of radiographic screening for an orbital foreign body before MR imaging. AJNR Am J Neuroradiol 2000;21:426–433
13. Shellock FG. Heart valve prostheses and annuloplasty rings. In: Reference Manual for Magnetic Resonance Safety, Implants, and Devices: 2007 Edition. Los Angeles: Biomedical Research Publishing Group; 2007:224–226
14. Gimbel JR, Johnson D, Levine PA, Wilkoff BL. Safe performance of magnetic resonance imaging on five patients with permanent cardiac pacemakers. Pacing Clin Electrophysiol 1996;19:913–919
15. Martin ET, Coman JA, Shellock FG, Pulling CC, Fair R, Jenkins K. Magnetic resonance imaging and cardiac pacemaker safety at 1.5-Tesla. J Am Coll Cardiol 2004;43:1315–1324
16. Pennell DJ. Cardiac magnetic resonance with a pacemaker in-situ: can it be done? J Cardiovasc Magn Reson 1999;1:72
17. Roguin A, Zviman MM, Meininger GR, et al. Modern pacemaker and implantable cardioverter/defibrillator systems can be magnetic resonance imaging safe: in vitro and in vivo assessment of safety and function at 1.5 T. Circulation 2004;110:475–482
18. Sommer T, Vahlhaus C, Lauck G, et al. MR imaging and cardiac pacemakers: in-vitro evaluation and in-vivo studies in 51 patients at 0.5 T. Radiology 2000;215:869–879
19. Kalin R, Stanton MS. Current clinical issues for MRI scanning of pacemaker and defibrillator patients. Pacing Clin Electrophysiol 2005;28:326–328
20. Kanal E, Borgstede JP, Barkovich AJ, et al. American College of Radiology white paper on MR safety. AJR Am J Roentgenol 2002;178:1335–1347

21. Shellock FG. Neurostimulation systems: general information. The effects of magnetic resonance imaging (MRI) on deep brain stimulation system (Activa) for movement disorders. Section II: MR procedures and implants, devices, and materials. In: Reference Manual for Magnetic Resonance Safety, Implants, and Devices: 2007 Edition. Los Angeles: Biomedical Research Publishing Group; 2007: 244–246

22. Shellock FG. Neurostimulation systems: deep brain stimulation. In: Reference Manual for Magnetic Resonance Safety, Implants, and Devices: 2007 Edition. Los Angeles: Biomedical Research Publishing Group; 2007:247–255

23. Shellock FG. Cochlear implants. Section II: MR procedures and implants, devices, and materials. In: Reference Manual for Magnetic Resonance Safety, Implants, and Devices: 2007 Edition. Los Angeles: Biomedical Research Publishing Group; 2007:186–188

24. Shellock FG, Hatfield M, Simon BJ, et al. Implantable spinal fusion stimulator: assessment of MR safety and artifacts. J Magn Reson Imaging 2000;12:214–223

25. Shellock FG. Bone fusion stimulator/spinal fusion stimulator. Section II: MR procedures and implants, devices, and materials. In: Reference Manual for Magnetic Resonance Safety, Implants, and Devices: 2007 Edition. Los Angeles: Biomedical Research Publishing Group; 2007:154–157

26. Hartnell GG, Spence L, Hughes LA, Cohen MC, Saouaf R, Buff B. Safety of MR imaging in patients who have retained metallic materials after cardiac surgery. AJR Am J Roentgenol 1997;168:1157–1159

27. Shellock FG, Shellock VJ. Metallic stents: evaluation of MR imaging safety. AJR Am J Roentgenol 1999;173:543–547

28. Teitelbaum GP, Bradley WG Jr, Klein BD. MR imaging artifacts, ferromagnetism, and magnetic torque of intravascular filters, stents, and coils. Radiology 1988;166:657–664

29. Pride GL Jr, Kowal J, Mendelsohn DB, Chason DP, Fleckenstein JL. Safety of MR scanning in patients with nonferromagnetic aneurysm clips. J Magn Reson Imaging 2000;12:198–200

30. Shellock FG. Section II: MR procedures and implants, devices, and materials. In: Reference Manual for Magnetic Resonance Safety, Implants, and Devices: 2007 Edition. Los Angeles: Biomedical Research Publishing Group; 2007:125–315

31. Tope WD, Shellock FG. Magnetic resonance imaging and permanent cosmetics (tattoos): survey of complications and adverse events. J Magn Reson Imaging 2002;15:180–184

32. United States Health Care Administration. Tattoos and Permanent Makeup. Rockville, MD: U.S. Food and Drug Administration; 2006

33. Chaljub G, Kramer LA, Johnson RF III, Johnson RF Jr, Singh H, Crow WN. Projectile cylinder accidents resulting from the presence of ferromagnetic nitrous oxide or oxygen tanks in the MR suite. AJR Am J Roentgenol 2001;177:27–30

34. Colletti PM. Size "H" oxygen cylinder: accidental MR projectile at 1.5 Tesla. J Magn Reson Imaging 2004;19:141–143

35. United States Health Care Administration, Center for Devices and Radiological Health. MRI safety. http://www.fda.gov/cdrh/safety/mri-safety.html.

36. Kanal E, Barkovich AJ, Bell C, et al; ACR Blue Ribbon Panel on MR Safety. ACR guidance document for safe MR practices: 2007. AJR Am J Roentgenol 2007;188:1447–1474

37. Shellock FG, Kanal E; SMRI Safety Committee. Policies, guidelines, and recommendations for MR imaging safety and patient management. J Magn Reson Imaging 1991;1:97–101

38. Dillman JR, Ellis JH, Cohan RH, Strouse PJ, Jan SC. Frequency and severity of acute allergic-like reactions to gadolinium-containing IV contrast media in children and adults. AJR Am J Roentgenol 2007;189:1533–1538

39. United States Health Care Administration. Information on gadolinium-containing contrast agents. http://www.fda.gov/cder/drug/infopage/gcca/default.htm.

40. High WA, Ayers RA, Chandler J, Zito G, Cowper SE. Gadolinium is detectable within the tissue of patients with nephrogenic systemic fibrosis. J Am Acad Dermatol 2007;56:21–26

41. Deo A, Fogel M, Cowper SE. Nephrogenic systemic fibrosis: a population study examining the relationship of disease development to gadolinium exposure. Clin J Am Soc Nephrol 2007;2:264–267

42. Broome DR, Girguis MS, Baron PW, Cottrell AC, Kjellin I, Kirk GA. Gadodiamide-associated nephrogenic systemic fibrosis: why radiologists should be concerned. AJR Am J Roentgenol 2007;188:586–592

43. Saab G, Abu-Alfa A. Will dialysis prevent the development of nephrogenic systemic fibrosis after gadolinium-based contrast administration? [letter] AJR Am J Roentgenol 2007;189:W169

44. American College of Radiology. Manual on Contrast Media. 5th ed. Reston, VA: American College of Radiology; 2004

45. Kubik-Huch RA, Gottstein-Aalame NM, Frenzel T, et al. Gadopentetate dimeglumine excretion into human breast milk during lactation. Radiology 2000;216:555–558

46. Brody AS, Sorette MP, Gooding CA, et al. AUR memorial Award. Induced alignment of flowing sickle erythrocytes in a magnetic field. A preliminary report. Invest Radiol 1985;20:560–566

47. Brody AS, Embury SH, Mentzer WC, Winkler ML, Gooding CA. Preservation of sickle cell blood-flow patterns during MR imaging: an in vivo study. AJR Am J Roentgenol 1988;151:139–141

48. Nelson KL, Gifford LM, Lauber-Huber C, Gross CA, Lasser TA. Clinical safety of gadopentetate dimeglumine. Radiology 1995;196:439–443

Index

Note: Page numbers followed by *f* and *t* indicate figures and tables, respectively.

A

Abscess
  of cervical spine, 259–262
  epidural
    of cervical spine, 259–261
    in pediatric patient, 341–342
    thoracolumbar, 303, 305*f*
  of foot/ankle, 216–217, 217*f*
  on postgadolinium T1-weighted images, 90, 92*f*
  of wrist/hand, 135–136
Acetabular labrum
  normal anatomy, 38, 40*f*, 42, 43*f*–44*f*, 147, 147*f*
  pathology, 147–148, 148*t*
  postoperative MRI evaluation, 151
  tears, 147–151, 148*f*–149*f*
    classification, 149, 149*f*
Acetabulum
  articular cartilage, normal, 147*f*
  normal anatomy, 39*f*–40*f*, 42, 42*f*–43*f*
Achilles tendinitis, 209–210
Achilles tendinosis, 209–210, 210*f*
Achilles tendon
  disorders, 209–210, 209*f*
  normal anatomy, 51*f*, 54, 55*f*
  repair, postoperative MRI findings, 221–222, 222*f*
  tear, 210, 210*f*
AC joint. *See* Acromioclavicular joint
ACL. *See* Anterior cruciate ligament
Acquired immune deficiency syndrome, 262, 264, 303
Acromioclavicular joint
  abnormalities of, 105
  capsular hypertrophy of, 105, 109*f*
  morphology of, 103
  Mumford procedure and, 114
  normal anatomy, 17, 22
  osteoarthritis, 109, 109*f*
Acromion, 17, 19*f*–20*f*
  morphology, types of, 103, 104*f*–105*f*
Acute transverse myelopathy, in cervical spine, 262

Adhesive capsulitis, of shoulder, 112–113, 113*f*
Adolescent(s), spine, normal anatomy, 339–340
AIDS. *See* Acquired immune deficiency syndrome
Alcohol abuse, and osteonecrosis of knee, 191
α angle, 157, 160*f*
Amyloidosis, cervical spinal involvement in, 265
Anatomy. *See* specific anatomical entity
Anconeus (muscle), 23, 24*f*, 25, 25*f*, 26*f*, 27
Aneurysm, 381
Aneurysmal bone cyst, 388, 389*f*
  spinal, 320*t*, 322–324, 323*f*
Angiography. *See* MR angiography
Angiolipoma, spinal, 327
Ankle. *See also* Foot/ankle
  sprain(s)
    lateral, 203–204, 204*f*
    medial, 204–205, 204*f*
    syndesmotic (high), 205, 205*f*
Ankylosing spondylitis
  cervical spinal involvement, 235, 236*f*, 264
  hip involvement, 160
Annular ligament, of elbow, injury, 121
Anterior cruciate ligament
  avulsion, 174, 174*f*
  cyclops lesion, 199, 199*f*
  graft, tunnel placement, 199*f*
  normal anatomy, 42, 44, 45*f*, 46, 47*f*–48*f*
  reconstruction, MRI findings after, 198–199, 198*f*–199*f*
  tears, 174–177, 174*f*–178*f*, 175*t*
Anterior tibial tendon, disorders, 214, 215*f*
Anterolateral ankle impingement, 215, 217*f*
Arachnoiditis, 311, 312*f*
Arthritis. *See also* Osteoarthritis
  cervical spine involvement, 264–266
  inflammatory, 362–363
  psoriatic, cervical spinal involvement, 265
  septic
    of elbow, 124
    of foot/ankle, 217
    of shoulder, 112

Arthrography. *See* MR arthrography

Articular cartilage. *See also* Osteoarthritis
    components, 353
    of elbow, 362, 365*f*
    of feet, 362
    gradient-echo image, 80, 82*f*
    of hands, 362
    of hip, 359–360, 362*f*–364*f*
    imaging protocols for, 353–356
    of knee, 356–359, 356*f*, 359*f*–361*f*
    lesions
        classification, 356, 357*t*–358*t*
        grading, 356, 357*t*–358*t*
    MR signal characteristics, 353
    repair, postoperative imaging, 363–367,
        365*f*–367*f*
    specialized pulse sequences for, 353–355,
        354*f*–356*f*, 355*t*
    structure, 353
    zonal histology, 353, 354*f*

Artifact(s), 14–15
    magnetic materials causing, 425–426
    metallic substances and, 425–426
    susceptibility, gradient-echo imaging and, 14

Astrocytoma, low-grade, spinal, 331–332

Atlantoaxial dissociation, 238, 239*f*

Atlantooccipital dissociation, 236–237

Atlas (C1), 62, 62*f*
    trauma, 237–238

Axis (C2), 62, 62*f*
    trauma, 238, 238*f*

B

Baker (popliteal) cyst, 193, 194*f*, 374–375, 375*f*

Bankart
    lesion, 82*f*, 98-99, 98*f*, 100*f*, 103
    repair, 114

Biceps brachii muscle
    anchor, 101, 101*f*, 102, 113
    normal anatomy, 22–23

Biceps brachii tendon
    anchor, 100, 101*f*, 102, 103*f*
    distal, injury, 121, 122*f*
    long head of, 22
        abnormalities, 109–112, 111*f*–112*f*
        in bicipital groove, 17, 18*f*
        normal MRI appearance, 109, 110*f*
    normal anatomy, 18*f*
    short head of, 22

Biceps femoris muscle, strain, 185, 186*f*

Bicipital aponeurosis, 23

Biopsy, musculoskeletal, MRI-guided, 410*f*, 411

Bone scan(s), 419–422, 420*f*–421*f*

Bone tumors. *See also* specific tumor
    benign, 386–389
    clinical presentation, 385
    diagnosis, 385–386
        MRI and, 370
    of foot/ankle
        benign, 220
        malignant, 220
    malignant, 389–393
    MRI, advantages, 385–386

Brachialis muscle, 22–23

Buford complex, 100–101, 101*f*

Bursitis, 379–381, 382*f*

C

Caisson disease, and osteonecrosis of knee, 191

Calcaneus, stress fractures, 207, 207*f*

Calcific tendinitis, of shoulder, 113

Calcium pyrophosphate dihydrate deposition disease, cervical
    spinal involvement in, 266

Capitate, occult fracture, 131*f*

Carpal bones, distal, occult fractures, 130–131, 131*f*

Carpal instability, 135

Carpal tunnel syndrome, 138–139

Cartilage, articular. *See* Articular cartilage

Cauda equina syndrome, 296–297

Cellulitis, of foot/ankle, 216–217

Cerebrospinal fluid
    in spine, normal MRI appearance, 63
    on T2-weighted image, 77*f*, 78

Cervical spinal stenosis, 241*f*, 244*f*, 247, 250–253, 251*t*,
    251*f*–257*f*
    absolute, 252
    causes, 250, 251*t*, 253*f*
    central canal, 250–251, 253*f*
    degenerative upon congenital, 250, 252*f*
    foraminal, 250, 251*f*
    grading, 253, 257*f*
    mild, 253
    moderate, 253, 256*f*
    objective measures, 252–253
    relative, 252
    severe, 253, 257*f*

Cervical spine, 229–268
    abscess, 259–262
    acute transverse myelopathy, 262
    ankylosing spondylitis, 235, 236*f*
    annular tears, 244–245, 245*f*
    anterior longitudinal ligament, tears, 235
    arthritides, 264–266
    C2 nerve root, 67, 70*f*
    compression fracture, 232, 232*f*
    degenerative conditions, 242–255

diffuse idiopathic skeletal hyperostosis, 235
discitis, 256–259, 261*f*
epidural abscess, 259–261
facet dislocations, 232–233, 233*f*–234*f*
flexion-compression injuries, 232–233, 232*f*
flexion-extension imaging, 242, 243*f*
imaging protocols for, 229
infectious conditions, 255–262, 261*f*
instability, characterization, 241–242, 242*f*
intervertebral discs
    avulsion from adjacent vertebral body, 235
    bulge, 245*t*, 246
    degenerative disc disease, 243–245, 244*f*
    displacement, 245–250, 246*f*
        and stenosis, 241*f*, 244*f*, 247
    extrusion, 245*t*, 246–247, 248*f*
    herniation, 235, 250, 251*f*
    horizontal rupture, 235, 235*f*
    injuries, 235
    pathology, 245, 245*t*
    protrusion, 245*t*, 246–247, 247*f*
    sequestration, 245*t*, 246
    "soft" *versus* "hard," 247, 247*f*
intradural infections, 261–262
intrinsic inflammatory myelopathy, 262–264
leptomeningitis, 261–262
ligaments, normal anatomy, 67*f*–68*f*
in multiple sclerosis, 262, 263*f*
myelitis, 261–262
neural foramina, normal anatomy, 67
neural structures, normal anatomy, 67, 69*f*
normal anatomy, 66*f*, 67, 67*f*, 68, 68*f*, 70*f*–72*f*, 71–72
pediatric, normal anatomy, 339–340
posterior ligaments
    edema, 235
    injuries, 233, 235*f*, 242, 242*f*
prevertebral hematoma, 235
specialized pulse sequences for, 229
subacute necrotizing myelopathy, 263–264
subdural abscess, 261–262
trauma, 229–242
    axial load injuries in, 230, 236, 237*f*
    classification, 230–236, 231*f*
    evaluation, 230, 230*t*
    hyperextension injuries in, 230, 233–235
    hyperflexion injuries in, 230, 232–233, 232*f*
    imaging protocols for, 230
    mechanism of injury in, 230
    penetrating, 238–241
    region of injury in, 232
    spinal cord injury in, 235
        characterization, 241
tuberculous involvement, 258
tumors, 262
T2-weighted images, 77*f*, 81–84, 83*f*–85*f*
vertebral bodies. *See* Vertebral bodies

vertebral osteomyelitis, 256–259, 261*f*
Chamberlain's line, 258*t*, 259*f*
Charcot neuroarthropathy, 218
Chemical-shift imaging, 403, 407*f*
Chiari malformations, 345
    with myelomeningocele, 344
    and occipitocervical stenosis, 253–254
    types, 254, 259*f*
Child(ren). *See also* Pediatric spine
    age 2 years, spine, 340, 341*f*
    age 10 years, spine, 340, 342*f*
    epidural abscess in, 341–342
    sedation protocols for, 338–339
    wrist/hand
        growth arrest, 131
        physeal bars, 131
        physeal injuries, 131, 131*f*
Chondroblastoma, 386, 387*f*
Chondrosarcoma, 393, 393*f*
    epidemiology, 385
    spinal, 325–326, 326*f*
Chordoma
    chondroid, 324
    spinal, 324–325, 325*f*
    typical, 324
Claustrophobia, 429
Clivus canal angle, 258*t*
Collagenous tissue, on T1-weighted images, 9, 10*f*
Computed tomography, 416–419, 417*f*–419*f*
Contrast-enhanced imaging, 14–15
    for MR arthrography, 397, 397*t*
    safety, 428–429
Conus medullaris, pediatric, 339*f*, 340–341, 341*f*
Conventional radiography, 414–416, 415*f*–416*f*
Coxa saltans (snapping hip syndrome), 153–154
Crowned dens sign, 266
Cryotherapy, MRI-guided, 411*f*, 412
Crystal deposition disorders, 126
CSF. *See* Cerebrospinal fluid
CT. *See* Computed tomography
Cubital tunnel syndrome, 125–126
Cyclops lesion, of anterior cruciate ligament, 199, 199*f*

D

de Quervain tenosynovitis, 135, 136*f*
Diabetic myonecrosis, 376–377, 378*f*
Diagnosis, arrival at, correlation of imaging findings with
        patient history and examination in, 90–93, 92*f*
Diastematomyelia, 344
Differential diagnosis, correlation of imaging findings with
        patient history and examination for, 90–93, 92*f*
Diffuse idiopathic skeletal hyperostosis, cervical spine
        involvement in, 235

Diffusion-weighted imaging, 403–404
Discitis, in pediatric patient, 341
Dupuytren contracture, of wrist/hand, 140, 141*f*
Dynamic (functional) imaging, 402–403, 403*f*–406*f*

E

ECU. *See* Extensor carpi ulnaris
Elbow, 118-128. *See also* Forearm
    articular cartilage, 362, 365*f*
    compression neuropathies, 125–126, 125*f*–126*f*
    degenerative conditions, 122–123
    epiphysiolysis, 119, 119*f*
    imaging protocols for, 118
    infectious conditions, 123–124
    lateral and medial epicondylitis, 122–123, 124*f*
    LCL complex injury, 121, 121*f*
    ligamentous structures, 25*f*, 27–28
    loose bodies in, 119, 120*f*, 126
    medial collateral ligament, injury, 119–121, 120*f*
    MR arthrography image, 399*f*
    neural structures, 25*f*, 27*f*
    neurovascular structures, 27–28, 27*f*
    normal anatomy, 22–30, 24*f*, 28*f*–29*f*
    occult fractures, 118–119
    osseous contusion, 118–119, 119*f*
    septic arthritis, 124
    soft-tissue masses of, 126–127, 126*f*
    specialized pulse sequences for, 118
    synovial disorders, 126
    tendons, 22–23, 24*f*–27*f*, 27–28
    trauma, 118–122
Enchondroma, 387, 388*f*
Eosinophilic granuloma, spinal, 320*t*, 324, 324*f*
Ependymoma, spinal, 331–332, 333*f*–334*f*
Epidural lipomatosis, 300–301, 301*f*
Epithelioid sarcoma, 385
Ewing sarcoma, 390–393, 392*f*
    epidemiology, 385
    spinal, 326–327
Examination, physical, findings in, correlation with imaging
        findings, 90–93
Extensor carpi ulnaris, 23, 25, 25*f*
Extremity scanners, 400–401, 402*f*
Extrinsic carpal ligaments, injury, 132–133, 133*f*

F

Fast spin echo imaging, 8–9
Fatigue fractures, in hip, 151
Fat pad disease (Hoffa disease), 187
Femoral head, osteonecrosis, 154–155, 155*f*

Femoral neck fracture, nondisplaced
    on short tau inversion recovery image, 79, 79*f*
    on T1-weighted image, 79, 79*f*, 86
Femoroacetabular impingement, 156–157, 157*f*–160*f*
FHL tendon. *See* Flexor hallucis longus tendon
Fibrous dysplasia of bone, 389, 390*f*
Fingers, muscles and ligaments, 33, 34*f*
Flexor hallucis longus tendon
    partial tear, 214–215, 216*f*
    tenosynovitis, 214–215
Flip angle, 5, 6*f*, 8, 13
Fluid-attenuated inversion recovery, physics of, 8
Foot/ankle, 202-225
    abscess, 216–217, 217*f*
    arthrodesis, postoperative MRI findings, 222–223
    bone contusion, 203, 203*f*
    bone tumors
        benign, 220
        malignant, 220
    cellulitis, 216–217
    Charcot neuroarthropathy, 218
    degenerative conditions, 208–216
    ganglion cysts, 219, 219*f*
    hemangioma, 219
    imaging protocols for, 202
    infectious processes, 216–218
    ligament sprains, 203–205
    normal anatomy, 51*f*–61*f*, 52–60
    osteomyelitis, 217–218, 218*f*
    postoperative MRI findings in, 221–223
        susceptibility artifact in, 222*f*
    septic arthritis, 217
    specialized pulse sequences for, 202
    sprains. *See* Ankle, sprain(s)
    stress fractures, 206–208
    tendons
        disorders, 208–215
        repair, postoperative MRI findings, 221–222, 222*f*
        tears, recurrent/new, 222, 222*f*
    trauma, 203–208
    tumors, 219–220
Forearm. *See also* Elbow
    distal, muscles, 32–33
    muscle architecture, 23–25, 24*f*
    muscles, classification of
        by compartment, 24–25
        by location, 23–24
FSE imaging. *See* Fast spin echo imaging

G

Gadolinium contrast, 14–15, 14*f*
    for MR angiography, 410–411
    for MR arthrography, 397, 397*t*

safety, 428–429
Ganglion cyst(s), 373–374, 374*f*
    in foot/ankle, 219, 219*f*
    in wrist/hand, 139–140, 142*f*
Ganglioneuroblastomas, intermediate-differentiated,
        spinal, 327
Ganglioneuroma, spinal, 327, 327*f*
Gaucher disease, and osteonecrosis of knee, 191
Giant cell tumor
    of bone, 388
    spinal, 320*t*, 322, 322*f*
    of tendon sheath
        of foot/ankle, 219–220
        of wrist/hand, 139–140, 141*f*
Glenohumeral instability, 97–100, 98*f*–100*f*
Glenohumeral osteoarthritis, 108–109, 108*f*
Glenoid, 17, 18*f*, 20*f*
Glenoid labrum
    inferior, 17–20, 20*f*
    normal anatomy, 17, 18*f*–20*f*, 20
    pathology, 100–103, 102*f*, 103*f*
    superior, 17–20, 20*f*
Glomus tumor, of wrist/hand, 140
Gout, cervical spinal involvement, 266
Gradient-echo images, 7–8, 8*f*, 9
    characteristics of, 9, 9*t*, 13–14
    recognition of, 80, 82*f*
    three-dimensional, 14
Greater trochanteric pain syndrome, 152–153

H

Hallux valgus, repair, postoperative MRI findings, 223
Hamartoma, of wrist/hand, 140
Hamstring strains, 154
Hand(s). *See* Wrist/hand
Hemangioblastoma, spinal, 332, 335*f*
Hemangioma, 372–373, 373*f*
    of foot/ankle, 219
    T1- and T2-weighted images, 86–87, 91*f*
    vertebral, 319–320, 320*f*, 320*t*
    of wrist/hand, 139–140
Hemangiopericytoma, spinal, 329–331
Hematoma, 375–376, 376*f*
    of thoracolumbar spine, 308–309, 311*f*
    on T1-weighted image, 10*f*
Herniated nucleus pulposus. *See under* Lumbar spine
High-resolution imaging, 400, 401*f*
Hip, 147–163
    abductors, 38
        tears, 153, 153*f*
    adductors, 38
        strains, 154
    articular cartilage, 359–360, 362*f*–364*f*

articular surfaces, 37, 39*f*
athletic, 147–154
bone marrow abnormalities, 154–156
degenerative conditions, 156–160
extensors, 38
external rotators, 38
femoroacetabular impingement, 156–157, 157*f*–160
flexors, 38
greater trochanteric pain syndrome, 152–153
idiopathic transient osteoporosis, 155–156, 156*f*
imaging protocol for, 147
inflammatory disorders, 160
intraarticular pathology, zone classification, 149, 150*f*
MR arthrography image, 398*f*
muscles, 38, 39*f*–41*f*
    strains, 154, 154*f*
normal anatomy, 37–42, 40*f*, 42*f*–44*f*
osteoarthritis, 158
pain in, differential diagnosis, 147–148, 148*t*
specialized pulse sequences for, 147
stress fractures, 151, 151*f*
synovial disorders, 160–161, 160*f*–161*f*
trauma, 147–154
traumatic posterior subluxation/dislocation/lateral
        impaction, 151–152, 152*f*
trochanteric bursitis, 152–153
History, patient, correlation with imaging findings, 90–93
Hoffa disease, 187
Humeral epicondyles, 24*f*–26*f*
Humeral head, 17, 18*f*
Humerus, 20, 20*f*
    capitellum, osteochondritis dissecans, 125, 125*f*
    greater and lesser tuberosity, 20*f*, 22

I

Iliotibial band syndrome, 191
Implant(s), metallic. *See also* Metallic object(s) or
        substances
    MRI in presence of, 406–408, 409*f*
        in pediatric spine, 347*f*, 348
    safety profiles, 426–427
Infant(s)
    age 3 months, spine, 340
    full-term, spine, 340
Infraspinatus muscle and tendon, 22
Insufficiency fractures, in hip, 151
Intervention(s), MRI-guided, 411–412
Intervertebral discs. *See under* Lumbar spine
Intervertebral osteochondrosis, of lumbar spine,
        277–278, 278*f*
Intraoperative MRI, 401
Inversion time, 8
ITB syndrome. *See* Iliotibial band syndrome

J

Jersey finger, 133
Joint fluid, 86, 90*f*
Juvenile rheumatoid arthritis, cervical spinal involvement
   in, 264

K

Kienböck disease, 136–137, 137*f*
Knee, 164-201. *See also* Anterior cruciate ligament; Posterior
      cruciate ligament
   acute hemarthrosis, 164
   adhesion formation in, 193
   anterior interval
      definition, 193
      scarring in, 193
   arcuate complex, injuries, 181, 181*f*
   articular cartilage, 356–359, 356*f*, 359*f*–361*f*
   Baker (popliteal) cyst, 193, 194*f*, 374–375, 375*f*
   bursitis, 190–191, 190*f*–191*f*
   collateral ligaments
      normal anatomy, 44, 48*f*
      tears, 179–180, 179*f*–180*f*, 181*t*
   degenerative joint disease, 193
   degenerative (nonacute) pathology, 187–195
   dislocation, 182–183, 182*f*
   extensor mechanism
      degenerative (nonacute) pathology, 187, 188*f*
      normal anatomy, 52
      traumatic injuries, 183–185
   gradient-echo image, 82*f*
   Hoffa disease (fat pad disease), 187
   imaging protocols for, 164
   infectious conditions, 193–194
   injuries, "terrible triad," 180
   loose bodies in, 185–187, 186*f*
   meniscocapsular separation, 166*t*
   meniscus/menisci
      allograft replacement, MRI findings after, 194–195, 198*f*
      degenerative, 193
      discoid, 188, 189*f*
      normal anatomy, 42, 50–52, 51*f*
      postoperative MRI findings, 194–195, 197*f*
      repair, MRI findings after, 194–195, 197*f*
      tears, 165–172
         bucket handle, 166*t*, 170*f*–172*f*, 171
         complex, 166*t*, 172
         displaced, 170*f*–173*f*, 171
         grading, 164*t*, 165–167, 165*f*
         horizontal, 165*f*–167*f*, 166*t*, 167
         morphologies, 166, 166*t*
         MRI characteristics, 165–166, 166*t*
         types, 164*t*, 165, 165*f*

      vertical longitudinal, 166*t*, 169–171, 170*f*
      vertical radial, 166*t*, 167–169, 168*f*–169*f*
   muscle strain at, 185, 186*f*
   neurovascular structures, normal anatomy, 50*f*, 52
   normal anatomy, 42–44, 45*f*–50*f*, 46–52
   Osgood-Schlatter disease, 188, 188*f*
   osteochondrosis(es), 188, 188*f*
   osteomyelitis, 193–194
   osteonecrosis, 191–192, 192*f*, 192*t*
   osteophytes, 193
   partial meniscectomy, MRI findings after, 194–195,
      195*f*–196*f*
   patellar dislocation, 183–184, 183*f*–184*f*
   patellar tendinitis, 187, 188*f*
   patellar tendon rupture, 184*f*, 185
   plicae, 188–190, 189*f*–190*f*
   posterolateral corner
      injuries, 180–181, 180*f*–181*f*
      normal anatomy, 44, 48*f*
      structures of, 180
   posteromedial corner
      injuries, 181–182, 181*f*
      normal anatomy, 44, 48*f*
      structures of, 181
   postoperative MRI findings in, 194–199
   quadriceps tendon rupture, 185, 185*f*
   septic effusion in, 193–194
   Sindig-Larsen-Johansson disease, 188
   specialized pulse sequences for, 164
   stress fractures, 187, 187*f*
   trauma, 164–187

L

Larmor equation, 3–5, 5*f*
Lateral ankle ligament, reconstruction, postoperative MRI
      findings, 222, 223*f*
Lateral collateral ligament
   of elbow
      injury (sprain, tear), 121, 121*f*
      normal anatomy, 28*f*, 29
   of knee
      in arcuate complex, 181, 191
      injury (sprain, tear), 179, 183
      normal anatomy, 44, 47*f*
Lateral collateral ligament complex, injury, 121, 121*f*
   injury, 121, 121*f*
   normal anatomy, 28, 29
Lateral ulnar collateral ligament, 27–29, 28*f*
   accessory, 121
   injury, 121, 121*f*
LCL. *See* Lateral collateral ligament
Leptomeningeal hemangioblastomatosis, 332
Lipoma, 371*f*, 372, 372*f*

of elbow, 126–127, 126*f*
of wrist/hand, 140, 141*f*
Lipomeningocele, 344
Liposarcoma, 382–383, 383*f*
Little Leaguer's elbow, 119, 119*f*
Longitudinal relaxation, 5
LUCL. *See* Lateral ulnar collateral ligament
Lumbar spinal stenosis, 287*f*–289*f*, 293–296, 296*f*
    anatomic changes causing, 295, 295*f*
    degenerative upon congenital, 294–295, 294*f*
    grading, 295–296
    mild, 295–296
    moderate, 296
    objective measures, 295
    severe, 296
Lumbar spine, 269-315. *See also* Thoracolumbar spine
    annular tears, 275*f*, 277, 277*f*, 282
    herniated nucleus pulposus, 282–287, 286*f*–289*f*
        central, 286, 286*f*–287*f*
        far lateral, 286–287, 286*f*, 289*f*
        foraminal, 286, 286*f*, 288*f*
        lateral recess, 286, 286*f*
        posterolateral, 286, 286*f*, 288*f*
    imaging protocols for, 269
    intervertebral discs
        anatomic zones on axial images, 286, 287*f*
        bulge, 278, 278*f*, 279, 283, 284*f*
        degenerative disc disease, 277–278, 280–281, 280*f*–283*f*
        extrusion, 278, 278*f*, 279, 279*f*, 283–285, 285*f*
        herniation, 277–278, 277*f*–278*f*. *See also* Herniated
            nucleus pulposus
            broad-based, 278*f*, 279
            contained *versus* uncontained, 280
            focal, 278*f*, 279
            generalized, 278, 278*f*
            intravertebral, 280
            localized, 278, 278*f*
            recurrent, 307, 308*f*
        migration, 279
        normal, 277, 277*f*, 280
        pathology
            classification, 277–280
            differentiating MRI features, 277, 277*f*
            nomenclature for, 277–280
        protrusion, 278*f*, 279, 279*f*, 283–286, 284*f*
            central, 286, 286*f*–287*f*
            far lateral, 286–287, 286*f*, 289*f*
            foraminal, 286, 286*f*, 288*f*
            lateral recess, 286, 286*f*
            posterolateral, 286, 286*f*, 288*f*
        sequestration, 278, 278*f*, 279
        "soft" *versus* "hard" pathology, 287, 290*f*
    intervertebral osteochondrosis, 277–278, 278*f*, 280
    intradural-extramedullary mass, postgadolinium
            T1-weighted image, 81*f*
    normal anatomy, 73–74, 73*f*–75*f*

pediatric, normal anatomy, 339, 339*f*
specialized pulse sequences for, 269
spondylosis deformans, 277, 278*f*, 280
trauma, 269–277
    systematic approach for, 270, 270*t*
vertebral bodies. *See* Vertebral bodies
vertebral end plates, degenerative conditions, 280–289
Lunate, idiopathic osteonecrosis, 136–137, 137*f*
Lunotriquetral ligament, injury, 132, 133*f*
Lymphoma(s)
    epidemiology, 385
    spinal, 327–328, 328*f*

M

Magic angle phenomenon, 15, 52, 135, 167
Magnetic dipole, 3, 3*f*
Magnetic field(s)
    metallic objects in, 426
    physiologic effects, 425
    static, physiologic effects, 425
    time-varying, physiologic effects, 425
Malignant fibrous histiocytoma, 385
    epidemiology, 385
McGregor's line, 258*t*, 259*f*
MCL. *See* Medial collateral ligament
McRae's line, 258*t*, 259*f*
Medial collateral ligament
    of elbow
        injury (sprain, tear), 119–121, 120*f*
        normal anatomy, 27, 28*f*
    of knee
        injury (sprain, tear), 179–180, 179*f*–181*f*, 181*t*, 183
        normal anatomy, 44, 45*f*–47*f*
Median nerve
    compression
        in carpal tunnel, 138–139
        at elbow, 125–126
    at elbow, 26*f*, 27, 27*f*
Meningioma, spinal, 328, 330*f*
Meniscus. *See* Knee, meniscus/menisci
Metacarpals, occult fractures, 131
Metallic object(s) or substances, 425–427
    artifact-producing, 425–426
    external, 427
    internal, 426–427. *See also* Implant(s), metallic
    in magnetic fields, 426
    superficial (skin surface), 427
Metastatic disease
    of bone, 385
    spinal involvement, 316, 332–335
Metatarsal stress fractures, 207–208, 208*f*
MFH. *See* Malignant fibrous histiocytoma
Microscopy, MR, 400, 401*f*

Morton neuroma, 221, 221f
Motion artifact(s), 15
MR angiography, 408–411, 409f
    images, recognition of, 80, 82f
MR arthrography, 14–15, 397–398
    direct, 14–15, 397, 398f–399f
        contrast for, 397, 397t
    images, recognition of, 80, 82f
    indirect, 15, 397–398, 399f
MRI study(ies), review, steps for, 77
MR microscopy, 400, 401f
MR spectroscopy, 405–406, 408f
MR venography, 411
Multiple myeloma
    epidemiology, 385
    spinal involvement, 324, 325f
Multiple sclerosis, cervical spinal involvement, 262, 263f
Muscle. *See also* specific muscle
    tear(s), 378, 380f
    on T1-weighted images, 9, 10f
Myelitis, cervical spine, 261-262
Myelomeningocele, 344, 344f
Myonecrosis, diabetic and idiopathic, 376–377, 378f
Myositis ossificans, 376, 377f

N

Navicular bone
    accessory, 211, 211f
    normal anatomy, 52f–54f, 53–54, 56f, 58, 59f, 60, 61f
    stress fractures, 207, 208f
Necrotizing fasciitis, of wrist/hand, 136
Net magnetization vector, 3–5, 4f, 7f
Neuroblastic tumors, spinal, 327
Neuroblastoma, spinal, 327
Neurofibroma, 377–378, 379f
    spinal, 329, 331f
Neutron(s), physical properties of, 3, 3f
Nonossifying fibroma, 389, 389f
Nuclear scintigraphy, 419–422, 420f–421f

O

Occipitocervical junction
    anatomic relationships, 258t
    injury(ies), 236–238
    lines for use with MRI and computed tomography, 258t
Occipitocervical stenosis, 253–255
OCD. *See* Osteochondritis dissecans
Odontoid fracture(s), 238, 238f
Olecranon bursitis, septic and nonseptic, 124
Osgood-Schlatter disease, 188, 188f

Os peroneum, 214, 215f
Osteoarthritis, 362–363
    Acromioclavicular joint, 109, 109f
    glenohumeral, 108–109, 108f
    of hip, 158
Osteoblastoma, 386
    spinal, 320t, 321, 321f
Osteochondritis dissecans
    of humeral capitellum, 125, 125f
    of talus, 205–206, 206f
Osteochondroma, 387, 388f
    spinal, 320t, 322, 323f
Osteogenic sarcoma, spinal, 326, 326f
Osteochondrosis(es)
    in intervertebral body, of cervical spine, 277-278, 278f, 280
    in knee, 188, 188f
Osteoid osteoma, 386
    spinal, 320, 320t, 321f
Osteomyelitis
    acute, 124
    differential diagnosis, 341, 342f
    of foot/ankle, 217–218, 218f
    of wrist/hand, 136
Osteonecrosis
    alcohol abuse and, 191
    of femoral head, 154–155, 155f
    in knee, 191–192, 192f, 192t
    of talus, 215–216, 217f
Osteosarcoma, 389–390, 392f
    epidemiology, 385
    spinal, 326, 326f
    subtypes, 390, 391f
Os trigonum, 214–215, 216f

P

Painful os peroneum syndrome, 214
Pain management, MRI-guided interventions for, 412
Parallel imaging, 399–400
Pathology. *See* specific anatomical entity
Pavlov ratio, 252–253
PCL. *See* Posterior cruciate ligament
Pediatric spine. *See also* Child(ren); Spinal dysraphism
    and adult spine, differences between, 340
    conus medullaris, 339f, 340–341, 341f
    fractures, 342–343, 343f
    imaging protocols for, 338
    with implants, imaging in presence of, controversies with, 347f, 348
    infectious conditions, 341–342, 342f–343f
    MRI, controversies with, 347–348
    normal anatomy, 339–341, 339f
    specialized pulse sequences for, 338
    trauma, 342–343, 343f

Periosteal chondroma, 386–387

Peripheral nerve sheath tumor
    malignant, spinal, 329, 331*f*
    of wrist/hand, 140

Peroneal tendon, disorders, 211–214, 213*f*–215*f*

Peroneus quartus muscle, 213, 214*f*

Pes anserine bursitis, 190, 190*f*

Phalanges, of hand, occult fractures, 131

Physical examination, findings in, correlation with imaging findings, 90–93

Pigmented villonodular synovitis, 378–379, 381*f*
    elbow involvement in, 126
    foot/ankle involvement in, 219–220, 220*f*
    hip involvement in, 161, 161*f*

Piriformis syndrome, 154

Pixel(s), 7

Plantar fasciitis, 220–221, 221*f*

Plantar fasciotomy, postoperative MRI findings, 222–223

Plantar fibromatosis, 219, 220*f*

Plasmacytoma, solitary bone, 324

Positron emission tomography, 422, 422*f*

Posterior ankle impingement syndrome, 214–215

Posterior cruciate ligament
    graft, tunnel placement, 199*f*
    laxity, grading, 179, 179*t*
    normal anatomy, 44, 45*f*, 48*f*, 49, 51*f*
    tears, 177–179, 178*f*

Posterior interosseous nerve, compression, 125–126, 126*f*

Posterior interosseous nerve syndrome, 125–126

Posterior longitudinal ligament, ossification, 247–250, 249*f*–250*f*

Posterior tibial tendon
    dysfunction, 210–211, 211*f*
    tears, 211, 212*f*

Precessional frequency (ω_0), 3, 5*f*

Pregnancy, 427

Prepatellar bursitis, 191, 191*f*

Pronator syndrome, 125–126

Proton-density weighted images, 8–9
    characteristics of, 8–9, 9*t*, 11, 12*f*
    fast spin echo, 11, 12*f*
    with fat suppression, 11–12
    spin echo, 11, 12*f*

Pseudoaneurysm, 381, 382*f*

Pseudomeningocele, 309–310, 312*f*

Psoriatic arthritis, cervical spinal involvement in, 265

Pulse sequence(s), 7–8
    advantages and disadvantages, 9, 9*t*
    available for review, determination of, 77–80
    characteristics, 9, 9*t*
    conventional spin echo, 7–8, 7*f*, 9
    fast spin echo, 8–9
    fluid-sensitive, 9
    gradient-echo, 7–8, 8*f*
    novel (advanced), 403–406
    signal-to-noise ratio of, 9

    specialized
        for articular cartilage, 353–355, 354*f*–356*f*, 355*t*
        for cervical spine, 229
        for elbow, 118
        evaluation of, 87–90
        for foot/ankle, 202
        for hip, 147
        for knee, 164
        for lumbar spine, 269
        for pediatric spine, 338
        for shoulder, 97
        for thoracic spine, 269
        for tumors of spine, 317
        for wrist/hand, 129
    spin echo, T1-weighted
        characteristics of, 9–10, 10*f*–11*f*
    standard, 8–9

PVNS. *See* Pigmented villonodular synovitis

R

RA. *See* Rheumatoid arthritis

Radial collateral ligament, 25*f*, 27, 29
    injury, 121

Radial head, fractures, 118–119

Radial nerve, 27*f*, 28
    compression, at elbow, 125–126
    at elbow, 25*f*–26*f*

Radial tunnel syndrome, 125–126

Radiography, conventional, 414–416, 415*f*–416*f*

Radius, distal, occult fractures, 130–131

Ranawat criterion, 258*t*, 259*f*

RCL. *See* Radial collateral ligament

Rectus femoris strain, 154, 154*f*

Rheumatoid arthritis, 126
    cervical spinal involvement in, 264, 265*f*
    hip involvement, 160
    and occipitocervical stenosis, 254–255, 260*f*
    wrist/hand involvement, 138, 138*f*–139*f*

Rice bodies, 135

Rotator cuff, 20, 20*f*, 22, 22*f*–23*f*
    tears, 106–108, 106*f*–108*f*
        MRI characteristics, 107, 107*t*

S

Safety, 425–429

Sarcoma
    epithelioid, 385
    Ewing, 390–393, 392*f*
        epidemiology, 385
        spinal, 326–327

Sarcoma (*continued*)
  osteogenic, spinal, 326, 326*f*
  spinal, 325–327
  synovial, 384, 384*f*
Scaphoid
  fracture/deformity, 129–130, 130*f*
  occult fractures, 129–130, 130*f*
  posttraumatic osteonecrosis, 137, 138*f*
Scapholunate ligament, injury, 132, 133*f*
Scheuermann's kyphosis, 288
Schmorl's nodes, 287–289
Schwannoma, spinal, 328–329, 330*f*
Scoliosis, 298–300, 300*f*
  MRI, controversies with, 347–348
Sedation, for pediatric patient, 338–339
Short tau inversion recovery
  characteristics of, 9, 13, 13*f*
  fat-suppressed images, evaluation, 87–90, 91*f*
  images, recognition of, 78*f*–80*f*, 79
  physics of, 8
Shoulder, 97–117
  adhesive capsulitis, 112–113, 113*f*
  calcific tendinitis, 113
  degenerative conditions, 103–112
  fluid in, 86, 90*f*
  imaging protocols for, 97
  ligaments, 20, 20*f*
  MR arthrography image, 82*f*, 398*f*
  neurovascular structures, 20, 21*f*
  normal anatomy, 17–22, 18*f*–23*f*
  osseous structures, 17, 19*f*, 20
  postoperative MRI findings in, 113–114
  septic arthritis, 112
  specialized pulse sequences for, 97
  trauma, 97–103
  vascular malformation, MR angiography, 82*f*
Sickle cell disease, and osteonecrosis of knee, 191
Signal intensity, factors affecting, 9, 9*t*
Signal localization, 5–7
Signal-to-noise ratio(s), 9
Sinding-Larsen-Johansson disease, 188
SLAP lesion(s). *See* Superior labrum anterior and posterior lesion(s)
Snapping hip syndrome (coxa saltans), 153–154
Soft-tissue tumors, 370–385
  clinical presentation, 370–371
  determinate lesions, 139, 371–381
  diagnosis, MRI and, 370
  at elbow, 126–127, 126*f*
  history with, 370–371
  indeterminate lesions, 139, 371
  malignant, signs of, 371, 371*f*
  physical examination with, 371
  in wrist/hand, 139–140
    benign, 139–140, 141*f*
Spinal cord
  atrophy, 251, 254*f*

bacterial infection, 264
cervical, 66*f*
  compression, 241, 241*f*
  injury, 235
    characterization, 241
    management, 241
cystic degeneration, 251
disease, acquired immune deficiency syndrome and, 264
granulomatous disease, 264
injury
  in cervical spine trauma, 235, 241
  in pediatric patient, 343
  without radiographic abnormality, in pediatric patient, 343
metabolic disease and, 264
necrosis, 251
normal MRI appearance, 64, 66*f*
parasitic infestation, 264
toxic disease and, 264
viral infection, 264
Spinal dysraphism, 343–347. *See also* Pediatric spine
  classification, 343, 343*t*
  definition, 343
  occult, 343*t*, 344
Spinal stability
  assessment, 270, 272–277
  definition, 272
  posterior ligamentous complex and, 270*f*, 273, 273*f*
  three-column concept, 272–273
Spinal stenosis. *See* Cervical spinal stenosis; Lumbar spinal stenosis
Spine. *See also* Cervical spine, Thoracic spine, Lumbar spine, Thoracolumbar spine
  dynamic (functional) imaging, 402–403, 403*f*–406*f*
  foramina, normal anatomy, 67
  normal anatomy, 60–67
  intervertebral discs, normal anatomy, 60–62
  ligaments, normal anatomy, 64–67, 67*f*–68*f*
  load-bearing imaging, 402–403, 403*f*–406*f*
  nerve roots, normal anatomy, 67, 69*f*
  pediatric. *See* Pediatric spine
  positional imaging, 402–403
  vertebral bodies, normal anatomy, 62–63, 62*f*–65*f*
Spin-lattice relaxation, 5
Spin-spin relaxation, 5
Spondylolisthesis, 297–298
  degenerative, 297, 299*f*
  iatrogenic, 297–298
  isthmic, 297, 298*f*
  Meyerding classification, 297, 297*f*
  pathologic, 297
  traumatic, 276*f*, 297
Spondyloptosis, 297
SPONK. *See* Spontaneous osteonecrosis of knee
Spontaneous osteonecrosis of knee, 191–192, 192*t*
Sprain, ankle. *See* Ankle, sprain(s)

Stener lesion, 133
Steroid use, and osteonecrosis of knee, 191, 192*t*
STIR. *See* Short tau inversion recovery
Stress fractures
    calcaneal, 207, 207*f*
    of foot/ankle, 206–208
    in hip, 151, 151*f*
    in knee, 187, 187*f*
    metatarsal, 207–208, 208*f*
    navicular, 207, 208*f*
Subacromial bursitis, 105, 106*f*
Subacromial impingement syndrome, 103–106
Subacute necrotizing myelopathy, in cervical spine, 263–264
Subscapularis muscle and tendon, 17, 18*f*
Superior labrum anterior and posterior, lesions, 100–103, 101*f*–103*f*
Supraspinatus muscle and tendon, 17, 19*f*–20*f*, 22
Supraspinatus tendon
    tear, 86, 90*f*, 108, 108*f*
    tendinosis, 105, 106*f*
Susceptibility artifact(s), 15
    gradient-echo imaging and, 14
Synovial cyst, 374–375, 375*f*
Synovial osteochondromatosis, 126
    of hip, 160–161, 160*f*
Synovial sarcoma, 384, 384*f*
Syringohydromyelia, 344–345, 345*f*
Syrinx, 251, 344–345, 345*f*

T

Talus
    osteochondritis dissecans (osteochondral defect), 205–206, 206*f*
    osteonecrosis, 215–216, 217*f*
Target sign, 378, 379*f*
Tarsal tunnel surgery, postoperative MRI findings, 222–223
T2 decay, 5, 7–8
TE (echo time), 7, 7*f*–8*f*
Tendons, on T1-weighted images, 9, 10*f*
Tenosynovitis, de Quervain, 135, 136*f*
Teres minor muscle, 22
Tethered cord syndrome, 345–347, 346*f*
    MRI, controversies with, 348
TFCC. *See* Triangular fibrocartilage complex
Thoracic spine, 269–315. *See also* Thoracolumbar spine
    disc herniation, 287, 290*f*
    imaging protocols for, 269
    normal anatomy, 72–73
    osseous structures, 64*f*
    pediatric, normal anatomy, 340
    specialized pulse sequences for, 269
    trauma, 269–277
        systematic approach for, 270, 270*t*

    vascular supply, 63, 65*f*
    vertebral bodies, 62, 64*f*
Thoracolumbar Injury Classification and Severity Score, 270, 270*f*
Thoracolumbar spine, 269–315. *See also* Lumbar spine; Thoracic spine
    arachnoiditis, 311, 312*f*
    burst fracture, 271*f*, 274–275, 275*f*
    decompression without instrumentation/fusion, postoperative MRI findings, 307, 308*f*
    discitis, 302*f*, 303, 304*f*
    disc pathology, 275, 275*f*
    epidural abscess, 303, 305*f*
    epidural hematoma, 275–277
    epidural lipomatosis, 300–301, 301*f*
    facet arthropathy, 291–292, 291*f*–292*f*
    fracture morphology, 270, 270*f*–273*f*
        evaluation, 270–272, 271*f*–273*f*
    hematoma, 308–309, 311*f*
    high-intensity zone in, 275, 275*f*
    infectious conditions, 301–304
    instrumentation/fusion, postoperative MRI findings, 307–308, 309*f*–310*f*
    neoplastic changes, 271–272, 272*f*–273*f*
    osteoporotic vertebral fractures, 270–271, 271*f*
    postoperative MRI findings, 304–312
    stability, assessment, 270, 272–277
    synovial cyst, 292–293, 293*f*
    trauma
        classification, 270
        neural compromise in, assessment, 273–274, 274*f*
        penetrating, 274, 274*f*
        role of MRI in, 270–277
    tuberculous involvement, 303–304, 306*f*
    vertebral osteomyelitis, 301–303, 302*f*
    vertebral translation or dislocation, 276*f*, 277
Thumb, ulnar collateral ligament injury, 133, 134*f*
Torg ratio, 252–253
TR (repetition time), 8
Transverse magnetization vector, 5
Transverse relaxation, 5
Trauma. *See* specific anatomic entity
T1 recovery, 5, 8
T2* relaxation, 5, 7–8
Triangular fibrocartilage complex, 33, 35*f*, 37
    components, 131
    injury, 131–132, 132*f*
    tears, 131–132, 132*f*
Triceps brachii muscle, 23
Triceps tendon
    distal, avulsion, 26*f*
    injury, 121–122, 123*f*
Trochanteric bursitis, 152–153
Truncation artifact(s), 15
T sign, 399*f*

Tuberculosis
  cervical spinal involvement, 258
  osteomyelitis caused by, 341, 342*f*
  thoracolumbar involvement, 303–304, 306*f*
Tumors. *See also* Bone tumors; Soft-tissue tumors; specific
      tumor
  bone, 370, 385–393
  foot/ankle, 219–220
  soft-tissue, 370–385
  spinal
    anatomic locations, 316
    cervical, 262
    classification, 316
    diagnosis, image evaluation for, 316
    differential diagnosis, 341, 342*f*
      by anatomic compartment, 316, 317*t*
      imaging modalities for, 316
      procedure for, 316
    extradural, 316–328, 318*f*
      differential diagnosis, 317*t*
      metastatic disease as, 318–319, 319*f*
      primary benign, 319–324, 320*t*
      primary malignant, 324–327
    imaging protocols for, 317
    intradural-extramedullary, 316, 328–331, 329*f*
      differential diagnosis, 317*t*
    intramedullary, 316, 331–335, 332*f*
      differential diagnosis, 317*t*
      metastatic disease, 332–335
    metastatic disease as, 316
    MRI, advantages and disadvantages, 316–317
    specialized pulse sequences for, 317
  wrist/hand, 139–140, 141*f*
T1-weighted images
  characteristics of, 8–10, 9*t*, 10*f*–11*f*
  conventional spin echo, 9–10, 10*f*–11*f*
    with fat suppression, 9–10, 11*f*
  evaluation, 79*f*, 86–87, 91*f*
  with fat suppression, 11–12, 13*f*
  postgadolinium, 9
    evaluation, 90, 92*f*
    recognition of, 80, 81*f*
  recognition of, 78–79
T2-weighted images
  of cervical spine, evaluation, 81–84, 83*f*–85*f*
  characteristics of, 8–9, 9*t*, 10, 11*f*
  evaluation, 81–86
    pattern recognition, 84–86, 90*f*
  fast spin echo, 10, 11*f*–12*f*
  fat-suppressed
    characteristics of, 9, 9*t*, 10, 11–12
    evaluation, 87–90, 91*f*
    recognition of, 79
  of knee, evaluation, 84, 86*f*–89*f*
  recognition of, 77*f*, 78–79, 78*f*
  spin echo, 10

U

UCL. *See* Ulnar collateral ligament
Ulna, distal, occult fractures, 130–131
Ulnar collateral ligament, 25*f*, 27–28
    of thumb, injury, 133, 134*f*
Ulnar impaction syndrome, 134–135, 135*f*
Ulnar nerve
    compression
      at elbow, 125–126, 125*f*
      in Guyon's canal, 138–139, 140*f*
    at elbow, 25*f*–26*f*, 27, 27*f*
Ulnar tunnel syndrome, 138–139, 140*f*

V

Vasculature, MR angiography, 80, 82*f*
Vector(s), magnetization
    longitudinal, 5, 6*f*
    net, 3–5, 4*f*, 7*f*
    transverse, 5, 6*f*
Vertebral artery(ies), 70*f*
    injury, 238, 240*f*
Vertebral body(ies)
    characteristics of, 81, 84, 84*f*
    edema, 230, 230*t*, 261*f*
    hemangioma, 87, 91*f*
    height loss, 232
    hyperextension injuries and, 233
    integrity, 230, 230*t*
    normal anatomy, 62–63, 62*f*–63*f*
    spine infections and, 256, 258, 259
    stenosis and, 247, 249*f*
    subluxations, 264
Vertebral compression fracture
    on computed tomography, 80*f*
    on short tau inversion recovery image, 79, 80*f*, 88, 91*f*
    T2-weighted images, 88, 91*f*
Voshell bursa, 190
Voxel(s), 7

W

Wackenheim's clivus baseline, 258*t*, 259*f*
Welcher's basal angle, 258*t*
Whiplash injury(ies), 235
Wrist/hand, 129-143
    compression neuropathies, 138–139, 139*f*–140*f*
    degenerative conditions, 134–135
    extrinsic carpal ligaments, injury, 132–133, 133*f*
    ganglion cysts, 139–140, 142*f*
    imaging protocols for, 129

infectious conditions, 135–136
interosseous ligaments, injury, 132, 133*f*
ligaments, 35, 36*f*
MR arthrography image, 399*f*
musculotendinous units, 30, 30*f*–31*f*, 33, 35, 35*f*–36*f*, 37, 38*f*–39*f*
neurovascular structures, 30, 30*f*, 32*f*
normal anatomy, 30–37, 30*f*–39*f*
occult fractures, 129–131, 130*f*–131*f*
osseous anatomy, 35, 36*f*–37*f*

rheumatoid arthritis, 138, 138*f*–139*f*
soft-tissue masses, 139–140
specialized pulse sequences for, 129
tendons, 33, 35*f*
    disorders, 135, 135*f*–137*f*
    injuries, 133–134
    overuse syndromes, 135, 137*f*
trauma, 129–134
tumors, 139–140, 141*f*
vasculature, 35, 36*f*